Comments from Readers

Your project sounds fascinating. Who knew there were so many ways to die or diseases to kill you? In centering health and its many facets as the prime-mover in history, you've opened an intriguing and (in many ways) novel perspective. You lay out the case clearly, and your discussion of the historiography spells out your differences with previous medical/scientific/biological interpretations. You've established your work as something new. *Health Matters* fits the rubric of "Big History." Big History does not specialize; rather, it is multidisciplinary and draws on the sciences, natural history, and the humanities to look at long-term—actually *very* long term—trends, trying to find common or unifying patterns in human history. Your MS would seem to fit in nicely.

Mark Lender, Ph.D.
Professor of History, Emeritus, Kean University, Union, New Jersey

This work represents a thorough and scholarly effort that provokes and challenges the reader to confront your proposition that (good) health is the key to a long and satisfying life. I could not resist seeing what you had to say on the topic of "lust," which I found to be an appealing read.

Alan Lippman, M.D.
Past President, Medical History Society of New Jersey

I was quite taken by your extensive knowledge and appreciation of not only history but also literature, art and music. Quite impressive for a scientist with special training and expertise in a number of medical fields. It does remind me of C.P. Snow.

Thomas Owsley, Esq., A.B. (Harvard), J.D.
Retired President, Crown Central Petroleum, Baltimore, Maryland

Health Matters is a timely subject and I suspect it will continue to be so through year-end.

William Allerton
Governor General, Order of the Founders and Patriots of America

The breadth of what you cover is striking, and you write in clear, straightforward prose without a touch of academic jargon that so often defines a work for a restricted audience. My guess is that it may fall in the zone between trade and academic presses. Medical schools offer first year courses in what is often termed humanities—at least that was the case a while back when I was editing Jared Diamond's *Guns, Germs, and Steel*.

Donald Lamm
Retired Chairman and President of W. W. Norton Co.

I think your thesis is excellent.

Wilbert S. Aronow, M.D. (Harvard)
Editor, *Cardiovascular Disease in the Elderly* (CRC Press)
Professor of Medicine, New York Medical College

I can clearly state that it is outstanding and a compelling read. Your grasp of detail is comprehensive, and the research is noteworthy.

Albert Byrd Crum, M.D. (Harvard), M.S. President, The Proimmune Company, LLC

It all looks very solid! All the information you included was perfectly accurate, but there is an interesting link between that species' extinction and the mastery of fire: cooking eliminates many of the anatomical advantages *P. boisei* possessed.

Donald Esker, Ph.D., Professor, Department of Geology, Marietta College

The book is full of wonderful detail references and anecdotes. Great fun to read and an amazing piece of work and scholarship. Thank you for sharing it. The book has remarkable scope. It seems ecumenical in its approach to religions which is refreshing!
           William B. Greenough, M.D. (Harvard)
         Professor of Medicine, Emeritus, Johns Hopkins University

I like the perspective and thesis of the book. It makes great sense to me. Other than books I have read about the effects of the plague on civilization or of the influenza epidemic of 1918, I have not seen much in the way of health perspectives in history. Seems long overdue and much to your credit to address it. Clearly, this is a tremendous undertaking. I like how you have laid out the "haves", "needs", "urges", and "wants" in the introduction. I understand that this is fundamental to the book and its structure. I think of early science and early religion/mythology as connected in an attempt to understand and explain nature, whether it was at the level of everyday existence and survival or of attempts to explain the cosmos. I like the lower portion of the second page of Part One. Sweeping in scope. Well done.
             Edward Charles Horton
         Past Marshal, Baronial Order of the Magna Charta

You are truly amazing. I was particularly interested in the section about bacteria and viruses.
             Michael Labowsky, Ph.D.
         Past President, Yale Club of Central New Jersey

It's inspiring. The content caught and held my interest, and I could see how you got from A to Z.
              Harry Redd
         Governor, First Maryland Company, Jamestowne Society

Re: Lust and Law and Lawyers in Health Care Industry – Both sections represent your thesis well.
             Megan Reynolds, J.D.

I think it is fascinating and is really a profound analysis for which you should be really congratulated.
            John J. Sciarra, A.B. (Yale), M.D., Ph.D.
         Professor and Chair Emeritus, Department of Obstetrics and Gynecology
           Northwestern University Medical School, Chicago, Illinois

I think your new book will be of interest to the historian of health and medicine.
             Richard Sher, Ph.D.
     Professor of History, Emeritus, New Jersey Institute of Technology, Newark, New Jersey

I hadn't known that Michael Crichton went to Harvard Medical School -- fascinating!!
            Caroline Grace Katz, A.B. (Harvard), author
           The Daughters of Yalta (Houghton Mifflin Harcourt, 2020)

Very nice!
              Christos Christou
         Governor General, Order of the First Families of Maryland

I have "surveyed" your m/s. WOW, what an undertaking!
              Garrett Power, J.D.
         Professor Emeritus, School of Law, University of Maryland-Baltimore

We would love to have you talk to the Harvard Club about your book- It would be such an honor for us!
            Karen Boyle, A.B., M.D., F.A.C.S.
          President, Harvard Club of Maryland

I read with interest your carefully researched Meditation on St Luke. Try as I might, I could find nothing heretical, or even unreasonable, in the text! I suppose one might question that Luke was the most famous physician in history on the grounds that his contribution to medicine has no parallel to Galen's. However, you are probably right in that ascription bearing in mind he was a doctor afield, more famous because of his effect outside the field of medicine. It is also worth noting the amount of attention Luke gave to Jesus' and the disciples/apostles healings in both his works.

Luke's closeness to Theophilus supports the contention Luke was a gentile. Ralph Major seems to undercut his own assertion that Luke was "an insignificant physician," because he acknowledges Greeks dominated medicine in 1st-century Rome, so Luke, being Greek, was hardly insignificant even though he is better known for his Gospel and the Acts.

Glad to see footnote argues that adoption by Joseph gave Jesus a double claim to be a son of David—in the eyes of Jewish law. That touches on the controversy over the virgin birth, though I realize that is not your concern here.

Your extract seems carefully researched. Thanks for giving me a peak.

Rev. Dr. John Bassett Moore Frederick
Clerk in Holy Orders, Church of England
Past Director, Church of England Children's Society
Governor Emeritus, Society of Colonial Wars in the State of New Jersey

I thoroughly enjoyed reading your book. Fresh ideas were stitched together in an easy-to-read outline that was well researched and cleverly crafted. Good theology always spurs discussion. Your points were well made and there will always be people to argue for another line of reasoning. My prayer is that whatever discussion proceeds from the reading of your book, be it positive or negative, will only serve to edify and challenge you.

Rev. Dr. Mernie Crane
Adjunct Faculty, Wesley Theological Seminary
Board of Directors, George Washington University Institute for Spirituality and Health

Health Matters

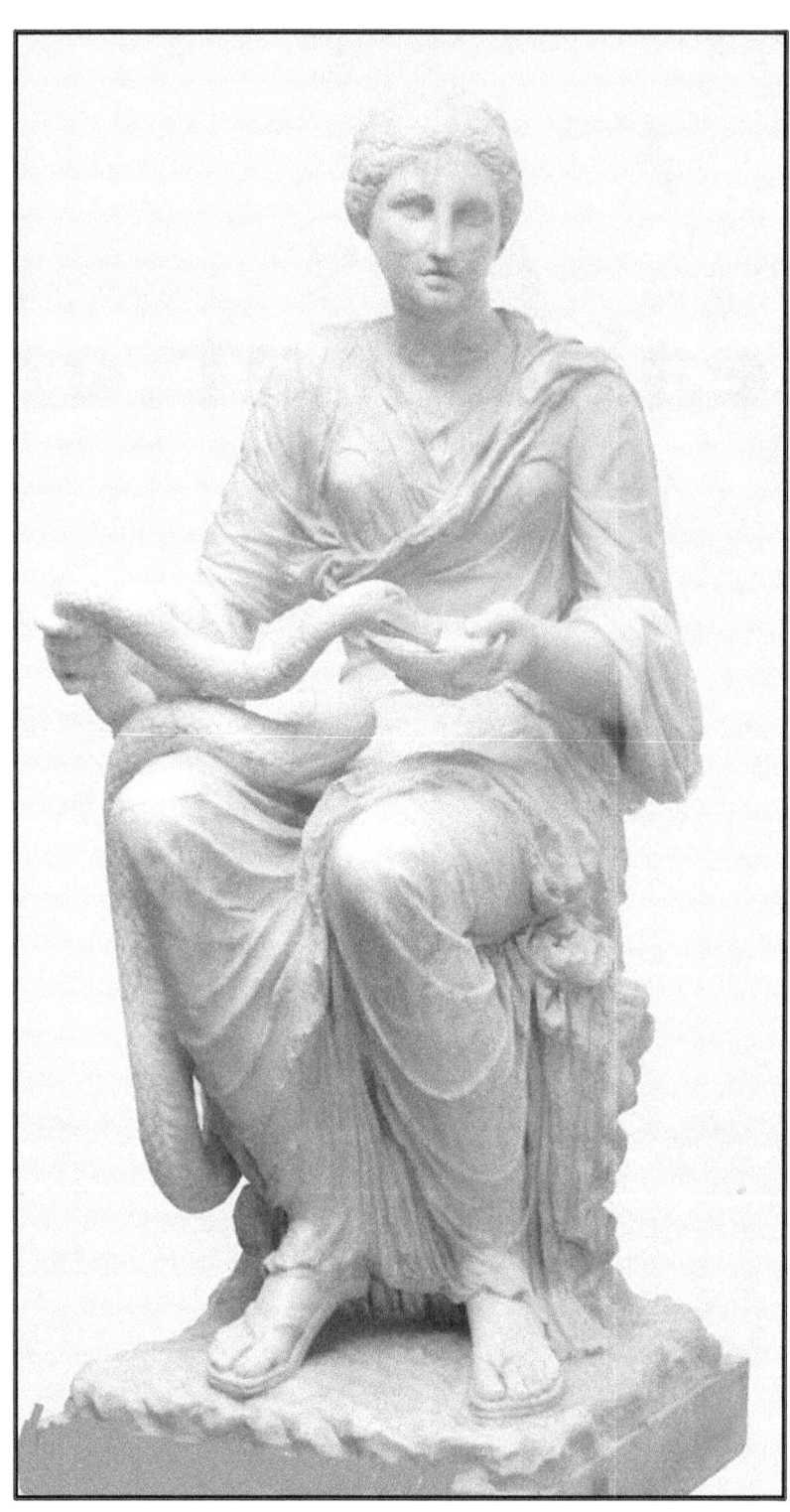
"Hygeia" in The Hermitage (from Google Images)

Hygeia

HEALTH MATTERS

A New View of Human History

By

George J. Hill, M.D., M.A., D.Litt.
Captain, Medical Corps, USNR (ret)

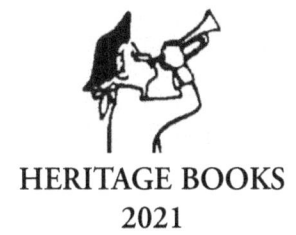

HERITAGE BOOKS
2021

HERITAGE BOOKS
AN IMPRINT OF HERITAGE BOOKS, INC.

Books, CDs, and more—Worldwide

For our listing of thousands of titles see our website
at
www.HeritageBooks.com

Published 2021 by
HERITAGE BOOKS, INC.
Publishing Division
5810 Ruatan Street
Berwyn Heights, Md. 20740

Copyright © 2021 George J. Hill, M.D., M.A., D.Litt.

Cover designed by Debbie Riley

All rights reserved. No part of this book may be reproduced or transmitted in any form or by any means, electronic or mechanical, including photocopying, recording or by any information storage and retrieval system without written permission from the author, except for the inclusion of brief quotations in a review.

International Standard Book Numbers
Paperbound: 978-0-7884-######

To Lanie,

with deepest thanks for your patience

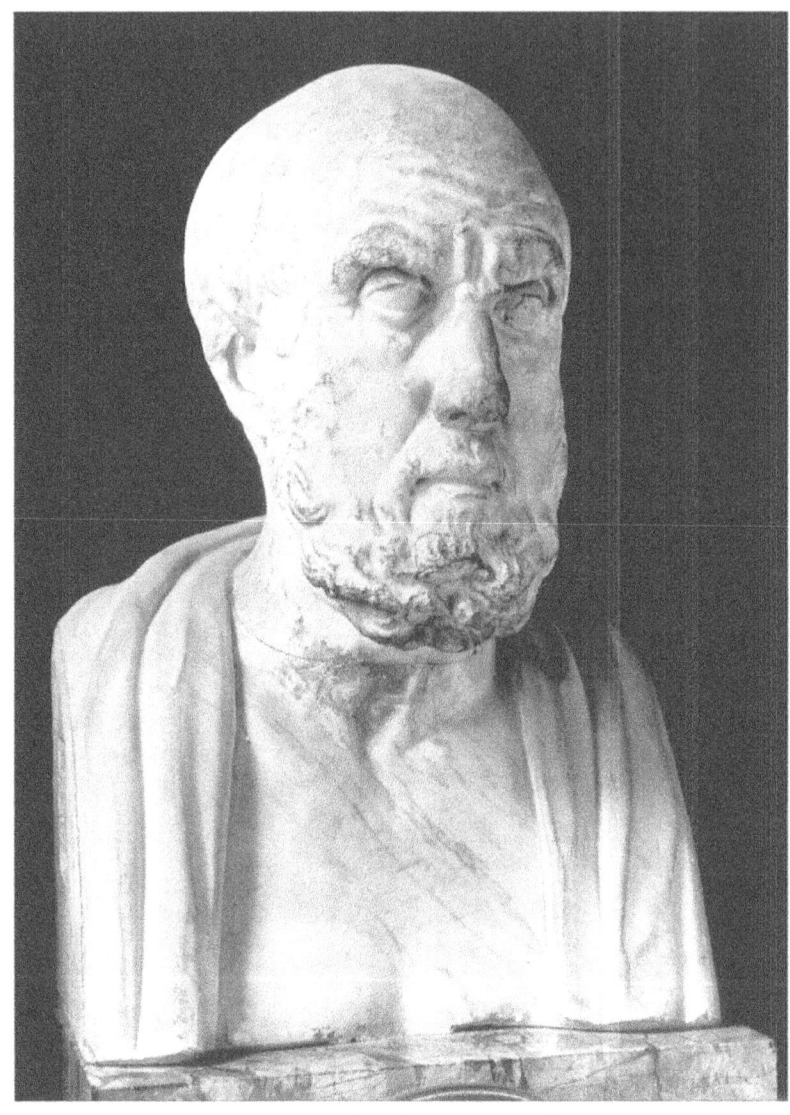

Hippocrates of Kos, from The Bridgeman Art Library

Hippocrates of Kos (c.460–c.370 B.C.)
Founder of Western Medicine

Contents

Illustrations x
Perspective – A Physician-Historian Views History through the Lens of Health xvi
Introduction – Overview of Health Matters 1
    Health and Life 3
Part One - Human Health – The Components of Health 4
    Humans' Haves, Needs, Urges, Wants, and Exceptions 5
    Chapter 1. The Haves 7
        A. The Body 8
        B. The Mind 10
        C. The Environment 12
    Chapter 2. The Needs 15
        A. Air and Breath 15
        B. Sun and Light 17
        C. Sleep and Dreams 19
    Chapter 3. The Urges 20
        Three Instincts for Survival 20
            A. Water 21
            B. Food 23
            C. Shelter 25
        Two Additional Urges 27
            D. Lust 27
            E. Social Connections 36
        Two Uniquely Human Urges 43
            F. Clothing – Personal Covering 43
            G. Fire 46
        Another Urge 48
            H. Dogs and Other Animals 48
    Chapter 4. The Wants 50
        A. Love 51
        B. Money 52
            Relationships Between the Haves, Needs, Urges,
            and Wants 54
        C. Enough 55
    Chapter 5. Other Considerations 57
        Pain, Exercise, Avocations 57
    Chapter 6. The Exceptions 59
        A. Unavoidable Exceptions 59
        B. Religion 59
            Needs, Urges, Wants 61
            Altruism 64
            Sacrifice 65
            Self-Sacrifice 66
        C. Irrational Behavior 67
            Search for Adventure 67
            Miscalculation of Risk 68
            Rejection of Science 69
            Neuropsychiatric Reasons 69
            Addiction 70

        D. Benefits from Disregarding the Exceptions 70
        E. The Dark Side of Medicine 70
    Chapter 7. Choices and Ambitions 71
        A. Choices and Decisions 71
        B. Ambition 74
    Chapter 8. Death 74
        A. Death with Dignity 74
        B. Immortality 76
    Chapter 9. Public Health 78
        A. Infectious Diseases 80
        B. Endemic – Pandemic 81
        C. Biology and Biochemistry 81
        D. Parasites 83
        E. Microbes and Viruses 85
        F. COVID-19 88

Part Two - Health Matters in Human History 89
    Chapter 10. Health and Illness in Medicine, Science, and Technology 90
        A. Human History from the Perspective of Health 92
        B. Developments in Human Health – Topical 95
            Rituals 95
            Plants 96
            Metals 98
            Beverages 98
            Addictive Substances 99
            Surgery 102
            Psychiatry 102
            Doctors Afield 103
            Saint Luke 103
        C. Developments in Human Health - Chronological 106
            4000 BCE to 323 BCE 107
            323 BCE to 11th Century CE 110
            11th Century CE to 16th Century 114
            16th Century CE to 18th Century CE 117
            18th Century CE to 19th Century 123
            19th Century CE to 20th Century 126
            20th Century to the present 138
    Chapter 11. Health Care Industry 148
        A. Health Care at Home 148
        B. The Health Care Industry, 1945-1975 151

Part Three - Discussion and Conclusion 156
    Chapter 12. Historiography 157
        A. Three Other Books 157
            Warfare Between Science and Theology 157
            The Structure of Scientific Revolutions 164
            The Whig Interpretation of History 169
        B. Telling the Story of History 170
            Famous People 170
            Making Choices 172

    An Argument 173
   C. A Driver of History? 173
   D. Intellectual History 174
 Chapter 13. Recent History 175
  The Last 120 Years 175
 Chapter 14. Discussion and Conclusion 178
  Final Thoughts 178

Acknowledgments 180
Appendices 181
 A. Death 181
 B. Parasitology and Microbiology 197
 C. More Doctors Afield 203
 D. COVID-19 Chronology 210
 E. Hippocratic Oath 215
Bibliography 217
Notes 248
Index 306
Other Books by the Author 321
About the Author 322

Illustrations

"*The Doctor*," by Sir Luke Fildes (1897) — Front cover
    In the Tate Museum, London (from Google Images).
    The background color of the cover is green, which is the academic color for medicine. The tradition of green was established by Harvard University and it has since been adopted in the academic community. The reason that green was chosen for medicine is unknown. The particular shade is now "Kelly green."

"Hygeia," Greek goddess of health — Frontispiece

Hippocrates of Kos — Page vi
Saint Luke, c. 800 — Page xi
Thomas Eakins, "The Gross Clinic" — Page xii
Thomas Eakins, "The Agnew Clinic" — Page xiii
Red Cross Nurse, World War I – Recruiting Poster — Page xiv
Coronavirus, schematic. — Page xv

Texas Medical Center, Houston, Texas — Page 155

George J. Hill, photograph of the author — Page 317

The Caduceus, symbol of Hermes — Back cover
    Hermes was a Greek god and herald of the gods. Adopted by the U.S. Army as a symbol of Medicine, from U.S. Army website: http://www.milbadges.com/corps/usa/med.

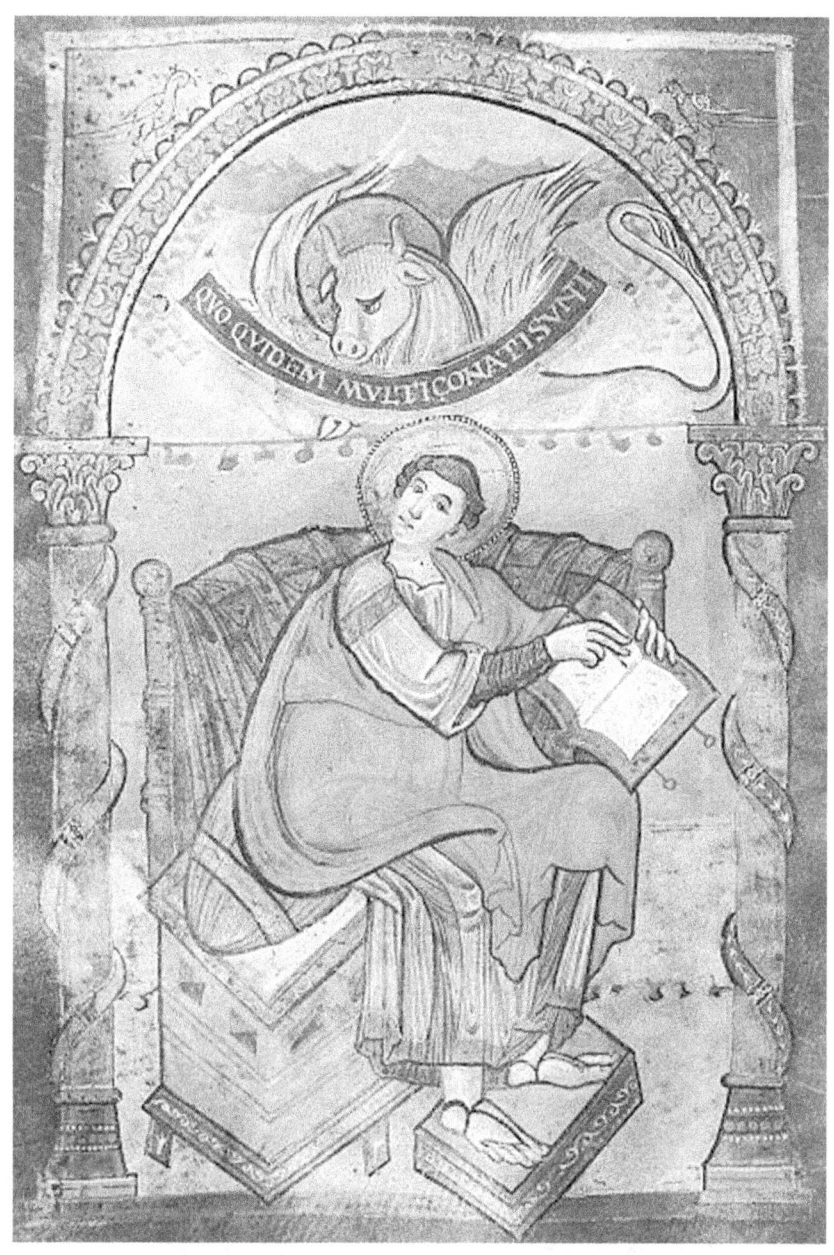

From the Gospel of St. Riquier or the Gospel of Charlemagne, Google Images

Saint Luke, c.800

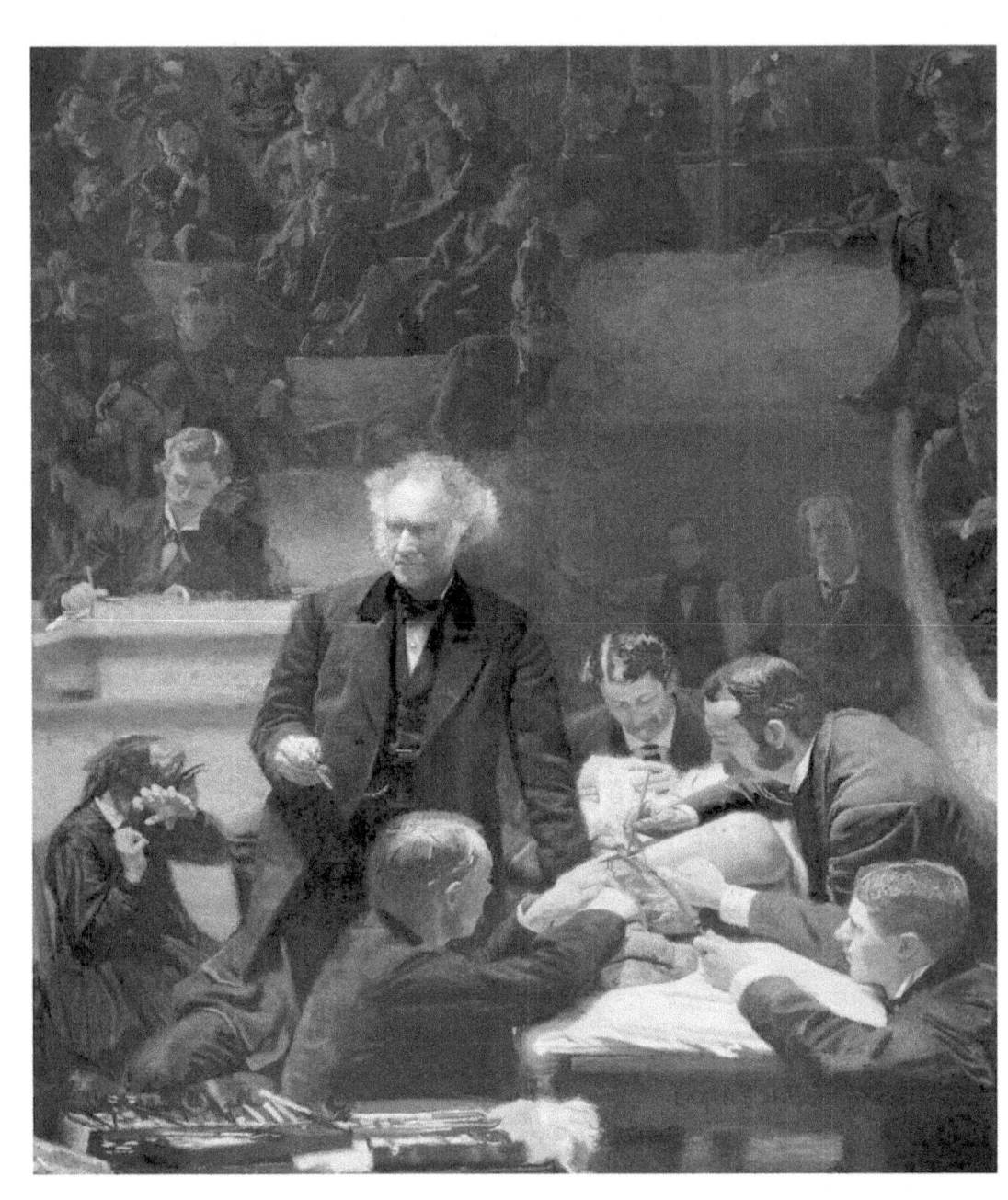

From the Philadelphia Museum of Art

The Gross Clinic
Thomas Eakins. 1875

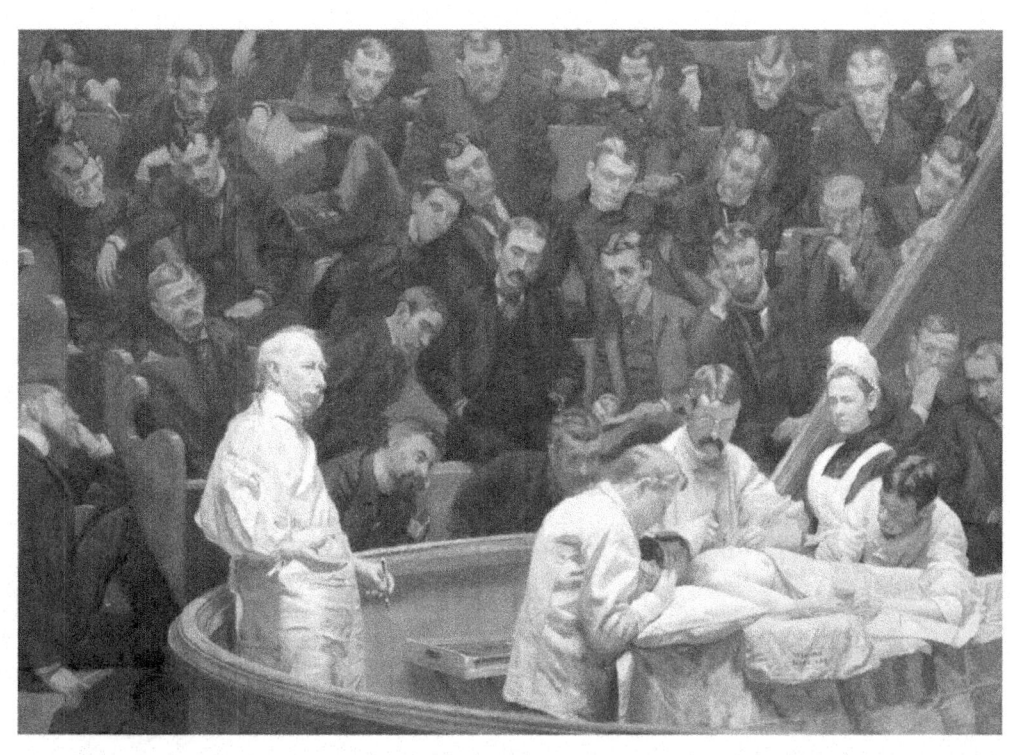

From the Philadelphia Museum of Art

The Agnew Clinic
Thomas Eakins. 1889

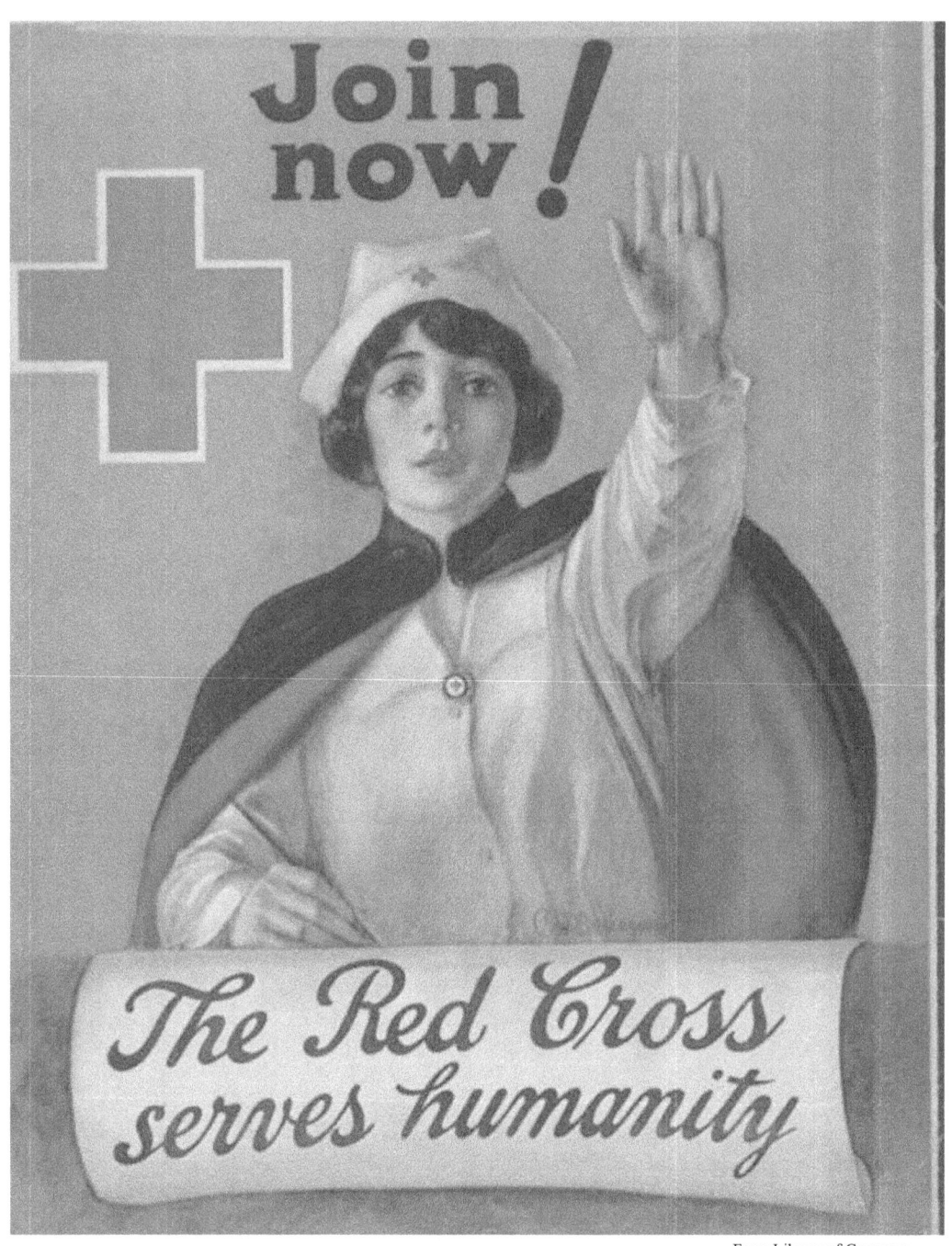

From Library of Congress

Red Cross Nurse
World War I
Recruiting Poster

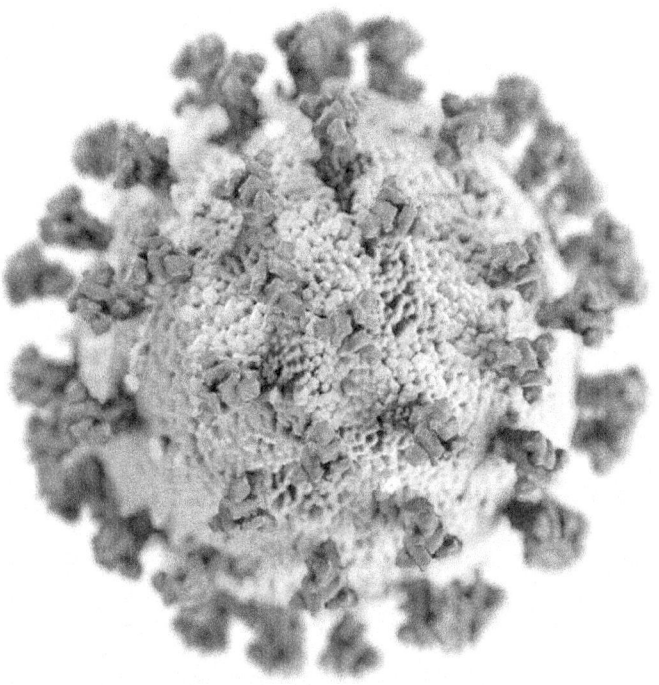

From World Health Organization

Corona Virus -- Schematic

Perspective

This book is about human history, viewed through the lens of health, written by a physician-historian. You are entitled to know about the writer of this book, and thus about the writer's personal perspective.

I am writing this at the age of 88, near the end of a long life. I am a Midwesterner by birth, with family roots in New England, and I have now returned to the Atlantic Coast. I am a fifth generation Iowan, descended from those who first broke the prairie soil in that state. I lived in a small town in Iowa during the Great Depression and World War II. We could feel the effects of the Dust Bowl. I am White, and until I went to college, I knew little about people of color. My generation is sometimes called the Silent Generation. This generation is largely forgotten. It is located between the famous Greatest Generation that won that war and their children, the Boomer Generation. In 1949, I volunteered to become a United States Marine. It was the start of a military reserve career which spanned 43 years and four wars. I was in the Marine Corps as a corporal, then in the Public Health Service as a lieutenant, and finally in the Navy, from which I retired as a captain in 1992. I went through "boot" camp during the Korean War, and I was on active duty for two years in the U.S. Public Health Service. I was in Bethesda, Maryland, in the tense days of the Cuban Missile Crisis. I volunteered twice for service in the Vietnam War, and I was recalled to active duty in the First Gulf War – Operation Desert Shield/Desert Storm.

Many people have helped me in life. With their recommendations, I received work-study scholarships for four years at Yale College. While there, I decided to become a doctor, and I received scholarships to attend the Harvard Medical School. I was a surgeon for forty years, and during that time I also was involved in primary care and emergency medicine as a Navy doctor. My work as a physician also included teaching, research, administration, and work in oncology and public health.

I was also a historian and a scientist. My social sciences teacher in eighth grade awakened my interest in history. She said that I was her best student in American history. My interest in history has always been very broad, but it has mainly been in the history of the last two centuries, and in the history of science and medicine. I was given a Gilbert chemistry set as a Christmas present at the age of 12, and I began to do experiments with additional supplies that I bought at a local drugstore. My interest in science eventually extended into the fields of biology, chemistry, and medicine. I developed a principal focus on cancer as the result of a chance assignment given by an instructor at Yale. I have studied Latin, German and Spanish, and although I am not fluent in these languages, I find that languages are useful skills for a historian. I was an active scientist for more than forty years, in both laboratory research and in studies with patients; in recent years, most of my publications have been in the field of history.

After retiring from surgery, but while still active as a physician, I earned a Master's Degree in history, and then a Doctor of Letters. My academic career includes appointments as professor of surgery, preventive medicine, oncology, and history. I have been president of a hospital's medical staff, chief of staff of a public hospital, chairman of many academic committees, president of the faculty of a medical school and of its faculty union, chief executive officer of several academic organizations, a faculty division chief, department chairman, associate dean, and acting college president. I am now an Emeritus Professor of Surgery at Rutgers New Jersey Medical School and an Adjunct Professor of Surgery at the Uniformed Services University of the Health Sciences. I am a Fellow Emeritus of the Explorers Club, a Life Member of the National Assembly of the American Cancer Society, and Emeritus Member of the Boards of the Frost Valley Y.M.C.A. and Sterling College.

My wife, Helene Z. Hill, Ph.D., has been a partner in my work in science. We first shared a laboratory in 1962, and we have published 26 papers as co-authors. Our family includes four children, three grandchildren, and three great-grandchildren. We have traveled to more than 50 countries and we have hiked on all seven continents. We trekked to the Base Camp of Mount Everest and along the Inca Trail to Machu Picchu, and we have climbed the 48 Four Thousand-foot Mountains of New Hampshire.

Introduction

"Health Matters" Is the Search by Humans for Good Health and a Long Life. It Is the Quest to Avoid Illness, Treat Disease, and Delay Death.

This essay proposes that health is the fundamental driving force in human history. Simply stated, human history has always been about health. I propose that human history is based on health and on beliefs about health, and that the ultimate goal of humans is the search for good health and a long life. The most important question that humans have always asked is: How can I be healthy? The answer is to avoid illness, to treat disease, and to delay death. This is what is meant by *"Health Matters."*[1]

Good health comes from good luck or making good choices. The opposite of good health – which Lewis Mumford called "illth" – comes from bad luck or making bad choices. Health beliefs are what humans think will keep them safe and well. Health beliefs were crucial to human society as it evolved.[2]

Part One of this book discusses the Haves, Needs, and Urges that are present in humans. Part One begins with what all humans have at birth: their body, their mind, and a surrounding environment. These are the three Haves. There are then three Needs, without which humans cannot survive. The first need is air to breathe, for without air, life is very short indeed. The second need is the sun, which is the primary source of all energy on earth, and which also is the principal source of light. The third need is sleep. Humans also have several Urges. The Urges derive from the search for health – for *Health Matters* – which means that if you don't prepare for the future, something bad will happen, and that you will have poor health and an early death.

There are seven (or possibly eight) urges or needs for preservation of health. These are the drivers of history of human beings. If you prefer the notion that history is based on choices, humans' decisions are made on the best choice for health in regard to these urges. The first three urges are Water, Food, and Shelter. These urges are necessary instincts for survival, and they are also seen in other animals. All animals need water and food, and most animals need shelter from predators. Water is a daily need. Food must be found and stored. Shelter is a hiding place for safety and protection. The next four urges are Lust, Social Connections, Personal Covering, and Fire. The last two of these are unique to the human species. Lust leads to procreation and thus to the preservation of the species, and which may take precedence over the urge for shelter. Social connections are seen in a family, or in a clan, or in a community. Personal Covering with clothing, to protect from cold, is something that no other species needs or has developed. The seventh urge is for fire and fuel, which is necessary to start a fire to keep it going – no other species can do this. I will add to this list an eighth possible human urge: the use of animals, especially the dog. Canines have a unique connection with humans, as companions and guardians, useful for work, and sometimes to be food. All of these urges are necessary for health.

There are also two things that humans Want: Love and Money. This essay discusses the relationships between the Needs, Urges, and Wants, and then the subjects of Exercise, Avocations, and what is Enough. There are three types of Exceptions to these urges. The first type of exception includes those that are Unavoidable, including genetic problems, such as Down syndrome and other birth defects. The second exception is Religion. This is an unusual exception, because many people believe that it is an urge rather than an exception. Religion, including mythology, is also involved in the early history of the health professions. This subject of religion includes Altruism and Self-Sacrifice, accepting risk for the sake of others, which is necessary to preserve the species. The third exception is Irrational Behavior, which is to say, some other reason that defies logic. Some examples are: to choose risk in the search for adventure; miscalculation of risk, as in the immaturity of childhood; careless behavior; or false bravery (especially in teenagers); rejection of science (such those who are opposed to vaccination); or psychological or neuropsychiatric reasons, such as sociopathic behavior, addictions (e.g., alcohol, nicotine, marijuana, opioids), alcohol, autism spectrum disorders, and adverse effects of drugs (e.g., antibiotics).

The essay diverges at this point to enumerate some benefits that accrue from disregarding the exceptions, and the ways that choices are made in making decisions about health. The next major topic is Death, which is inevitable, even if the Haves, Needs, Urges and the Wants are perfectly satisfied, and the Choices are selected.

We will then see how these components of health – the Haves, Needs, Urges, Wants, and Exceptions – led to the development of the modern world. Medicine and science arose from the search for health: how people learned to improve their health and their chances for a long and healthy life. First came self-trained men and women who had "the gift" of the ability to treat the sick and care for wounds; and midwives, who helped women in childbirth; and then the early herbalists – men and women who could find plants with useful effects. These early health care workers found apprentices who also had "the gift" of healing, and who passed their skills to the next generation. Some of them had special skills. They became the "barber surgeons" who developed techniques for procedures using their hands – manipulation of the body, treatment of fractures, wounds, and abscesses. In this way, modern internal medicine and surgery developed, and also the fields of pharmacy and nursing. Religion also evolved from the same impulse. Some of the early healers were gifted in caring for peoples' emotional needs.[3]

Medicine became the dawn of science; it was the first scientific profession. The fields of chemistry, physics, biology, preventive medicine and public health developed in the search for medicines and a safe environment. Early humans needed food, water, and shelter, which were the first three primal urges. These urges are instinctive in mammals. Hunter-gatherers soon found drinking water, and they searched for food on land and in water – in streams, lakes, and the ocean. Water and food were the first two urges, and they were the most important. Hunter-gatherers' searches for water and food, and their need to return to shelter, required understanding of the world about them. And thus, from those early searches, geography and astronomy developed. The hunter-gatherers on land and those who lived near water, early fishermen, were followed many generations later by farmers, who domesticated wild fruits and vegetables and created agriculture. Some farmers and fishermen lived near each other for protection, as an advanced form of the urge for shelter. From such small communities, towns and cities developed, in which individuals could specialize in production of useful crafts. In this way, engineering, architecture, and trade gradually evolved. The alphabet, mathematics, philosophy, and the various art forms – visual, performing, musical – also developed as these skills arose and flourished in human societies. The martial arts can also be traced to the desire of humans to have a safe and productive environment.[4]

Part Two of this book is entitled "Health Matters in Human History." In Part Two, I will show the effects that serious diseases and deaths have had on human history, and the effects that have occurred in societies which have tried to ameliorate or prevent illness, diseases, and deaths. The devastating effects of illness and death on human history will be additionally emphasized with examples of contrasts, in which good health and longevity enabled some individuals or groups to survive. I will discuss the points from two perspectives: first, by topic; and secondly from the aspect of chronology, from earliest humans to the present time.

Part Three includes a section on Historiography, additional Discussion of all of the previous subjects, and a Conclusion. In Historiography, I examine the subject of human history, looking again at the question of how history can properly be defined and written. There are many ways to look at the subject of history. For example, I compare *Health Matters* with Thomas Kuhn's *Structure of Scientific Revolutions*. My view is that *Health Matters* is not a new paradigm in science; it is instead more appropriate to think of *Health Matters* instead as a new way, another way, to look at human history. Also, is it possible to say that there is a driving force in history? That was proposed by Alfred Thayer Mahan in *The Influence of Sea Power upon History*. The Discussion returns to the many ways that religion and science have impacted upon human health. Medicine, the field of health care, incorporates aspects of both religion and science. Religion, science, and medicine have changed over the long history of the human species. I also propose that *Health Matters* is based on both the activities of specific individuals and on choices made by communities of peoples. I once asked the eminent historian Professor Robert Darnton the question "What is history?" He immediately replied, "History is informed argument." I argue that *Health Matters*, as discussed in this essay, is the driving force in human history.[5]

Health and Life

Skol
"Good Health" Toast in Danish, Norwegian, and Swedish

The argument proposed in *Health Matters* is that the ultimate goal of humans is the search for good health and a long life. That health and life are connected should be obvious, but the relationship has heretofore been recognized infrequently. *Health Matters* is intended to correct this defect, and to show that there is indeed a close relationship between life and health, and that this relationship has been the dominant role in human history.[6]

"Life" appears in *Encyclopedia Britannica* as both a noun – living matter – and as a verb – a process. Living matter has several attributes, such as responsiveness, growth, and energy transformation, but the principal ones are reproduction and metabolism. Reproduction is required for a species, but not for an individual. However, metabolism is crucial to life of an individual. It is the *sine qua non* of life. Metabolism in *Britannica* is "the sum of the chemical reactions that take place within each cell of a living organism and that provide energy for vital processes and for synthesizing new organic material."

No connection between the words "health" and "life" appears in *Webster's Unabridged Dictionary* or in *Encyclopedia Britannica*, and it is rare to find it anywhere else except in medical books. In *Webster's*, the word "health" does not appear in connection with the derivatives of the word "life," such as "live," "living," and "alive." No less than 50 other words derived from "life" appear in *Webster's* as nouns, verbs, adjectives, and adverbs; and with dozens of uses derived from the concept embedded in the word "life." For example, there are the words "lifeguard," lifeless," lifelike," lived, and lively." Health does not appear in any of these definitions of life. The word "health" and 22 congeners of this word are in *Webster's Unabridged Dictionary*, but the word "life" does not appear in any of Webster's definitions of these words.

The paucity of connecting the words "health" and "life" in *Webster's* is also present in *Encyclopedia Britannica*. The *Britannica* article on "Life" by Carl Sagan, Lynn Margulis, and Dorian Sagan is a brilliant discussion of the definition of life and of its possible origins. The authors issue a disclaimer, stating that "life is complex and difficult to briefly define." Nevertheless, their long article does cover the topic thoroughly from the point of view of science. They do not discuss the many other ways that the word "life" appears in the modern world in literature, philosophy, and the arts. It is interesting that the word "health" does not appear even once in the long *Britannica* article on Life.

The Bible was examined for any possible connections between the words, "health" and "life." The search was almost fruitless. In the Concordance to the *King James Version*, there are 409 citations of "life," 231 citations of "live," 86 of "alive," and 19 of "health" (17 in the Old Testament and two in the New Testament). The two words, health and life, appear together in only two places in the *King James Version*: Genesis 43:28 ("Thy servant our father is in good health, he is yet alive"), and Proverbs 4:22 ("For they are life unto those that find them, and health to all their flesh"). In the Old Testament, most of the early references are to bodily life, while the later citations refer to other uses of the word, such as "years of life." Most of the references to "life" in the New Testament are metaphorical, such as to "eternal life" and "everlasting life." Day by day life counted for much in Biblical times. There are 57 references to "all the days of his/her/my/our life," or to the life of a specific person. However, there is scant connection between life and health in the Bible.

In contrast to *Webster's*, *Britannica*, and the *King James Version* of the Bible, the word "life" appears in more than 200 places in *Health Matters*, and it is found in nearly every chapter of the book. The word "health" appears in 547 places, and "health" is in every chapter of *Health Matters*.

Health Matters

Part One

Human Health

The Components of Health

Humans' Haves, Needs, Urges, Wants, and Exceptions

This essay argues that *Health Matters* – the search for health – involves the knowledge that if you don't prepare for the future, something bad will surely happen, and that you will have poor health. The goal of *Health Matters* is to delay the ultimate end point of life, which is Death. Stated another way, it is to prolong Life. Most of us take life for granted, but we often think of death. This essay will discuss the requirements for life, while death is always lurking in the background.[7]

In our species – *Homo sapiens* – awareness of the existence of a future is more advanced than in other animal species. Other mammals, such as elephants, appear to show emotional responses to death, and they may be aware of the future. Knowledge of the existence of a future, and how to prepare for it, may also be greater in *Homo sapiens* than in other previous species of the genus *Homo* which are now extinct.[8]

There is a double meaning in the title of this essay, *Health Matters*. The word "health" is used both as a noun and as an adjective; and "matters" is used both as a verb and as a noun. Health (as a noun) means what is important, when matters is a verb. On the other hand, when used in sequence as "health matters," health (as an adjective) and matters (as a noun), is what this essay is all about.[9]

****

Part One of this book shows how society has evolved from the ways that humans have utilized the three "haves" of health that they had at birth, and how they worked with their two needs, the seven or eight urges, and the three exceptions. The further development of the modern world is the subject of Part Two of this book. The modern world has evolved on two paths, although the paths are not completely separate: One path is based on science, the other is non-scientific. Medicine, which is both an art and a science, is a good example of a bridge between the two paths of science and non-science. History may be another example of a bridging field, because it is based on both facts (science) and opinions (non-scientific). Religion is the quintessential non-scientific field, although admittedly many clergymen have made advances in science.

Science is based on the assumption that there is an answer to every question about nature. A scientist searches for answers to questions, based on the belief that for every question, there is only one best answer. Technology, which is applied science, is based on the same assumption. Art has long been present in human history, and it is present in the modern world, in many forms, although it defies classification as either science or non-science. The same can be said for music. Art and music probably arose with the incantations of the witch-doctors, with painted faces and dances. Art and music now utilize input from imagination and technology. In some ways, the world of art and music is similar to that of the world of science. There is in art and music a search for perfection. However, in art and music, it is not a search for a single best answer. As some humans began to think of the world and its future, their imagination led to speculation. And from these thoughts, we have philosophy, mathematics, the alphabet, and law. It would be interesting to trace the development of all of these fields of human endeavor from their earliest origins, but that would take us far beyond the scope of this simple essay on *Health Matters*.

The modern world thus includes science and technology, medicine and religion, art and intellectual activity. The history of the modern world, of modernity, is like a motion picture which is seen through different lenses, depending on the perspective of the viewer. Sometimes it seems to be replayed, but, as with all of history, and as with time itself, it is continuously moving forward. Toward infinity. The early modern world developed methods of water storage, of fishing and agriculture, and of the use of animals. Then humans began to use fibers, woven on looms; and then architecture, weaponry, walled cities; and the later attributes of civilization, such as the use of sketching and writing, and discoveries in geography and geology. Curious minds developed philosophy, mathematics, and astrology. Biology, chemistry, physics, geology, and astrology began as observational sciences; and astrology then morphed into astronomy. It is usually said that observational science was followed by experimental science, and that this became the modern method of science. However, technology played an important role in the development of experimental science, because humans tried various ways to develop fishhooks and methods of weaving. Technology and science have always worked hand-in-hand. Humans tried the use of different materials in these early experiments, looking for what worked best. Experimental methods led to great advances in the first four of these "hard" sciences that were mentioned above. Astronomy has recently become an experimental science, too. And then the so-called "soft sciences" of psychology and sociology appeared, in which the experimental method has also been applied, cautiously, and warily. Most of the experiments on humans, or on groups of people, have significant ethical issues. Humans later developed other forms of technology, including power – first water power, then steam power, electricity, and atomic power.[10]

Death is something to study, to try to understand, and to avoid as long as possible. Death cannot be, and is not, an exception to the urge to preserve health, for the urge to preserve health inevitably ends with death. All living things must die. Death is the *sine qua non* of life. Some exceptions to the urges to preserve health are Unavoidable, but the first major exception to these urges is Religion. For example, the belief that "God wills it." Some believe that this is not an exception, for they would say that religion itself is actually a fundamental urge for preservation. The second exception is Altruism and Self-Sacrifice, for the sake of others, and thus also to preserve the species. Altruism and self-sacrifice are included under the rubric of religion, because these behaviors are often based on religion. The third exception is Irrational Behavior, which is some other reason that defies logic. Some examples are the search for Adventure; or Miscalculation of Risk, as in immaturity, carelessness, or bravado; or Rejection of Science, as in the denial of benefits of vaccination; and Neuropsychiatric reasons, including mental illness, dementia, brain tumors, addictions, autism, and adverse effects of drugs. It is also clear that some of the exceptions have been beneficial, either to individuals or to society. A few examples will be provided for the exceptions that have been made by choice, and some that have been accidental.

We begin by remembering what humans have: a body, a mind, and the environment that surrounds us.

Chapter 1

The Haves

What Humans Have

Everyone is born with a body and a mind, into an environment. The human body and its environment are physical things, whereas the mind is but a figment of the imagination. In this essay, the term environment refers to the external environment, which surrounds us, rather than the interior environment (*milieu intérieur*), a term that is used in medical science to represent the fluidic mass of which the body is composed.[11]

It is an interesting challenge to compose brief sections of this essay on the Body, the Mind, and the Environment to introduce the subject of *Health Matters*. These three terms are already understandable, and nothing is required to justify the proposal that they are essential components of human history. Nevertheless, a discussion of each is necessary to clarify their connections to this essay on *Health Matters* in humans. There are also important connections between these three topics, which suggest that more interactions between them are likely to be seen in the future. We will first examine a few aspects of the human body and mind, and then interactions of the body and mind of humans with the environment.[12]

A. The Body

When nature, being oppressed, commands the mind
To suffer with the body
–Lear, in William Shakespeare, *King Lear*, Act 2, Scene 4[13]

The history of the body of a person, and thus of all people, begins at the start of life. A person's history is usually reckoned from the date and time of birth, which is also called parturition or nativity. Biologically speaking, a person's life actually begins several months earlier, at the time of conception, when sperm and egg are conjoined, or perhaps even a bit earlier, when the sperm and egg are released to begin their passage. If this is true, all sperm and eggs should be considered as signs of life. However, not all fertilized eggs normally produce a living child, for there are many ways that the process may end before birth. One of the saddest endings is when it is a child is found to be dead at birth – a stillbirth.[14]

The precise definition of "birth" is also problematic. The moment of birth could be when a child exits the birth canal, or it could be the moment when a newborn baby is free of its mother. This is either when the "cord is cut," but with the placenta still in the uterus, or after both baby and placenta have appeared. In some instances, and in some cultures, the umbilical cord may be allowed to wither, instead of being cut. There is also an earlier period, of pre-natal life, which started several months earlier. At that time, for every baby, this was the moment after a man and a woman came into intimate contact, and then soon, one sperm and one egg met and conjugated inside the woman. No one knew that this had happened at that time, and the silent development of the embryo, which became a fetus, an unborn child, was called a miracle by some.[15]

Some scientists call the baby's time in the uterus the pre-natal period, which has three stages. The first stage, known as "pre-embryonic," which occurs in the first few days, is a time of cell division and cell maturation. This is followed by the "embryonic" period of organ development, which lasts from the third to the eighth week of development; and then the "fetal period" in which the tissues and organs continue to mature until birth, which occurs about nine months after conception.[16]

The climax of the union of sperm and egg is known as fertilization, which normally takes place in the Fallopian tube. The egg had moved into the tube from the ovary in which it had resided, taking its turn in the menstrual cycles that began with the puberty of the mother. Fertilization results in (1) a reassociation of male and female sets into a full set of 23 pairs (n=46) of chromosomes, (2) establishing a mechanism for sex determination, depending on whether the male set of chromosomes included the X or the Y chromosome; and (3) activation of the zygote, which contains all that is needed for the new individual. The zygote, about 0.1mm in size, would be just barely visible. For reference, note that the head of a straight pin is approximately 2mm in size, and the pin itself has a diameter of about 0.8mm. The zygote is formed in the Fallopian tube, but within about four days, the enormous cell of the zygote has divided into smaller cells of normal size that are known as blastomeres. The cohering blastomeres are transported downward into the uterus for further development. Dividing and enlarging, the blastomeres develop into a blastocyst, which attaches to the interior of the uterus. An inner cell mass, called a trophoblast, develops into a placenta and fetal membranes, through which the mother nourishes the fetus, and transports its waste products. The inner cell mass contains the cells that will form the embryo. Three layers of cells are formed, which will form all of the tissues and organs of the body: the ectoderm (outer layers, such as the skin), mesoderm (middle layers, such as muscles), and endoderm (inner layers, such as the gut). At this time, the tiny developing embryo of a human looks much like the embryo of any other mammal. By the fourth week, it has developed a C-shape, with head and tail close together. The heart can already be seen, and the tail will eventually vanish. At five weeks, the embryo is 8mm in length, and it would be easily visible were it not deep within the uterus. However, it soon can be seen with ultrasound. At eight weeks, it can respond to delicate stimulation. "During the third month the young fetus clearly resembles a human being, although the head is disproportionately large. ... At four months individual differences between the faces of fetuses become distinguishable. ... At five months downy hairs (lanugo) cover the body, and some head hairs appear. ... Fetal movements ("quickening") are felt by the mother. At six months eyebrows and eyelashes are clearly present. ... At eight months fat is depositing beneath the skin. The testes begin to invade the scrotum [in boys]. At nine months the dull redness of the skin fades and wrinkles smooth out. The body and limbs become better-rounded. ... At full term (38 weeks) the body is plump. ... The average time of delivery is 280 days from the beginning of the last menstrual period ... Pregnancy may extend to 300 days or even more, in which case the baby tends to be heavier. Premature babies born under 27 weeks of age are less likely to survive ... whereas those more than 30 weeks old usually do survive."[17]

After it passed through the birth canal and entered the world, the baby's first purposeful act is instinctive: to breathe and to inhale air, even while it was still attached to its mother. The baby's environment had changed, however, from complete darkness to light. Its first actions were reflexes – it moved its arms, legs, and body. The baby sought for and found the maternal breast, for milk to satisfy its urges for water and food; and for its mother's arms, to provide safety. The baby then slept, and in its brain, its mind began to have thoughts, to think. The baby's survival depends on the mother's social connections, because the world is a harsh place, and the mother could not do it alone.[18]

Anonymous said, "The child is the father of the man" in Hindi (aka Urdu), and this metaphor has since been repeated many times. The baby develops into a child, the child grows into an adolescent who then becomes an adult. The adult matures physically and then it slowly declines. If long-lived, the adult ages and dies. Death may occur at any time; it is the body's only certain outcome. The transit of every person through each of the stages of life may be interesting, or challenging, or tragic. Humans have observed the body in themselves and in others, in each of these stages, and as the body is represented in drawings, paintings, sculpture, and photography. The depiction of the body may be nude, or covered, but the imagined body is still there. If the nude body is visualized through imagination, it is by a function of the mind. The nude may be chaste, but the view may be imagined as lusty, even pornographic.[19]

We all know that the body is composed of organs, but we rarely think about them unless we are ill. A specific organ comes to mind when we have a toothache, a headache, stomach pains, a broken leg, a kidney stone, a skin rash, a heart attack, or if the doctor says, "it's a problem with your liver." The number of organs is often said to be 78, but the count varies depending on where you look. Some say 100 organs, from the largest (supposedly the skin) to the smallest (perhaps the pituitary gland). Organs have also been grouped into eleven organ systems. They range from the slimy interior of the intestine to the hard-bitten fingernails at the skin's tip. From the beating heart to the steadfast liver. The solid bones and hardy muscles which pull them, the soft spleen and lymph nodes, the receptive bladder, the organs of reproduction and the nervous system which activates them. The endocrine glands, and the lungs which sustain everything. We do not live alone, though, because within and around the body are saprophytes and parasites, and examples of communalism, mutualism, and symbiosis. Think of the passage of food. Chopped into pieces and ground by the teeth, food is sprayed with a mildly alkaline enzyme in the mouth to begin digestion. Food is then partially liquified by the stomach's acid (and that acid is really strong), and churned with more enzymes in the intestines. The good stuff slips invisibly through the intestinal walls into lymphatic tubules and blood vessels, which carry the nutrients to where they are needed. The liver is a major factory for this type of work. What is left is liquid slop. More nutrients are extracted during the passage as it winds though more than twenty feet of small intestines. Near the end, the intestines squeeze most of the water from the slop, extracting the water for reuse. It has been called "the economy of the body." The slop is moved inexorably onward through the colon, where with helpful bacteria waiting to enjoy their meal, it is finally turned into a semi-solid mass of you-know-what for daily output. Many bacteria accompany the final passage. Some are dead, but many are alive, and their descendants usually find a way to return to the duty in someone's large bowel.[20]

The body is a wondrous thing. It is all derived from the three components of the original inner cell mass, the trophoblast, mentioned above. These are the outer layer (ectoderm), the inner layer (endoderm), and the middle layer (mesoderm). And such different courses these three layers take. From the ectoderm, we have both skin and brain. Anyone who has been to a butcher shop knows what a brain looks like. Compare that big mushy vital organ with leathery skin, will you? The endoderm develops into many organs, including stomach, pancreas, and the bowels. In the butcher shop, these are tripe, sweetbreads, and chitlins (or offal). Not only do they look different, they are indeed very different in their functions. One function is in their secretions, which ranges from very acidic in the stomach to nearly neutral in other parts of the intestinal tract. Stomach acidity ranges from pH of 1.0 to 3.5; neutral (distilled water) is pH 7.0. How does the lining of the stomach cope with secretions as acidic as hydrochloric acid, which is more acidic than vinegar? That's a good topic for a biology class. In fact, the stomach doesn't always cope with this high acidity, and then you get a peptic ulcer. Peptic ulceration is abetted by a germ called *Helicobacter pylori*. From mesoderm, we have muscles of three types: striated muscles, such as the biceps and the tiny muscles of the hands; smooth muscles in the intestines; and cardiac muscles. The first two types are motionless except when stimulated through their nerves, but the heart has a natural beat that continues even when it is isolated from its nerves. Isn't that amazing? Fat isn't usually listed as one of the organs, but it certainly functions as one, though it is dispersed throughout the body. Adipose tissue (fat) is derived from mesoderm. There are two types. One type is the familiar white fat (slightly yellow in color), which is mostly lipid. White fat is used by the body as an efficient way to store calories. The other type is brown fat, which is rarely seen, but it has a special function – it is packed with mitochondria. Brown fat is helpful in maintaining body temperature in the cold.[21]

This brief section on the Body shows that the life history of a person connects with many of the other topics that are covered in *Health Matters*, including the mind, the environment, air, light, sleep, water, food, shelter, social connections, lust, and love.[22]

B. The Mind

je pense, donc je suis = cogito, ergo sum (I think, therefore I am)
–Descartes, *Discourse on the Method* (1637)

The brilliant scholar of the Enlightenment, René Descartes (1596-1650), formulated the modern version of mind-body dualism when he developed a "new science grounded in observation and experiment." Descartes dismissed knowledge that was based only on "authority, the senses, and reason."[23]

Humans nevertheless continue to think in older ways, and to believe what they learn from others, especially those in authority, and what they perceive, and what they believe is reasonable. Although science should be based on observation and experiment, as stated by Descartes, scientists are human; they are trapped by what they know and believe. In the 1950s and 1960s, dozens, or perhaps hundreds, of students and young scientists at the Harvard Medical School saw a sentence posted above a window in a professor's conference room: "We only see what we look for, we only look for what we know."[24]

Consider the brain and the mind: Thinking occurs in the brain, as the mind works in its unpredictable ways. Some behavior is instinctive, such as responses to the urges for food and water and to be with other people. Flight responses are instinctive from some apparent dangers, such as loud noise or flashing light. Other dangers must be experienced or taught, such fire, or the top of a flight of stairs.[25]

Consideration of the future is a matter of the human mind. "Imagine this?" we think. "Or that." It is the knowledge of a future, and to use this knowledge to prepare for the future, that is one of the things which distinguishes humans from other mammals. Thinking of the future, and using tools to create the future that we want, is something that no other mammal can do. The first tool is the creation of a cover, at first just a skin or something made from large leaves, but then woven cloth and a weapon.[26]

"To be, or not to be, that is the question," and "I'm thinking of it …" Thoughts such as these pass through our minds, often uninvited. When we try to think of something, we often fail, and then, suddenly the answer appears in our mind. The mind is mysterious. As we let our thoughts wander, we think of instinctive behavior, of learned behavior, of imagined behavior, of trial and error, learning from mistakes; of the id, ego, and superego; of "muscle memory" in dance, and of practicing on the piano while inserting a personal note on the keyboard. The left hand plays the bass, which sets the rhythm. We appreciate the illuminating thoughts of Oliver Sachs, who wrote *The Man Who Mistook His Wife for a Hat* and several other books about disorders of the mind, and of both the book and the movie, *A Beautiful Mind*.[27]

We think of the many ways that wisdom is expressed: "bright" or brilliant or gifted; and the sadness of the slow development of senility in our parents and grandparents, or the rapid onset in a young person of Alzheimer's disease; of the loss of memory in amnesia, and the inability to communicate in Parkinson's disease. We know of patients whose minds are paralyzed with anxiety – a neurosis – or terrified with unreasonable paranoia – a psychosis. We think, what are the odds for me? Day dreaming, planning, making choices, remembering, weighing risks, making choices – all of these are processes of the mind. Imagination of things unseen has continuously propelled us to the future. Happiness, sadness, and other emotions are complex subjects, but they are largely reflections of the ways that people think of events, not of the events themselves. Joseph Henrich believes that the human mind evolved in the West in different ways than in the rest of the world. In his book, *The Weirdest People in the World*, he argues that people who are WEIRD (Western, educated, industrialized, rich, democratic), the prohibition "Don't marry your cousin!" is responsible for changes that "created states to replace tribes, science to replace lore, and law to replace custom." Looking to the future, which is not something that a historian is supposed to do, we can ponder about artificial intelligence (AI) and what might happen to *Homo sapiens*. Will our species be succeeded by a living species, or will there be a robotic future?[28]

The mind can be put at ease in several ways. Sleep can do it, but sometimes that is difficult, as we all know. A pleasurable experience can put the mind at ease, such as listening to a favorite piece of music, or with prayer, or when someone smiles. Some folks remember the song that began with "Pack up your troubles in your old kit bag and smile, smile, smile." Habit is another way to put the mind at ease. Habit is a way of doing things without thinking, and the mind can rest. This may be useful, or it may be harmful. There are good habits and bad habits. There is habitual behavior, repeated day after day. There are habitual responses to a signal, such as when the odor of cooking comes from the kitchen. Ivan Pavlov wrote about that. When food is expected, dogs bark, and humans' mouths water. Breaking unwanted habits can be a painful experience. We will have more to say about habits at a later point in this essay, when I discuss how habits conflict with conscious thinking in making choices.[29]

One final thought about the mind. Returning to the subject of wisdom, or its opposite – a dull mind. Can wisdom be measured? Should intelligence be measured? What to do with people who are just "average" or below average? These become social questions, when we recognize that the environment plays a vital role in determining success, by whatever method is used to measure it. The highest scores on IQ tests, on pre-college testing (SAT, PSAT, and so forth), for admission to medical schools (MCAT), and in financial success, measured in so many ways, are all achieved by those who start with the greatest advantages. The issue is framed by the question of "nature versus nurture." Genetics surely plays a role in a person's success, but the environment also matters a lot, and that is what we now need to examine.[30]

C. The Environment[31]

> Wherever the factories went, the streams became foul and poisonous: the fish died or were forced, like the Hudson shad, to migrate, and the water became unfit for drinking and bathing.
> –Lewis Mumford, 1934[32]

The final outcome of human history is dependent on the interactions of the body, the mind, and the environment. A good outcome is what humans seek. This is what is meant by the words, *Health Matters*. The environment is that which surrounds. The word environment is derived from the French *environ* (surrounding), and from Old French, meaning "enclose" or "encircle." The word *vir* (man, or hero = Latin) might seem to be the appropriate root of *environ*, but that is a false cognate.

The natural environment contains four interlinking systems: the atmosphere, hydrosphere, lithosphere, and biosphere – or simply: air, water, earth, and living things. Air and water are discussed in some detail below – air, as a human need; and water, as a human urge.

Earth is one of the four elements that were described by the Greeks, and it is also one of the five Buddhist elements. Earth is a word that represents both the planet and its soil. In Latin, Earth is *terra* or *terra mater*, named for Terra, the goddess of Earth. We recognize her name in French as *terroir* (soil) and in English in "terrain." In Greek mythology, Terra was Gaia (Γαῖα), mother of Uranus (god of heaven) and Pontus (god of the sea). The unitary concept of these elements (earth, air and sea) in Greek mythology has been incorporated into an ecological hypothesis, the so-called "Gaia principle," proposed by Lynn Margulis and James Lovelock. This is a notion that all components of the earth are one symbiotic organism – a self-regulating system. They would probably agree that a healthy earth, both organic and inorganic, would be necessary for people, as I propose in *Health Matters*.[33]

Humans, of course, are living things. We are included within the biosphere, and we relate to the other three components of the environment in a unique way. That is to say, we can alter our personal environment in ways that are unimaginable to other animals and plants, and we can also alter the environment of the world. Not only that: we have begun to dabble with the environment of the solar system, with human footprints on the moon and an unmanned motor vehicle, left on the planet Mars.[34]

This part of the essay on *Health Matters* begins with a discussion of human actions on the environment of the earth, its water, and its sky. The essay continues with an outline of the unnatural environment that is produced by the interactions that humans have with each other. What humans have done to the earth, water, and sky is intolerable; and what we do to each other is inhumane.

History tells us that there are some environmental catastrophes that cannot be specifically predicted or avoided. Some of these events occurred before humans existed, such as the extinction of the dinosaurs and many other species, which appears to have been caused by the strike of an enormous asteroid 65 million years ago. Volcanoes erupt, sometimes by surprise even to those who are experienced in spotting the warning signs, as Mount St. Helens did in 1980. In theory, we have the ability to strike and destroy an asteroid before it hits the earth, but not every asteroid is spotted, and terrible storms occur unexpectedly, in spite of modern methods of tracking weather patterns.[35]

Global warming has been occurring inexorably for at least 12,000 years. Scientists have proposed various ways to retard or perhaps even to reverse the warming trend. This would be a historic accomplishment. However, there is no concerted plan to attempt to do this. Instead, the danger continues to increase, and it now appears to be accelerating. There are many reasons for this. Some people deny the existence of global warming, in spite of the disappearance of many glaciers in the last few decades; and the earth has become measurable warmer. A major accelerant of global warming is the continued release of gases such as carbon dioxide, methane, and chlorofluorocarbons (CFCs) into the atmosphere, which produces a "greenhouse effect" on the earth. The "greenhouse effect" can easily be understood, if you stand in a greenhouse on a cold winter's day, with the sun warming the flowers and vegetables that are growing there. The damaging effects of global warming are greatest on those in the poorest areas of the world. Without understanding the cause of the problem, the people in these areas suffer from blazing heat where they live, from drought where they farm, and on land that is flooded from the rising ocean.

The earth now must support nearly eight times the population that existed 200 years ago. Much of the earth's surface has been converted from natural forests and grasslands to uses that satisfy human needs and desires: pastures for animals that are intended for human consumption; land that is need for agriculture; and space for people to live on, in houses, towns, and cities. The habitats of many other animals are threatened, or have been destroyed. Hundreds of species of insects, birds, and small animals have become extinct. Think of the dodo and the passenger pigeon. These are only two species, but millions of individual animals are gone forever. The existence of the honey bee is threatened, for unknown reasons, but all of the theories include the handiwork of humans. Amphibians are dying throughout the world, probably also as the result of unintended mischief by humans. Coral reefs are dying rapidly as the result of global warming, although pollution plays a role in that extinction, too. The rivers, estuaries, and oceans that formerly teemed with edible fish, shellfish, and aquatic mammals, are now barren and polluted. The earth, air, lakes and oceans are covered with pieces of plastic, which range in size from microscopic bits to huge pieces that can kill even a whale or a shark, when ingested or trapped. There must be a limit to the ability of the world to produce enough food to satisfy an increasing population. Many of these endangered species are hunted by humans for food and pleasure. A delicacy known as frog legs (*cuisses de grenouilles*), is especially popular in France and China. Hunted as food for humans, the honey nectar bat *(Macroglossus minimus)* is a threatened species in southeast Asia. A trophy head of a rare white tiger is displayed with pride by an American hunter. Humans almost killed the last American bison, and they drove wolves, panthers, and beavers out of much of their normal habitat. Will the growth in population cease only when starvation occurs, or will population growth be slowed into a steady state? It is difficult to estimate what the ideal population should be. It is even more difficult to imagine how the diverse societies in the world would achieve such a goal, when there is little agreement on issues that are simpler than population control.[36]

In spite of the enormous problems that are mentioned in the preceding paragraphs, the subject of the environment is now being seriously discussed, and some corrective actions have been undertaken. There are two major aspects in environmental studies: the physical environment, and the social environment. Recent efforts have shown some success in both of these aspects of the environment. The challenges have been: First, to decrease rate of deterioration of the environment; second, to stabilize it; and third, to improve it. It appears that "progress" in the environment has heretofore been downhill. Applying the law of gravity as a metaphor, it is hard to stop the slide. It is then a bit easier to stay in place, but very hard to turn upward. To turn the clock back, so to speak. And this is true with the degraded environment. The most important task is to recognize a problem and to stop it. The Great Smog of London in December 1952 led to the passage of the Clean Air Act of 1956. Another step forward in the environmental movement was the publication by Rachel Carson in 1962 of *Silent Spring*. Carson had been studying the problems caused by the wide use of pesticides in agriculture and of DDT (Dichlorodiphenyltrichloroethane) used to eradicate disease-carrying mosquitos. There was tremendous opposition by the chemical industry and its allies in government, but *Silent Spring* is now recognized as one of the most important books ever published. The silence that Carson described was from the absence of birdsongs, because birds were killed by eating insects that had been sprayed with DDT. Birds' eggshells are especially vulnerable to DDT. Another good example was the accomplishment in the 1970s, when a world-wide ban was accepted for aerosolized chlorinated fluorocarbon propellants, which were destroying the protective layer of ozone in the atmosphere.[37]

For the physical environment, the actions would require setting aside some beliefs, such as "it's a beautiful lawn," and instead accepting the warning, "Don't mess with Mother Nature." A beautiful lawn requires chemical pesticides and fertilizers, which ultimately penetrate into ground water, or proceed on the surface of land into a lake or ocean. Some of these chemicals are dangerous to humans, and also to other plants and animals that are unseen innocent targets. 2-4D (2,4-Dichlorophenoxyacetic acid), a herbicide, was later used in "Agent Orange" in the Vietnam War, along with a related chemical known as 2-4T. Quality control was poor, and "Agent Orange" was contaminated with another chemical, dioxin, which has caused a variety of diseases, including cancer.[38]

Humans have polluted the world's environment with many other toxic materials that are discussed in different parts of this essay. These toxins include substances that are elements, compounds, poisons, and radioactive wastes. Elements such as arsenic, cadmium, chlorine, fluorine, lead, mercury and nickel. Simple compounds, such as phenol and tetraethyl lead, and complex compounds with long chemical names, including polymers based on carbon and silicon. Poisons such as phosgene, ricin and anticholinesterase inhibitors, and runoffs from tear gas ingredients such as CS and MACE. Radioactive wastes from plutonium and radium. The list is formidable.[39]

An important step in the environmental movement has been to find a natural environment, and then to preserve it. This is not an easy task, because so little of what was once a natural environment is still present, except in the deepest jungles. Humans have intentionally or unintentionally been the conduit for plants and animals from one continent to another. Endogenous in one continent, exotic in another. Animals such as the rat and mouse assisted in this world-wide transportation of many species, carrying seeds and insects as they traveled with sailors. Our species, *Homo sapiens*, has been called "Earth's preeminent predator," because we have harvested wild animals for meat and destroyed their environment. This has enabled the passage of many bacterial and viral diseases to humans. The coronavirus known as SARS-CoV-2, which causes the disease COVID-19, is believed to have been transmitted from cave bats in Hubei Province, China. An intermediate animal host, the pangolin (a scaly anteater, eaten in China), is suspected. The disease first appeared in humans in the late fall of 2019 in the city of Wuhan, Hubei, on the Yangtze River. It was reported that the first patients were probably exposed to the virus when they were shopping at a "wet food" market in Wuhan at which wild animals are sold for food. The origin of the virus is uncertain, however, because of the possibility that this virus had been isolated and cultured in the laboratory of Dr. Shi Zhengli at the Wuhan Institute of Virology (WIV). Dr. Shi's laboratory is said to have "the world's largest collection of horseshoe bat viruses." The World Health Organization has been attempting to trace the infection to its source, but with limited success to date.[40]

The conservation movement has had a beneficial effect on the environment, by stabilizing the population of animals that are hunted, such as game birds, some fish, deer and elk. Conservation has also stabilized the environment that these animals need for food, shelter, breeding, and migration. The game animals are, however, not necessarily present in the original balance that was in that area. For example, the population of elk has increased dramatically after the wolves were removed; and the much-admired ringtail pheasant is exotic, not native to America. To restore the original balance of much of North America would require re-introducing the beaver; and then allowing beavers to construct their dams. Beaver dams convert rapidly flowing streams and small rivers into ponds, with the effluent trickling into small brooks and wandering creeks. The beavers' ponds eventually become pastures, when the beavers move to other locations in search of more trees, which is their favorite food. The farms and pastures in much of the United States were created as a result of removal of the beavers.[41]

Changes have also occurred in the social environment. The three steps have been progressive: meritocracy, equal opportunity, and affirmative action. The first, meritocracy, was believed to be an improvement over opportunities that were given to those who had power, prestige, and money, or were born into families with all of them. Equal opportunity was intended to give a chance for success for women, and for those who didn't have as much; it was supposed to level the playing field. Affirmative action sought to address ancient wrongs, by seeking to give opportunities for the poor, for people of color, and even those who had gone astray and were willing to return. All three of these attempts to change or correct the social environment have been challenged. If two people are competing for one position, one will win, but if affirmative action is applied, the loser may argue that the selection process was unfair. There can only be one winner, and the other will be a loser. Unfortunately, for one person in such a pair who are in competition, it must be a zero-sum game. In the long run, society may be benefited by affirmative action, but it will always be painful for those who lose because of the failure of meritocracy and of equal opportunity. The issue now is to ensure diversity, to recognize it, and to embrace it. The task is long overdue. One of the shocking examples of the need is the elitist approach to medical education that was accepted as the norm in the early 20th century. The Flexner Report in 1910 prompted the closure of five Black medical schools at a time when Black students were unable to enter most other medical schools. And as a result, few Black men and women were able to become physicians. The deficit has been estimated to be approximately 30,000 Black physicians over the past century.[42]

Thomas Malthus said that population would increase until it was stopped by starvation, war, or pestilence. The "pestilence" problem will be discussed at a later point in this essay, for it is a subject that is close to the heart of any physician. The human history of wars took a distinct change in August 1945 with the use in World War II of two atomic weapons, dropped by the United States on Japan. Before that time, as the weapons were being prepared and tested, and on many occasions since them, radioactivity has been released which has caused the accidental or unintended deaths of thousands of people. The cover of *The Bulletin of the Atomic Scientists* shows the Doomsday Clock, the hands of which are nearly together, pointing toward 12:00. In consideration of the deleterious effects of humans on climate change, on January 22, 2020, the minute hand was moved closer to midnight than it ever has been: it is now 100 seconds from the meridian. The physical environment of the world is still dangerous.[43]

Chapter 2

The Needs

The colorful Buddhist prayer flags that fly in Nepal and Tibet in the Himalayas, and in many places elsewhere in the world, are reminders of the Needs of humans. These five flags have identical inscriptions that show Lung-ta, the Windhorse, who is surrounded by prayers in Tibetan characters. The flags are intended to fly in the wind. The colors represent the five elements – blue (earth), white (water), red (fire), saffron (space), and green (cosmic winds). The Greeks also had a concept of the elements. Empedocles taught that there were four – earth, air, fire, and water – which were opposed to each other, but which were also combined into the four qualities: dry (fire + earth) cold (earth + water), wet (water + air), and hot (air + fire).[44]

Our use of the word "element" has different meanings than it does in the Buddhist religion and to the Greek philosophers, but there is a commonality here that is useful in thinking about the needs, urges, and wants in the health matters of humans. Earth, air, fire, and water appear in both traditions, and the gold prayer flag (saffron, for space) must refer to the sun and sunlight. It is perplexing that green represents "cosmic wind" and blue represents "earth," inasmuch as earth, which is turned green as it is drenched with water (and colored blue by reflection from the sky), would represent the food that is necessary for life to exist. There is nevertheless enough in these two traditions, Greek and Buddhist, to allow us to acknowledge the thoughts of many others in the past regarding the basic human needs.[45]

Sleep must also be added to the group of needs. Humans need to sleep, and while sleeping, they dream. There are the human needs: air to breathe, sun and sunlight, and sleep to rest, recover, and dream.

A. Air and Breath

> And after these things I saw four angels standing on the four corners of the earth, holding the four winds of the earth, that the wind should not blow on the earth, nor on the sea, nor on any tree.
>
> –Rev. 7:1[46]

"As I live and breathe!" It is a mild epithet, but it shows the intimate connection of life to the act of breathing, and thus to air. The word, air, has many meanings, but for this essay on *Health Matters*, the principal use of the word is in respect to what air means to life on earth, especially to human beings. We must think first of the definition and composition of air, but at the same time, we cannot refrain from thinking of air as an image, a meme, in slang, and in literature, film, and music. The act of breathing air begins with the act of inspiration – to take a deep breath. Inspiration is also a word with a psychic meaning: to inspire, to impart a truth, or motivate to action.[47]

Scientists specializing in biology think of air in connection with its contribution to the balance of life, which is the cycle known as photosynthesis and respiration. Photosynthesis by plants produces oxygen that is utilized by animals; and in respiration, animals produce carbon dioxide, which is the necessary ingredient for photosynthesis. Excessive amounts of oxygen would be poisonous for plants, but the amount of oxygen in air is well balanced at the level needed by plants. On the other hand, carbon dioxide would be poisonous for animals, except for its consumption by plants. Neither plants nor animals can exist without each other. An exquisite example of the borderline between plants and animals is the single-celled organism known as *Euglena*. This organism contains chloroplasts, which during daytime hours are transformed by sunlight and produce chlorophyll. At that time, *Euglena* becomes green and utilizes the process of photosynthesis and produces oxygen. At night, it loses its chlorophyll, turns white, and no longer produces oxygen. The ability to balance between producing oxygen in the light, and resting in the dark, uniquely enables *Euglena* to exist within earth's normal atmosphere.[48]

Breathing is the key to the transfer of oxygen from the atmosphere into the body of animals, such as humans. The process appears to be simple, but it is not. One can study the anatomy, physiology, and biochemistry of the organs involved. Buried in the mass of detail, and often forgotten, is the statement that "Carbon dioxide is one of the most powerful stimulants of breathing." One might think that oxygen deprivation would be the stimulus to breathe; but instead, if breathing stops for a minute or longer, breathing is mainly stimulated by a slight increase in acidity of the blood as the level of carbon dioxide increases. Nevertheless, breathing is also stimulated by low levels of atmospheric oxygen, such as occurs in mountain climbing, and in acute pulmonary diseases, such as bacterial and viral pneumonia (e.g., COVID-19), and in chronic obstructive pulmonary disease (COPD), which can produce dangerously low levels of oxygen in the blood. The normal range of oxygen saturation of arterial blood gas (ABG) in adults is from 94 to 99%, according to the Lung Health Institute. Some internet sources suggest that saturation ranges from 60% to 80% may be acceptable. However, it is ridiculous to suggest that saturation levels that low are normal. At 90% or less, it is impossible to walk rapidly or climb up steps. The rate of breathing, in breaths per minute, in one of the vital signs that are monitored by medical personnel in hospitalized patients, and as a matter of record at the time of most visits to a physician. The usual rate is 15 per minute, with a range from 12 to 18 being acceptable. The patient's appearance during breathing is also important. Does it seem to be difficult? And are the accessory muscles of respiration used, such as elevation of the shoulders with each inspiration? The bed of the fingernail is also observed. Is it pink, or is it slightly blue – cyanotic – which is a tell-tale sign of poor oxygenation of the blood? Non-cancerous pulmonary diseases have in recent years been the third leading cause of deaths in the United States. Respiratory problems are a major cause of disability and misery in debilitating chronic obstructive pulmonary disease, seasonal allergies, other allergies, bad colds, and non-fatal influenza.[49]

By the time a student enters middle school, a teenager would have little difficulty in answering a question about a burning candle that is placed in a jar: Why does the candle's flame begin to flicker and then die? The student answers: Because the burning candle used up the oxygen in the air. That answer would not have been possible before oxygen was discovered. It was in about 1790 that Antoine Lavoisier, in France, challenged the view that an invisible substance, phlogiston, was liberated when combustion took place – such as the burning of a candle wick. But not even Joseph Priestly, one of the discoverers of oxygen, could accept that this newly discovered element was responsible for burning. It took about 30 years for the phlogiston theory to be replaced by Lavoisier's oxygen theory, which is that burning, as in that candle in the jar, consumes oxygen instead of liberating "phlogiston." The oxygen theory had the advantage of simplicity, which in philosophy is called "Occam's Razor."[50]

A few other uses of the word "air" or of its derivatives, and "wind" should suffice to illustrate the important place that air has in human life. We think of Aeolus (Αϊολος,), Greek god of wind, who controlled the Anemoi, (Greek = Ανεμοι), the minor gods of the winds, and Boreas (Greek = (Βορέας), the god of the north wind. Aeolus, Anemoi, and Boreas have never left us; they are memes. From Aeolus, we have the wind harp, known as the aeolian harp. From Anemoi, we have a variety of windflowers, such as the buttercup. The rarely seen but delightful Northern Lights are known as aurora borealis, combining aurora (Latin = dawn) and borealis (Greek). The phrases, "hot air," "bad air," "air head," and "on the air" immediately call specific images to mind. The following uses of "air" are easily understood: *Into Thin Air*, an "air of complacency, the "flute's air," "Air Force," the National Air and Space Museum, and the cheerful ditty, "I'm forever blowing bubbles." And when bubbles appear in movies such as *Titanic* and *Jaws*, you know that for someone, the end is near.[51]

B. Sun and Light

And God said, "Let there be light," and there was light. God saw that the light was good, and he separated the light from the darkness. God called the light "day," and the darkness he called "night." And there was evening, and there was morning—the first day. And God said, "Let there be a vault between the waters to separate water from water." So God made the vault and separated the water under the vault from the water above it. And it was so. God called the vault "sky." And there was evening, and there was morning—the second day. –
Genesis 1:3-8

The sun is the source of all of the energy in the solar system, and thus of all the energy in and on the earth. All living things – both plants and animals – depend on the sun for their being and for their continuation. These are grandiose statements, to put it mildly. In order to take a humbler approach, we should look at some of the things that the sun does in the course of daily life. The words light and sun may be conflated, because all light is directly or indirectly derived from the sun. This commentary concludes with a few comments about sun + light (sunlight) as it appears in the non-scientific world, in the hope that the reader may pause to consider what memories "sunlight" conjures in his or her mind.

We see in the opening passage from Genesis that some of the earliest thoughts of humans have been about light – the light of day – which, of course, comes from the sun. The Bible says so, and so, too, does science. It's the same for both. It is the same if a person believes the Bible and disregards science, or if one simply tries to understand the scientific argument and regards the Bible as fiction. But the similarity soon stops. The story in the Bible makes it simple: Darkness and light, earth and sky and water. All in seven sentences. Some people believe that this statement is metaphorical, and the first steps in creation are not intended to be two, 24-hour days. Nevertheless, it's still rather straightforward. The scientific story is much more complicated. In fact, the scientific theory of formation of the earth is still in flux. What was once called a theory was downgraded to become a hypothesis, and is now simply known as a "model." The present "model" began in 1755 with Immanuel Kant, who was a philosopher, "neither highly versed in either physics or mathematics," and certainly not an astronomer. After more than 250 years, the language is scientific instead of Biblical, and it is uncertain: the "model" just "appears basically correct." That is somewhat of a let-down. The expert who composed the essay on the solar system in *Britannica* wrote, "The current approach to the origin of the solar system treats it as part of the general process of star formation. ... the theory of Laplace incorporated Kant's idea of planets coalescing from dispersed material, their two approaches are often combined in a single model called the Kant-Laplace nebular hypothesis. ... Although a number of such problems remain to be resolved, the solar nebula model of Kant and Laplace appears basically correct."[52]

The uncertainty regarding the origin of the sun (and earth and the moon) suggests that humans should go forward with what they can see, regardless of the theory of how it all started. "Look on the bright side" was good advice. And that's what we should do. A crash course in physics could be considered, from its earliest beginnings to the discovery of the laws of gravity and motion and also thermodynamics, discussions of the concepts of entropy and infinity, and the theory of relativity. This enormous task must be truncated to summarize only what scientists have learned about the sun and light, and to suggest what is still unknown.[53]

The sun is a star in the galaxy known as the Milky Way, which seen in the sky at night. It is a bit weird, to be inside the Milky Way, yet also looking up at it. The sun is about midway in size of the stars. The sun is composed mainly (90%) of hydrogen. It burns continuously, forming helium, which amounts to 9.9% of the sun. The remaining 0.1% of the sun's mass is composed of the heavier elements such as iron, calcium, and so forth – in a very different ratio than appears on earth. The burning sun emits the full spectrum of electromagnetic rays, from the shortest – gamma and x-rays – to longer rays in the invisible ultraviolet range, and then the longer rays that are visible to us, and then even longer invisible rays of infrared and radio waves. The sun has been burning for about 4.6 billion years. It is expected to follow the way of other stars and get brighter before it dies in about 10 billion years. The sun revolves about once a month (every 25-29 days, with the poles revolving faster than the equator). Yes, the sun does revolve, though you can't see that. The earth revolves on a daily basis, and in the far distant future, the rotation of the earth is expected to match the rotation of the moon, "turning once in 30 of our present days." Can you imagine that? Our world, our moon, and our sun are constantly spinning, but we don't feel it at all. Scientists now believe that the universe, the cosmos, began with a "big bang" some 13.8 billion years ago, at a moment called Planck time. There is no scientific theory (yet) about what existed before Planck time, which leaves us only with the non-scientific statement in Genesis.[54]

A word about light, as viewed from the perspective of science: Light is a form of electromagnetic radiation. As explained above, the electromagnetic spectrum ranges from short gamma rays and x-rays to long radio waves. The visible part of this spectrum is what is known as light. To the human eye, light is colorless, but if light is passed through a prism, or through droplets of rain that act in a similar way to scatter it, colorless light becomes a rainbow of colors. The science of light is known as optics, which studies the dispersion, refraction, and reflection of light. These phenomena are understandable because they are part of common language. It is, however, difficult to grasp the notion that light is both a particle and a wave. That light travels at a speed of about 186,000 miles per second is a mantra that is learned and recited by school children, although it seems rather fantastic. It is also taught, and repeated on tests by students, that according to quantum mechanics, light has a dual nature. Quantum theory describes light as consisting of discrete packets of energy, called photons; and also, that light is a wave. The wave-particle duality is shared by all primary constituents of nature. This theory – and note, this is only a theory – is difficult to grasp, and most people wouldn't try to believe it or to understand it. A student must answer the question correctly, and then perhaps move on to other things.[55]

The medical aspects of sun and light are usually positive for humans, but sometimes the reverse is true. Sunlight is necessary to prevent rickets. It is a complicated matter, involving activation of Vitamin D by sunlight, and then Vitamin D enables calcium to be incorporated into bone. Otherwise, the bones are soft and bend easily. It is especially debilitating in children. Rickets was especially common in the northern hemisphere in winter, and it has been reported in women who immigrated to London from the Indian subcontinent and who were, for religious reasons, forced to remain indoors. Sunlight is believed to be the cause of a high incidence of melanoma in people of Scottish origin who live in tropical zones. In Scotland, where the sun isn't as bright, and people are more heavily clothed, the incidence of moles that are transformed into melanoma is much lower than in Australia. The discovery of the method of treating babies with neonatal jaundice by exposing them to ultraviolet light was one of the recent triumphs of pediatric medicine.[56]

Sun and light and sunlight are easier to consider from the perspective of ordinary life. Think of the many ways that we speak of them. In song: "You are my sunshine / You make me happy." In love: "You are the light of my life." In fiction: Ernest Hemingway, *The Sun Also Rises* (1926), which finally became a Hollywood movie thirty years later, in 1956. Before that movie was made, there was *Sunset Boulevard* (1950). The movie cowboy traditionally rides west, into the setting sun, as the film ends. We have sunbeams, sunburn, and lightning strikes. We put up our hand or turn down the brim of our hat, when "the light is in my eye." We still say that the "sun rises in the east and sets in the west," an observation that doesn't accept the heliocentric theory of the universe. It's time for drinks when "the sun crosses the yard arm." "Light's out!" is the command to children from their parents at bedtime.[57]

Enough of that. Whatever would we do without sun and light? Yet life has what is known as a circadian rhythm, a 24-hour rhythmic cycle. It is the earth's cycle of light and darkness, which is, at the equator, 12 hours of sunlight, and 12 hours of darkness. Dark is the time to sleep.

C. Sleep and Dreams

To sleep, perchance to dream
—Shakespeare, *Hamlet*

Sleep is difficult to define, though everyone knows what it is. We know what it means to sleep, as a verb, or what sleep means as a noun. All humans need to sleep, although the length of sleeping time is variable from person to person. Ordinarily, the longest period is for several continuous hours of sleep, perhaps six to nine hours. The time varies in duration from infancy to elderhood; and it is often supplemented with additional naps. During sleep the muscles relax, and responsiveness to external stimuli is diminished. The sense of danger is blunted. Odd things can happen however, such as sleepwalking, known as somnambulism, and sleeping with eyes wide open and appearing to be awake. That's really weird. Humans are usually recumbent when sleeping, in a favorite position.[58]

Sleep is different in other mammals; whales sleep with half of the brain active, so they can rise to the surface to breath; and bears hibernate. Chickens immediately fall asleep in the dark, and during the daytime, a disagreeable old hen can be pacified by putting her head beneath her wing. The hen thinks it is night, and she becomes quiet. Roosters crow when the sun rises or when an eclipse ends; wags say that the rooster believe he is responsible for the sunrise. Sleep is usually a nighttime activity (incongruously speaking). In that way it is associated with an opposite Need for Sun (and Sunlight), which is the epitome of daytime activity. Some people have the ability to waken and react instantly, whereas others are groggy when awakened and then have a difficult time returning to sleep. In the first category we think of firefighters, special forces military personnel, most physicians; and in the 19th century, telegraphers, such as Thomas Edison. The telegraph operator awoke, received a message from the clacking machine, tapped out a response, and then immediately fell asleep again. In the other category, I think of my wife. She would stay awake long after I answered the phone at, say, 1:00 a.m. I would say to the surgical resident, "Call me again after you get the lab result." I would then fell asleep again immediately, while she tossed and turned, unable to return to sleep.

When thinking of sleep, we remember diverse subjects such as hypnosis, sleep apnea, drug-induced sleep and caffeine-induced awakeness, sleep deprivation, insomnia, jet-lag, and narcolepsy. And hallucinations, somniloquy (sleep talking), enuresis (bed-wetting), nightmares, panic attacks, and restless legs. Scientists speak of REM (Rapid Eye Movement) sleep as being the time of dreams. The mind is the connection between dreams and the imagination.[59]

Dreams are mentioned in other ways that emphasize the importance of dreams in human affairs. The most famous use of the word "dream" in the 20th century was the moment when Martin Luther King, Jr., spoke on the steps of the Lincoln Memorial to an immense crowd on the Mall in Washington, D.C., on August 28, 1963. To 250,000 people, King shouted, "I have a dream!" And as a great orator with an important message, he repeated the phrase again and again. And then, "Free at last!" After recalling Dr. King's words, it almost seems trite to mention other ways that "dream" and "dreams" have entered our imagination. However, some of us can remember songs, such as "I dream of Jeanie with the light brown hair" and "I'll see you in my dreams." There is Dreamworld and DreamWorks. We can dream of a long life, hoping mostly to have good dreams (think rainbows) and few bad dreams (nightmares). Shakespeare said, "We are such stuff / As dreams are made on," although we usually remember it as, "The stuff that dreams are made of" from the movie, *The Maltese Falcon*. Shakespeare reminds us of the magic of sleep in his unforgettable play, *Midsummer Night's Dream*. Could it be that dreams are the key to human development? Not necessarily to progress, but to imagine what could be, and then to do it. Sometimes we dream of the past to imagine the future, as Shakespeare said: "What's past is prologue."[60]

We now turn to the Urges. To reiterate, there are seven, or possibly eight. The urges can best be thought of in three groups: the basic instincts for water, food and shelter; the additional urges for lust and social connections; the uniquely human urges for clothing and fire; and also, the human urge for the dog.

Chapter 3

The Urges

Dans les champs de l'observation le hasard ne favorise que les esprits prepares
"In the field of observation, chance favors the prepared mind."
–Louis Pasteur[61]

This part of the essay on *Health Matters* speaks about what humans must have to survive, as individuals and as a species. Knowing they must have for survival is important, but knowledge is insufficient without action. This is driven by the urges. It is important to prepare for action to locate and utilize the needed items. Preparation is needed for survival. The motto of the Boy Scouts is "Be Prepared."[62]

Three Instincts for Survival – Water, Food, and Shelter

All mammalian species require water, food, and shelter. The order in which these three requirements must be satisfied is variable, depending on the species, the time, and the environment. Humans have an urgent, daily, need for water. Acquisition of food can be delayed in order to find a secure location, especially in a dangerous environment. One can imagine various possibilities.

One scenario is what many people are facing at this moment, staying in their homes, with social distancing imposed due to COVID-19. In a detached house, a water source is essential, food must be obtained and stored, and security is needed – with locks on doors and windows. In an apartment house, the requirements are the same, but the principal source of security is the exterior of the building.

Now think of other scenarios that are less likely, but which could happen to anyone, even on a commercial airliner or a cruise ship. Imagine this: You are on the ocean, a guest on a sailboat, far from land. The boat is suddenly hit with a strong wind, and is blown over. The skipper is forced to abandon ship, and you, too, must go off of the vessel. What will be in the life raft, and what to do next? Was a May Day signal sent and acknowledged? If not, you are in serious trouble. For a vivid, though fictional, depiction of this problem, see Robert Redford in the movie, *All is Lost* (2013).

Or you could be a passenger in a small airplane flying over a remote part of the world. Imagine that you are somewhere over northern Alaska, sightseeing, and the engine fails, and the plane crashes, killing the pilot. You're suddenly alone in the wilderness. No May Day signal was sent. Another possibility: What if you miss seeing a signpost and now you are lost while hiking in the late fall in New Hampshire. Or if darkness falls when you are hunting alone, without a trail, in a wilderness area in Colorado? Someone may miss you, and help may be on the way, but you need to find a place for shelter, for safety, before nightfall, and also water and food.[63]

A. Water

And the Spirit of God moved upon the face of the waters. (Genesis 1:2)

And Moses lifted up his hand, and with his rod he smote the rock twice: and the water came out abundantly, and the congregation drank, and their beasts also. (Numbers 20:11)

Water has a profound meaning for all living things. But even before there were living things on earth, there was water. Most of the surface of the earth is covered with water. The canyons of the oceans are deeper than the highest mountains, and sunlight does not reach the ocean depth. Water was one of the four elements of the world that were the basis for life, in company with earth, air, and fire.

Water has three phases – liquid, solid, and gaseous. Crucial changes occur in water when it freezes – at the freezing point, 0^0C. or 32^0F. – and when it boils – at the boiling point, 100^0C. or 212^0F. Water is a chemical, with a symbol of H20. This symbol shows that water is a molecule combining one part (one atom) of the element known as oxygen, and two parts (two atoms) of the element known as hydrogen. The word "salt" in this essay also means a molecule; it refers to equal parts, chemically combined, of the element sodium – a positive ion – and chlorine – a negative ion. Sodium is a soft silvery metal and chlorine is a yellowish green poisonous gas, and combined they form the familiar white granules that we know as salt. We have a taste for salt, and we of want more of it than is good for our health. It is a minor exception in *Health Matters*. This information about water and salt is unknown to many people, and it is of little help to a person who is looking for a source of water to drink.

There is, nevertheless, much that everyone knows about water, and it is so important that it is worth repeating here. Ocean water is salty. Most of the water on land contains little or no salt. If it is free of salt, we say that it is fresh water, especially if it comes from a pure spring or comes down as rainwater. However, it may be polluted or brackish, and it such cases it usually will have a noxious appearance, odor, or taste. Humans are mostly composed of water, but the water of the human body is not "fresh," nor is it as salty as the ocean. That is the result of a slow change that has occurred in ocean water, a process of evolution which also is of little interest to a thirsty person. In the interior of continents, far away from the oceans, salt water is rare, and many people cannot imagine salty water.[64]

Humans have an inborn desire to add salt to their food. Salt (sodium chloride; NaCl) brings out the tastiness of what otherwise might be a bland dish. We savor salt, meaning that we enjoy it by eating it slowly. We must achieve a balance in intake to replace the loss of salt in perspiration, urine, and bowel movements. The human body contains very little sodium and chlorine, only 0.2% of each element, in comparison to oxygen (65%) and carbon (18.5%). The amount of salt in the body is carefully regulated through a process of nature which developed early in the process of evolution. It is wise to eat salt slowly, and to add little to food, because dietary salt is an easily overlooked cause of hypertension and premature death from heart disease, stroke, and peripheral vascular disease. Food served in restaurants, packaged as frozen meals, and for take-outs is generally high in salt, because it enhances taste and it aids in food preservation. Salt is insidiously added to most canned goods, especially vegetables and soups. Meat is terribly bland without salt, but it can be cooked carefully without drenching it in salt. It is best to cook with fresh vegetables, instead of canned foods, and to add salt warily. Normal dietary needs have been the subject of argument for many decades, with debates between physicians, dieticians, and the food industry. The best estimate at this time is that the maximum daily amount of salt should be 2,300 mg per day (about one teaspoon). Most of that is now included in prepared food, which would allow very little to be added from the salt shaker. The best plan seems to be this: take a sip or a bite of the soup or food, and think about it. If it needs salt, sprinkle just a little on it.[65]

Several things are important to anyone who seeks to find a secure, daily, source of fresh water. Ice is usually a good source of fresh water, and it is buoyant, so it floats above the surface of fresh water, and it floats even higher on the surface of ocean water. Ice can also be hazardous: "On thin ice" is a metaphor for danger; we slip on the icy sidewalks; and icebergs are dangers to ships. Ice has long been used to preserve food. Some plants, such as some cactuses, concentrate and store potable – drinkable – water. Many species of fish and mammals that live in the ocean are also good sources of fresh water. The reasons for these attributes are interesting to scientists, but they are of little practical interest to a person in desperate need of fresh water. People have used many techniques to locate good sources of drinking water, in different parts of the world. Palm trees growing in the desert suggest a place to dig for water. Coconuts from coconut palm trees can be cracked to yield a white liquid in the center known as coconut milk, but the "milk" is usually made from grinding the flesh of mature coconuts. As a vegetable product, it is not really milk, which is the proteinaceous liquid secreted by the mammary glands. The interesting taste of coconut milk is caused, in part, by its high content of saturated fat. Whether it is good for health, or bad for health, is contested, but the majority view at this time is that it is beneficial. Limestone caverns in Central America become entrances into caves known as *ceynotes*, where water can be found during the dry season. Also, water flows always flows downhill, so a tiny stream can be followed until it joins another stream, and then together they flow into a creek, and then into a river. If the river disappears into an underground cave, it will probably reappear somewhere, either into a lake, the ocean, or another river. The third phase of water – of steam – becomes important when humans employed fire for cooking. Water that is hot enough to boil can occasionally be found in nature, in pools near geysers, as in Iceland and in Yellowstone Park. However, steam is otherwise rare in the natural world. Water vapor, as seen in clouds, is composed of tiny particles of either liquid water or ice; it is not steam. Natural boiling water was rarely used by humans, in contrast to the common use of fire for cooking and preserving foodstuffs.[66]

Humans have a love affair with water, and it is much more than simply the urge to consume water, to quench thirst, and to find a source of water to drink. The many other ways that humans love water are also important for health. Most humans enjoy water on their skin. They bathe in it for cleanliness ("Cleanliness is next to godliness"). They swim in it for recreation or for necessity ("Jump in, the water's fine" or "It's sink or swim"). And they soak in it to soothe aches and pains ("Oh, doesn't that feel good!"). It is probably not a coincidence that humans also enjoy looking at water. It may be still water in a pond, a rippling brook, or a seashore with crashing waves. Fresh clear water, or salty ocean water. Meat, vegetables, and fruit are prepared by washing before eating them raw or cooked. By this simple act to cleanse food from dirt, for aesthetic purposes, humans have inadvertently reduced the bacterial contamination of their diet. Raw foodstuffs thus contain less than the minimal infective dose (MID) of many bacteria. Boiling in water reduces bacterial content even more, and humans can be happy with the final product. It is another use of water for human health.[67]

Water is a crucial element in most religions. It certainly is for Jews, Hindus, Muslims, Buddhists, and Christians. Zoroastrians, who are famous for their fire temples, include water (*apo, aban*) and fire (*atar, azar*) as the two agents of ritual purity. The Hebrew Bible tells of God's punishment by the great flood for humans' bad behavior, sparing Noah and those that he brought into the Ark; and of the rock that Moses struck for water in the wilderness. That miracle saved them. The Hindu belief in reincarnation utilizes the mystic power of the Ganges River, which carries the ashes of the faithful downstream to the ocean and into a new life. The ablutions with water that are performed by a devout Muslim are a beautiful way to purify both body and soul. The Buddhist prayer service, *puja*, does not usually include water, but water is needed for the Buddhist's ceremonial tea made with sour butter, and the beer, known as *chang*. Water drives Buddhist prayer wheels that spin endlessly, carrying tiny pieces of paper on which are written the sacred words, *On mani padme hum*. Water is necessary for the tea ceremony of Japan. The baptismal ceremony of Christians is central to their belief. One baptism is usually accepted by every denomination, although some require rebaptism by immersion as adults. Consecrated holy water applied by a priest or some other member of the clergy is preferred, but in an emergency, such as impending death of an unbaptized person, anyone can do the job with whatever water is at hand.[68]

Many other uses of water are important for human health: Think of boundary waters for protection, of water for growing crops from rain or irrigation, of solutions made by pharmacists of water-soluble drugs, of tool-making by quenching red-hot metals into water to strengthen them. No wonder that farmers study the clouds to decide when to plant and when to harvest. The chance of rain governs their plans for the yearly cycle. Humans will stop work to watch a hurricane or a rainbow, both of which depend on water. Water is the subject of art, in music, in paintings, and photographs. We remember "Singing in the Rain," "A gentle dew from Heaven," and a day at the beach with our family. Natural springs were converted into baths by Romans in many places such as in Bath, England. The waters there were warmed by nature, as they are in the geysers of Iceland and Yellowstone Park. The hot water springs that became baths in German-speaking countries are named with the suffix "-bad," as in Marienbad (Mary's bath), Czechoslovakia.[69]

What humans have done with water is a long, sad story. It started well, when humans began to use water for drinking, as other animals had done. But although water is our most important natural substance, we have wasted water and polluted it with garbage and chemicals, especially plastic. Many other forms of life – both plants and other animals – that use it and live in it have also suffered greatly, and their suffering continues to increase. The *Silent Spring* is emblematic of this problem.[70]

B. Food

Man shall not live by bread alone.
–Deuteronomy 8:3, Matthew 4:4[71]

Hunger and thirst are urges that are required to satisfy what the body must have for food and water. These urges and their satisfactions are regulated through the nervous system and hormones. This is what Walter Cannon meant when he wrote about "the wisdom of the body." Many other parts of the body are also involved. For example, the capacity of the gastro-intestinal tract plays an important role in feedback, signaling satiety ("I'm full") to end consumption of food. As it is with all mammals, the first food that humans consume is milk, and milk is almost the perfect food for humans.[72]

Food for humans consists of four major components: carbohydrates, proteins, fats, and trace substances. The first three of these compose the caloric requirements of the body – what the engine of the body needs for fuel. The body needs calories – fuel – on a continuous basis, so the urge for calories is usually satisfied by food eaten every day. The fourth component, trace substances, includes vitamins and minerals, which are not needed on a daily basis. The minerals in the body were originally found in the ocean – sodium, potassium, some calcium and a bit of magnesium. The amount and concentration of each mineral is automatically regulated, are they are stored within the body – another example of the "wisdom of the body." Dietary deficiency in trace substances is not evidenced by a specific urge, but a diet that includes all three caloric components is usually sufficient to protect against this deficiency.

Humans are omnivorous, meaning that they can eat and digest food that originates from either plants or animals. A normal diet may be either vegan (including both vegetables and fruits, but no animal products), or omnivorous (including meat, fish, dairy products, and eggs). A "vegetarian" diet would supposedly be vegan, but many vegetarians, known as ovolactovegetarians, consume dairy products and eggs. Humans originally ate anything they could find to satisfy their craving for food, for they could not be fussy when they were hungry. Children need calories from newborn babies through their teenage years. Humans, like other mammals, provide young children with milk. It is a dietary miracle. Milk provides the nursing child with all of the necessary components, provided by the breasts of the lactating mother. Nature's rules, exercised through hormones, say that nursing must stop long before a child is able to obtain its own food. However, each child must be weaned so its mother can prepare to have her next child.[73]

Everyone must always be looking for food. Parents must teach their children how to find food. Scavenging among plants, looking for what may be edible. Looking in the water for a motionless shellfish, such as an oyster, that might be picked up and tasted. Small fish and birds, and little animals of any kind that might be edible, even insects and worms. Early humans would have tried to do this – eating wild plants and animals. This approach would also be needed for a person who suddenly becomes lost in the wilderness. Prepare, look carefully, taste warily, and be satisfied. Save something for the next meal.

As humans developed tools and techniques for hunting and fishing, some found a carnivorous diet to be best. Eskimos typically ate only meat, mostly fat – blubber – during the winter. One of nature's wonders is that the body is usually able to break the three main components of the diet into smaller molecules and recombine them into what is needed. Proteins, from both meat or vegetables, are composed of many amino acids, which can be repurposed into carbohydrates or stored as fat. This aspect of "the wisdom of the body" was needed for survival. Other humans domesticated plants and animals and they then developed a varied diet. Such a diet includes eggs – another miracle of food – because eggs provide virtually all dietary components. Still other humans became strict vegetarians – vegans – most notably the Jains of India, who believe in reincarnation and practice non-violence. Jains eat only fruits and vegetables that grow above the ground, thereby protecting insects and worms that live in the earth. Many humans became fishermen and farmers, although some have remained as hunter-gatherers, in the Kalahari, in the tropical forests of the Amazon basin, in New Guinea's valleys, and in Australia. In the evolution of modern society, fishermen probably came before farmers, because the waters of the ocean, the lakes, and the rivers were teeming with edible animals. These animals were originally eaten raw, but techniques were then found to prepare them for food – drying in the sun, softening with rot; or by cooking on rocks before the fire, and stewing in pots made from bark or clay.

Methods for storing food were developed from chance observations. Accidental freezing of meat, fruit, and vegetables (frozen foods); dried food (such as fish); food that is tolerant of long storage (potatoes and squash); storage in salty water or sprinkled with salt (known as "margination"); fermentation (from storage at ambient temperature); storage in alcohol (beer in various forms is common throughout the world); in mild acid (e.g., vinegar, from apple juice); and in spices. Once food was found to have been preserved by accident in any of these ways, some humans would think of ways to repeat and enhance the effect. Every kitchen had vinegar, a mild acid, and also a bottle of ammonia, a mild base. The cook didn't know anything about acid or base; she just knew that they were different, and that the difference was important. And there would be storage bins for onions, beets, and other hardy vegetables.

Agriculture developed as plants were chosen for edibility and the best strains were selected for propagation. Grasses produced seeds that could be harvested, and from these, several strains of wheat were developed across the northern parts of the Old World, from Asia to Europe. Wheat was prepared for food by grinding the seeds into powder, and then by heating it to form various forms of bread. Now wonderful varieties of bread have been developed, ranging from the delicious tubular baguettes of France to the mouth-watering forms of *pan* and *naan* of western and central Asia. These breads are usually baked and eaten every day, as described in the words "daily bread" in the Lord's prayer. Italian pasta, which can be stored before it is cooked and eaten, is also made from a variety of wheat. The absence of bread becomes a metaphor for famine: "When I have broken the staff of your bread … you shall eat, and not be satisfied" (Leviticus 26:26). The "staff" in this phrase refers to the board on which bread is baked.

In the southern parts of the Old World, the seed known as rice was developed in the same way. Many different strains of rice exist, which indicate that the domestication of rice occurred in different places. Wheat, rice, and other plants, such as legumes, all produce varieties of a complex digestible carbohydrate known as starch. Starch is a polymer; it is a complex combination of molecules of carbon, hydrogen, and oxygen. The last two of these are familiar from the structure of water; the first, carbon, is recognized as the key element in living things. A simple combination of these three elements, known as a monomer, is sugar. One form of sugar, glucose, is a common building block of starch. A combination of two molecules of glucose is known as glycogen. The body's supplies for immediate energy are mainly stored as glycogen, which can be rapidly degraded into glucose. This is another example of "the wisdom of the body." Other forms of sugar exist, such as fructose, which is common in fruit. Legumes are especially useful because they produce edible beans, such as lentils, combined as *dal*, in India. Legumes have nodules containing nitrogen-fixing bacteria on their roots, and they self-fertilize the land on which they are grown. Other grasses were developed that provided food for newly tamed and domesticated animals, especially cattle. Some of these, such as clover and alfalfa, are also legumes. In the American continents, domestication of crops began much later, after humans arrived at the height of the last Ice Age. The first Americans developed many different forms of other starchy vegetables, such as potatoes and corn. Europeans call it maize, because in the Old World, corn means wheat. Europeans who settled in America learned to utilize many other species of plants that were not found in the Old World. Some plants were medicinal, others were herbs or spices, and others became edible vegetables and fruits. Medicines were derived from quinine and cocaine; anti-oxidants from black tea; edible hot peppers and sweet peppers; many varieties of tomatoes; and sweet corn, popcorn, and field corn.

Some aspects of food production have had an effect which could be considered marginal, and some have been harmful. Sugar is commonly overused, because humans need very little, yet much is consumed because it is tasty. Marketing of sugar and sugary products is very effective, and consumption is high. Sugar consumption can produce terrible effects on individuals – diabetes and prediabetes, for example – and at a high societal cost. The cultivation of sugar was also the principal use of the transatlantic trade in enslaved African people, with effects that have continued long after that form of slavery was abolished. Coffee and tea are mildly addictive, and have little benefit, but are produced at great cost. Think of the arable land that is used, and the labor of people involved. Tobacco is worse; it has no benefit to humans, and it causes enormous depletion of fertilized land. Useful medical products are obtained from poppies (morphine and other opioids), hemp (marijuana), coca (cocaine), and mushrooms (peyote) – but it is an understatement to say that these products have also been misused. Fermentation of fruits and vegetables has long been used to produce mild alcoholic beverages, and then to distill it to a higher concentration. The useful properties of alcohol as an industrial chemical must be balanced against the deleterious effects on people: the temporary mind-altering, permanently addictive, life-endangering, and destructive behavior of alcohol upon individuals.[74]

The chemistry and biology of foods is of little interest to hungry people, although food science has been employed successfully to feed the world's growing population. This is, however, a subject with a *double entendre*. Food is a basic requirement for life, and it therefore becomes an urge for human health. As the population of the world increases, it needs to be fed, and more of the natural environment must be converted to agricultural land. The so-called Green Revolution is based on ways to induce genetic mutations in plants, especially in wheat and rice, and thus to increase the yield of crops – with dramatic effects in Pakistan, India, and elsewhere in the world.[75]

We will have more to say about food at a later point in this essay, when food is prepared and eaten as an important aspect of the human community. It is the process of digestion, in which raw materials such as milk, eggs, fruit, vegetables, and meat, are transformed and rearranged into new substances which are distributed throughout the body. The process of transformation of food into energy is known as metabolism. Each of the major religions has rules for food, including the time of daily meals, which may vary within the week and with the season. There are also religious rules about what is edible and what is proscribed.[76]

C. Shelter

Ein feste Burg ist unser Gott, ein gute Wehr und Waffen.
—Martin Luther, "A Mighty Fortress"[77]

A shelter is a place of safety that one can venture from, and return to, and defend. Shelter is one of the three great urges that must be continually satisfied by humans. The human need for shelter, for a safe place, is deeply embedded in the instinct for survival. It is a biological phenomenon that occurs in both plants and animals. It is seen in trees, as they bend before the wind and protectively curl their leaves as the sun rises, to avoid the loss of water. And it is present in many species of animals, as ticks scurry into the shadows, and earthworms squirm to reach grass at the edge of the sidewalk. Squirrels nest in hollows of trees, and bears find caves in which to hibernate. The urge of humans to find shelter is an instinct which is driven largely by fear. One of the important word-stems in the Proto-Indo-European languages is "Kae-id," meaning "to strike." It appears in words meaning "to kill," such as homicide and suicide, and it also appears in important actions such as decision, incision, and excision. Humans need to balance the perpetual need for shelter against the occasional requirement to strike.[78]

The biological basis for responses to emotions, such as fear or pleasure, begins with the senses. The principal senses are five: smell, sight (vision), hearing, taste, and touch. The first four of these senses are transmitted through seven of the twelve cranial nerves, whereas the sense of touch – which includes the sensations of pain and pressure – is transmitted by peripheral nerves. Four of the cranial nerves have both sensory and motor functions. Motion, both voluntary and involuntary, is due to muscle contraction as the result of impulses carried by cranial and peripheral nerves. The autonomic nervous system also plays a vital role in responding to emotions. Other senses include those required for balance, and some say there is also a "sixth sense," intuition. The feeling or sensation of fear may be triggered by any of the senses, and it may result in both voluntary and involuntary responses. The feeling of fear may be a physical threat, such as the unexpected odor of smoke, or a loud noise; or it may be emotional, as when a mother suddenly realizes that her child is missing. The responses include transmissions through any or all of nine cranial nerves, such as blinking the eyes, from contraction of the oculomotor nerve; the peripheral nerves, causing contraction of the muscles of the back and hand, arching the back, and making a fist. And through the autonomic nervous system, with a sweaty palm, or stimulation of the gastro-intestinal tract and the bladder, accidentally releasing urine or stools, described in graphic barnyard language.[79]

Stimulation of the autonomic nervous system by fear also triggers the "flight or fight" response with release of hormones from the adrenal gland. These hormones include epinephrine (also known as adrenaline) and nor-epinephrine from the adrenal medulla, which is the smaller, interior part of the gland; and cortisol (also known as cortisone) from the larger outer part – the cortex – of the adrenal gland (the relationship is identified by the prefix "cor."). The "flight or fight" hormones are released by the cells of the adrenal gland into the bloodstream. The adrenal hormones circulate throughout the body and cause many secondary effects through the production of other hormones, such as cytokines. These secondary hormones are intended to be used by the body to be useful and to aid in recovery from shock and stress, but if the body does not, or cannot, respond properly, cytokines have deleterious effects which cause contraction of blood vessels, loss of organs, and death.

The word, "shelter," is probably derived from *sheltrum*, a word meaning "roof" or "shield" – a weapon of defense – in Middle English. Many of the words that mean "safety," and which are familiar to humans, have connotations that derive from the notion of shelter. In Martin Luther's thunderous hymn, the first lines mention *Burg* (castle, fortress), and *gute Wehr und Waffen* (good barrier and weapon), which is translated into English as "bulwark, never failing." The idea that protection will come from *unser Gott* (our God) invokes the idea that this *Burg* is a holy place – a sanctuary (Latin = sacred). From *burg* we have Hamburg, the second largest city in Germany, and Magdeburg. And then in Anglo-Saxon English, *burg* becomes Edinburgh, and "boro," as in the borough of London.[80]

Shelter and safety are connoted in German by the word *Schloss*, which has several meanings, including castle, lock, bolt, and bar. For this reason, Franz Kafka's, *Das Schloss*, translated into English as *The Castle*, has a more complex meaning in the original. Many other common words can be traced back to words meaning safety – a harbor or haven is a safe place, a port, for ships. *Copenhagen*, capital of Denmark, means "merchant's harbor." Bremerhaven, Germany, is "Bremen's harbor." New Haven, Connecticut (Latin = *novum portum*), is etymologically identical to Newport, Rhode Island.[81]

The top predators in any region are usually large animals or birds that are carnivorous or omnivores. The top animals in the food chain have less reason to feel fear than those that are below it. They have less need for a safe place to retreat to than smaller animals. However, all animals need safe places for nesting, for birth, and for protection of their young. The presence of humans alters the natural ways of other animals' behavior, because humans developed tools – including weapons – and they learned to use these weapons to hunt animals and in combat with other humans. Humans learned to be fearful of the top predators – bears, lions, rhinos – and of poisonous snakes, and of other dangers in nature. Humans therefore sought carefully for caves and cliff ledges in which they could live, cook, and rest; and from which they could venture for hunting, scavenging for food, and to explore the world around them. The caves and cliff dwellings of Avignon, in France, perhaps 30,000 years old, and the dwellings of Mesa Verde, in Colorado, about 3,000 years old, are reminders of how humans found safe places to live, many centuries ago. A human who seeks to explore the wilderness, or who is suddenly thrust into it by chance, has the same need for safety. Especially if he or she is lacking in a weapon. For several centuries, men in America were always expected to have a sharp knife in their pocket – a pocket knife – and they began to carry a knife as a youth. It is a matter of religious faith and tradition that a Sikh male, anywhere in the world, will always carry a knife. It may have a large, curved, very sharp blade, or it could be a tiny symbolic dagger, in order to pass a security check at the airport or a courthouse.[82]

One of the interesting connections that humans have with nature is the relationship between humans and trees. The three Urges mentioned here – water, food, and shelter – can be found in trees. Water can be found in some trees such as coconuts, and in sap, transported in cells of xylem and phloem. Water drips from cuts into the bark (as with sugar maples) or cuts from branches (in birch trees and *Ficus* trees). Water is located in arid areas where trees are growing, as in oases in the Sahara or along streams in the American west. The most useful immediate shelter for humans is built from branches and logs; stones may be stronger, but wood is easier to utilize. Wood is essential for the one quality that is unique in humans, and which distinguishes humans from all other living things: Fire. But first, we must consider two more human urges: lust and social connections, which are vital in humans' search for health.

Two Additional Human Urges – Lust and Social Connections

D. Lust

> For each man kills the thing he loves.
> –Oscar Wilde[83]

This part of the essay on *Health Matters* could be entitled "Sex and History: From the Bible to the Kinsey Reports." It could be the title of a course in college. Or of a book, with the additional subtitle, "Helen of Troy, the Wives of Henry VIII, and More." We must tread lightly while writing on this delicate issue, to avoid vulgarity and to treat both genders as equally as possible. The word "lust" is chosen to emphasize the potentially dangerous nature of the act of heterosexual and homosexual conjugation in humans. I do not intend at this point to discuss other forms of lust, such as the lust for power.[84]

The definition given for "lust" in Merriam-Webster's dictionary as "usually intense or unbridled sexual desire: lasciviousness." The origin and dissipation of lust will be described as the process develops in rather bland scientific terms. The reader may wish to substitute synonyms in lay language, or with commonly used slang words, for a more entertaining description of lust, from start to finish – or, if you will, from beginning to end. Shakespeare was always looking for a *double entendre.* These double meanings include epithets, which grandmothers called "strong language." They refer to three components of health as it appears in this essay: Religion, the Body, and Lust. In Religion, the epithets are usually violations of the Fourth Commandment. What a difference two letters makes! Leave out "s" and "h," and eschatology becomes scatology. For instance, the word "darn" appears to be innocent, but in this case, it does not refer to repair of clothing; it is a substitute for "damn." Other epithets refer to the Body in graphic terms, with comments on body parts that are usually kept hidden, such as "peter" (penis), and to waste products of digestion, such as "shoe dirty" (not a job for a cobbler). And in Lust, many choice epithets call attention to both normal and abnormal acts and positions of the sexual act; for instance, when "screw" is a verb, it can be viewed either as a carpenter's tool, or as the male organ doing a job.[85]

In contrast to other urges, lust is commonly episodic; it is pathological if it is continuously present. Lust is evoked by the neuro-endocrine system, which was mentioned above in connection with the response to a cold environment. The stimulus for lust arises at some point in the nervous system, and it continues by activity of the endocrine system and other parts of the nervous system. The stimulus may arise in the cerebral cortex, in the form of imagination, or by reception through the cranial nerves – especially those that receive and transmit sight, smell, and touch on the face – or through peripheral sensory nerves, as in the hands or elsewhere in the body, especially in the erogenous zones of the skin. The endocrine system is stimulated to respond with a cascade of hormones from the adrenal gland and other organs, activating blood vessels in various parts of the body. The cascade that began with lust continues with feedback to the brain and stimulation of the musculo-skeletal system. A large amount of movement is the usual result. The forebrain may say "stop" or the amygdala may say "proceed." What Sigmund Freud called the "id" will usually prevail, however, and unless the process is interrupted, it continues to the familiar climax. Orgasm. Then lust usually, quietly, recedes.[86]

In mammals, as in all vertebrates, successful completion of sexual conjugation is necessary for propagation of individuals, and thus for continuation of the species. Methods to achieve success are therefore embedded in the genes. The two potential partners in the sexual act often have different views on the subject, and lust by one or the other is sometimes required to bring the act to completion. Failure may occur as the result of impotence in the male, or physical or emotional inability of the female to participate. Time and place are important factors in achieving success. If lust is aroused prematurely and cannot be controlled, danger may ensue. If mutual attraction is insufficient, the male may nevertheless succeed. In humans, this may be known by a variety of euphemisms, some delicate, some vulgar, but it is best defined as rape. In domestic animals or those in zoos, the male may need coaxing, or stimulation, first to become aroused, and then encouraged to finish his work. These tasks are necessary for owners of costly but potentially lucrative bulls and stallions, and for veterinarians who care for propagation of reluctant pandas and giant turtles.[87]

Historians have usually avoided the role of sex in human affairs, except when it is absolutely necessary to mention it. Sex (as a verb) by Helen of Troy and Paris was the initiation of action in Homer's semi-fictionalized *Iliad*. Whether there was mutual consent, or not, heightens the drama, but sex was the spark that started that epic fire. Homer's *Odyssey* was a lesson in ancient geography and adventure, but the story revolves around lust: in the Sirens' temptations of Ulysses, who is saved when he is warned by the goddess Circe; the anger of the courtiers who try to seduce his wife, Penelope; and the dramatic conclusion when Ulysses returns to take her to bed. There are also many episodes of temptation, gratification, and unrequited love in the third book of the trilogy: Virgil's *Aeneid*.[88]

Sexual issues underlay much of Charles Darwin's work. You can't have biological reproduction in the *Origin of Species* without sex, and sex drive can be exhibited in humans in many ways. Few readers of *Alice's Adventures in Wonderland* know of the possibility that Charles Dodson (aka Lewis Carroll) was a pedophile. Did you know that Dodson/Carroll had an uncanny interest in nude pre-teenaged girls? He took many risqué photographs of them. His book of nude and partially clothed young women is no longer listed in Dodson's on-line biography, and it has been purged from the internet.[89]

If you look for sex in history, it's abundant. For example, look for sex in the history of literature, art, politics, religion, intellectual history, geographic history, and the history of science and medicine. Sex by mutual consent is there, or by grudging consent, by force (usually by the male), or sometimes even, allegedly, by accident. Most venereal diseases are contracted in sexual encounters, and one of them, the "great pox" – syphilis – altered world history. The adjective "venereal" is indeed derived from Venus, the Roman goddess of love and beauty. Sex can be a problem in psychology – a fetish of many types – or in psychiatry, either as attraction (nymphomania) or aversion (delusional fearfulness).[90]

The examples are literally countless. The Bible is a good place to start. The geography is the Middle East, in the Fertile Crescent. There are so many stories based on sex that it's easy to begin: Adam and Eve discovered their nakedness, and soon they began to have children. No surprise there. The city of Sodom has become a metaphor for male homosexual sexual encounters; God disapproved, and Lot left town. Although Lot lost his wife (she became a pillar of salt) when they left Sodom, his two daughters took her place; they got him drunk, had sex with him, and they had Moab and Ammon. Incest, but on this occasion, women initiated it. Noah took the world's beasts, two by two, for later coupling. Samson was destroyed by Delilah's entrapment; that was for sex, of course. The beautiful story of Ruth is about marriage – i.e., sex. Rachel and Leah both had sex with one man, Jacob. Rachel hid the jewels that she stole from her father by hiding them under her skirt at the time she was menstruating, saying "the custom of women is upon me." It's all about sex. The details aren't told to children, of course. About five hundred years after the Jewish Bible concluded, politics roiled throughout the Middle East, and then the Christian era began. In the New Testament, the purity of the Virgin Mary is a contrast to the Old Testament. Her conception is a miracle, Joseph accepts this (good fellow that he is), and the fact that Mary had many other children, presumably in the usual way, is rarely mentioned.[91]

The sexual activities of ancient Greece and Persia now seem a bit bizarre. Men with boys, men with men, women with women. Infidelity. Slaves for sexual playthings. Eunuchs, believed to be harmless, and certainly fruitless, were in the harems. Men with eunuchs, both enjoying sex. Much of that is told in elliptical fashion in their plays and in fragments of writings. Perhaps not much change in the next century, though, in the world of Alexander, so-called "The Great." He took a wife, Roxanna, in what is now northern Afghanistan, and then died suddenly, mysteriously, in Baghdad. Alexander is said to have loved men more than women, but who knows? Alexander's empire was divided after he died, and Ptolemy took Egypt. His descendant, the last Pharaoh of Egypt, Cleopatra VII, is famous for wooing and wedding Julius Caesar, and then Mark Antony, as well as her younger brother, Ptolemy XIV. Perhaps she wasn't a seductress, but she obviously understood men; and she had at least four children. Caesar's wife was the one who is still portrayed as the symbol of purity. Julius Caesar also bedded Cleopatra, who bore him a son, although that presumably wasn't the reason that he was stabbed in the back (Shakespeare wrote, "Et tu, Brutus?"). Caesar's death was due to a political conflict; it was not about women., though he apparently had plenty of experience in that area, too.[92]

Elsewhere in the Roman Empire, in the time of Nero, an entertaining conversation can be found describing the varied sexual activities of men and women. Translated from Latin, it is *The Satyricon of Petronius the Arbiter*. These scenes, if not the oblique language of the *Satyricon*, could be of San Francisco, California, in the 1960s, when hippies were enjoying their freedom and sex: To Petronius, the woman shrieked, "You have slaughtered the delight of Priapus, a goose, the very darling of married women!" And he answered, "I'll give you an ostrich in place of your goose! … Cruel Eros himself had never dealt leniently with me, loved or lover, I am put to the torture!"[93]

If we move to the 12th century in central Asia, Genghis Khan (1162-1227), the Great Khan, was ruler of the Mongol Empire. His many wives and consorts produced many sons and daughters. His descendants are literally countless. It has been calculated that he could be an ancestor of perhaps 0.5% of the people of the world. The name and title of Khan could afterward be taken only by a descendant of Genghis, so Timur, aka Tamerlane (1336-1405), whose empire was even larger than Genghis, adopted the title of "Padshah," but after marrying a descendant of Genghis, his sons could be called "Khan." It's all about sex and power. And dangerous, too. The Khan family is still associated with power in Asia.

In early medieval Europe, documents are a bit scanty, but there is no reason to believe that there was a lag in interest in sexual activities. The record of the English monarchs and their companions stretches back to King Arthur and his fictionalized castle, Camelot, in the late 5th and early 6th centuries. The story of Camelot is a shining example of duplicity, posing a high moral tone against lusty reality, as told in the love story of Sir Lancelot and Queen Guinevere. Most of the monarchs of England after Arthur have been Kings, though several have been notable Queens. The line was nearly broken in 1066, but a distant cousin in the Royal family – William, Duke of Normandy – won the Battle of Hastings, and thus kept the English Royal line intact. However, King William I introduced French customs, and new methods of courting, into England, and better record-keeping – the Domesday Book – in which details of property and marriage can be found. There is abundant evidence of the importance of sex in the British aristocracy since the Conquest, and no doubt these activities were widespread throughout the realm.

Some of Geoffrey Chaucer's fictional Canterbury Tales, written in the 15th century, are stories of ordinary people, a few of whom are coarse but all are interesting. Many of the tales are about sex; for instance, the "Miller's Tale," which revolves around infidelity and revenge. The bawdy ways of the French in 16th century France were revealed in the novels, *Gargantua and Pantagruel*, by the eminent and knowledgeable (wink, wink) physician, François Rabelais. In the next century, the English began to settle in North America, bringing with them a variety of social and religious norms. The prudish Puritans of New England and the devout Quakers of Pennsylvania sought to control all aspects of life, both public and private – including sex. The *Mayflower* Pilgrims had a Royal bastard, but he was an exception to the general rule in that colony. Men and women who violated the rules about sex were shunned, or worse. The norm was portrayed by Nathaniel Hawthorne in *The Scarlet Letter*, and bestiality and sodomy were hanging offenses. The customs in Massachusetts differed from those of the wealthy aristocrats who settled in Virginia. In that colony of cavaliers, life was often eased by a more liberal attitude toward sex. Men had sex with their wives, and also with enslaved women. There was also space enough in the New World to permit those who wanted to escape from constraint. Rebels from Boston and Salem could move west or south, to relocate in Rhode Island, or in the Dutch colony of New Amsterdam, and later in Appalachia. Women had more control of their own assets in Dutch territory. They could inherit, save their money, and choose a mate. The West became a place for those who did what they wanted to do, not what someone else said they should do. Including how and when to do IT.[94]

"Bundling" was common in New England to ensure compatibility between the prospective bride and groom. They would share a bed, but be separated by a sheet – the young man on one side, the girl on the other side. However, if the two appeared to be compatible, another step could be quietly taken to ensure that the marriage would achieve the desired product – a child. We can assume this, because many of the first children born legitimately in New England were "premature," less than nine months after the ceremony. And sometimes the ceremony had to be rushed; this was called a "shotgun" marriage. Quakers, on the other hand, insisted on announcing the pending marriage at two successive monthly meetings. Both sets of parents needed to approve the marriage, and if no objections were raised by others at the meetings, and if "carnal knowledge" was not demonstrated by a growing waistline of the young woman, the ceremony would take place after the second announcement. All who were present would sign the document in a precise order, including the newly married couple. If the couple couldn't wait, they would have to marry without permission, and then accept being "read out of meeting." In many Asian cultures, the marriage would be arranged by the parents, and sometimes the couple would meet for the first time at the ceremony. Depictions of the act of sex in various forms, and performed by strange creatures, may produce wonder and perhaps were intended for pre-nuptial guidance of Hindus in South Asia. A loving, productive, relationship probably occurs as frequently after an arranged marriage as one in which the couple meets and decides to marry for love, with or without parental consent. Lust and whatever else is needed to make a marriage successful, or not, appears to follow either way.[95]

The works of Shakespeare are an important source of knowledge about sexual attitudes in England in the late 16th century. Shakespeare's beautiful sonnets are still appreciated by lovers, and some of his lusty characters are still with us. Their language is archaic, but their behavior is strangely familiar. Kings, princes, jokers and fools are all there. Shakespeare's conflation of "maid" and "made" in *Romeo and Juliet* is a good example of his sexual puns. *Midsummer Night's Dream* is one of Shakespeare's most popular plays, telling of sexual relationships involving gods, humans, and animals. Shakespeare lived in the Elizabethan Age. This was a time when accusations of misapplied sexual encounters could be very dangerous. Elizabeth I was the daughter of Henry VIII and Ann Boleyn. Whether Ann was unfaithful to the King, or not, is unproven, but he wanted to be rid of her because he wanted a son. She was accused of fornication with another man. Infidelity to the king was treason in those days, and she was soon beheaded. What happened to her paramour was worse. Her daughter Elizabeth, as Queen, dallied with many men, but she apparently resisted temptation, or was coldly indifferent. Some men and women are disinterested in sex, for various reasons. Sir Walter Raleigh was famous for the myth of casting his cloak in front of Queen Elizabeth as she was about to cross a gutter.

He wooed the Queen, yet he was beheaded by her successor, King James I. Both Sir Walter and Queen Elizabeth are remembered in the geographical nomenclature of North America. Elizabeth, the Virgin Queen, gave her name to the colony of Virginia, while Raleigh is the capital of North Carolina.[96]

Another odd sequence in the British Royal family begins again with Queen Victoria (1837-1901) and continues to her great-granddaughter, Queen Elizabeth II. During her lifetime, Victoria was the model of decorum, faultlessly faithful to her husband, and mother of nine beautiful children. All of the young princes and princesses appeared to have appeared almost spontaneously, in some strange sexless manner. She was the eponymic leader of the strict Victorian Age. However, in later years, long after the death of Prince Albert – who was her husband and also her first cousin (incestuous?) – the Queen had an uncommonly close relationship with a Scotsman named John Brown. This was, of course, known to the nobility at the time. As a Scot, he is always shown wearing a kilt and a dirk. The dirk that dangled from his belt was sheathed, but no one knows whether he wore dirk, so to speak, sheathed under his kilt. Most historians of the English Royal family now think Victoria and Brown had an intimate relationship of some kind. Victoria's son, King Edward VII, had been a notorious womanizer as Prince of Wales, but his son, George V, and grandson, George VI, were models of propriety. Dull, that way. The long-lived Queen Elizabeth II has followed the same path, dutifully delivering babies without apparent emotion. However, many of the men and some of the women on side branches of the Royal family tree have come to grief as a result of their sexual impulses. The list is long, but we may remember especially Mrs. Wallis Simpson and the Prince of Wales (who was for 10 months, King Edward VIII). The Prince was famously fond of many women before he found Mrs. Simpson, and she also had her favorites. That was acceptable in those days, and before and since then, too. Elizabeth's sister, Princess Margaret, had a life that was definitely not straightforward. Elizabeth's son Charles, Prince of Wales, has married twice, although rumor has it that he wavered from the first, Diana, before he divorced her to marry Camilla. And while she and the Prince were still married, Diana also had uncommonly close friends of the opposite sex. The troubled monarchy is, however, still supported by a majority of Brits. It may be that the common folk can see that lusty imperfections are only beauty marks when they are displayed by Royalty.[97]

The fact that lust can lead to danger is well known. True stories of events that began with lust and led to a fatal climax titillate the readers of current events and history. The association of lust with danger, and the consequence, lust and loss, thus becomes a subject for biographies, history, and documentary movies; and in imagination, in the form of romantic and gothic novels, paintings, *film noir* movies, and opera. Think of lust and loss in novels: *Wuthering Heights* and *Tess of the d'Urbervilles*; the movies, *Double Indemnity* and *Rosemary's Baby*; and in operas, such as *Aida, Don Giovanni, La Traviata, La Bohème,* and *Romeo and Juliet.* Ironically, the faithful Romeo of the opera has become a meme representing an ardent suitor of many women; and the elegant but amoral Don Giovanni, translated into English, has been degraded to mean "the john" who is "serviced" by a prostitute.[98]

Three examples in American history will suffice to illustrate the potential danger of lust. In 1859, Philip Barton Key II was shot in Washington, D.C., by Congressman Daniel Sickles, who discovered that Key was having an affair with his wife. Key was not an insignificant person. He was the son of "Star Spangled Banner" poet Francis Scott Key, who had transgressions of his own that are largely forgotten. Pleading temporary insanity, Sickles was acquitted, and he became a general in the Civil War. The "fair sex" can also play the same game, as Jean Harris showed in 1980, when she shot her ex-lover, Dr. Herman Tarnower, for having affairs with several women. She pleaded that it was an accident, and that she had planned to commit suicide, but she was convicted of murder anyway. The event made national headlines because Harris was the headmistress of the prestigious Madeira School for girls, and Tarnower was a well-known author of *The Complete Scarsdale Medical Diet.* Former governor and vice president Nelson Rockefeller died in 1979 of a "heart attack" in his town house in New York City. It later became known that he was with a woman who was not his wife, and the presumption has since been that he died during intercourse. Whether or not the act was completed is unknown. Tabloids implied that he "Died between her legs." It was later revealed that Rockefeller had many affairs, before and during both of his marriages. These examples show that lust can lead to the death of both the reputation and the body.[99]

The temptations of lust have led to attempts to enhance or depress it. Chemical methods have been most effective aphrodisiacs (enhancers): capsaicin ("Spanish fly") used topically on the female genitals, or orally as cayenne pepper; and mood or mind-altering substances, especially alcoholic beverages and chloral hydrate (the "Mickey Finn"). Also, substances from mushrooms (peyote); drugs, such as barbiturates, notoriously Quaaludes, cocaine, and addictive derivatives of the opium poppy (heroin and oxycodone [Oxycontin]); and other toxic substances, such as lysergic acid (LSD), and methamphetamine ("meth"). On the other hand, anaphrodisiacs have been used in attempts to depress the urge for sex. Saltpeter (potassium nitrate) was used for many years in a vain attempt to discourage sexual impulses and closet masturbation in boys and men. British servicemen have long believed that bromide was added to tea to curb sexual desires. Estrogens suppress testosterone, and are effective in blunting libido and arousal, but at a risk of producing untoward side effects. Drowsiness produced by alcohol consumption or barbiturates may inadvertently depress the impulse, but alcohol also inhibits clear-headed consideration of the sexual impulse. A drunk man may push, the lady doesn't clearly say "No," and the show goes on. This list is incomplete, but it shows the great interest in the subjects of lust and sex.

Some of the most famous men in America are the 46 presidents. Several of them have displayed remarkable dexterity in negotiating political success while also finding ways to enjoy sexual relationships that might have, at the time, destroyed their careers. Perhaps in some cases, the challenge was to rise to the occasion. The letters of George Washington show his deep affection, perhaps unrequited, for Sally, the wife of his neighbor, Lord Fairfax. But George soon married Martha Custis, while Sally stayed with Fairfax. The second president, John Adams, had a trusting wife, and he appears to have deserved her trust. But he only lasted for one term. Thomas Jefferson, like George Washington, had two terms in office, in spite of the rumors that he was having children with an enslaved servant. He was, indeed, but that was never proved until the twentieth century. In the next century, the United States also had a two-term president who had a well-deserved reputation as the father of an out-of-wedlock child. As the song went, "Ma, Ma, where' my pa? Gone to the White House, ha, ha, ha." The president was Grover Cleveland, and his two terms were not sequential, but he was the only president (thus far) to be successful in that way. In the twentieth century, we see both contrast and similarities in two distant cousins – Theodore and Franklin Roosevelt. Theodore, a Republican, and Franklin, a Democrat, shared many aims and they occupied many of the same political offices. But they differed in respect to their family lives. Theodore, tragically widowed, remarried and never wavered in his affection; nor did his wife. His eldest daughter, Alice ("Blue Gown"), was an interesting character in Washington. She may have been promiscuous, but the rest of Theodore Roosevelt's children were as straight as arrows. Cousin Franklin, on the other hand, was cheerful with his many affairs (secret at the time), and Eleanor, too, was happily intimate with a lady friend. Franklin and Eleanor continued to be partners in politics, but their children followed in the wayward ways of the parents, with too many wives and sweethearts to enumerate.[100]

In the period between the two Roosevelts, Woodrow Wilson was president. He, too, was a man who loved women, and not only his wife, although he had two of them. Most of what he wrote and did in regard to women was never imagined by others in his lifetime. He was a passionate man in private, and in his personal life, although he always showed a rather dull looking, top-hatted, dignified image to the public. After FDR came Harry Truman, who like Teddy Roosevelt, was a man who was devoted only to his wife, although he had a mother-in-law who thought he wasn't worth much. Then came Dwight Eisenhower. Ike is said to have been a bit too close to his lady driver in Europe, but nothing much came of that. After Eisenhower, John Kennedy won a close race to beat Richard Nixon. Jack and Jackie Kennedy seemed to most of America to represent the fictional Camelot, which coincidentally was a Broadway musical at that time. Insiders in Washington knew that there was a swinging back door, so to speak, to the East Wing of the White House, but most of America wouldn't know about it until much later. And that there were probably two back doors at that time, because Jacqueline Kennedy apparently had her own lovers, too. The Kennedys were followed by two rather sexless presidencies, the Johnsons and the Nixons. Lyndon Johnson and Richard Nixon were incredibly vulgar in private conversations, but none of their inappropriate talk was about sex. Betty Ford, who married Gerald as her second husband, was the first divorcee to become the First Lady. Ford was followed by the epitome of rectitude, Jimmy Carter, who failed to be re-elected. Carter was embarrassed even to think of lust. The first divorced president, Ronald Reagan, lasted two terms. He became famous in Hollywood, where swapping partners in the evening was an important part of life. His First Lady, Nancy Davis Reagan, brought astrology to the White House. Reagan was followed by the Honorable George H. W. Bush, who was thought to be a gallant man, a bit "handy," but nothing more than that. We then arrive at the Clintons. The pleasures and travails of President Bill Clinton and First Lady Hillary. His ejaculate on the dress of Monica Lewinsky, and lying under oath about not having sex with "that woman," led to his impeachment. Morals have changed over the past two centuries, however. Bill Clinton actually rose in popularity during the trial, and he was not convicted. The attempt to remove him from office failed, and he continues to be popular. Another of the Bushes and then the Obamas – eight years with nothing to gossip about. The 45th president was Donald J. Trump, who famously bragged about his exploits with women before he became president. He was taped saying that he'd grab them by the [nether parts]. It is an understatement to say that there is more to be revealed about that. Joe Biden narrowly won the election in 2020, and once again, the U.S. has a president without a wandering eye. He is said to have been a bit handy, but that's a politician for you. Nevertheless, although many Americans disapproved of some of these presidents, it would be difficult to show that any president failed as the result of his sexual activities.[101]

In the past century, changes have occurred in sexual activities throughout the world, enabled by discoveries in embryology, pharmacology, and gynecology. Women can now prevent conception with "the Pill" instead of the age-old methods of refusing or choosing the date of intercourse. Termination of pregnancy became possible with sterile abortions and pharmaceutical interventions, instead of coat hangers and abortifacient herbs. And couples have been relieved of the need for coitus interruptus and condoms. These changes have not been universally accepted. There is great reluctance in some religious groups, such as Evangelical Christians, Roman Catholic Church doctrine, and traditional Muslims. On the other hand, in 1979, the leaders of the Peoples Republic of China instituted birth planning in an attempt to control the rapid growth of the country's population. The so-called "one child" policy has been modified several times, most recently in 2015, when a "two-child" policy was announced. Many people now believe that "safe sex" is the best sex, or at least it is better than no sex at all.[102]

The differing roles of men and women throughout history begins with lust. But it is not only lust. Men and women have biological differences, which give them different roles in the family and in society. The other needs of humans also play a part in the ways that men and women interact. The need for social connections includes a division of labor in the group, and thus the male and female are assigned to different roles. The need for shelter includes personal protection, and that means a search for power. Dominance, maximizing power, is usually exerted by males – the physically stronger sex – over females; and in the urge for lust, in sexual intercourse. There nevertheless have been some powerful women in history, and their power sometimes (but not always) derived from their use of gender, as in the "wiles" of women. If time and space permitted, we could speak of women from the legends of Eve and of the Amazons to the present time. Think of the different types of power exerted by individual women: Pharaohs Hatshepsut and Cleopatra; the Biblical Esther and the Queen of Sheba; the Virgin Mary and Joan of Arc; Elizabeth I and Catherine the Great; Prime Ministers Golda Meier, Margaret Thatcher and Angela Merkel; Mother Teresa in Calcutta (Kolkata), India, and Aung San Suu Kyi in Myanmar. And the matriarchal Sherpa women of Northern Nepal. Some were never married, some were courtesans, some were faithful mothers; and all were exceptions to the general rule. In a matriarchy, the women choose their husbands and may be polyandrous; and they inherit property. The trend in recent history in financially "developed" countries, is for women to become empowered, with equal rights, even though they have biological differences that make it difficult for men and women to have true equality.[103]

Science has also intruded into the discussion of sex and population control in another way, but it was unfortunate. The modern movement known as eugenics traces its beginning to Darwin and its end with Hitler. Briefly, Charles Darwin's *Origin of Species* is taken (incorrectly) as the starting point for the notion of "survival of the fittest." This idea was given another boost by Darwin's cousin, Sir Francis Galton, who coined the term "eugenics." Galton suggested that the fittest would be descended from those who were from the best families. The idea caught the imagination of the elite in America, including such notables as Theodore Roosevelt. Some of the outcomes now seem monstrous, such as the sterilization of "mental defectives." Oliver Wendell Holmes wrote the U.S. Supreme Court decision in 1927, in which he stated the "three generations of imbeciles are enough," authorizing the state of Virginia to sterilize Carrie Buck. Adolph Hitler did not need to mention the word "eugenics" when the Third Reich confined and executed mentally ill men and women (the word was not German). The idea of eliminating "degenerates" had become acceptable. It is largely forgotten now that Hitler was supported by such men as the Prince of Wales (later King Edward VIII of England) and Charles Lindbergh, the famous aviator. Lindbergh coined the political phrase, "America First," that came back with a roar in Donald Trump's campaign for the presidency in 2016.[104]

Many other changes have occurred in attitudes toward sex and gender over the past century. Some of these were apparent changes but had previously been unrecognized or had been hidden. Sexual deviants – hidden homosexuality, pederasty, and false professions of chastity – were discovered, hidden among the priests, bishops, monks and nuns of the Roman Catholic Church. These shocking revelations have led to findings of duplicity that existed for centuries within monasteries, convents, schools and churches, and also in other denominations. It appears that interest in sex was always there, just out of sight. Harems have existed in many places in America, too. They are usually dominated by males, but sometimes with common consent and no permanent partners. Hidden away, sometimes in cities, but more often in lonely places. In the theatre, subtle changes in attitude were subtly introduced with interracial romances in *South Pacific*, and then, suddenly, nudity in *Hair* and gaiety of *La Cage aux Folles* brought the burlesque of "La Moulin Rouge" from Paris to Broadway to Hollywood. Thousands of movies on Netflix and Hulu now feature nude scenes of wild love-making, regardless of the genre of the movie, whether comedy, drama, crime, or adventure.

Most Americans still profess to believe in the typical monogamous family, persisting unendingly ("until parted by death"), while allowing that a few men and women may choose, without fault, individually, not to marry and live alone. Such solitary behavior is considered, nevertheless, to a bit strange. During the past decade, however, there has been a remarkable change in attitude in America, and to some extent in other parts of the world, toward those who are in various ways different from the majority group in gender. Attitudes have changed from time to time in the past regarding minority groups, depending sometimes on income and social status. For example, those who were wealthy could cross-dress, if they chose to do so. And perhaps, it may have been more acceptable for women to be very close to other women than it was for men to show affection to other men. Whispers of lesbianism were not as dangerous to reputations as was the career-ending rumor of homosexuality.[105]

This issue is both biological and sociological. The biology is exemplified best by the existence of a variety of conditions called "intersex" in humans. One example is hermaphroditism. Rare, but clearly obvious at birth, such a baby has a male organ, but who also appears on close examination to have a vagina. Therefore, the baby is also a girl. What to do? Giving an ambiguous name to the baby could delay the answer for a little while, but the gender needs to be put on the birth certificate. Physicians worried about this. Some physicians recommended surgery to eliminate traces of one gender or the other; sometimes amputation of the little penis. It was not a happy solution, but it was done, quietly and rarely discussed again. The baby may still have undescended testicles, which later will become a problem. There are many other forms of anatomical bisexuality, and for every such baby, parents agonized over their choices and how to prepare for the future. If a child showed an uncommon interest in clothing and activities associated with a different gender, it was an issue for the parents, the extended family, and their social group. A recent change, however, has now occurred in some parts of American society regarding previously undiscussable differences in sexual orientation: of attitudes toward homosexuality, bisexuality, transsexuality, uncertain gender, alternating gender, no gender, and the happy display of an alternate gendered appearance. We may see a young man with a wispy beard, dyed purple hair, wearing a skirt, walking to his class in college. The change has spawned, so to speak, the ever-changing informal movement known as LGBTQX (and more), for lesbian, gay, bisexual, transsexual, queer, and gender neutral. These issues have affected all aspects of society, including family life, schools, playgrounds, public toilets, churches, politics, government laws and regulations, and the armed forces.[106]

At the same time, women have been empowered by Title IX in the U.S. code, which requires equal treatment of men and women in colleges that receive federal funding; and by the social network inspired by the Me Too (or #MeToo) movement which arose in response to reports of flagrant sexual abuse of women by men who had powerful positions in the entertainment industry. The problem for women still is the risk of reporting the incident: shame, disbelief, loss of future opportunity; or difficulty of proof: "she said" versus "he said," or "it was mutual consent" or "it never happened." DNA recovered can be helpful, but DNA may nevertheless beg the question of consent.[107]

The presumption of lust has long been presumed to be sufficient cause for lynching in America. An African American boy, Emmett Till, fourteen years old, was accused of offending a white woman. He was lynched in Mississippi in 1955. Leering was sufficient cause for the lynching of many others. Torture and a slow death, by hanging and burning, cheered on by white men, women, and children, with photographs taken during and after the event. As if it were a picnic. Harper Lee's novel, *To Kill a Mockingbird*, was believable, for it placed the deadly burden on a Black man, even if he was entrapped, or falsely accused, or if the affair may have been with mutual consent. Sexual relations between men and women of different races, known as miscegenation, was illegal, and interracial marriage was prohibited by law in many states in the United States until 1967.[108]

Venereal disease can be miserable or fatal, or both. The group of sexually transmitted diseases (STDs), commonly known as venereal disease (VD), are caused by a variety of microorganisms, including bacteria, parasites, and viruses. STDs include syphilis, gonorrhea, chlamydia (trichomonas), and genital herpes. Secondary diseases caused by STDs include acquired immunodeficiency syndrome (AIDS) from human immunodeficiency virus (HIV), and cancer of the cervix from human papilloma virus (HPV). These secondary diseases are well known to be fatal, and need no further elaboration.

Two examples illustrate the misery and potentially fatal outcome from a sexual encounter. One example is syphilis, which was formerly known as the "great pox" to distinguish it from smallpox, and with the euphemism, "bad blood." Syphilis presents as a small, itchy sore, called a chancre, which is usually in the genital area, but wherever lust induces sexual activity to begin. This is called "primary syphilis." The sore recedes spontaneously, but in most cases, if syphilis is not diagnosed, the disease presents again with a fleeting rash. This is secondary syphilis. Again, the rash recedes spontaneously, and if treatment is not given, a third phase develops. This phase, tertiary syphilis, is the slow killer.

Tertiary syphilis can be devastating, as the tiny spiral-shaped bacteria invade the brain, spinal cord, aorta, and other organs. Tertiary syphilis is known by the diseases it causes: general paresis (psychosis and dementia), tabes dorsalis (a painful disease of the peripheral nerves), aortic aneurysm, and ugly lumps called "gummas" in various parts of the body. Syphilis can be treated with antibiotics, but if not treated in the first or second phase, it can be transmitted through intercourse, or to innocent children during pregnancy or at birth. Tertiary syphilis is devastating to the patient, but supposedly the disease is not infectious in that stage. African American men with syphilis were followed for many years without treatment by the U.S. Public Health Service in the so-called Tuskegee experiment. The study started before treatment with penicillin was known to be effective, but it drifted along without oversight after penicillin became available. We still do not know if penicillin would have helped the men at that time, but the damage was done. The reverberations of this unethical study continue to affect relationships between the African American community and the Public Health Service, and to sour many African Americans on the subject of vaccination.[109]

Gonorrhea, known for centuries as "the clap," can also be treated with antibiotics, although resistance to penicillin and other primary antibiotics has gradually emerged, and the future may be bleak. Gonorrhea is sometimes just a nasty irritation, especially in men, who may only experience pain in the genital area and a yellow discharge ("the drip") from the penis. Promptly treated, a sailor may return again to the same prostitute on his next leave, renewing his acquaintance and his problem, and be treated again. For the woman, however, the story can be very different. Infection with the gonococcal bacillus passes up the vagina to her uterus and fallopian tubes. She often develops a raging fever, and may die of septicemia if untreated; and the infection often causes lasting damage to the fallopian tubes. She may become sterile, or have an ectopic pregnancy, with a high likelihood of hemorrhage as the fetus develops outside of the uterus. She has an increased risk of cervical cancer and of other sexually transmitted diseases (STDs). Unless treated promptly, her baby can be blinded by gonorrhea in the birth canal.[110]

A virtually endless list of other side effects – some intended, some unintended – of lust could be listed, but one more deserves to be mentioned before this chapter ends. It is divorce. If both husband and wife are unhappy with their marriage, and have no children, or their children have matured, separation may be mutually satisfying, and may be beneficial to both. Love and attraction for each other may have faded. In this event, lust may not be a consideration. Lust, however, often plays an important role in the decision to divorce. It may be that one or the other has lost the urge, or one the other has found a different outlet for the urge. For example, a new partner, or a change in sexual orientation. Many marriages are held together because of the children, and lust or the lack of it must therefore occasionally be suppressed. Sad but true. Financial entanglements may overcome lust, and hold a marriage together as a partnership, without love. The danger of social ostracism may hold an unhappy marriage together, as in some religious communities. However, in the end, as it usually does, lust fades away. However, as we shall soon see, humans are kept together by social connections, and procreation continues.

E. Social Connections

Some type of social connection is seen in most multi-cellular organisms, in order to ensure diversity in reproduction. Scientists call this phenomenon "strength through hybrid diversity," in order to enhance adaptation to an environmental challenge. The importance of hybrid diversity has long been known by farmers and animal breeders. Exceptions to this general rule occur in many plants and in a few animal species, which are self-fertilizing or hermaphroditic. In these species, genetic diversity is ensured by stimulation of cross-pollination or cross-fertilization.

In mammals, social connections are needed for procreation, which is to say, for breeding purposes. A social connection has an additional role in most mammalian species. An individual in a social group – whether it is a pack, herd, family, or clan – derives protection as a result of being a member of a group, and the individual is expected to make a contribution to the group's success. In this way, there is a reciprocal relationship between the health of the individual, and the health of the group. Not all members of the group are the same. There are three major differences: age, gender, and skill. The youngest members need to be fed, clothed, and protected; and then to be trained to assume their roles as adults. The older members of groups are usually treated respectfully, and their advice is appreciated – although, sad to say, more so in some societies than in others. The burden of work falls on those who are in the middle years, between very young and very old. Different roles are assigned by nature to men and women, because only women can give birth. In addition to bearing and nursing children, women's work usually consists of additional activities related to young people and the homeplace. Men's work therefore becomes the other necessary tasks – finding water and food, providing security for the home, and participating in protection of the group. As societies evolved, women became bearers of water from its source to the home, and they assumed responsibility for food production, preparation, and storage. It was soon seen that cooperation would be useful, and "many hands make light work" must have been recognized early in human life. Some jobs cannot be done alone. Every able man would participate in barn-raising in early New England, and everyone who was available would help with the harvest of a field of oats. Women had quilting parties and they helped the men in harvesting oats and flax. The spirit of cooperation led to the notion of the Golden Rule of reciprocity in many religions and cultures: Do unto others what you would have them do unto you. Exercises in bridge building that require teamwork are used as problems for outdoor leadership courses.[111]

Preparation and consumption of food is an important aspect of communal living. Of many possible examples, one must suffice to illustrate this point. It will be recognized by many readers, because it is recent American history. In the early 20th century, the daily pattern of life in America was different from what is seen in the 21st century. Similar changes have also occurred throughout the world.

At the time when most of the people in the United States lived on farms and ranches, or near agricultural land in small towns and villages, the routine was a simple one. For much of the year, it would be up with the sun, to eat and work; and when the sun went down, it was time to work indoors – for instance, sharpening tools – and sleep. This daily pattern would continue through the year, although the hours of sunlight were shortened by winter or lengthened by summer. There were three meals every day: a hearty breakfast, a large meal at noon – called "dinner" – and a light meal at about six o'clock, called "supper." The only difference would be on Sunday, when baked or fried chicken would be the center piece of the noon meal. Sunday breakfast might include pancakes with maple syrup. The weekday breakfasts would usually consist of eggs, starch, and meat. A couple of fried eggs, a side of corn grits or fried potatoes, one or two pieces of sliced bread with butter and jam, a dish of oatmeal or dry cereal with milk and sugar, and fried bacon, ham, or beefsteak. Coffee for the parents and a glass of milk for the children. Some fruit, such as apples or pears, after they were ripe enough to eat. The noon meal was called "dinner" because it was the big meal of the day. Typically, roast beef with mashed potatoes and gravy, vegetables – peas, beans or carrots – on the side, and a large slice of pie or cake for dessert, with cream on top. Milk for the children, coffee for the adults. For supper, a small plate of leftovers from the noon meal; or milk toast, consisting of a bowl of warm milk with two slices of bread, toasted and cut into bite-sized pieces, with a spoonful of butter slowly melting on top and sprinkled with salt. No coffee after supper, because it would keep you awake. There will be more to say about this simple menu later, but it is important to consider it briefly at this point, because it relates to the process of digestion. A healthy society is one in which everyone has enough to eat, and can assimilate it.

    The choices for breakfast, dinner, and supper were traditional, and they were passed from one generation to another. The menus varied from one part of the country to another, depending on what raw materials were available. But they all had this in common: Unknowingly, it was good for health. After a large breakfast, there was time to line up for the outhouse or the potty or toilet in the indoor bathroom. The body's autonomic nervous system energizes the "gastro-colic reflux," and this ensures that the day will get off to a good start. Food in the stomach stimulates the colon to get to work. All that is needed is some toilet paper to finish the job. And then a light meal in the evening enables the stomach to empty promptly. It is pleasant to lie down after supper and not feel bloated, or have regurgitation as a reminder of what has just been consumed. This, too, is a normal response of the autonomic nervous system. A heavy meal, especially one containing fatty meat, stimulates a hormonal response which closes the outlet from the stomach. The duty of the pyloric sphincter, as it is called, is to give the stomach about two hours to grind a fatty meal and churn it with acid. If a person lies down before that action is finished on a large, fatty meal, the result will be belch, burp, or vomit. Milk, Pepto-Bismol, Maalox, or Tums can be tried. But the best choice was made long ago: it was a light meal in the evening, called supper.

    Another aspect of communal life is based on the gendered roles of humans – of men and women – which are clearly defined in some cultures, although less so in others. Physical strength plays an important part in the role of men, and male dominance, referred to as patriarchy (the father is ruler), is present in most cultures. The history of Henry VIII and his six wives is a tale of male dominance. Henry VIII became an enormous man, gigantic in size, with overwhelming physical power as he aged. Males are thus the dominant sex in many societies. More kings have been rulers than queens, though a woman may be the "power behind the throne" of a man. A Muslim male can have four wives. He can divorce any with a simple utterance, no reason needed, and then take a new wife.[112]

    A society led by women is somewhat unusual, yet history records the emergency of matriarchy in many places. In Nepal, near Mount Everest, Buddhist women select their mates, and they can choose to have more than one – that is to say, to be polyandrous. In the Khumbu region, women are the owners of property, and they are responsible for their homes and their communities, while their men are often absent, working in the mountains as Sherpas, or elsewhere, far from home. Women generally lack the physical strength of men, but in legend and history, women have achieved agency in other ways. The "wiles" of women have been mentioned since Eve tempted Adam. Empowerment of women may be enabled by mutual choice, as it probably was for George and Martha Washington, and James and Dolley Madison. Or it may be the result of chance, as when Edith Bolling Wilson assumed control of the office of the president in 1919 when Woodrow, her husband, was incapacitated by illness.[113]

In biology, it had long been believed that many sperm competed to fertilize an egg, and the battle was won by the strongest sperm. This view of male dominance has been upended by research which shows that perhaps the egg chooses which sperm to accept. In birds, the preening of many males – such as roosters – allows a thoughtful hen to make her selection. Some women have achieved power through inheritance and ruled with great success. Examples include the Egyptian pharaohs, Hatshepsut and Cleopatra; Elizabeth I, Queen of England; and the Empress of Russia, Catherine "the Great." Elizabeth and Catherine not only inherited power, they defended it, cleverly and sometimes ruthlessly. The Book of Esther tells of a beautiful Jewish woman who achieved power through marriage to a Persian king, and then exercised it on behalf of her people. It is probably a fable, but it is a memorable one and it is celebrated in the Feast of Purim. Women have also achieved prominence in legend and history for virtuous leadership, rather than for power. To name a few, some of whom were mentioned previously: The Virgin Mary, St. Joan of Arc, Clara Barton, and Florence Nightingale.[114]

The balance of power between women and men is sometimes tilted unexpectedly, as exemplified in the fictional tales of Scheherazade and Turandot. In the tale of *One Thousand and One Nights*, the virgin Scheherazade tells a new story each night to the monarch of Persia, defying death, and finally winning his love. In Puccini's opera, on the other hand, the powerful Chinese Princess Turandot yields to the love of Prince Calaf when he correctly answers her question, "What is like ice, and yet burns?" He replies, "Turandot." However, occasionally, power and fame are shared equally by men and women. William II and Mary II were successful when they were King and Queen of England after the Glorious Revolution of 1689. The most successful family in science is that of Pierre and Marie Curie, and their daughter Irène and her husband Frédéric Joliot, all four of whom received Nobel Prizes for their work.

The gendered aspects of history, described above, are relationships of biology and history. Biology is the fundamental science of health. In this way, human history is derived from the search for health. This is the argument of *Health Matters*. C. P. Snow (1905-1980) considered that the scientific revolution was the "only method by which most people can gain the primal things (years of life, freedom from hunger, survival for children)." Snow believed that social connections were crucial in achieving these primal things: "the social condition is with us, we are part of it, we cannot deny it. … we are members one of another. [In] primal things. It seems to me better that people should live rather than die; they shouldn't be hungry; and that they shouldn't have to watch their children die." Snow believed in the importance of protecting children, and in "sharpening the concern of rich and privileged societies for those less lucky," based on his experiences as he grew up in a poor family in England.[115]

There is a need in human society to feed and protect children. Care is important. Nevertheless, caring for children should not be counted as a separate primal urge, for child care it is a consequence of living in social groups. Some will be primary caregivers to children, whereas others will find food, water, and clothing for them. Some will not give birth to children, or father them, but as Snow emphasizes, members of human social groups are responsible for ensuring that all children are safe and have enough to eat. Care and safety are partners in this endeavor.[116]

Humans inherited methods of communication from their animal predecessors which were important in their social groups. By sounds and signs – speech and non-verbal language and gestures – humans have enhanced their social group performance, peace between groups, and sexual activity. Humans may also have had an advantage over their humanoid ancestors, with anatomy of the larynx that favored the ability to speak. The word "communication" begins with the Latin prefix, *com* = with. Togetherness. Communication is usually peaceful, a term of health, although the word stem is also present in communicable diseases. There can also be angry or warlike communications. It reminds us of the social groups known as communes and Communists, which have a mixed record in history. When verbal communication is difficult to understand it is sometimes called babble, which paradoxically calls to mind both the Biblical Tower of Babel (Genesis 11:1-9), when groups could not communicate with each other, and the 20th century translating tool, Babel Linguistics. However, "babble" can be pleasant – as in a babbling brook. Non-verbal communication can be with body language (a wink or a shrug), or American Sign Language for the deaf. Or with hand signals, as in Tribal sign language, or as a salute or a hug of affection. To extend a hand, to curtsy, or to bow are signs of respect. They are healthy indicators. We say, "Hello," *Guten morgen* (good morning), or *Shalom* (peace), and to be "soft-spoken" is taken as a sign of good health. Warnings come when "Mayday" crackles over the radio, or when SOS appeared in Morse Code: dot dot dot - dash dash dash - dot dot dot. Flag signals can communicate bad news or good news: The pirate's skull and crossbones, or a red pennant with a white diagonal stripe that signals that diving activity is underway. Or the yellow flag of "Q" for quarantine. It's good news to see the blue signal flag with a square white center for the letter "P." It is the Blue Peter, for "Sailing from Port" or "Outward Bound." At a yacht club, it means "Come aboard. It's time for cocktails."[117]

When a community grew to become larger than a small family, differences inevitably appeared that required mediation for a peaceful settlement. Arguments occurred over ownership of personal property, territorial rights, and in situations involving violence. These disputes were originally settled by meetings of the tribal elders, who would sit and talk until concurrence was achieved. The agreement was often ratified by a ceremony, such as smoking peace pipe or clasping hands. In time, spokesmen appeared who were most eloquent and could argue a point of contest from either side. These men had the ability which is now seen in lawyers. It was the beginning of the legal profession. Conflicts which ended in death or injury would require consideration of how to punish the miscreant and how to deter others from similar misbehavior. These issues would now be considered as criminal charges and the outcome would be some form of corporal punishment. Here, too, a spokesman would be called upon to defend the accused person. And thus, the practice of criminal law emerged. In some societies, a presiding officer or a small group of men would be chosen to make a decision; they would evolve into judges. At a later time, juries of men of similar status to the accused would make the decisions. In every instance, lawyers would be involved. We will have more to say about these tribal meetings and associated ceremonies at other points in this essay, and we will return at the end to comment on the professions of law and medicine as they relate to each other at the present time.

As social groups evolved and increased in size, the groups also considered different forms of government. Space in this essay does not permit a full examination of the types of government that have existed in human history, ranging from tiny bands of migrant hunter-gatherers and small villages along the waterfronts, to larger villages and small cities with the development of agriculture. The hierarchy of leadership and sharing of responsibility evolved into systems ranging from hereditary oligarchies at the right side of the governance spectrum to communal democracies on the left. The spectrum of governance, whether hierarchical or communal, also relates to the economic impact that the mode of government has on individuals. The need to retain personal possessions was soon accompanied by the urge for money. The proper means for distribution or redistribution of wealth then became an issue for each social group. The market described in Adam Smith's *Wealth of Nations* is a sharp contrast to Karl Marx's *Communist Manifesto*. A middle ground is seen in many social groups, with moderation in the form of sharing or giving to those who are less fortunate, which is taught or required by many religions, or with a form of altruism, such as socialism, that is based on ethics and morality instead of religious doctrine.[118]

The discussion of the human need for social connections includes the issue of "the self" and "the group." It is a paradox, expressed in the words, "alone" and "together." The biological need for "the group" is the focus of this chapter. The scientific study of "the self" is the domain of psychology; "the group" is the subject of sociology. We now examine "the self," and the occurrence of "self" and "group" in human history. The "self" and the "group" appear in many genres: in memoirs, poetry, novels, and scientific works; and in depictions in photographs, paintings, and music. Two books that are especially instructive in thinking about this paradox are *Alone* and *The Lonely Crowd*. In *Alone,* Admiral Richard Byrd describes spending six months alone in Antarctica in the winter of 1934. Byrd sought to satisfy a dream of adventure, but instead, it was nearly a disaster. Imagine the contrast to Byrd's *Alone* in large gatherings of people, such as in Times Square, on New Year's Eve; or at the Prom concert in London. The world's largest-ever crowd may have been that in Rio de Janeiro, Brazil on December 31, 1994, when 4.2 million gathered to hear the rock concert by Rod Stewart and the fireworks on Copacabana Beach. The risk of acquiring COVID-19 did not dissuade 460,000 motorcycle riders to gather for their annual Biker Rally in August 2020 in Sturgis, S.D. And the fact that the Rally spread the disease to hundreds of people in more than twenty states is not mentioned in the announcement for the planned 2021 Rally on the Sturgis website. A middle ground between the sense of loneliness and the sense of the crowd is described in *The Lonely Crowd* (1950) by David Reisman and two colleagues, which argues for the need to find a balance in inner-directed and outer-directed thought and activity.[119]

Everyone feels the need to be alone at times, and most humans also have the urge, at other times, to be with other people. These impulses are deeply rooted in biology, and they also are seen in other mammalian species. The young male "lone wolf" is admired for his hunting ability, but he must obey "the law of the pack." The connection with other people often includes a sense of place, known as topophilia. This memory of geography may be expressed in many ways: in song, "Home on the Range," "My Old Kentucky Home"; and in thoughts, "homesickness" and *Heimat* (German = homeland).[120]

Some of the interesting aspects of "the self" involve the contrasting feelings of loneliness and the need to be alone. A human who is alone is more likely to feel fear than a human who is in a group. Fear, however, can be a two-edged sword; it can either propel a person to search for safety, or it can lead to paralysis and even death. This, too, is not something that is unique to humans. A mountain lion drops down from a cliff into the midst of a band of elk. The elk scatter, confusing the lion, and they run toward a place of safety. This is the biologically useful response to fear. On the other hand, we see, but find it hard to understand, how a cat stalks a bird that watches the cat, but the bird does not move. The expressions, "a deer caught in the headlights" and "scared to death" are untoward responses to fear, and thus of the variable responses to this emotion. Humans have a conflicted attitude toward safety. A Safety Officer must be obeyed by school children, but naughty boys are often trying to escape from surveillance. A "Cassandra" has been a term of derision since the first Cassandra attempted in vain to warn her fellow Trojans about the wooden horse that the Greeks left when they departed for home. Americans admire "Braveheart" and "Oh, Pioneers," but only reluctantly will Americans acknowledge the benefits of *Crossing to Safety*.[121]

The need to be alone appears to be in conflict with the urge for social connections. I will discuss the needs of humans to be alone, at times, and the some of the consequences of solitude. This discussion considers both the positive and negative aspects of the concepts of "the self" (alone) and "the group" (together), and of what I believe is, in the search for health, a balance between these two positions. The search for balance between "alone" and "together" is expressed by the motto of the United States. The Latin phrase, *E pluribus unum*, meaning "out of many, one," is a goal, though imperfectly achieved.

A person may be alone for one of many reasons, and sometimes for a combination of one or more of them. Perhaps the most common reason is simply the desire for privacy, such as for intimate personal functions (to dress or bathe), to meditate, to avoid or surprise someone, or to work alone. "Solitary" may refer to a punishment, or it may be mean an assignment in military service. A person may be alone as a test of self-reliance, or it may occur as an accident, while sailing or swimming. Most artists need to work alone at times, and at other times, to be with others. Writers compose, artists paint, actors and musicians need to practice alone; and then they work with others – agents, publishers, casts, and orchestras – to display, perform, and sell their art. Athletes often train alone – shooting baskets, long-distance running – but they usually do their best when coached and as members of a team. Surgery is a "team sport"; a surgeon practices alone, but must lead a team in the operating room. Scholarship is a lonely profession, but a scholar of language or history must find an audience to read or listen to the product, whether it is written, spoken, or displayed. On the other hand, solitary confinement of a prisoner is correctly perceived as being a great punishment. Prisoners in "solitary" are known to welcome small creatures, such as mice and ants, for companionship. The "Birdman of Alcatraz," Robert Franklin Stroud (1890-1963) is an example of a self-taught ornithologist. Stroud was in solitary confinement for 42 years for murder.[122]

Religion can be the cause of either solitude or of group connections, or – at times – of both. The argument that religion evolved in the search for health will be discussed at a later point in this essay. However, at this point a few examples should suffice to show the many ways that humans use religion as the reason to be alone, or with others. The hermit, in many faiths, lives alone; a Christian monk or nun may live in a monastery or convent, but in some orders, they never speak with others. The Buddhist monk lives apart from the world, wearing a simple saffron robe, and begs for food. On the other hand, thousands of people gather to worship together in Christian cathedrals, in Hindu festivals, and at the end of the Muslim pilgrimage – the Hajj – to circle the Black Stone of the Kaaba in Mecca. Confession, conscious, and conscience have meanings that relate one person to other people; these words begin with the Latin prefix "con" (together). Conscience, indeed, is the highest function of the three aspects of the psyche that were described by Sigmund Freud. The id (instinct, the pleasure principle), the ego (from "I," myself; the realistic principle), and the superego (conscience; internalization of social norms; the "ethical component of the personality").[123]

The social groups that gather in religious ceremonies, such as those mentioned in the preceding paragraph, are similar in many ways to the groups that gather for non-religious purposes. People who are not related to each other in any known way will gather for celebrations (as mentioned earlier, Times Square on New Year's Eve, the Prom concerts in London, and the Fourth of July on the Esplanade in Boston), for athletic events (huge crowds at the Superbowl and the World Series), and to dine indoors at crowded restaurants and outdoors in parks. In these cases, it is often possible to meet people who are standing or sitting nearby, and thus to develop new friendships and extend the social connections. Some of these gatherings occur with ominous intent, or become dangerous: the mobs in Paris during the Revolution, and the mob that invaded the U.S. capitol building on January 6, 2021. The popular "TED talks" encourage learning about technology, entertainment, and design, and they depend on connections between people who have similar interests. The internet with virtual imaging, such as Zoom, has made it possible to be connected with others in ways that in previous centuries were unimaginable except in science fiction. We can ponder the health aspects of these actual and virtual connections. The absence of a desire to congregate with others is pathological, a sad neurosis known as agoraphobia. It is a word that traces its origin to the Greek word *agora* – the marketplace – which teemed with people. Physical and mental health can either be improved or hindered in many ways in social connections between people.[124]

Altruism and egoism are the two opposing poles in the spectrum of the social connections of humans. Altruism is "unselfishness, devotion to the welfare of others." It is the "opposite of egoism." A feeling of altruism – the altruistic spirit – enables humans to bond, to work together, to have happiness, and to succeed in endeavors which one person alone could not accomplish. Altruism enables humans to grieve for others' losses, and for the loss of others. Altruism is inconsistent with a simplistic notion of Darwin's theory of natural selection, expressed in Herbert Spencer's words, "survival of the fittest," because perfect altruistic behavior may end in the death of an unselfish person on behalf of another. The death of an altruistic person may even be as a sacrifice to save the other. Altruism is an important aspect of personality, of the self of a person, because it enhances social connections. Altruism is normal human behavior, and it is probably transmitted genetically. Otherwise, altruism must be an epigenetic passage from one generation to another, a process that is still a conundrum. A discussion of Altruism reappears in the section on Death, and then definitively in Religion, after a discussion of suicide and self-sacrifice.[125]

The field of health also encompasses many aspects of solitude. The notion of the "Other" includes those who are excluded, or who feel excluded, from the main stream of society. For instance, a feeling of solitude or of true loneliness may exist in those with disabilities, such as with bodily defects of nerve, muscle, and bone, causing difficulty in ambulation, grasping, hearing, or speech. And in others who cannot see or hear; or those with special needs, including the autism spectrum, Asperger's, and Down syndrome. Or those who must interrupt their daily life for injections or other treatments. The "Other" may be subjected to violence – as in the imprisonment, expulsion, or marginalization of religious dissenters; in the torture and lynching of people of color in the United States; and in the mass executions of Jews and others deemed to be "defectives" in the Holocaust. The "Other" may be a person who is excluded from the group in less dramatic ways – poor, homeless, speaking with a foreign or different regional accent, or lacking in formal education. Or in subtle ways, as when a boy is always the last to be chosen to play on a team; or by the failure of a teen-aged girl to be accepted into the clique of a "Queen Bee," or by her failure at the end of "rush week" to be "pledged" by her mother's sorority at college.

The notion of having "ins" and "outs" has long been a characteristic of society. Even societies that seem to be homogeneous usually have some type of rank order. The order may be maintained so silently that it is impossible for an outsider to recognize the means by which it is achieved. When the social order is manifestly unfair, the issue may be addressed by methods ranging from education and law, to violence and displacement of those who previously were privileged. The outcome in societies has ranged from silently increasing the "quota" of those previously excluded, to laws demanding affirmative action, and eventually to rebellion and warfare between the classes.

There are also psychological and psychiatric reasons for the feeling of loneliness, or for wishing to be alone. For many, being alone, or the feeling of isolation, causes fear. On the other hand, the feeling of uneasiness of being with other people – agoraphobia, mentioned above – is rare. It may have affected Emily Dickinson, who wrote many volumes of poetry while rarely venturing out of her room. Untreated paranoid schizophrenia, with delusions of persecution, can lead to fatal withdrawal from other people.[126]

Those who are interested in health have for many centuries believed in the use of isolation and quarantine to prevent transmission of infectious diseases. In the Middle Ages, some patients with leprosy were driven out of towns in Europe to fend for themselves, alone. Ships arriving in ports in the Mediterranean Sea were required to fly the quarantine flag, a yellow pennant, until they were proved to be free of disease. The most dreaded disease was smallpox, which had occurred in epidemics in the Old World for thousands of years. It first appeared in America after the voyage of Columbus in 1492. The yellow flag, for the letter "Q" (signal "Quebec"), is the oldest flag in the International Code of Signals.[127]

We are now in the midst of the greatest test of human solitude in the history of the world. The situation is unique. Although it is said that a historian should not attempt to predict the future, the events of the past few months are perhaps a grim glimpse of what may be ahead. A novel coronavirus, SARS-CoV-2, first appeared in Wuhan, China, in December 2019. It is believed to have originated in bats. This virus is the cause of the disease in humans known as COVID-19. The disease spread quickly to many other continents. It was declared to be a world-wide health emergency by the World Health Organization on January 30, 2020, and as a pandemic on March 11, 2020. The major route of transmission of the virus is by inhalation of droplets spread by coughing or sneezing, although the virus has also been found in stool samples. As a result, in the first months of 2020, border restrictions were created that increasingly separated the world's countries, and in most countries a recommendation or requirement for social (and physical) distancing of people has since been in effect, in every continent. Intercontinental travel largely came to a halt, and in many countries, people have been confined to their homes, except for travel or work that is deemed to be essential. Face masks are now being worn by millions of people when out-of-doors, and many meetings are now being held as video conferences. We are learning new ways to show a pleasant connection, while still exhibiting social and physical distancing. Some people now greet by placing the palms together and bowing slightly – *namaste* – as in India; or by placing the left hand over the heart, as is common in Central Asia; or by bumping elbows.[128]

The problem of COVID-19 has spawned a large new field of literature, with articles such as "How the Pandemic is Turning Us Inward," "The Courage to Be Alone," and "Why Zoom is Terrible." The COVID-19 pandemic led to recalling the history of previous epidemics: "What Plague Novels Tell Us" and "History's Deadliest Pandemics, from Ancient Rome to Modern America." However, that list was incomplete, and more past pandemics were soon added to the list. There are also many reports in recent newspapers of problems in the food chain, and of civil unrest. The most serious travail in the United States occurred on January 6, 2020, when a mob invaded the Capitol in Washington, intent on preventing Congress from voting to accept the results of the Presidential election. Most of the men and women who participated in that riot were not wearing masks, except those who disguised themselves or it was part of their pseudo-military uniforms, whereas the law enforcement personnel that attempted to defend the Capitol were wearing masks to protect against the virus. How the COVID-19 pandemic will evolve or when it will end is impossible to forecast. However, Thomas Malthus comes to mind. In 1798, Malthus opined that, unless it is checked by other means, such as moral restraint, population will grow until it is stopped as the result of starvation, war, or pestilence. In the meantime, we await the coming of the Muses to inspire writers and artists. Will it be Melpomene, the muse of tragedy; or Polyhymnia, hymn's muse; or epic poetry, from Calliope? But surely it will be Clio, the muse of history.[129]

Two Uniquely Human Urges – Personal Covering and Fire

Many animals have an instinctive need for social connections, but only humans require personal covering and fire. Personal covering is an immediate need for most humans. The need for personal covering may in some instances even precede food, water, and shelter. For instance, imagine that you are suddenly cast into the wilderness on a cold rainy night. You are driving alone in a car that hits a deer and your car spins off of the road and crashes. You will be lucky to have a blanket in the back seat to wrap up in. After you have stopped shivering, you may begin to think of how to satisfy your other needs – for food and water – and how to find your way back to the road to look for help.

F. Clothing – Personal Covering

> And the eyes of them both were opened, and they knew that they were naked;
> and they sewed fig leaves together, and made themselves aprons.
> –Genesis 3:7

The usual depiction of Adam and Eve's discovery of their nakedness shows them with fig leaves over their private parts. However, the author of Genesis continues to say that they made garments – aprons. Indeed, something like an apron – a blanket or a cloak – is what would be needed, not just a simple fig leaf. This garment, for personal covering, would be a necessity in many parts of the world. Not to cover nakedness, but for warmth, especially at night, although not during the daytime in warm regions such as the Kalahari in Africa, the Amazon basin and the jungles of New Guinea. For more than a century, the *National Geographic* has shown images of people in remote parts of the world who have little body covering. Cups and sheaths made from gourds cover their genitalia for symbolic purposes, not for warmth. These are ceremonial coverings, as it was with Adam and Eve. However, when night falls, men, women, and children huddle together in the dark for warmth, and personal cover is good for health.

Personal covering probably evolved from the urge to seek shelter. It is the result of humans' knowledge of the future. The urge to seek shelter would be instinctive, but the choice of shelter, and of how to enhance it with personal covering, would be based on thought, on imagination, and clever use of tool-making ability. Humans make things. Useful things, decorative things, and playful things. Personal covering of various types – large leaves, bark, strips of wood, and clothing – were tools that allowed shelter to be portable. Personal covering could then be protective, and it would also serve as a disguise for the hunter. No other mammalian genus than *Homo* has used personal covering for warmth and protection, and it must have been intentional work by hominids to create these early forms of garments. Covering of the body with various forms of disguise are seen in some non-mammalian vertebrates, such as birds and fishes, and as camouflage in invertebrates, including insects and cephalopods. In these species, disguise and camouflage usually serve either one or the other of two purposes: pretending to be a predator (in order to hide successfully), or not to be a predator (to enhance unwary prey). Some mammals exhibit spectacular camouflage – the zebra's stripes are known as "dazzle" in military terms – but these coverings are inbred in the species, and not chosen or worn as external covering.

Personal covering from the elements of nature allowed humans to migrate and live successfully almost everywhere on earth. The ability to find shelter and create personal covering has enabled humans to live for many centuries in some of the world's highest mountains and driest deserts. Safety was a major consideration in both the search for shelter and proper clothing. And for more than one hundred years, with shelter and clothing, humans have lived on the coldest continent – Antarctica.

Instinct has enabled humans to confront the four great challenges of the natural world – cold, heat, wind, and precipitation. Human skin color plays an important role in this conflict with the elements.

Skin color and health are related in many ways. For example, black skin absorbs heat better than white skin, and it is also more tolerant of the sun than white skin. White skin is especially sensitive to damage from exposure to the sun, and for this reason, it should be protected with clothing. Sun burn is not caused by visible sun light, but rather from the spectrum of invisible rays that emanate from the sun. These characteristics of the skin are useful for Black people living in Africa. North of the Mediterranean Sea, the sun's rays strike the earth less directly, radiation is weakened, and white skin is now seen in humans.

Humans have learned to exploit their natural strengths, and to overcome their weaknesses in order to deflect nature's environmental challenges. Their methods include thoughtful behavior (avoiding the heat of mid-day and the cold of night) and artifice (shelter and personal cover).

The greatest environmental challenge is cold temperature, which is exacerbated by wind and precipitation. The deadly combination of cold and wind has been known by humans for millennia, and it can now be computed using the so-called wind-chill index. The aggregative effect of cold air and rain has also been known for a very long time. As a result of conduction, convection, radiation, and evaporation, a four-fold greater rate of increase or decrease occurs in water than in air. In most circumstances, however, conduction plays the dominant role in the environmental danger posed by a combination of cold and rain.

Most mammalian species originally developed in a specific environment. Each species is therefore well adapted to its usual environment, although each can be troubled by an environmental challenge, such as change for several years in precipitation or temperature. Humans, on the other hand, are different from other animals. They have evolved with the capacity to adapt to a change in the environment. Humans also change their personal micro-environment – their shelter and clothing – in order to live in a new environment. The protective responses to a cold environment that are seen in mammals include effects on many body systems. These responses are intended to alert the body to danger, and to conserve the body's core temperature. The body must preserve its core temperature, even if skin temperature falls below freezing and must be lost. Shivering is one response to a cold environment. Shivering serves as a warning to the individual, and as an effect of the muscles to produce and maintain body heat. Shivering is accompanied in hairy mammals by pilo-erection (bristling hair), enabling the body to have the insulating effect of a blanket of air above the skin. Pilo-erection also occurs as the result of fright, as a mixed effect of the endocrine and nervous system. It is seen in the "fight or flight" reaction of the neuro-endocrine system which Walter Cannon called "the wisdom of the body."

Another effect of a cold environment is called "cold diuresis," meaning increased urination, as the result of stimulation of the hypothalamus by receptors in the skin. The hypothalamus, a tiny region in the brain near the pituitary gland, secretes anti-diuretic hormone when the receptors send the signal, "I'm cold!!" Cold diuresis encourages consumption of water, with the intended effect being to preserve blood flow to vital organs, especially the kidney. Whatever the intended response is, however, it requires the availability of plenty of water, at a time and place where water may be difficult to obtain. The most important response that humans can make to a cold environment is the healthy one: to seek and succeed in a search for shelter, cover, warmth, and water.

In the search for health, humans have used personal covering of many types, which are grouped together under the term "clothing." This includes the use of personal covering for symbolic purposes, such as garments worn in religious ceremonies. Some of these symbols of covering and clothing are useful for mental health, and will be discussed later.

"Clothing" for physical health began with nothing more than what was readily available in nature: hairy skins from animals, feathers from birds, and vegetable matter. Plants provided leaves and bark for clothing, as with Adam and Eve's fabled fig leaves. Originally humans just used cloaks and blankets for clothing, with one layer at first, and then more. And then foot and head coverings. Clever people figured out how to join bits of hair and products of vegetation. And how to tie and fasten the pieces into parts that fit more closely together, and which could be divided into separate parts. Hand coverings probably came later, and they had to be removed in order for thumb and fingers to work as needed. Mittens at first, and then gloves. Some humans made garments from shells, strung together.

Humans developed, in many different places, methods to join threads together to make cloth, by felting, knitting, and weaving. Felting was probably the first, in which animal hair is matted by moisture.

Humans then began weaving on primitive looms, by crossing strips of material. We call them warp and weft. The first weavers must have used strips of skin and bark, and then they began using coarse grasses and reeds, and then animal hair. Knitting is more complicated; it utilizes loops of yarn which are joined together with a knitting needle. The principal natural fibers now used in making cloth are the vegetable fibers of cotton and linen (from flax); silk, from silkworms; and wool, sheared from many animals, such as domesticated sheep, goats, rabbits, and dogs, and occasionally wild animals such as reindeer. Fibers are also obtained from many other plants, and in some parts of the world jute and hemp are commonly used. Insulation of clothing with kapok (from seeds) or down (from young birds and animals) improves its ability to protect against the cold.

Clothing also had an important use in the personal protection against enemies, whether they were dangerous humans or animal predators. This form of clothing must be thick and heavy, a good shield. It would thus serve a double purpose, for it would also be good protection against the elements of nature. Human hands, with opposable thumbs and fifth fingers, and fists, were weapons that were used in offense and defense. A weapon is therefore often an added, inseparable, component of clothing. There are countless examples of this ancient partnership of personal covering with something held or carried: the shepherd has his staff; the hunter his blade; the cook her stirring stick; the fisherman his line and hook; and the cowboy his lariat. Personal covering has often had a metaphorical role in history. For instance, see the powerful images of clothing in the story of Joseph and his "coat of many colors" (Genesis 37:23-4), and of his father's despair: "Israel in mourning girded his loins with sack cloth." And the sequel in Genesis 38, which tells of Joseph's brother Judah, and Tamar, Judah's daughter-in-law. Tamar wore "widow's garments [that] covered her with a vail," which we now spell "veil." This led Judah to believe that she was "a harlot, because she had covered her face." At the time that passage was written, unlike today, a woman's face was not supposed to be covered in the lands of the Fertile Crescent.

Useful parables are derived from stories about clothing. The soldiers cast lots for the robe of Jesus (John 23:4) and thus fulfilled the prophesy of Psalm 21:18-19. Jesus' robe was recognized as precious because it was seamless, and it should not be divided. This contrasts to the legend of St. Martin of Tours, who used his sword to divide his cloak, giving half of it to a cold beggar, clad in rags.

The characteristic image of John the Baptist is easily recognized in paintings and in church windows because of his primitive appearance. "John was clothed with camel's hair, and with a girdle of skin about his loins" (Mark 1:6; also, Matthew 3:4). In images of John, his hair is unkempt, and he is barely covered, wearing a hairy garment or skin, with a belt. His garment is usually brown. The belt is significant, because it is an example of a way that a hand-held object is added to clothing.

Clothing has also been used as an additional way to distinguish the appearance of men and women, and to define the role of gender in society. In most societies, more restrictions have been placed on the actions and dress of women than on men. *Feme covert* ("secret woman") described the role and place of a married woman in much of Europe for many centuries. The term refers to the expectation that women would be expected to be silent and modestly dressed, and thus invisible in public. This is also known as *purdah,* for women to be out of sight, or to be totally covered in the presence of strangers. Throughout Asia, since antiquity, women have often been covered with garments that reached the ground and that hid the head and face and the shape of the body. This custom is older than the two thousand years of the present era, and is present in many religions. In various parts of the Islamic world, observant women today wear the headscarf, known as the *hijab*; some women also wear full body covering, the *burka,* and the *niqab,* in which only the eyes are visible. Religious customs and social traditions in the Christian world have also emphasized head cover for women. A headscarf or hat is expected to be worn by all women in Catholic and Orthodox churches, whether they are worshipping, or just visiting. Covering of the head has morphed into fashionable hats and veils, as in the cheery song that begins, "In your Easter bonnet, with all the frills upon it." Many unique personal coverings have evolved as clothing for women and men in different parts of the world. For example, the flowing, gracious (and expensive) silk *ao dai,* worn by women in Vietnam; the elegant and deceptively simple appearance of the Indian sari; the ancient kimono of Japan; and the sarong of women in Indonesia, Polynesia and Hawaii. The grass skirt, the hula dance, the lei, and the aloha shirt have become emblematic of Hawaii. Buddhist monks, regardless of their financial status, display uniformity in their orange robes. Some men formerly preened in a three-piece suit, a starched shirt, and a top hat. Mahatma Gandhi, on the other hand, identified himself, and his political cause, by dressing as a peasant, wearing a loincloth known as a *dhoti*.

Some clothing styles have come and gone: the girdle and constricting layers of dress worn by Victorian-era women; the intentionally humble style of dress which was demanded in America in the 17th century for Puritan and Quaker women; and the wide, starched, flowing coronet of the Sisters of Charity. In the late 20th century, nurses in America took off their distinctive caps. Caps had been proudly worn by nurses for many decades. The cap identified the wearer as a nurse, and it linked her with the institution – usually a hospital – where she was trained, or with an organization, such as the Navy Nurse Corps.

In the present era, clothing is sometimes made from metal (as in armor, and cloth of gold) or woven from polymers of silica (glass) and carbon (plastic), and clothing has become decorative and symbolic in many other ways. For more than a century, the physician with a stethoscope in the pocket of a long white coat was the ultimate symbol of health. Then times changed. Doctors, nurses, and others in the health professions wear various colors of "scrubs" in hospitals, and even on the street. Now the stethoscope is draped around the neck. Cotton "scrub suits" with short-sleeved shirts and string-tied pants were once worn only in the operating room, and were left there to be washed. Times changed again. The symbol of the health professional is now an invisible inhuman figure in PPE – Personal Protective Equipment – which serves to isolate the wearer from the patient.

G. Fire

The use of fire distinguishes humans from all other animals, and also from all of other forms of life. The importance of fire in human history cannot be overstated. In this section of my thesis that human history is the search for health – because health matters – I will now discuss fire: how and why humans used it as a vital tool, and how it now affects all of life on earth. I will begin by proposing what early members of the genus *Homo* must have thought of fire; and how they used it, fed it, and kept it alive for the sake of their health. We will next discuss the chemistry of fire, and show how it has become part of our daily life.

It was sometime in the Stone Age – probably the Middle Neolithic Period – when early hominids saw that a sustained fire could be useful. Most of the fires that they would see were caused by lightning strikes. Lightning strikes still cause annual fires in Australia. Natural fires occurred on the earth's surface only as the result of lightning, spontaneous combustion, volcanic eruptions, and meteorites, and the latter three causes were rare. Animals had long been aware of fires, of course, but every other species had tried to find ways to escape from fire. Even the closest relatives to humans – the great apes and their cousins – avoided fire. Theoretically, apes could have done what humans did with fire. However, for some unknown reason, they did not. About two million years ago, or perhaps less than that, some hominids recognized that fire could be beneficial in two ways. They recognized that fires provided warmth, supplementing the need for personal covering; and the residue left after fires included edible foodstuffs – animals and wild vegetables that had been cooked. Early humans also saw that danger from animal predators was reduced by the presence of fire; it kept the wolves at bay. And for the first time, humans could see at night. They could carry light deep into the caves that they used for shelter.[130]

Some humans, braver than others, cautiously moved into a fire zone and saved embers and used them to create fires which they could control. The aborigines of Australia still do this. It was how Tierra del Fuego (Land of Fire) got its name. It is likely that it happened when a fire started from a lightning strike, and the indigenous people kept the fire burning for as long as possible. Wind direction and geography would be important to the early users of fire. They would have recognized that it was best to stay upwind and downhill from an active fire. The early humans immediately knew that fuel was needed to keep their small fires alive. That was the beginning of the eternal human search for fuel, which continues today. The search for fuel became a constant requirement, akin to the search for water, food, shelter, personal covering, and companionship. Fuel is not shown as a separate urge, however, because it is secondary to the need for fire. A safe source of fire, and a safe place to store fuel to feed it, is the sixth urge in human's search for health.[131]

In Greek mythology, the method by which humans acquired fire is subsumed by the legend of Prometheus, the supreme trickster, a master craftsman, a god of fire. He was a clever fellow; his name means Forethinker. Prometheus is said to have tricked Zeus, who as a result hid fire from mortals. However, Prometheus stole fire and returned it earth. As punishment for humans, Zeus created Pandora and her eponymic jar which had a great lid. In spite of Prometheus' warning, Pandora married Epimetheus (Hindsight), and she took the lid off of the jar. Out flowed all of the miseries of humans: evils, hard work, and disease. Hope alone remained within it. Prometheus, however, brought the arts and sciences to humans, as well as fire, the means of survival. The reader may see some similarities in this Greek legend to the story of Adam and Eve in Genesis. The methods by which fire could be maintained, fueled, and restarted is a matter of archeology and anthropology, not of this interesting legend.[132]

In chemistry, fire is said to be the product of rapid oxidation of material in the process of combustion, which releases heat, light, and other products. Oxidation is the loss of electrons. In combustion, the weak double bond in molecular oxygen, O2, which joins two single oxygen atoms, is converted to stronger bonds as it produces carbon dioxide and water. The process is exothermic, meaning that energy is released in the form of heat. When sufficient heat is reached, at what is known as the ignition point or the flash point, visible flames are produced. Flames consist mainly of carbon dioxide (CO2), vapor of water (H2O), and nitrogen (N); the atmosphere surrounding a fire is notably lacking in oxygen. Animal life is therefore imperiled by both the heat of fire and the lack of oxygen. The color of the flame and its intensity will differ depending on many factors, including the substances that are being burned, and the distance in the flame from the source of heat. The spectrum of light in flames includes visible light, ranging from white and yellow to orange and red, and then to black smoke. Invisible infrared light and ultraviolet light are also emitted. Fire begins when the temperature of carbon-containing material is raised to the ignition point in the presence of oxygen. Fire is maintained by a continuous supply of heat, oxygen and fuel, in a chain reaction, known as the fire tetrahedron. A lightning strike, volcanic eruption, or meteorite may deliver energy sufficient to reach the flash point, and then there is fire. Spontaneous combustion occurs when piles of wet grass or leaves ferment, generating sufficient heat to reach the point of ignition.[133]

The ability to maintain fire was crucial for those who first discovered its usefulness. Branches, leaves, dry limbs, and grass would have been gathered and stockpiled; and a watch was carefully kept to keep the fire going. Humans soon found that some forms of wood would be especially useful; this would also be tinder which could be used to bring an almost dead fire into life again. Clever thinking and restless hands soon found that warmth resulted when sticks were rubbed together. Pursuing this clue, several ways to rub two pieces of wood together to make fire were developed in different parts of the world. In a similar fashion, Neolithic people struck stones together, making tools, and on some occasions, sparks were seen – similar to those in fires. Further exploration led to discovery that striking some stones – flint or pyrite – against each other, would produce a useful spark that could, with a gentle puff and a bit of tinder, burst suddenly into fire. This was magical. Maintaining a fire became a family responsibility, and was an important aspect of the education of children. Fire soon became a part of rituals, and a warm stone was a useful medical treatment for an ailing part of the body.[134]

Over a period of many centuries, humans have discovered many uses for fire. Fire and its many derivatives, in one form or another, are now part of daily life for every person in the world. Cooking was improved from simple roasting in an open fire, to frying on a hot rock and baking beside the fire (after grass was domesticated into wheat), and boiling (after pottery was fashioned). Fire was probably was next used to clear forested land for agriculture, and at about the same time it was used for signaling and for cremation. In later periods, fire was used for smelting and forging metals – the so-called Bronze Age and Iron Age – and it was used in various forms as a weapon, and for propulsion (the first steam engine was Hero of Alexandria's aeolipile), and for nefarious purposes, such as torture and execution.

A further word about fire and the urge for personal covering. Some forms of clothing are naturally protective against fire. Wool and cotton are far less likely to burst into flames and cause injury to humans than synthetic plastic clothing such as polyester, which melts and burns. Clothing incorporating the mineral asbestos, or which is made from fine sheets of asbestos, is highly resistant to flame and fire, and it is also insulative against heat. However, inhalation of asbestos fibers results in a debilitating and often fatal disease known as pulmonary mesothelioma. The useful properties of asbestos are now outweighed by the risk of using this substance for insulation and in clothing. Fire retardant and flame protective clothing has been developed using a chemical known as Tris, which is a short version of Tris(2,3-dibromopropyl) phosphate, and with other similar chemicals with acronyms such as PFAS, PBDEs, and EHTBB. Unfortunately, these chemicals are toxic when worn or consumed by children, and environmental scientists have been trying to eliminate their use in clothing.[135]

Any discussion of clothing and fire should mention the distinctive garments and tools carried by firefighters. These First Responders must have the ability – the unnatural urge – to rush toward and into a dangerous place – a fire – instead of recoiling from it, as most people would. A firefighter's dress uniform, proudly worn, is usually dark blue, of a hue slightly lighter than so-called Navy blue (which is almost black); a distinctive billed cap, a brass-buttoned coat (called a blouse), and trousers. The firefighter's work uniform, also proudly worn, consists of a number of protective garments that differ depending on the assignment, but there is a fireman's hat, sloped at the back to permit water to run off, a heavy yellow rubberized coat, a respirator, oxygen tank, and tools, carried in the hands and on the back.

The human use of fire has had many other unintended consequences. Forest land has been consumed, originally for subsistence agriculture, and for fuel and lumber, and more recently for industrial farming and to land on which to settle the world's growing population. Consumption of forests and grass lands has contributed greatly to the increase in global warming, with the production of greenhouse gases, melting the ice throughout the world, a rise in sea level, and to world-wide pollution. Yet fire can also be beautiful. We love the warmth and companionship of sitting by a camp fire. A family gathers around the fireplace, the hearth, on a winter's evening. Jack London tells of the poignant anguish of losing fire in his unforgettable story "To build a fire." We pause to think, but we cannot imagine a world without fire.[136]

Jack London also told a memorable story about "man's best friend," the dog, which is the next subject in this essay. If you haven't read London's "White Fang," you should find the time to do so now.

Another Urge

H. Dogs and Other Animals

Of all the animals, dogs and humans have long had a special relationship, told in expressions such as: The dog is "Man's best friend." "If you want a friend in Washington, get a dog." "Give the dog a bone." "Dog is God spelled backwards." The Canaanite woman said to Jesus, "Even the dogs eat the crumbs that fall from the master's table." The relationship between humans and dogs is the longest cooperative relationship that exists between humans and other animals. We call it domestication of the dog, but the dog may look at it from the opposite perspective. Who knows?[137]

Animals probably should not be called an "urge" that is in the same category as the seven urges that are discussed above. However, human interaction with animals has been so extensive, and this interaction has existed for so long, that animals should be mentioned in connection with *Health Matters*.

Perhaps it was about 12,000 years ago when a curious wolf, maybe hungry or for some other reason, and lacking the usual sense of fear, slowly crept up toward a man who was sitting by his campfire. The wolf's eyes glowed with reflection from the fire, and the man watched the wolf. For some reason, perhaps aroused by curiosity, the man tossed a scrap of meat toward the wolf. The wolf took it, and waited for more. The man saw this, and he thought that it was good. This evening was followed by more of such encounters. The curious man and the unusual wolf gradually developed a relationship, and it flourished. This event was not singular, for it must have occurred in similar ways in many other places at about the same time. Jack London told something like this in his fictional short story, "White Fang," about a hybrid wolf-dog in Alaska more than a century ago. The animal was initially wary, but curious. The fictional wolf-dog, White Fang, gradually became friendly, and eventually was the savior of the man. Or perhaps the modern dog is descended from a wolf pup, brought into a cave 12,000 years ago, not yet afraid of anything, and was raised by a man who treated the pup well as he grew older. The pup grew to be a wolf. And that wolf, by chance, was slightly different from other wolves. It was somewhat compatible with humans. It parented that difference into a new breed, and the descendants of that breed became a new species – the dog, *Canis lupus familiaris*.[138]

Humans and dogs have generally had a good, companionable, relationship. However, the relationship has often been tilted in favor of humans. Humans have worked dogs to death, some have cruelly tormented dogs, and many dogs have been subjected to pain, without anesthesia, in research. Some early Antarctic explorers made plans to use their sled dogs for as long as they were needed, and then to survive by eating them. Dogs have also been crucial for medical experiments, including development of the pump-oxygenator for cardiac surgery and organ transplantation. The great, loveable, Saint Bernard dog is famous as a rescue animal in the Alps, and trained guide dogs have given new life to those without sight. Law enforcement agencies use dogs that have been trained to detect illicit drugs and to sniff for living bodies and cadavers. Sadly, some have been trained to attack, and the movies showing German shepherds biting Black protestors are painful to watch. Alsatians and Doberman pinchers are the most common police dogs. Faithful "service dogs" are now commonplace in grocery stores, restaurants, and on airplanes. A dog's friendship may be the only companion for a person who lives alone.

The dog is but one of several animals that have been used by humans for thousands of years. Many other animals have been selected by humans by selective breeding over a span of many generations. The horse, the chicken, pigeon, and other poultry; the pig, rabbit, sheep, goat, cow, llama, cat and other animals have been domesticated, to serve a variety of purposes. Some have been bred to work, while others were bred to be producers of food, clothing, protectors, and pets. The dromedary, elephant, and reindeer are wild animals that have been put to use by humans. Domesticated animals that escape or are returned to the wild must re-adapt to survive. After a generation or two, some of these previously domesticated animals, such as the pig or dog, can become aggressive. A cat may exhibit friendly behavior inside the house, but feral instincts quickly return when the cat is outside. A safe relationship with domesticated animals requires constant attention, especially large ones with teeth, horns, strong legs, or a body that can crush. All animals may harbor dangerous parasites that can affect humans.

Although humans' most common animal companion – or pet – is the dog, humans also have developed a warm friendship with many other domesticated animals. Knowing looks are often exchanged between humans and animals, suggesting facial recognition and empathy – a sign that true friendship exists in this relationship. After the dog, the horse was probably next to be domesticated, and then cats, pigs, rabbits, sheep – and many others. And not just domesticated animals; humans have adopted and cared for many animals who were injured or abandoned; and after treatment, the animals have been returned to the wild. The list of wild animals rescued in this way is long, and it includes diverse creatures including mammals, raptors, sea turtles, sharks and whales. Other primates have been allowed into homes: monkeys in Asia and America, and chimpanzees. Some of these relationships have been tragic. Monkeys are playful, but they can introduce disease into a human home. Chimpanzees have suddenly turned sour and maimed or killed their owners.[139]

Domestication, meaning "belonging to the house" (Latin), began after the peak of the last ice age (the Last Glacial Maximum, also known as the height of Wisconsin glaciation), about 20,000 years ago. At the peak of the Wisconsin Glacial Episode, the Laurentide Ice Sheet covered North America with glaciation as far south as the Ohio River. As the glaciers receded, humans gradually moved north into previously glaciated areas. As previously mentioned, the first animal to be domesticated was the wolf (*Canis lupus*), about 15,000 years ago, during the period known as the Pleistocene. A severe cold spell, known as the Younger Dryas, then intervened, but warming gradually resumed. The present epoch, known as the Holocene, began about 12,000 years ago. Since then, except for several short-lasting cold periods, world temperatures have continued to rise. The first plants were domesticated about 12,000 years ago, as humans slowly made a transition from hunter-gathering to agriculture. This was the beginning of the Neolithic Period, when humans began to work creatively with stone. Domestication of plants and animals showed a rapid increase beginning about 11,000 years before the present era. Over the next six millennia, many species of plants and animals were domesticated in Europe, Asia, and the Americas. The cat was domesticated about 4,000 years ago in Egypt.[140]

Domestication has also been accomplished for other animals, including several species of birds, the honeybee, silk worm, and land snails. Selective breeding of plants produced many varieties of crop plants that are the basis for agriculture and flowering plants that are bred for domestic beauty and pleasure. Some rat and mouse species, both of the genus *Mus*, have become domesticated, although not always by humans' choice, and as both pets and pests they have profited from this biological adventure.[141]

Ethical questions arise about humans' use of zoos, in which wild animals lose privacy and lose their ability to roam, yet are protected. However, there can be no question about the human misuse of wild animals that are maimed or killed for their body parts, such as ivory tusks and gall bladders, or poached and sold for what is believed to be medicinal purposes. Some species have been driven nearly to extinction by this type of illegal, immoral harvesting. In the past, humans have thoughtlessly, or even intentionally, caused many species to become extinct. The list is long – the great auk of New Zealand, the passenger pigeon of North America; and almost, too, the American bison, known as the "buffalo." Some species have been driven away from their traditional hunting grounds, and they are troubled. That list is very long; it includes the wolf, the prairie dog, many species of birds.[142]

The steadily rising temperature of land and ocean threatens many animal species. The rise in temperature started at the end of the last Ice Age, when, as noted above, the period known as the Holocene began. However, although the slow rise in temperature began before humans had an effect upon the environment, humans have now contributed to the rising temperature of the world in many ways, including destruction of woodland habitat and with emission of greenhouse gases. The increase has been accelerated by a steady increase in the world's population. There is also the so-called "fusion" or "melting" effect when ice becomes liquid. It requires 80 calories to melt one gram of ice, without a change in temperature. The temperature of ice and water remains at 32°. But only one calorie is required to raise the temperature of one gram of water by one degree; from say 32° to 33°. It is not surprising that as the world's ice melts, the world's temperature will rise more rapidly. When ice melts in Greenland, fresh water pours into the North Atlantic, and the ocean gets steadily but surely warmer and less salty.

Chapter 4

The Wants

Love and money are the most prominent of all of the things that humans want. They are different in many ways, but humans nevertheless recognize their intimate connections. Think of someone who says, "I wouldn't do it for love or money," or the ultimate rejection, "Not for love or money!" These expressions show the high esteem in which both love and money are held, in spite of their differences. Love, with many definitions, is the ultimate intangible quality, whereas money is the opposite. Love is evanescent. The word is both a noun and a verb, and it easily transforms into an adverb or adjective. Money is the opposite. It is something to grasp. The word is most frequently used as a noun, though it can be transformed into an adjective. The opposite qualities of the two words are recognized in the loftiest thoughts of humans, in which everything can be loved, and in the depths, in which everything is fungible with money. Both of these wants, love and money, have important connections with *Health Matters*.

A. Love

Love is a Many Splendored Thing.[143]

It is difficult to place Love into the categories of human Needs, Urges, and Wants. It appears at times that Love is a Need, and it is often an Urge, and it seems always to be a Want. With that disclaimer, Love is discussed as it relates to the subject of *Health Matters*. Of the many ways that the word love is used, the most important is that love represents affection, as in a mother for her child, and in sexual attraction. Both are necessary for the continuation of the species. In order to place some limits on this aspect of *Health Matters*, we will focus on the word "love" and not on its many synonyms and derivations. It is tempting to digress with comments on qualities such as compassion, forgiveness, and mercy. Mentioning only one of these before returning to the subject of love, in Shakespeare's memorable words,

> The quality of mercy is not strained.
> It droppeth as the gentle rain from heaven
> Upon the place beneath. It is twice blest:
> It blesseth him that gives and him that takes.[144]

When love is reciprocated, the effect of love is enhanced. Both mental and physical health can be improved, but constant attention is needed to achieve and maintain this relationship. Love is often expressed in poetry. The sonnet is a form that has often been chosen for a love poem, as in Elizabeth Barrett Browning's *How Do I Love Thee*,

> How do I love thee? Let me count the ways.
> I love the to the depth and breadth and height
> My soul can reach, when feeling out of sight
> For the ends of being and ideal grace.

Alfred, Lord Tennyson wrote,

> 'Tis better to have loved and lost
> Than never to have loved at all.[145]

Some of the other uses of the word love are derived from its meaning of affection and attraction. For instance, in Britain, "Hello, Love" can start a conversation. Love is also used as a synonym for an amorous affair, or copulation, which may lead to more. For some strange reason, "love" in a tennis match means less – zero. The uses of love as a verb are related to its use as a noun – to cherish, to feel passion, to caress, and so forth. Or to express an innocent desire, as in "I'd love to go with you," or platonic love, which is a deep friendship without sexual intent. Speaking of platonic, Plato may have preferred a more active role in sex. The myths about Greek gods, who persisted with Roman names, provide examples of unworldly sexual behavior that was the norm at that time. For instance, there is beautiful Adonis, born of incest, who is the favorite of Aphrodite (the Romans' Venus); and Eros (Cupid), her son. Aphrodite is the daughter, perhaps by Zeus, or one of the other gods. The gods played the field in those legends.[146]

Throughout the Bible, the word love is used to mean many of the definitions that are given in Merriam-Webster's dictionary. Forty-nine books of the King James Version of the Bible contain the word "love," and "love" appears in 267 verses. The quotations are shown on eleven pages of the Concordance. The word "love" appears in five pages in the Hebrew Bible, known to Christians as the

Old Testament (OT), and six pages in verses in New Testament (NT). The Old Testament is about three times the length of the New Testament, and we can estimate that "love" therefore appears about three more often in the NT than in the OT. The first two citations are in Genesis, and in the second of these verses, love appears in the meaning of sexual attraction. The last citations appear in the final book of the Christian Bible, and it is in the penultimate citation that love also appears as a sexual attraction. For Christians, the most important statement about love is expressed in Matthew 22:37-39: "On these two commandments hang all the law and the prophets … Thou shalt love the Lord … and … Thou shalt love they neighbor as thyself." However, the First Commandment, given to Moses, is not expressed in the words that are spoken by Jesus, "love the Lord." All versions of the OT instead show variations on the theme of a Commandment: "Thou shalt have no other gods before me" (KJV). In the Torah, the statement is longer, but it begins: "I the Lord am your God" (Exodus 20:1). Love is not mentioned. The Koran mentions "love" in 83 verses. Most of these are statements about the love of Allah, or of the love of Allah for humans, as in "Allah will bring a people, He shall love them and they shall love Him."[147]

Another meaning for love comes from the Greek word *agape*. We can think of this as a person's adoration to a supreme being – God – or as a person's loving relationship and concern for others. The word *agape* in the New Testament means both the fatherly love of God for humans, and the reciprocal love of humans for God. It also is the God-like affection of one person for another. Many of the meanings of *agape* Love are connected to health, to *Health Matters*. These meanings include affection for others, especially for helpless babies and those who are unable to care for themselves, and sexual attraction. We have seen above that humans have an Urge to form groups, starting with families; and they also have an Urge for Lust, which leads to procreation. The helpless baby and the looks exchanged between potential lovers are expressed in this meaning of love. Darwin's theory of the origin of species does not articulate a reason for the altruistic behavior of love that cares for others. Could it be *agape*?[148]

B. Money

> For the love of money is the root of all of evil.
> –1 Timothy 6:10

Money is easier to place than Love within the category of human Wants. Money is certainly not a Need, and it is not an original Urge. It has become a Want only with the development of early civilization. Money is, however, a factor in *Health Matters*, because it can produce either a positive or negative effect on Health. It is sad to say, but in general, wealth is more likely to lead to health and a long life, while poverty leads to illness and early death. The unequal division of wealth, and the progressive separation of rich from poor, was noted two thousand years ago. The relationship of humans to money is often influenced and mediated by religious leaders. Paraphrasing Jesus, who is reported to have said twice, with some irony, that to him who has, shall more be given, but from him that has not, shall all be taken away. As the saying goes: "He who has, gets."[149]

Wealth is thought of as having a great amount of money, or of its equivalent. Poverty is the reciprocal of wealth. We usually admire wealth, and we pity poverty. However, we are also taught to beware of wealth, and to assist the poor. Some of the most admired individuals in history are those who have forgone wealth, and who have advised others to follow the same path. The legend of Midas is set against the Christian virtue expressed by the widow who gave her last pennies, and of Buddha, a Prince, who gave away everything. We see admirable images of St. Martin, cutting his cloak to clothe the beggar, and of St. Francis, the playboy who gave everything away and cared for wild animals. The images of ostentatious and beautifully clothed and bejeweled emperors, kings, queens, and generals are stark contrasts to the simple cloaks of the Franciscans and the plain white cotton dress of Mother Teresa. Money can also be a risk to health, if it is stored where a robber may become a killer.[150]

In the modern world, money now is at the center of the issue of *Health Matters*. Who will pay for health care, and how much should it cost? And while money's relationship to health care may seem to be an evil consequence of modernism, also known as modernity, the issue is older than money itself. Money was created as human civilization developed, as towns grew into cities, and as cities became grouped into countries. Before there was money, there was something of value that could be exchanged; for instance, cowrie shells in Native American trading. And before there were items of value for trading, there was barter: something made by one person, exchanged for something that was possessed by another. Indeed, barter was the method used in the twentieth century in thanks for a doctor's service: "Here's a dozen eggs, doc, and thanks for the delivery of my baby son." A healer-priest always expected and received something appropriate for doing the job. It was originally a token – a gift, expected, but given freely, to the medicine man in a tribe. It has since become transactional, a fee to be paid to a physician. There were many steps along the way from token to fee, and there is space here only allude to a few. The token given to early healer-priest would soon be standardized, and it would become expected.[151]

The Hippocratic Oath says nothing about a fee or payment that would be expected of the physician. However, the practice of medicine surely was a commercial enterprise at that time (460 BCE), because the physician promised in the Oath that he abjured from charging a fee to teach the sons of his own teachers. Medical education was already a business, and so was the practice of medicine.[152]

Physicians are usually well compensated, whether they work on a fee-for-service basis, or are employed, or are on a variable salary (perhaps with additional benefits, such as stock options or based on performance rating), or are on a strict salary (such as from a government agency), or if they volunteer their service and are compensated by simply feeling good about what they do. We see high titles, such as William Harvey, named "Physician Extraordinary" to King James I, and others after him who were Sir and Lord in England. Great wealth has been accumulated by physicians who developed drugs and surgical implants and dietary products, such as Drs. William E. Upjohn, Homer Hartman Stryker and John Harvey Kellogg. The term "leech" was for many years a *double entendre*, because leeches were used for treatment, and some physicians were called leeches because of their avarice. Money is the subject of the topics of fee-splitting, fee-setting and anti-trust suits against medical societies, negotiated fees, sliding scales for fees, fees waived; charity care, without fees; and insurance, both for health care and to protect physicians against loss in lawsuits claiming malpractice.[153]

Proper compensation for a physician has undergone a gradual change over the past seventy years. The main reward was formerly the wonderful opportunity to serve as a physician. The rewards are now more complicated to understand, and they are unevenly distributed. In developed countries, humans invest an enormous amount of time and money in matters relating to health. Previous sections of this essay have shown the indirect effects of the several Needs and Urges in humans' search to secure and preserve health. The quest is a costly one, and it is a cost that is growing. In ancient days, there was little available except herbs and magic, but the rise of scientific medicine has changed all of that. The search has been successful in many ways, as life expectancy continues to increase, and the other metrics for health are also rising. The details in the annual reports of the World Health Organization and the World Bank show opportunities for improvement in outcomes, by country and by region; and in efficiency, as measured as the ratio of outcomes and cost as a proportion of per capita income.[154]

Costs may be controlled to some extent, and allocated more fairly, but it is likely that the upward world-wide curve of health care costs will continue to rise. Health matters so much in human affairs that it trumps everything else. The costs involved can be examined in many ways, but there are four principal categories: (1) health care personnel, (2) pharmaceuticals, (3) facilities, and (4) ancillary personnel. Health care personnel includes physicians, nurses, and many other groups who work closely with patients, including physician assistants, emergency responders, physical therapists, laboratory technicians; the educators of health workers – medical schools, nursing schools, and so forth; and those who provide close support, such as secretaries, chaplains, and social workers. The category of pharmaceuticals includes the industrial costs of research and development; formulating, transporting, and dispensing drugs and other products of the pharmaceutical and implant industry; and the personnel costs in all of these activities, such as workers in the laboratory, pharmacists, the sales force, and administrators. Facilities include hospitals, extended care facilities, rehabilitation centers, nursing homes, free-standing clinics, and services rendered by airplane and motor vehicles in remote areas. Ancillary persons include those who arrange for compensation and payment for health care personnel, pharmaceuticals, and facilities; healthcare administrators in branches of government; those who work in the insurance industry, providing health care and coverage for tort claims; adjacent fields such as the legal profession, advertising, lobbying, food services, office supplies, computer management, and waste disposal; and the many non-profit organizations that have been created to support health research and treatment. As the health industry has grown, the profit motive creeps in to leverage health matters for personal gain.[155]

Relationships Between the Needs, Urges, and Wants

The search to satisfy each of the various needs, urges, and desires is not a simple one. The two absolute needs – air and sunlight – must be satisfied. There is no question about that. Air is breathed. Humans must have access to the sun, at least for part of each year; humans need light, whether from the sun or fire, or from other sources; and humans need sleep, which is usually best achieved in darkness. The epithet, "As I see and breathe," is a reminder that light and breath are partners in life. The circadian cycle, of light and dark, is one of the cycles of life itself.

Even when one of the urges is foremost, the others are still kept in mind. As chance favors the prepared mind, when the search is for food, and new source of water is found, both food and water may become available. Food and water are often found together. Furthermore, the desires for love and money may momentarily, and detrimentally, overtake all of the necessary urges.

Many other connections occur as humans search to satisfy their urgent requirements. The search for personal covering – clothes and their accessories – may account for the greatest number of the connections with other urges. Human searches for food and water involve the use of containers to carry these needed substances back to a place of shelter. We see animal skins and woven baskets in their hands or on their backs as they search for what they need, and then return to homes that they share with others. In this way, water, food, shelter, and personal covering, and social connections are intimately related. It is in the shelter where fire is built and fuel is stored to maintain it. In most cases, fuel for the fire will be firewood. Baskets or ties made from animal skins or vines will be used to transport branches and leaves. This is a form of tool, which I refer to as an extension of personal covering.

Social connections are often seen in the use of distinctive clothing. Health and its opposite, unhealth, often appear simultaneously. Think, for instance, of Nazi officers in impeccable black uniforms sitting on horses in Poland in World War II, looking down on Jews who are trudging along the streets. Each of them is wearing a yellow Star of David on the coat. Or prisoners in the concentration camp at Auschwitz, in shabby uniforms, striped with alternating shades of dark and light gray. A similar scene appears in photographs of chain gangs of prisoners in America, as white overseers on horseback, wearing broad brimmed hats, look down on chain gangs of Black inmates at labor in striped prison uniforms.

Other types of unhealth are illustrated by various forms of clothing. The straight jacket is a garment that was invented to control psychotic patients; the term "straight jacket" has since become a meme for any form of restriction. The ultimate form of unhealth, which is death, is recognized by distinctive garments throughout the world. A simple burial shroud is used in much of the Islamic world. Funeral clothing of the embalmed corpse, lying in a coffin, seen in much of America, is sometimes pre-selected by the impending decedent. Funeral clothing of the dead in the Western world is a dramatic contrast to southern Asia, in which an unclothed body is left on a mountain peak, to be consumed by vultures; or burned on a pyre beside the Ganges, with ashes left to drift to the sea. The ultimate use of distinctive clothing and accessories that are associated with death, is that of a military funeral at Arlington National Cemetery. A solemn procession is headed by slowly marching troops, a horse with empty saddle, boots reversed in stirrups, accompanied with flags and music. A fallen warrior or an old soldier is buried in a grave, dressed in uniform with medals and badges, in a casket that is slowly lowered beneath the ground. The American the flag is folded and carefully presented to the next of kin. Or after cremation, when the veteran's ashes are ceremonially interred in a columbarium. Or is buried at sea in an ancient ritual, in which the old sailor's body, covered with a flag, is brought to the edge of the ship's main deck and is slipped into the ocean, as the flag is pulled off and retained for the family to save.

In the last century, the combination of shelter and personal protection reached astonishing new levels, enabling humans to descend to great depths in the ocean, and to survive and walk on the surface of the moon, and in outer space, tethered to an orbiting spacecraft. Social connections now exist even in these faraway places, as humans travel in small groups into the depths of the sea in bathyspheres, and for months, living and working while cocooned in gravity-free space capsules.

C. Enough

As a conclusion of the discussion of the several Components of Health, it is necessary to examine the question of how much of each is enough of each. The powerful needs and urges for survival must be balanced to achieve the desired effects. Too little is not enough. Too much produces discomfort, ill health, or death. For each urge, there must be a feedback mechanism that, at an appropriate moment, gives a warning sign or acts as a brake. The goal is to achieve balance – harmony – a happy median. Failure to recognize the warning signs is discussed below in Exceptions. Failure includes young children, or those who choose to take risks, or who for psychiatric reasons are unable to understand danger. We must realize when enough is enough.[156]

For the two needs, air and sunlight, "enough" is what is commonly achieved. For air, which humans need as a constant companion, a few extra breaths can be taken without ill effect, but rapid deep breathing – hyperventilation – immediately causes side effects which bring a halt to it. The reason for this is that a hyperventilation produces a low blood level of carbon dioxide, which in turn produces a feeling of light-headedness, and panic. For excessive exposure to sunlight, the punishment of sunburn can serve as a warning, and hyperthermia of the entire body is a punishment or a tragedy. Blindness is a rare consequence of directly staring at the sun, as in a mystical or hallucinatory trance, or by observing a partial eclipse of the sun without protective eye covering.

The first three urges are water, food, and shelter. The need for water is recognized by thirst. When this need is fulfilled, thirst disappears, and it is said that thirst has been slaked. Excessive water intake causes water intoxication, which produces hyponatremia (a low level of salt – NaCl – in the blood), and this can be fatal. The need for food is recognized by hunger and it is aroused by the aroma of cooking. When hunger has been rewarded sufficiently, we say that we are satiated. If temptation leads to excessive consumption, the result may be a midsection of the body that is engorged with fat, Type II diabetes, and eventually morbid obesity. If for any reason, such as a desire not to offend the host, or as the result of ingesting too much alcohol, a second, third, or fourth helping may be taken. The result of drunken gluttony may be vomiting and aspiration of food and beverages, or rupture of the stomach and esophagus; in either event, the result may be death. The neuroendocrine system of the body is responsible for recognizing the loss of thirst when enough liquid has been consumed, and the recognition of satiety, which triggers the loss of appetite for food. The desire for shelter usually leads to a sense of fulfilment, as in "My Home Sweet Home," but when taken to greater lengths, as in a recluse or hermit, it can become a pathology. The home of a recluse becomes a fortified castle, into which none but Death may enter.[157]

The next two needs are lust and social connections. Lust is usually satisfied with orgasm in one or both partners. If it happens first in the man, libido passes, relaxation occurs, and then sleep. The man is usually in control, so the woman must accept what happens. The moment passes. However, if libido is excessive, uncontrolled behavior may follow, with serious injuries to many parts of the bodies, and even by death. A messy business for the coroner. It is better when "enough" is recognized by both parties. Love is the harmonious solution. Love is the happy feedback of lust. The need for social connections is somewhat different, except when group sex is the issue, which involves only a few people. The social connection list in an orgy is much smaller than in a multi-generational family, or a clan, or a tribe. The decision about whether a group is large enough is decided on the basis of several factors. For example, the amount of space that is readily available for group habitation; for water and food and protection from other groups; and by personalities – especially the group's leadership and traditions. If the group's size is stable throughout successive generations, all may appear to be well. The extended stable family is still characteristic of many groups in Asia. However, if there is a physical or psychological challenge, the social group may split apart, with disastrous results. Love (*liebe*, in German; *amor*, in Spanish; *amour*, in French; 爱 [*Ai*] in Chinese and Japanese), which is easily understood, though difficult to define, plays a significant role in determining the size and composition of social groups. The leader of a small social group, or the leaders of a large one – a clan, tribe, or nation – are responsible for success or failure of the group. The emergence of a leader is not unique in humans; a group of hens in the chickenyard have their pecking order, and a wolf pack has its alpha female. The dominant bull elk has a line of cows that trail along after him, while weaker bulls stand aside. In humans, social caste has often played a significant role in the hierarchy of group leadership. Caste may be detected by skin color (lighter is usually "better"), or by the mannerisms of speech, or by known genealogy. The determination that "good can be better" leads to choices of mutually attractive breeding partners. It can then lead to pious social Darwinism, placing blame on those who fail to achieve success. This leads to the ominous conclusion of righteous eugenicists, who seek to marginalize or exterminate those who are unsuccessful.

The two uniquely human needs are clothing (personal covering) and fire. Feedback in regard to both of these needs provides guidance about whether sufficiency has been obtained, whether more clothing or fire is needed for possible use, and when excessive amounts of one or the other may lead to disaster. Think of clothing: One layer after another, with cost and bulk and warmth increasing with each layer, and with each purchase. No one wants to be without enough clothing, but too much can lead to social exclusion ("she's too haughty for words"), to debt, to hoarding behavior, and even to hyperthermia. And fire: We usually know when we are warm enough, and we can bank the fire or turn off the furnace, and get under the covers, in order to avoid the possibility of a conflagration. The potential danger of fire may be recognized as an instinct, but it is quickly learned, as by a child who touches a candle flame or gets close to a burning campfire. It must, however, be taught early – "Don't play with matches" – because if the danger of fire is not experienced at a young age, the result of learning it later may be death.

Feedback is a mechanism to achieve the desired result of a steady state, in which enough is achieved, but without excess. In a child or in the youth of any species, the feedback mechanism is partially suppressed to allow for growth to occur. The ravenous appetite of an adolescent, for example, is necessary. The feedback mechanism switches to a different mode in an adult – to a more or less steady state, followed by the decline of an elder. This could be considered as a literary metaphor, analogous to the Laws of Thermodynamics in science, which describe the conservation of energy (with feedback, ensuring a steady state), and then entropy.[158]

The urge to have domesticated or wild animals living nearby is perhaps an unusual human need; or perhaps it is a want. In any event, there is a feedback mechanism in the relationship between animals (for example, the dog) and humans, which tells the human when there are enough animals in his domain, and if there may be too many. The issue is largely food and shelter for the animals, but also the possibility of danger, especially if the animals (say, boars or bulls or stallions) are large and aggressive, or if they may escape and become feral, or if they are in a large group, such as a pack of wild dogs. The decision must be made in time to avoid a confrontation that could lead to serious injury or even death.

The two wants, love and money, have well-known feedbacks which are intended to produce a happy median. For love between humans, the desired outcome is bliss, although jealousy, anger, and other emotions play roles in solving the problems of affection. For money, the balance between penury and hoarding is a constant concern. The legend of King Midas and his gold is remembered as a perfect example of excess, whereas vows of poverty – as exampled by St. Francis and St. Ignatius – have been taught as examples of goodness, or of good sense, for hundreds of years.

This concludes the discussion of the basic Components of Health. We now will examine some other aspects of human health: the role of exercise and of avocations.

Chapter 5

Other Considerations

Pain, Exercise, Avocations

Pain

Pain is a signal that something is wrong about health. Restating the words from the beginning of *Health Matters*: the goal of humans is to prevent or cure illness, and to live as long as possible. We can add to that, "without pain." The complex nature of the normal nervous system, which signals pain, and of the many causes and treatments of pain, are important concerns for physicians. The evolution of the ability to perceive pain is of interest to the biologist. However, for a human with pain, these scientific questions pale in importance to the issues of "What is the matter with me?" and "What can you do about it?" Pain cannot be placed in one of the categories listed above, for it is not a "Have" or "Need" or an "Urge" or a "Want," for pain is not always present, nor is it obviously needed or wanted.[159]

Pain is not a unique requirement of humans; other animals are also able to perceive pain. But the ability to perceive pain is crucial to survival. One can be born with or lose the other senses, such as sight, hearing, taste, and smell. And although loss of pain perception in one part of the body, perhaps in an arm or leg, is not necessarily fatal, the rare condition known as "congenital analgesia" (no pain perception) would be a terminal condition without constant attendance by people with normal pain perception. A child without the ability to perceive pain might bite off its tongue. Therefore, we have physical pain to indicate that something is wrong, and the prospect of suffering from pain is a useful warning sign for avoidance. Pain is also a metaphor for suffering in a mental sense. In Spanish, *dolor* and *duele* are words that derive from the same stem, but *duele* is also used to signify "hurt" (as in suffering) instead of physical pain. Physicians quickly learn to ask the patient to point to the place of pain: In Vietnamese, it is *dau*, and in German it is *Schmerzen*. Other European countries all have variations on *dolor* (Latin): The word for pain is *la douleur* (French) or *dolore* (Italian). When pain develops, the goal for *Health Matters* is to find the cause and treat it. If pain persists and the problem cannot be cured – as in widespread cancer, or rheumatic joint disease – the physician must continue to treat the pain.

Surgical procedures may be justified to ameliorate the pain, and topical anesthetics can be useful, but long-term judicious treatment with oral opioids is often needed. Pain was added in 1997 as the fifth vital sign to be monitored, along with heart rate, respiratory rate, blood pressure and temperature. The goal was to use a patient's self-assessment of pain, on a scale of 1-10, as a guide to pain management. The opioid crisis developed at about the same time, probably not coincidentally. As a result of this crisis, the Joint Commission (formerly the Joint Commission on the Accreditation of Health Care Organizations or JCAHO) began to re-evaluate the use and abuse of standards in pain management. In 2017, The Joint Commission made a decision to remove the "fifth vital sign" of pain from the assessment of a patient's status. Physicians and patients nevertheless must find ways to achieve the elusive goal of a pain-free life that is lived for as long as possible.[160]

Exercise

Daniel Lieberman says in *Exercised* (2020) that "humans age uniquely ... This unique behavior is strongly linked to our exceptional longevity in which we typically live beyond the age at which we cease to reproduce." Liberman begins with a statement similar to the argument in *Health Matters*, in which he says that, "Everyone wants to live long, but no one wants to get old. So, for centuries people have sought ways to slow aging and defer death." And that, "there is more to health than not being dead." *Health Matters* is comfortable with that thought. Lieberman says that "Hippocrates wrote 2,500 years ago that 'Eating alone will not make a man well; he must also take exercise'."[161]

The uniquely long life of humans is, according to Lieberman, the result of "what human grandparents – alone among species – have been doing for millions of years: feeding their grandchildren." Lieberman points out that chimpanzee mothers cannot have offspring more than once every five or six years, because they can forage only for one until it has been weaned. Human hunter-gatherers, he says, may have one or two babies before the first one is weaned. This requires the assistance of middle-aged and elderly people who are no longer having children. Lieberman cites an example of the Hazda people of northern Tanzania, in which a typical grandmother begins her working day soon after dawn, building a fire and digging tubers from the ground to cook for her daughter and her daughter's children. Lieberman marshaled evidence from Kenneth Cooper's studies of aerobics, which showed that physically active men and women had a lower mortality rate than those were not as fit. Lieberman says that humans avoid what Peter Medawar called the "shadow of natural selection" as "the older we get the less natural selection cares about fighting the accumulation of wear and tear that comes with age." Although "the shadow eventually comes," the "arrival and severity can be reduced by physical activity."[162]

Lieberman continues with a thoughtful scientific discussion about the physiology of exercise and the repair of exercise-damaged bodily tissue that is told in language that may be accessible to a recent Harvard graduate, although perhaps not for others. It is puzzling to try to understand the need to have grandmothers work so that their daughters can have many more offspring than other species, such as the chimpanzee. What have the fathers been doing (we only are told that they "continue to try to collect honey into old age"), and why is it so important to have more children?[163]

I accept the proposal that Lieberman attributes to Bengt Saltin, "Humans were meant to move." And also, Lieberman's conclusion that "our species never evolved to diet or cope with jetlag," and that "we never evolved to counter many aging processes to the same degree without physical activity."[164]

Avocations

After assuring that the needs, urges, and wants were satisfied, on many days, especially in winter, there has been time for other things. How humans decided to spend their discretionary time – their "spare time" as we now call it – has been of enormous importance in the lives of humans. We may think of a new vocation, a hobby that leads to invention, or that adds to the life of the community. Some people are unable to stop working, and some choose to withdraw for contemplation. Most people enjoy talking or working with others in non-essential activities. Having a hobby, whether it is handiwork or creative thinking. Endlessly talking, while sitting around campfires, in breakfast groups at a local diner, playing bridge, or sitting with others in a tavern. Coffee hour after church. Having fun with others. Even then, in the background, it's all about Health. *Health Matters*. These activities are mentioned because they are so important in the lives of humans, in every part of the world. They cannot be classified as a Need, or Urge, or Want. The need to spend time talking with others and having a hobby is somewhat like exercise. It is discretionary, yet it also often a necessary part of everyday life.[165]

Chapter 6

The Exceptions

We have now examined the fundamental components of the health of humans – what humans have and what they need, what their urges are, and what they want. It is now time to examine the various ways that humans fail to do what they should in order to avoid death for as long as possible. Many of these failures are due to exceptions to the components described above in *Health Matters*. Some of the exceptions are the result of choices made by humans, whereas other exceptions are unavoidable.

A. Unavoidable Exceptions to the Needs, Urges and Wants of Humans

In spite of our best intentions, it is sometimes impossible to choose the way toward good health and a long life. Some problems are apparent at birth, having occurred during development of the fetus, or as the result of genetic issues. For example, hydrocephalus, cranial synostosis, spina bifida, cystic fibrosis, congenital heart disease, and Down syndrome. Some are correctible with surgery and others can be ameliorated, but the impact on the child and the family may nevertheless be profound. Other genetic problems appear tragically later in life, such as Tay-Sachs disease, and Huntington's chorea. Accidents can happen unexpectedly, without warning, and everything changes. A person's life may end suddenly, or the accident may be a tragedy for someone else yet it impacts on many others. The accident may not be fatal, but it may cause disability and expense that alters the future. An unpredicted "act of God" may occur, such as an earthquake, a tornado, or a volcanic eruption, and this, too, may have profound sustained effects on the health of many people. A person's social group, whether family or clan or country, may require unplanned and dangerous duty. Each of these situations may lead to death, or injury, or the risk of ill health. Another exception is an obligation that is imposed by religion.[166]

B. Religion

Much of the guidance in respect to matters of health has been given by the religious leader. In earliest times, this was the priest or priest-healer, sometimes called witch-doctor, or shaman. The religious leader's guidance included the ways and means for humans to strive for, and hopefully thereby to achieve, their needs and urges and desires.

In health matters, religion has played a pivotal role in human behavior. In a positive role, religion warns about excesses in responding to each need, urge, and want, and it offers guidance to be satisfied when enough has been obtained. Religion thus can show the correct path to the median. In the vernacular, it is the happy midpoint. Religion also plays an opposite role in respect to the exceptions, by saying that some exceptions may be necessary or can be excused. Religion is also used as a means, or an excuse, by which individuals choose to act against the exceptions, and which are contrary to the search for health. By playing potentially both a positive and negative role in the quest for health, religion is a classic example of a double-edged sword.[167]

Two aspects of religion will be discussed in this essay on *Health Matters*. The first aspect is a discussion of the role of religion in respect to the urges and wants and the exceptions. The second aspect is the role of religion in the development of medicine and science, which will be discussed in Part Two of this essay. These two roles are connected by theory and practice, but they can be considered separately. This is not a review of the entire subject of religion (or of the many religions) throughout human existence, and in various parts of the world. It is impossible even to describe in detail the narrower role of religion in respect to the urges and exceptions. Nor is there space and time to examine the role of religion in the later development of medicine and science. The essay will only show the beginning, which is with health care. It will show that as it began, health care in humans was intimately associated with magic. From this early beginning in human society, health care and magic gave rise both to religion and to medicine. Medicine was the first science, the original science, and the resultant details of the history of medicine, science, and technology can be assumed to follow sequentially as they have already been written by others. Whether the history of science, medicine, and technology has been progressively upward – Whiggish history – or not, is also an interesting question. This will be discussed in Part Three of this essay on *Health Matters*.[168]

Religion developed as humans gathered in their earliest social groups. After satisfying their immediate urges for water, food, and safety, they produced families and gathered into social groups. In every social group, whether in a single family or in a larger clan, from earliest times, one or two people, a man or a woman, were able to handle issues involving the movement of the group and of the health of its members. The unique aspect of humanity, which separate hominids from other mammals, is humans' ability to develop new methods for health care. Other mammals show health care in various ways, such as grooming for lice in gorillas, and by the maternal instinct in many species to lick a newborn infant or one with an injury. In humans, the health provider in each group is a specialist. It is a person who is able to withstand the sight of blood, and who enjoys helping others. That person becomes the health provider. That person must also have the "gift" of healing. That person becomes the healer.[169]

The leader of the social group must have a view of the future, to organize the group in its search to find the urges, and to protect the group from danger. The healer must also have a view of the future. In either case, the vision of the future is often best expressed to others in the community in mystical language. For the leader, this vision can be used as a mandate for action: "Follow me, I can see the way." For the healer, it can be transmitted as the image of success when treatment is given: "You're looking better already." For both the leader and the healer, the mysterious image is enhanced by mystical performances. Magic is mystical. What you see is not necessarily true, but it is believable. The words "magic" and "mysticism" have many meanings. These two words are used more or less interchangeably, with "magic" referring to the illusion and "mysticism" referring to the mindset that accepts the illusion. Magic and mysticism lead easily to religion, which is concerned with unseen or spiritual issues. Two aspects of modern science have their origin in magic: from alchemy, modern chemistry has developed, and from astrology, we now have astronomy (although there is a powerful, irrational, human desire to continue to believe in astrology). These two aspects of science are discussed in Part Two of this essay.[170]

The person who can speak of the future is the religious person, one who is "invested with spiritual or moral authority." That, too, is a "gift," which involves understanding of the minds of people, and skill in communication. It may be one person who is the leader and who also deals with both the health and the spiritual issues of the community. That person is sometimes called "witch doctor" and "priest," but preferably as "healer" and "spiritual leader." Both healer and spiritual leader could be the same person, but only if the spiritual leader could stand the sight of blood. That person could also be the community's political leader, but that would require having the "gifts" both of healing and of speaking of the spirit.[171]

This section of *Health Matters* focuses on the spiritual leader, whose role becomes crucial in religion. If the spiritual leader is also a healer, that is to say an early physician, this section also pertains to that person. However, the further development of the role of the healer – the physician – will be discussed later, in Part Two, in the context of the history of medicine. The subject of religion, which is discussed here, follows the spiritual role of the leader. The leadership positions in any group also includes defense of the community, but the specific role of the military leader (say, captain) or of the previously mentioned chief (say, governor) of the community are not topics for further consideration in *Health Matters*.[172]

Religion and the Needs, Urges and Wants

The spiritual leader uses religion to guide the people in the community into the correct ways to respond to their needs, urges, and wants, and to utilize the various exceptions as guides to avoid, or to be excused, or to act upon as if they are not to be considered as dangerous or prohibited behavior. First, let us consider the relationship of religion to the three absolute **Needs** of humans: air, sunlight, and sleep. Air, to breathe, day and night, in and out. Perhaps ceasing for a few seconds, and then catching up with deep breaths, returning to a normal rhythm, without thinking about it. Inspiration and expiration. These words that are so familiar, "inspiration and expiration," have, at their roots, a spiritual meaning.

The Urges

Sun and sunlight: The most important act that the ancient Inca priest performed was at high noon on the day of the winter solstice. He stood at the stone altar and brought down a ceremonial axe, cutting the invisible bonds that had drawn the sun lower and lower each day throughout the autumn season. In the southern hemisphere, the sun traversed the northern sky, though rising in the east as it does in the northern hemisphere, and setting in the west, also as it does in the northern hemisphere. The Inca priest had been taught by his elders that he should watch the sunrise each morning in the eastern sky as sunrise moved further to the north to a point at which it would begin to move back toward the south. The Incas believed that if the priest didn't reverse the trend – the sun rising was rising later, and lower in the sky – the sun would disappear into the northern sky, and that would be the end of life. On the day of the winter solstice – June 20 or 21, in the southern hemisphere – in Machu Picchu, about a thousand miles south of the Equator, the sun would appear to rise in the center of a stone arch on the eastern side of the mountain range that surrounded the city. The priest would know that on that date, he could sever the bonds, and the sun would begin its slow climb out of darkness. It would still rise in the east, but it would gradually rise further to the south, in its inexorable cycle. As sunrise moved further and further to the south, spring would appear. The warmth of spring would allow potatoes to be planted, the llamas would mate, and the summer sun would shine overhead again. The Inca priest thanked the god, and the people knew it was god's gift.[173]

Sleep and darkness are associated in most religions with whatever is unhealthy, in mind or body. A relationship is assumed to be present. However, from the ancient Greeks and Roman gods to the ungodly witches of Hallowe'en, the image of humans and darkness, in legend and myth, is not a good one. The connection between religion and sleep (and darkness) in *Health Matters* thus often seems to be a negative one. However, as darkness approaches, the cycle of day and night takes its turn with the service of Evensong in the Christian church; and darkness is always followed by the break of day. It is said to be God's will that this should be, and that it is not bad for humans to have night and to sleep.[174]

Water: The urge for water needs little assistance by religion, but reverence for water is common to many religions. This would be a way to ensure that a source of potable water, and for protection of it, is always high on the list of priorities for any society. Water is also used for cleansing of the body, for cleaning of the environment (the shelter) and of clothing, and for cooking. These uses of water extend beyond consumption and involve other Urges. Baptism by application of holy water or with total immersion in sanctified water is a ritual that is common to all Christian traditions, and it is especially emphasized in some denominations.[175]

Food: The urge for food also needs little assistance by religion, although it appears that a priestly duty in all religions is to specify which foods are good, which are bad, and when and how they should be prepared and eaten. A modern public health message can be read into the dictum, although in most cases the subject of health is subsumed by the duty to observe the ancient guidance of the religion. Good food and good health are thus duties to god. Fasting during the month of Ramadan is one of the five pillars of Islam, and there are strict rules for other aspects of the Muslim diet. Christians ask their Heavenly Father for "daily bread" in the Lord's Prayer, and many Christians bow their heads and pray before each meal. Children are taught to say, "God is great, God is good, and we thank Him for this food."[176]

Encouragement can be expressed in tangible ways, such as: "You can be the 'first fruits' of the Lord's harvest"; or in promises of rewards in the future: "If you do that, you'll go to Heaven." Discouragement or prohibition is expressed in religious taboos, such as the injunction against consumption of pork, which is common to Jews and Muslims; and as aspect of the protection of many animals amongst Hindus; and of all animals by Jains, including even insects that live on roots of plants.[177]

Shelter: The urge for shelter is so great that religion follows the crowd, so to speak. The Ark must be sheltered, and by sheltering the Ark, the people are safe. Metaphorically, when the Ark is lost, "all Hell breaks loose."[178]

Lust: The lusty urge needs little assistance from religion, although some sects appear to relish the thought of sex more than others. The urge for lust is so pervasive that it offers great opportunities for ceremonies to honor the act or the products of sex; and to offer prohibitions that are intended to tantalize or to be disobeyed, and thus to be followed by acts and gifts of penance. A formal ceremony of marriage is the prelude to sex in many religions, and in many Christian denominations – such as Roman Catholics, Anglicans, and Methodists – each successful product of conception is welcomed with baptism as soon as possible, in a ceremony known as "baptism" that has profound religious meaning. Religion and the rules of society generally cooperate in prohibiting incest (although it was considered to be a way to keep power in some societies, such as ancient Egypt), but there is disagreement in various religions regarding sex between cousins and more distant relatives. Charles Darwin married his first cousin, and he worried that their daughter's poor health was the result of consanguinity. The Roman Catholic Church formerly acknowledged three types of relationships, each with five degrees: consanguinity (blood relationship), relationship by marriage (in-laws), and a spiritual relationship (Godparents and their descendants). The prohibitions on marriage were weakened with each degree of separation; i.e., with each generation. Permission for marriage could be given by an appropriate donation, which was calculated on the basis of the degree of separation.[179]

Social Connections: The nearly universal urge for connections in family groups, clans, tribes, and countries is reinforced by religion. Boundaries are established which reinforce religious differences. Some religions proselytize, however, and thus allow for increasing their borders. Others restrict their religion to those who are born within it, or to the caste in which they are destined to live, and thus protect both their lands and their genealogy. Religions depend on the social connections between believers. Think of the crowds in Hindu and Buddhist temples, and the crowds in the great mosques in the lands of the Muslims, and in Christian cathedrals and churches. It is believed by many Christians that the worshippers are the "church" and not the buildings. Worship in large groups, in the open, is characteristic of Muslim worship, most notably at the climax of the hajj, when the men prayerfully circle the Kaaba in Mecca. Smaller groups are typical of worshippers in Hebrew synagogues, but Jerusalem welcomes large crowds of Jews at the Western Wall, also known as the Wailing Wall. Muslims gather nearby at the golden Dome of the Rock on Temple Mount in the Old City of Jerusalem. The COVID-19 pandemic in 2020 has revealed the desperate need that many humans have for personal contact, especially in religious ceremonies. Great anxiety has been caused by the necessary abandonment of the usual touches, hugs, and kisses when welcoming a new baby. Grief is increased by interruption of the care of bodies after death.[180]

Clothing and Weapons: Clothing is a useful tool of Religion, as modes of dress can be described in elaborate detail by priests, religious customs, and sacred texts. Violations of religious canons of proper dress or behavior can offer opportunities for penance, forgiveness, and even penury. A "hair shirt" can be ordered to be worn by the penitent, or sandals may be worn instead of boots, to show dutiful obedience. Weapons are mentioned in connection with clothing, because clothing in many religions includes implements that are carried by the priests, and which are symbols of power. Some of these are tools that derive from weapons, which are intended to show strength. Some are intended to display tender leadership, such as the crosier, a "shepherd's staff" carried by an Anglican or Episcopal bishop. It is curved at the top to hook sheep, and symbolizes the Good Shepherd. A Sikh male always carries a small dagger which is hidden in his clothing, as a symbol of piety. The distinctive garments of many Jewish men and women are based on the Torah and customs that derive from ancient Israel, and from customs that arose during their diaspora from the Holy Land.[181]

Fire: The use of Fire in sacred ceremonies can be found in ancient records of most religions. Archaeologists find ashes, excavated in the center of dwelling places, and we can but wonder what ceremonies there might have been beside those campfires. After a family finishes the evening meal, a ceremony of some kind often takes place today. We see ancient firepits of the Zoroastrians in central Asia, and in ceremonies that still continue in those regions to the present time.

Dogs and Other Domesticates: The dog and other domesticated animals appear in religious traditions. The Jewish Bible tells of Noah's choosing pairs of animals to save from the Flood, and the "scapegoat" is mentioned in Leviticus. In the New Testament, we read of "crumbs under the table" that should be given to the dog, and a flock of sheep is the metaphor for the people of Christianity. The "fatted calf" is a delicacy. The "sacred cow" wanders fearlessly as it plods through the streets of India, protected by religion. It also provides useful service, converting brush and leaves (inedible for humans) into dung that is used for fuel and fertilizer. Although humans must be wary of the horns of zebuine cattle, the cow can be milked if care is taken. The elephant is the symbolic head of Lord Ganesh.[182]

The Wants

Guided by the religious leader, with ceremonies and texts, religion and its companion, mythology, interprets the two wants – love and money. Religion shows humans how the wants are to be incorporated into their lives. The two wants are associated with humans in social groups; neither love nor money has an attraction for a solitary person. To recapitulate a portion of the previous discussion of love as a want: the word "love" is mentioned in 49 books of the King James Version of the Bible. Love appears in the Bible as both sexual attraction and lust, and as a non-sexual form of love which is derived from the Greek *agape* – as love, reciprocated, with God; and also, as altruistic love for other humans. Love is mentioned in 83 verses of the Quran, in a manner similar to *agape*. Most of the references are to the reciprocal love of Allah for man, and of human love of Allah. Looking at the other human want – money – there is some similarity to the human desire for love, and here, too, religion and the religious leader offers guidance. Guidance from religion is not necessarily free of conflict of interest, however, for since earliest times, the priest or priest-healer would expect to be compensated for his advice. Especially, if the advice appeared to lead to a favorable outcome. When religion became organized, it required financial support for the hierarchy of priests, bishops, rabbis, mullahs, and lay leaders; and support for religious structures, such as synagogues, temples, cathedrals, mosques, monasteries, and other sacred places. Think of the Vatican, the Belz Great Synagogue in Jerusalem, the Washington National Cathedral, the Potala at Lhasa, the Bibi-Khanym Mosque in Samarkand. Appropriate gifts have been expected from Jews to support their synagogues; tithing on a regular basis has been encouraged in the Christian church; and giving alms (*zakat*) is specified in the Quran as one of the Five Pillars of Islam. One of the principal issues raised by Martin Luther, which led to the Protestant Reformation, was the requirement for payment of indulgences to secure waivers from behavior that was proscribed by the Roman Catholic Church.[183]

The religious leader's most important role in human society is to confront death. The principal duty of the priest, or the healer-priest, is to prevent or delay death. And to interpret death, so it can be understood and accepted, and sometimes appreciated. That is what *Health Matters* is all about. If the priest is also a healer, the healer-priest will have other tools that will be useful. However, the priest's duty and opportunity are to assist everyone in the group to believe that an unseen spirit is present to assist in the struggle with death. The subject of death will be elaborated upon at some length in a later section of this essay, and it is time to put it to rest, so to speak. One comment may serve as a segue way to the topic of religion. The passage across the River Styx, in Greek mythology, and continued by the Romans, is still a one-way trip. Prometheus did make the trip twice, but he is the only one who accomplished this, and he, too, eventually returned to Hades. Fine tuning the promise of Christianity, it is said that that some may not be as fortunate. Some Christians believe that the fires of Hell await those who haven't been good enough (in their charitable work), or sufficiently faithful, or (sad to say) are destined to go to the underworld.[184]

Altruism

I will take less, so you can have more.

The subject of altruism was mentioned previously in *Health Matters* in connection with social connections. Altruism will appear again in respect to death in instances which resulted from altruism – either intentionally or accidentally. Altruism is unselfishness. Altruism is probably a more primitive aspect of human behavior than the earliest forms of religion. We think of altruism as being a form of empathy, and also as humanism. However, altruism has become solidly incorporated into religious beliefs, and it is therefore appropriate to elaborate on it in connection with religion in *Health Matters*.[185]

Altruism is an immediate consequence of the urge for humans to have social connections. The individual must be concerned about both himself or herself and the others who are in the family and in the extended family – the social group. Concern for others is what defines altruism. It is fair to ask whether this behavior is the result of education (teaching and learning), or whether it is genetically transmitted. It might not appear that unselfishness – altruism – would be consistent with the Darwinian notion of natural selection, sometimes known as "survival of the fittest" or "nature, red in tooth and claw." However, it is clear from studies on twins who are separated at birth, and raised independently, that many aspects of human behavior are transmitted from parents to children. We must conclude, therefore, that altruistic behavior is heritable, and that education in the methods and purpose of altruism is intended to enhance something that in many people is already present, and that it can be enhanced. Whether altruism is transmitted genetically or epigenetically is still a debatable subject. Also, it cannot be said that altruism naturally extends to a concern for all other humans; we know that isn't true. Nor is the spirit of altruism evenly distributed, for some individuals are gratified by ruthless selfishness.[186]

A few examples should be mentioned of altruistic behavior that have become principles of religion. The last five of the ten commandments of Hebrew Bible demand proper behavior in respect to others; not to kill, or to commit adultery, to steal, to bear false witness, or to covet. These legalistic expressions are elevated to become a moral or ethical issue at a later point in the history of the Near East, as the Christian New Testament instructs each person to "love thy neighbor as thyself" and that the greatest reward is to "lay down thy life" for another. The Koran, or *Qur'an*, instructs the faithful to "give to the poor." The philosophy of Buddhism highlights the sacrificial poverty of monks and nuns, begging for food. They repeat, *"Om Mani Padme Um"* – "Hail to the jewel in the lotus" – as they travel on "The Way" together to nirvana. Religion has thus co-opted and enhanced the spirit of altruism that has existed since the time that humans first came together in social groups.[187]

Altruism has been displayed in many ways throughout history in ways that are based on either religious or secular customs, but often there is no easy way to categorize the altruistic acts as either one or the other. Some acts are reflexive, such as offering a bite of food or drink to another family member. However, it would be very different if it were to look for a homeless family and then to invite them to dinner; this could be based on religious training, or it could be done by any generous agnostic. Every member of the Boy Scouts promises to do a "Good Turn Every Day." A Scout is also expected to "Do my duty to God" in the Scout Oath. And to be Reverent – it is the twelfth Scout Law. Therefore, one might say that the altruism expressed in the "good turn" is also an aspect of religion. But the borderline between altruism and religion is blurred, isn't it? An altruistic event may be the result of honorable planning by a wealthy man, or it may be a sudden life-saving event performed by a hardened criminal. The former may be well-planned, advertised, and rewarded with praise; the latter could be deeply appreciated, but with little publicity, and forgotten.[188]

Those who are old enough to remember World War II appreciate the altruism that appeared during the war. Many heroic acts in that period are unknown, because they were never recorded, or never discussed, or because all of the people involved have died in silence. A few examples of true stories of altruism in the war that are emblematic of many others: the Dutch family in Amsterdam that sheltered the family of Anne Frank; those who tried to help each other in Auschwitz, as told in the movie, *Schindler's*

List; and the difficulty and suffering of those who lived through the Nazi occupation in Poland, seen in the movie, *The Pianist*. Also, the redemption of the tortured hero, who forgave his Japanese captor, in *Unbroken*. The fictional movie, *The Best Years of Our Lives*, summarizes it well. Many who volunteered for service in World War II died in combat or later, from wounds of body and mind. Most would never be known, but one memorable one can be mentioned: The movie actor, Jimmy Stewart, who flew B-17 bombers from England over Germany and who returned to America with terrible depression (now called PTSD, post-traumatic stress disorder).[189]

Sacrifice

Religion, at times, either encourages or excuses exceptions, or it merely dodges the issue of exceptions. Religion can turn a "blind eye" to what is going on in the real word, as it is principally otherworldly. Men and women of all religions have participated in all of the exceptions, guided by their religious leaders.[190]

The most important task of the ancient religious leader was to help his or her people deal with their greatest concern, which was death. It may not have been an immediate concern, but adult humans knew that death always happened, and children soon learned about death, too. So, the question was, what to do about it? The early religious leaders thought of a way. They imagined another world, a spiritual world, which ordinary people could only imagine, but to which only the priest or shaman had a special connection. The priest would suggest that a gift could be made to the spiritual world, as a bargain for what was needed to prevent death, or at least to postpone it. For instance, to ask the spiritual world, for rain, when water was needed; or success on the hunt, when the store of food was nearly gone. The religious leader would suggest that a gift should also be given as thanks for what had been received. An appropriate moment would be when a baby appeared safely; or after victory in battle with a neighboring tribe. The gift would be a sacred tribute, a sacrifice, given to the unseen force that controlled human destiny. The gift would be accepted on behalf of the unseen spirit by the mediator – the priest – who would prescribe the form and method of the sacrifice. The word "sacrifice" has a religious origin, as it is derived from "sacred."[191]

The history of sacrifice by humans is long and often rather unpleasant, and it is unnecessary to review it in detail in this essay. Definitive articles on "sacrifice" and "human sacrifice" have already been written by other historians. Sacrifice has probably been performed from earliest times by humans, using animals and other human beings. Sacrifice was originally sponsored by religious authorities, and sacrifices have been practiced widely, in all continents, and in almost every religion. The most vulnerable have been the easiest to sacrifice, whether they were children, women, prisoners, or the poor. Some of these sacrifices were so willingly accepted that they might be called self-sacrifices, but instead they would now be called conditioned responses. The vulnerable persons being sacrificed simply accepted it as their fate. These practices have been codified in religious texts, and sacrifice eventually has become secularized; i.e., without religious significance.[192]

One thing more to add about sacrifice is the subject of cannibalism, which is usually dodged in discussions of the sacrifice of humans. Human cannibalism illustrates the profound importance that religion has had on human behavior. Evidence for human cannibalism shows that it was often performed in religious rites, or as respect for the dead. For many years, it was argued by many historians and anthropologists that there was no good evidence that cannibalism accompanied the sacrifice of humans. Yes, other animals were dismembered, and the parts were placed on altars, to be burned and eaten. But did not that also happen when humans were sacrificially killed? That question can be asked rhetorically, because in ancient times, in, say, the area of the Near East, a sacrifice of meat, placed on an altar and burned, would be consumed. When the meat was from a human sacrifice, would it have been treated differently? Probably not. One of the most important aspects of the development of the Hebrews was the way that they differentiated themselves from their neighbors in respect to sacrifice. The Hebrew God, whether known as Jehovah, or with an unspoken name, did not permit the type of sacrifice that was required by the Canaanite god, Baal. This difference, which was a dramatic step forward in civilization, has largely been forgotten. Even now, the tragedy of Jephthah's daughter is sanitized. Her father had promised that whoever came first out of his house would be sacrificed. It was his daughter. In those days, that meant, to be killed, dismembered, burned on the altar, and eaten. Why the girl would have come running out of the house to greet him, and what happened to her is never told – except that she asked for permission to spend two months in the wilderness "to bewail her virginity," and that he did with her "according to the vow he had made."[193]

Self-Sacrifice

One of the curious problems of the exceptions is Self-Sacrifice. The discussion of sacrifice is the background for the issue of self-sacrifice. The most notable self-sacrifice in the history of any religion is that of Jesus of Nazareth. His death is said to have been foretold by him, spoken of in advance by him, and then willingly accepted, following several hours of expected humiliation and torture in public. His death was said to provide a means by which the rest of mankind could rise from their present miserable condition (which derived from the Fall, which was caused by Adam's failure to obey God), and thus to receive the promise of other things that were almost beyond imagination. The close followers of Jesus, except for one miserable turncoat, Judas Iscariot, then set about spreading this fantastic story, knowing that it would be at the peril of their own lives – as it was. The death of Jesus thus spawned many additional generations of Christian saints, who felt obliged to follow the same path of self-sacrifice for two thousand years, and still counting. It is notable that no one has ever been able to confirm the promise of life in Heaven after death, or of resurrection of the body (which is yet to come). Memories of the ancient practice of cannibalism, which was abhorred by observant Jews and then by Christians, nevertheless persist in the tale of the Last Supper, which has been retold in the ritual of the Mass. It has been the high point of worship for millions of Christians for more than two millennia. When Jesus had his final meal in Jerusalem with the twelve Disciples, he solemnly offered a cup of wine and bread, saying that this is my body and blood, and he asked them to share it with him. This is symbolic cannibalism.[194]

Some other notable self-sacrifices will serve as examples of this exception to the usual human belief expressed in *Health Matters*. Not all of these are for religious reasons, though many are. We remember the Masada, overlooking the Dead Sea, where more than 900 Jews are said to have leaped to their death as a matter of faith when besieged by the Romans in the first century of the Common Era. There was Roland, memorialized in the *Song of Roland*, who chose to die defending the Roncevaux Pass in the Pyrenees Mountains. That self-sacrifice allowed Charlemagne to escape with his main army in 778 AD. We think of Giordano Bruno, who would not recant, and was burned at the stake in Rome in 1600. And Joan of Arc, who met the same fate, for a similar reason, at Rouen, France, in 1431. Countless numbers of the Society of Friends, called Quakers, endured suffering and death for their religious faith in England and New England. In Salem, Massachusetts, in 1692, John Proctor defended his wife, who was accused of witchcraft, a religious crime, knowing that he might face the same fate. Both were convicted and sentenced to death. She was pregnant and her hanging was postponed until she gave birth. The hangings stopped and she survived, but he was hanged. He sacrificed himself so that she might live.[195]

Many Hindu women have allowed themselves to be burned with their deceased husbands in a ceremony known as *suttee*. It is a religious self-sacrifice. The Shinto honor code known as *bushido* has led many *samurai* warriors to commit a particularly gruesome form of self-sacrifice, by disembowelment, known as *seppuku* or *hari-kari*. It was not difficult, therefore, in World War II for the Japanese Navy to recruit many young aviators as *kamikaze* pilots who would be trained to crash their planes into American warships, on behalf of their faith. Self-sacrifice was not limited in that war to the Japanese. In December 1941, an American B-17 pilot, Captain Colin Kelly, saved his crew by keeping his doomed aircraft on a steady course as the others bailed out. He was posthumously awarded the Distinguished Flying Cross. Many American Marines have dived onto grenades to save others. The devout Muslims who hijacked four commercial airliners and then perished on September 11, 2001, were motivated by faith to learn to fly the planes, and then to carry out their carefully coordinated attacks. They were organized by Osama bin Laden, in the Islamic militarist organization that he created which was called al-Qaeda (Arabic = "the base"). We also remember the firefighters who rushed into the burning World Trade Center buildings and died there; and the passengers on Flight 93 on that same day, who knowingly brought the hijacked airliner down into Pennsylvania, saving the lives of others who they believed were targets in Washington, D.C. No one knows the motivations of the firefighters and the airline passengers, but it was probably by selective recruitment of willing workers as firefighters, and also by the instincts of the passengers to save other people, not specifically because of their religious faith. However, many of the Christians who died must have remembered, perhaps subconsciously, being taught that "Greater love hath no man than this, that a man lay down his life for his friends." and "You shalt love your neighbor as yourself." These two Biblical verses would be highly motivational at the time that they faced danger. The Buddhists who continue to immolate themselves in public in defense of their religious faith in Tibet and the western provinces of China are performing a dramatic form of self-sacrifice.[196]

Others are credited with self-sacrifice when it was not their intention to die. They took risks on behalf of others, and they failed in the game of chance. Remembering one of them: Clara Maass, a contract nurse with the U.S. Army in Cuba, who allowed herself to be a subject in Captain Walter Reed's experiments on the method of transmission of yellow fever. She was not a usual volunteer, for she received extra pay for participating in the experiments; and she did not intend to die. She chose to be a subject for the experiments because her family in New Jersey needed the extra money that she planned to send to them. But she did contract yellow fever, and she perished in 1901. She is rightly remembered as a hero, and her name was memorialized in the Clara Maass Hospital in Belleville, N.J. Walter Reed used the information about the infection of Clara Maass and other volunteers to show that yellow fever was transmitted by the bite of an *Aedes* mosquito.[197]

Many advances in medicine can be credited to the use of self-experimentation. Procedures that would be considered unethical if performed on others have been performed on themselves by physicians and scientists for hundreds of years. Curiosity and the possibility of making an important discovery are at the top of the list. There's a lot of ego in some of these self-experiments. The idea of helping people is in the mind of most self-experimenters, and at least five Nobel prizes have been given for discoveries made as a result of self-experimentation. However, many self-experimenters have suffered from temporary or permanent injuries, and some have died. It appears that some of these experiments were irrational and were probably intended to be harmful to the experimenters – the same type of irrational behavior that is involved in "suicide by cop." Many articles have been written by and about individuals who have experimented on themselves, in fields ranging from infectious disease to hematology, pharmacology, and surgery. The subject was reviewed in detail in 1987 by Lawrence Altman in his book, *Who Goes First: The Story of Self-Experimentation in Medicine*, and again in 2012 by Allen Weisse in an article entitled "Self-experimentation and Its Role in Medical Research."[198]

C. Irrational Behavior

The human requirements for health are the needs, urges, and wants that are described in the preceding sections of this essay. These requirements are not always met. If the needs are not met, a fatal outcome will soon follow, and this also is true for three of the urges: food, water, and shelter. Exceptions to the other urges and desires may imperil health and longevity. Some exceptions are unavoidable, because they occur as the result of unplanned events or are imposed by others. The requirements may also be disregarded intentionally, or accidentally, or unknowingly. These are forms of irrational behavior. Irrational behavior includes four other ways in which the human requirements for health have been disregarded. These are the search for adventure, miscalculation of risk, rejection of science, and neuropsychiatric reasons.

Search for Adventure: Why did George Mallory climb into the mist near the top of Mount Everest, and disappear forever? He said simply, "Because it is there," as if that would provide a sufficient explanation for a risk of almost certain death. Perhaps it does, especially to those who also yearn for adventure. Perhaps it is just purely for the spirit of the game of chance, or for the possibility of fame or for the possibility of money: for publication of a book, or future employment, or discovery of a hidden treasure. Some families are notable for seeking adventure. The heroic and even reckless children of President Theodore Roosevelt, President Franklin D. Roosevelt, and Ambassador Joseph P. Kennedy show many examples of daring, fame, misfortune, and death. They were always photogenic, sometimes grim, but usually smiling. They have inspired many others, lesser people like you and me.

There is no simple separation between a search for adventure and miscalculation of risk. Something that was proposed to be only a bit adventuresome can suddenly turn sour, and bad luck can strike even when risk appears to be low. Famed adventurer Steve Fossett took off alone in a single-engine plane on what he expected to be only a low risk, short flight from a ranch in Nevada on the morning of September 3, 2017. Fossett had circumnavigated the globe several times, and was the first to do this in a balloon and also in a fixed wing aircraft. Many of his records still stand. But that morning, he crashed, only 90 meters below the crest of a ridge line in the Sierra Nevada mountains. The attempt to find Fossett was the most expensive in American history, but it failed. It was not until October 2018 that the wreckage of the plane was accidentally discovered, with two of his bones and his wallet near it.[199]

Some professions are riskier than others. For example, consider a firefighter and a grocer; both are needed in society, but one is certainly risker than the other. Choosing to train as a first responder shouldn't be thought of as a foolish venture, nor need a grocer's life always be dull. It takes a spirit of adventure to choose a career in the armed forces, and then it is even more adventuresome to become a Ranger or a Navy SEAL. Ordinary civilians can exhibit unusual bravery when circumstances demand it, especially when their action is in concert with others. A business man or a grocer might go sailing or hunting in spite of the rare risks, even when all safety precautions are taken. Life cannot be risk free. The most important thing is to remember that if you're planning to do something that is dangerous, you should do it as safely as possible.[200]

It is easier to fall into the adventure trap if it appears there might be something beneficial that could result from the experience. It is a form of rationalization.[201]

Miscalculation of Risk: The risk of any situation should be considered in relationship to the potential seriousness of the outcome. It is the potential outcome that is important to consider, not simply the risk. If death or serious disability is a potential outcome, the risk ought to be very low, or – if possible – zero. The decision made by an expert American skier to ski down a black diamond trail may be reasonable in the United States, when skiing at a resort for the first time. The ski trails in America are usually standardized and well-marked. Potentially high danger, but low risk for an expert skier. To do the same in Switzerland would be foolish, where the trail markings are different, and they are not marked in the same way as in the U.S. The American skier would soon learn that risk had been miscalculated.

Courage is important in facing danger, but courage alone, without planning and skill, would require luck to succeed, and that would be a serious miscalculation of risk – to depend on chance, to whistle "Luck, be a Lady Tonight." The title of Stephen Ambrose's book, *Undaunted Courage*, implies that it was the courage of the Corps of Discovery that led to its stunning success as it crossed the Rocky Mountains from east to west, and returned, crossing the mountains again, with a job well done. And that this was a contrast to the tragedy of the Donner-Reed group, which failed in its attempt to cross the Continental Divide. But consider the difference: Lewis and Clark were supported by the President of the United States, and it was a carefully planned military expedition. In every way, the Donner group was different; it had poor leadership and insufficient logistical planning. Courage was indeed abundant in the expedition of Lewis and Clark, and they did enjoy some lucky breaks, such as having Sacagawea for a translator, but they did not miscalculate risk.[202]

Fear of being thought of as a coward has led many people to do dangerous things that they were unprepared for. Some may even have preferred to choose death instead of accepting a "white feather" or being called a "yellow coward." Or to choose a high risk to achieve a high reward, even though the outcome could be fatal. Rudyard Kipling's story of "Gunga Din" is emblematic of that choice: "You're a better man than I am, Gunga Din." Most of the women who die on their first parachuting jump have chosen to take the leap with a man. The men are well-trained, but not the women. Bravery replicates itself in each generation of admirable fools. The decision to perform a brave act in public, if successful, may lead to enormous rewards, as we know from the feat of David when he slew Goliath.[203]

If a decision about any problem must be made, it is important to weigh all of the factors before making a decision. There are two issues. The first issue is to try to avoid being in a predicament that may lead to a dangerous or fatal outcome; and the second is to obtain all of the information that would help make the best decision. Sometimes this is easier said than done, but it's worth trying to plan ahead.

Rejection of Science: The anti-vax movement is the most recent example of the rejection of science, but there have been many examples in the past. In the seventeenth century, prominent non-scientists refused to accept the Copernican hypothesis – that the sun is the center of the solar system, not the earth. Some astronomers were not immediately convinced, although that has long been forgotten. Many people probably still believe that the earth is the center of the solar system, as it is implied in Genesis. And this is confirmed by what they see. The sun must revolve around the earth, because everyone knows that the moon revolves around the earth, and both sun and moon appear in the east and disappear in the west. And there is a small population known as "flat earth" people, even though this is not stated in the Bible. Blood-letting used to be a routine method to treat many illnesses, until the early nineteenth century. Patients would request to be bled, and doctors obliged them. And some drugs that were in common use in the early twentieth century, such as mercurial diuretics, are now recognized as poisons. Confusion has resulted from beautiful images of flights in space that are shown on television and in movies without distinguishing between true images and those that are realistic simulations. Hollywood-type models of space ships. What is the layman to believe? One of the most difficult problems that the public has with scientists, especially medical scientists, is also that scientists don't agree on everything. And then sometimes well-established beliefs are shown to be wrong. Understandably, the public is confused about the disputes and changes in scientific theories. This confusion produced chaos in the era of COVID-19, as the issue became politicized in the United States.[204]

The pandemic known as COVID-19 is caused by the virus SARS-CoV-2. The two groups of actions proposed by public health professionals are (1) mitigation, or (2) containment. There are six components included in these two actions. Mitigation includes social distancing (separation of people by six feet, whenever possible); wearing face masks; and hand-sanitizing. Containment involves identification of cases, contact tracing, and quarantine. These six components are accepted in principle by more people in the United States who identify as Democrats than those who identify as Republicans. The difference is particularly obvious in mask-wearing. For example, a well-dressed middle-aged woman is seen walking alone, wearing a mask, in a suburb of Baltimore, which is in the Blue state of Maryland. In contrast, a young man, wearing a leather jacket with a flag on the back, wearing a black helmet but no face mask, is driving his motorcycle close to many others in the Red state of South Dakota. (In the United States, Democrats are associated with blue; Republicans with red.) The woman is likely to have a college education, and the motorcyclist is probably only a high school graduate, if that. The Maryland lady has a much lower risk to contact or to transmit COVID-19 than the motorcyclist. It is difficult to assess compliance with the five other public health recommendations, but it is likely that similar differences persist in those areas, too.[205]

Neuropsychiatric Reasons: Three groups can be defined, although there is some overlap between the groups: Impaired judgment, addictions (including some drugs), and other drugs.[206]

Impaired judgment may result from brain dysfunction; Alzheimer's disease, senile dementia, and other dementias; other causes of organic brain dysfunction, such as trauma, brain tumor, inherited or traumatic birth defects such as Down syndrome; functional brain dysfunction which includes autism spectrum (Asperger's), attention deficit hyperactivity disorder (ADHD), obsessive-compulsive disorder (OCD), schizophrenia (catatonia; fixed delusion; paranoia); organic psychosis (e.g., tertiary syphilis); bipolar disorder (formerly known as manic-depressive disorder), which can manifest itself as religious fanaticism; depression (including senile depression and post-partum depression); phobias and fetishes (e.g., allurophobia [terror of cats] or "tree-hugger:); posttraumatic stress disorder (PTSD), formerly called "shell shock"; sociopaths (e.g., serial rapists); and profoundly anti-science anarchists.[207]

Addiction to substances and behaviors, for example: tobacco – nicotine; opioids (especially Oxycontin in the U.S., heroin in England and the U.S., and opium and other derivatives of the poppy flowers in the East); cocaine (especially "crack" cocaine, in contrast to low-dose cocaine used as a non-addictive stimulant in Andean countries); other addictive mood-altering agents, such as methenamine ("crystal meth") and LSD (lysergic acid); gambling; hoarding; and purchasing.

Other drugs, especially alcoholic beverages; marijuana (which can be habit forming, though not truly addictive); unintended side-effects of other drugs, such as Valium or Contact, side effects of antibiotics, especially tetracyclines; and mood enhancing drugs and non-narcotic pain relievers: e.g., Darvon, Soma; and plant compounds (e.g., mandrake, nightshade, ricin, jasmine, licorice, and capsaicin).

D. Benefits from Disregarding the Exceptions

An impulse or a carefully considered plan may lead a person to follow a different path than would ordinarily be followed by what I have called the usual needs, urges, and wants of humans. The choice to make an exception to these usual activities may be in order to benefit the individual, or it may be made on behalf of the social group. The potential benefits from the exceptions were embedded within a discussion of the exceptions, but a few of them will be mentioned again at this point.

Religion is an exception which appeared early in social groups. Religion, with priests and priest-healers and ceremonies, provided necessary spiritual and physical guidance to humans. The origin of the physician can be traced to the priest-healer, and from the physician we have the beginnings of science and technology.

Heroism and courage have been demonstrated on countless occasions throughout history. These acts are sometimes difficult to explain, but they are nevertheless very important. Sometimes they have been performed anonymously, with a spirit of altruism, while at other times they have been accompanied with a flagrant proclamation of importance, as if to say: "Look at ME!" In either event, they have inspired many others to do likewise. We recognize that some professions are riskier than others, and courage is important in facing danger. Society is grateful that some are willing and able to take these risks, and the risk takers are often (though not always) rewarded for their successes.[208]

It is somewhat more difficult to see benefit from exceptions that I have defined as neuro-psychiatric. But there are a few that should be mentioned. Some skepticism is appropriate when statements by scientists are conflicting, or when a physician or another scientist advises something that seems to violate common sense. The anti-vax movement has charlatans behind it, but there is reason to be wary because both safety and efficacy of vaccination must be well established before a new vaccine is introduced to the public. Sad to say, safety and efficacy of some vaccines, such as the inactivated polio virus (IPV) vaccine, have failed in the past, and even now, the oral polio vaccine (OPV) is not completely free of risk. Yellow fever vaccines went through several stages to improve efficacy and reduce risk before a final yellow fever vaccine evolved. On another subject, we can learn much about possible interactions of humans with each other in the future by observing the benign, cheerful, optimistim of many children with Down syndrome. And the medical uses of narcotics are important for the relief of both severe acute pain and of chronic pain. The problem with narcotics has largely been laxity in prescribing and illegal dispensation of opiates, and patients suffering from addiction and deaths from overdoses should be cared for, not shunned.

E. The Dark Side of Medicine

When misbehavior occurs in physicians, it may have especially serious consequences. Physicians are humans, and for this reason, they sometimes exhibit irrational behavior in the same ways that are seen in lay persons – in the search for adventure, miscalculation of risk, and for neuropsychiatric reasons. If the problem is sociopathic, the result may be more serious than would be seen in a non-physician, for several reasons. The physician is granted the expectation of honor and honesty, and this implies that whatever he or she does must be for the good of someone else. This "free pass" can lead to temptation, to mischief, and then to something worse. It may be submitting to temptation in what is known as "false billing," meaning to inflate the time spent with a patient, or to divide one surgical procedure into several parts, each of which can be billed separately. And then to serious criminal behavior. Physicians also understand science well enough to be able to manipulate data and to hide evidence. If no autopsy is done, and the body is cremated, the *corpus delicti* has lost its voice. "Dead men tell no tales." If a physician becomes psychotic, with paranoid delusions, the problem is enhanced. In this case, the misbehavior of a physician may be boundless.[209]

The Dark Side of Medicine includes a long list of issues. It could begin with physicians who have hidden the cause of death when it could be embarrassing, and it could continue with those who have committed murders on a small scale or as serial killers. This compilation also includes sexual assaults by male physicians upon female patients, by performing unnecessary genital examinations, or by impregnating unsuspecting patients, or by posing as an anonymous sperm donor. The problem is magnified when a physician is acting in concert with other adults as coaches for adolescent girls and boys. To mention but one example: Dr. Larry Nassar (b. 1963) was sentenced to 40-125 years in prison for sexual assaults on scores of young women as the team sports physician for USA Gymnastics. Nassar fingered and fondled the girls, pretending this was part of a normal physical examination. His crimes were facilitated by other men in power, including the Dean of Osteopathic Medicine at Michigan State University and the gymnastic coach at USA Gymnastics. Physicians have been intimately involved in torture, assisting in cases of "harsh" interrogation, in cannibalism, in development of poisons and deadly infections for government agencies, and in false billings for individual patients and on a large scale as part of group practices. Physician aid in dying (PAD) is now allowed in some states and foreign countries, but when a physician is involved physician-assisted-suicide (PAS) or euthanasia in other jurisdictions, it is an illegal act. Physicians were involved in confinement and mistreatment of "hysterical" women in psychiatric institutions. The enormous problem of opioid addiction began with physicians, many of whom had good intentions, and the medical profession is not yet free of complicity in its perpetuation.[210]

We now examine the Choices that individuals and groups must consider in their search for health.

Chapter 7

Choices and Ambitions

A. Choices and Decisions

Time and tide wait for no man.[211]

Choices are the inevitable consequence of human intuition, curiosity, imagination, and dexterity. A choice must be made when any of the urges require a decision to be made. Sometimes the decision will be made by instinct, especially if the choice must be made immediately; but if there is sufficient time, the choice will be made after giving thought, and weighing the various options. In some cases, the decision will be to take the safer course; in others, the safe course will be rejected in favor of a potentially higher yield. For some choices, the individual may benefit; the alternative option might benefit the family or the group. The choice may be different for one person than another. The urges are universal, but the decision is personal. In either event, whether by instinct or by thoughtful consideration, the choice will be made that appears to be best for the health of the individual or the group. The choice for health is given in the title of this essay: *Health Matters*.

Decisions must be made. The decisions that humans make in regard to their essential requirements, our needs – for air, to breathe; for sun and sunlight; and for sleep, to dream, are automatic, and do not require much decision-making. However, even for these essentials, choices are usually made. For instance, we seek the best place to breathe, and then say "Ah, fresh air." And, "It's a sunny day, let's go outside." Or, "Make hay while the sun shines," either as a farmer would do it, or perhaps as a metaphor meaning, "Let's get to work." For sleep, we ordinarily find a good, safe, soft place to lie down, preferably in the dark. The child's prayer, "Now I lay me down to sleep …" recalls the proper preparation for bedtime.

The responses to the urges are usually automatic, by instinct. Responses are usually made by choices with little risk, but sometimes the choice requires careful consideration. Some examples are: Do I go for a bucket of water now, as usual, or after it stops raining? It's snowing today, but we're almost out of meat. Will this wretched day be a good day to go hunting for deer, or should I wait until the weather is better? Water is dripping into the cave. It's a safe place, but uncomfortable. Should I go looking for a better cave now? My wife isn't happy today. Is this the right time to sleep close, or should I wait? What shall we do with the cousins? Our families don't get along well together, but I really need to work with my brother-in-law on the next fishing trip. We can imagine these innocuous questions regarding choices to be made about the other urges – about clothing, fire, and animals – and about the wants, for love and money. However, the choices may require decisions that clearly affect health. A wrong decision, or an unlucky one, could have a disastrous or even a fatal outcome. It is therefore worth considering how choices are made.

Sometimes choices are made without thinking of the consequences. These choices may be based on habits. Some people are especially prone to make snap judgments; they may sometimes be lucky, or they may be perpetually unlucky. In some circumstances, a perfect decision is important. Nothing but perfection will suffice. The common expression is "Life or Death," although it usually doesn't mean such a dire outcome. It's just an expression. But for an architect or a tailor, perfection is truly expected. The apprentice tailor learns to "Measure twice, cut once." In the world of physics or physical chemistry, exactitude is required. Calculation of doses of radiation given by x-rays or radioactive isotopes must be very precise. Enough to kill the cancer, but not more, in order to prevent damage to the surrounding normal tissue. In astronomy and in managing objects launched into space, absolute precision is demanded, though time and distance are unimaginably large. Calculations made for NASA are based on exponential values, ranging into the billions, trillions, and beyond; yet the results must be perfect.

People often say "What are the odds?" without thinking that the expression means a calculation, based on real numbers, known or estimated, with a probability score. However, in biology and medicine, decisions are often based on probabilities. The gold standard, so to speak, is a probability of 95%. Even better is 99%. These percentages are referred to by scientists as "p = .05" and "p = .01." The percentages are based on calculations based on the mean – the average – of an array of numbers and a calculation known as the standard deviation. Another method of estimating the odds in science is known as X^2 (Chi-squared). This is a method that requires a complex calculation, but it leads to a workable conclusion. Formerly a laborious task, calculation of the odds by the method of Chi-square now can be performed with an app on a hand-held phone. A decision can be made on the basis of probability, depending on whether a "p" value of 0.5 or 0.1 is desired. In the end, it can be simplified. For example, if a new drug is tested 14 times and it has a positive outcome in one patient, the drug is considered to have passed the ".05" test, and it will be continued for further testing. Bridge players, poker players, roulette players, and other gamblers must have some way to "roll the dice." In most of these decisions, concern for health is not in the foreground, but it is always there in the background. Decisions may be based on weighing many factors, and also while acting swiftly, without the possibility of turning back. A surgeon often has to move quickly, keeping these three things in mind: Do I operate on this patient? When shall I operate? And where do I make the incision? If possible, the surgeon would surely ask the patient or a surrogate for permission, and would explain the plan for the operation in simple terms. But sometimes, such niceties are impossible. A dying patient brought in to the emergency room requires immediate action.[212]

In politics, different rules apply, but there are always rules to follow that determine the result. The outcome may be a plurality, or a majority, or a two-thirds majority. Or a "black ball" may be tossed into the ballot box, when one negative vote will defeat a proposition that requires a unanimous vote. Different sets of rules are followed by various political and social groups, but *Robert's Rules* is the one that is most frequently used.

One of the most agonizing decisions is rarely faced, but it is worth considering because of the impact that it has had on others in the past. Anyone might face it. The decision is one that must be made, when a choice has to be made about who can live and who must die. For example, if there are ten people on a sinking ship, and there are only life jackets for nine of them. Do you draw lots? Or perhaps one person simply says, "I can swim. You take mine." Morbid jokes begin with, "We need to bail out of this airplane, but there are not enough parachutes for all of us." It does happen, however, and then it's not a joke. A man can only save some of his children when the family is ordered to board the train to a concentration camp. Some can stay behind and be sheltered. How to decide which ones to save?

Al Capp's "Li'l Abner" comic strip featured a man named "Joe Btfsplk, who walked under a dark cloud. He always had bad luck, and he brought bad luck to others. He was the "world's worst jinx." Other people have a difficult time making decisions. Sometimes they wait too long, and the moment of opportunity passes. Gone forever. There are two principal ways to make an informed decision. Each method requires developing the problem into a simple statement. The question is then posed as either a binary problem (answered by 0 or 1 – as yes or no), or on a sliding scale from best to worst (e.g., a Likert scale of 1-5, with 1 being poorest, and 5 being best). Governmental agencies and businesses prefer the binary proposition, whereas most individuals and social groups prefer to use a sliding scale. A military Surgeon General was told that one of his hospitals was located on land that had recently been found to have a geological fault line. An earthquake could devastate the hospital. He asked, "Will it happen in, say, the next three years?" The answer was, "Not very likely." He said, "Well, then it won't be on my watch, so we won't abandon the hospital and rebuild it somewhere else." That was a binary decision, based on two factors: (1) assessing risk (very low) and (2) cost (very high). Business school teaches that one can make a decision in the same way, balancing potential risk versus potential gain. If a fixed sum of money is available for discretionary use, the decision can be either choosing a modest risk with a modest potential yield, or from a choice to take a high risk/high yield. The big winners are those who make the latter choice, and it turns out to be successful; but woe to the ones who take the high risk/high yield option and it is not successful. It is important nevertheless to make a decision. One of the most important decisions in the twentieth century was the decision made by General Dwight D. Eisenhower to launch the Allied invasion of France on June 6, 1944. At 4:30 p.m. on June 4, there was heavy rain outside Eisenhower's headquarters in England, but at 9:30 p.m., the weather report suggested a brief spell of better weather for the morning of June 6. Eisenhower decided to take the risk and said, "We'll go," and the order was given: D-Day will be June 6. It was the largest seaborne invasion in history.[213]

The pandemic of COVID-19 has made decisions necessary throughout the world to a degree that is without precedent in human history. The interconnection of the world's people in the twenty-first century has placed the entire human population of 7.8 billion at risk. Many have the opportunity to make choices, although most of the world does not. Wealth favors the ability to choose. In developing countries, most people do not have a choice about how to reduce their risk of developing COVID-19. They simply have to continue their daily life, trying to find enough to satisfy their basic needs – for water, food, shelter, and protection of their community. The risk of COVID-19 is far down on their list of concerns. In developed countries, and in the upper classes of countries in the mid-range of gross national products, choices are available for some people. There is, however, significant disagreement about what to do. There is a reduction in the opportunity to choose for some groups of people, such as health care workers, first responders, and those who are dependent on others for their daily existence. Even in developed countries, wealthy people have a much greater opportunity to choose than those who are poor. And what to do? The mantra of three recommendations to reduce the risk of COVID-19 – called mitigation of risk – includes face mask, hand sanitizer, and social distancing. The economic and social impact of the three mitigation procedures has been enormous, especially in the travel industry and in education, with secondary impacts on the welfare of millions of people and thousands of institutions. Some countries, such as Sweden, chose to take a less restrictive approach to implementing the mitigation procedures, although the results have not been as beneficial as were hoped for. Other countries, such as New Zealand, have implemented strong requirements, with success. But in much of the world, including the United States, Brazil, and India, there has been much less success in implementing the mitigation procedures. In the United States, there has been much debate about individual rights versus the need for community participation in controlling COVID-19. The "individual rights" point of view of many Americans is expressed in many ways: masses of people in close proximity in political rallies for Republican candidates, an enormous gathering of motorcycle riders in South Dakota, college students lined up at their favorite bars, and individuals who proudly reject wearing masks in public. There is also ruggedness in the American backbone. "Don't fence me in," was once a favorite tune. When students returned to the campus of the University of Iowa in Iowa City in August 2020, a student was asked about COVID-19. She replied, saying that she "resented the city's 'ridiculous' restrictions that were intended to protect against COVID-19." She said, "We're all farmers and don't really care about germs, so if we get it, we get it and we have the immunity to it."[214]

B. Ambition

There is much variability in humans with respect to setting goals. Humans may plan to be leaders, or to be followers, or they may just take what is offered, "to go with the flow," as the saying goes.
A leader may wish to be a Napoleon or a Mother Teresa. The final outcome will depend on ability, luck, circumstances, and health. If the first three of these are aligned toward success, the final determination will be determined by health – whether health is good, or not. Good health can result from making good choices, or from good luck. Bad health may result from bad choices, or bad luck. There can be a mixture, however, and the end is unpredictable. Good choices may be followed by bad luck; or vice versa. Bad choices, such as some of the exceptions listed above, may be followed by good luck, and the goal may be reached. For an example of a mixed end to ambition, remember Alexander of Macedon, so-called Alexander "the Great." In his ambition, he chose a life of exceptions. He choice was to accept danger in spite of risk, and he won battle after battle; but in the end, he suddenly died, prematurely. *Health Matters*.[215]

We now leave the subject of health for the time being, as we turn to examine the issue that is always in the back of our minds. Something that we hope to postpone for as long as possible. It is death.

Chapter 8

Death

A. Death with Dignity

Each of us is solitary; each of us dies alone.
– C. P. Snow[216]
Death be not proud.
– John Donne[217]

This section expands on some of the ways that death appears in the previous chapters about the various urges and the exceptions to these urges. The subject of death is then considered from the point of view of science, concluding with an overview of infectious disease and the pandemic of COVID-19. The ultimate question here is: What is death?[218]

Death is one of the most prominent themes in intellectual history and entertainment. Death sometimes appears in the plot as a surprise, or is disguised, or it may appear in a dramatic climax. The ending may be suggested by signposts given to the reader or viewer, but it is hidden from the actors. Some literary works about death are intended to serve as warnings, while others titillate the morbid senses. Some are ridiculous, although readers or viewers find them to be exciting or even amusing. Death or dying or temporary escape from death is the subject in fields that include music, literature – both fiction and true stories – poetry, religion, dramatic productions, projections in movies, music with hymns and instruments, opera, art and sculpture, cartoons and folk art, fantasy and fairy tales, newspapers and television, general history, the history of medicine, the history of science, and science fiction. Death may arrive unexpectedly, or it may be planned. The variations range from suicide to execution, from wars and infectious diseases, and deaths of many types, for different reasons, including assassination, beheading, deaths that are unexpected or unintended, duels, poisons, and medical accidents. Most are from "natural causes," but some are hastened as the result of "medical aid in dying." The list is long, and there is more about the ways of Death in the Appendix.

Death with Dignity: From "Scared to Death" to "Code Blue"

One of the duties of a licensed physician is to sign death certificates. The words written by a physician on the death certificate can determine the way the body of the deceased person is handled, how large his or her estate may be, and what happens to many other people who are still alive. The form of the death certificate varies from state to state, but in general terms, the physician is asked to state, to the best of his or her ability, (1) the primary cause and time of death, (2) any conditions that contributed to the death, and (3) any additional conditions that are important. The physician may not have known the patient at all, yet he will be asked to write answers to these questions and to sign and date the certificate. Many copies are made of the death certificate, for the hospital or nursing home, the funeral director, family members, attorneys, life insurance companies, and sometimes the federal government and the police department. A copy that is filed with the state health department is a source for statistics for the year of death, and for planning purposes in years to come. If someone challenges what is written on the death certificate, the physician who signed it may be overruled, but it is usually difficult to change it.

The most important decisions that are based on the death certificate are (1) Was this a homicide, for whom someone other than the deceased is responsible? Or (2) Was this a suicide? If both of these questions are answered in the negative, it still may a homicide, but no person or organization will be charged with the offense; and if it was not a suicide, burial can be made in hallowed ground, with full financial death benefits. Most deaths are categorized as being from (3) "natural causes," including accidents. Some may be accidental homicides, for which the deceased is responsible.

A few hypothetical examples will illustrate these points. A man dies of a cerebral hemorrhage, due to a clotting deficiency, caused by chemotherapy for pancreatic cancer. It is death from a "natural cause" (cancer), with a secondary or contributing cause: chemotherapy. On the other hand, suppose a college student on vacation becomes intoxicated, climbs onto the railing of an apartment house, and falls to his death. His death is an accident (a natural cause), but it could also be called a homicide. If he is under the legal age to consume alcohol, whoever supplied him with drink may be charged; and if the railing was not secured, the apartment house management may have a problem. Otherwise, it is just a sad event. If a patient dies who is suspected of having COVID-19, but who was not tested for the disease, should COVID-19 be entered on the death certificate? Sometimes it is, and sometimes it isn't.[219]

The techniques used in cardio-pulmonary resuscitation (CPR) have evolved over the past sixty years. Hospitals now have "crash carts" with equipment, supplies, and medications that are rapidly wheeled to the bedside of almost every patient who dies within the hospital, or even in the driveway or nearby parking lot. As a team appears, someone takes charge and all commence the sequence of activities that they have rehearsed in BLS or ALS (basic or advanced lifesaving courses). Usually, although not always, the team leader asks about the patient's diagnosis, and whether an Advanced Directive has been signed that allows death to occur without CPR. If no one knows the diagnosis, and if no one says, "No, this patient has an Advanced Directive to prohibit CPR," the "Code Blue" proceeds until the patient's heart beat and respirations have returned, or until the team agrees that the patient has "coded" (died).

When CPR was later extended to the lay community, the rules changed, and rescue breathing was then supposed to be "mouth-to-mouth" or "mouth-to-nose & mouth." If a health care provider is trained to insert an endotracheal tube, and is wearing personal protective equipment (PPE), CPR can be done with a reasonable degree of safety. But it is hazardous work. In recent years, an AED (Automatic Electric Defibrillator) can be found in many public buildings and in airport terminals.[220]

Assisted suicide, also called "death with dignity," or Medical aid-in-dying (MAID), is gradually winning converts. It may be requested by a patient who is dying with cancer, or with intractable neuro-muscular illness such as Parkinson's disease, or a person who sees senility – Alzheimer's – inexorably advancing. The patient requests a prescription of a lethal dose of a drug, usually a barbiturate, and takes it personally, though some assistance may be needed. This is often done in the presence of a family gathering for the purpose of saying farewell. As mentioned above, assisted suicide is now legal in several states in the United States and elsewhere, including the Netherlands and Colombia. Medical aid-in-dying now has legal status in the District of Columbia and in eight states, including New Jersey, which legislated it in 2019. A physician formerly gave an Oath not to provide a poison, even when requested to do so. Recent versions of the Hippocratic Oath have eliminated that prohibition, and allow physicians to have discretion in this matter.[221]

B. Immortality

The Opposite of Death

For many centuries, humans have conceived in various ways of a spiritual world, and of some form of "life after death"; of the possibility of immortality, of resurrection, and reincarnation. The spiritual world cannot be seen by ordinary humans, nor can its existence be proved. This spiritual world often includes belief in an afterlife – of the existence of purgatory, heaven, and hell – and beliefs in the reincarnation or the resurrection of the body, or simply of rebirth.[222]

Immortality is the opposite of death; death does not exist for an immortal person. Immortality requires life; a stone cannot be immortal. The concept of immortality is antithetical to science, which holds that all living things must die. Resurrection is a belief that a human's death is not permanent, and that a dead body can rise and return to its previous state. Even a decayed or destroyed body may be resurrected and rise from the dead. Reincarnation is somewhat different. Reincarnation is a belief that at the time of death, the spirit persists, and an individual is reborn in the form of a different animal, and that the process of death and rebirth continues unendingly. A human may be reincarnated as a fly. A cow may die and be reincarnated as a human. Reincarnation after death continues again and again; it is infinite. Although the concepts of resurrection and reincarnation are theoretically different, many who believe in one or the other confuse the details, and refer to each of them in similar ways. Both resurrection and reincarnation are inconsistent with science.[223]

Readers of the Christian Bible are familiar with the concept of resurrection, from the dialogue between Jesus and the Sadducees, who did not believe in resurrection. Jesus does not answer directly the question posed to him about resurrection, but instead gives a parable, which confounds the questioners. Many Christians say that they believe in the resurrection of the body, without fully understanding the meaning of the term. Nor is it easy to describe, for Jesus didn't explain the details. The concepts of immortality, reincarnation, and resurrection have now morphed into "rebirth" which can mean many things: an idea, which is restated after having been forgotten; or a field of blossoms in the spring.[224]

Death and Immortality in the Modern World

Developments in biology, medicine, surgery, technology, biomedical ethics, and law in the latter part of the twentieth century raised new issues regarding life and death. To mention a few, all too briefly: The question of mortality and immortality arises, as cancer cells derived from a long-deceased patient named Henrietta Lacks have become "immortalized." As "HeLa" cells, named for her, they are grown in prodigious amounts in tissue culture in laboratories throughout the world. Normal cells progress through a fixed number of cell divisions and they then normally fail to divide; the end of this process is known as apoptosis, or programmed cell death. The death of cells can be hastened by tumor necrosis factor (TNR) and it is modulated by the ubiquitous protein, p53. But for reasons still incompletely understood, HeLa cells continue to divide and thus her cell line is immortal.[225]

The notion of "brain death" was proposed in the United States, in order to make it possible to remove vital organs for transplantation while they were still functional. However, "brain death" is not a simple solution to the legal and biological definition of death. In addition, it also begs the question of who should receive a heart or liver or kidney, when there are more potential recipients than there are organs available. Another question is a troubling conundrum: Is the heart that is transplanted, and beating in another person, the heart of the dead donor, or is it now the heart of the fortunate recipient? A parent of the deceased donor may think of the recipient as giving additional years of life to their child. This issue is both emotional and philosophical. A different question arises in cases of liver transplantation, in which some transplanted livers undergo changes in which their cells incorporate enough of the recipient's genetic material to allow the recipient to stop taking anti-rejection drugs. In these cases, the transplanted liver has become a so-called "chimera," comprised of cells representing both donor and recipient. The death of the donor has allowed the recipient to continue to live. But are both donor and recipient still alive in some way? If a brain were to be transplanted from a living person into a cadaver, who is now alive? The donor or the recipient? It is a philosophical question. Bionics present another challenge in the issue of life and death. As various parts of the body are replaced by artificial parts, a person who might have died may live on for many years. At present, the body parts that are replaced are mainly those of the musculo-skeletal system – the muscles and bones. They are related to movement, such as arms and legs. However, miniaturization of functioning replacements of vital organs has become increasing successful. The goal to have an implantable artificial heart may be near at hand, and then perhaps a similar goal can be achieved for lungs, liver, and kidneys.[226]

A comment about new technology and the uncertain future: Cloning has made it possible to create almost identical copies of an animal. Did the original animal die? Are the cloned animals immortalized forms of the original animal? This is a conundrum for both philosophers and biologists. Another question arises with insertion of deoxyribonucleic acid (DNA) from one animal into the nucleus of an embryo from a similar animal. When it gives birth, it produces what is known as a transgenic animal. DNA is very durable. It can be recovered from animals that have long been dead and even from scrapings in ancient burrows. This technology may allow extinct birds and reptiles to be replicated as living forms, which are similar, though not precisely identical, to those seen in museums or buried in permafrost. The transgenic reproduction of the extinct animal is not a perfect copy of the original because inheritance involves more than what is transmitted in the classic sequence of DNA to ribonucleic acid (RNA) to protein. The reason for the difference is what is known as "epigenetic" transmission of inheritance. A long dead species may have its DNA extracted and brought to life again by transgenic methodology, but it would not be exactly the same as the original. Is such a species dead, or has it been brought back to life? There are also enormous ethical implications involved in the possibility of cloning or altering the genome of humans. The history of the eugenics movement shows the dangers of attempting to meddle with natural selection. It is clear that scientists need to worry before proceeding with this type of work in the laboratory, and that society must insist on a pause.[227]

Chapter 9

Public Health

We shift at this point to examine death from the perspective of public health, looking at deaths from various causes throughout the world. This is not a lively topic. In fact, many people would think it is boring. It was not even taught in most medical schools in the 1950s. Students were taught about infectious diseases, but not about all of the other subjects that are now considered under the rubric of public health. The discipline – the subject matter – of public health has been continuously changing over the last sixty-five years. As the world has changed, there have also been changes in science and medicine people have changed. Think of the ways: some are good, and some are awful. The world's temperature has risen, glaciers have been disappearing, the oceans are rising and are filled with pieces of plastic, and fish and coral reefs are vanishing. Population has gone from about 2 billion to nearly 10 billion. Much of what was forest land has been converted to agricultural use, and toxic products pollute the earth.

Scientists have discovered things that were smaller than could then be imagined; humans have travelled into space; and the telescope has shown a universe that is ever expanding. Medicine has broadened. It now is science-based in a way that it never previously had been, and medical students now study public health as a serious discipline. Medical students now learn careers which range at the same time from research at the laboratory bench, to the bedside and clinic, and to visits in the homes of patients and their families. And medical students now study public health as matters of policies that are based on mega-numbers of illnesses and deaths in populations.[228]

Public health is population-based, and public health is closely related to economic health; to both the economic health of the country, and of its people. The world's population can be divided into the haves, the have-nots, and those who are somewhere in between. Some of the "haves" are the group of developed countries, known as the G-6 or G-7 or G-10. It is like a country club. The "have-nots" are those at the bottom of the economy, including the so-called "third world" countries of the Cold War. Most of the countries between the "haves" and "have nots" are called "developing" countries, though that category also includes the manufacturing behemoths of China and India. There is no perfect way to rank the countries' economies, but Gross National Product (GNP), per capita, is as good as any. The United Nations' World Health Organization monitors the health of its member nations, using many metrics, and it displays the results on a yearly basis. The endpoint that is the most important is life expectancy. All of the other metrics, such as efficiency of health care funding and infant mortality, are necessary guides to achieving the goal of *Health Matters*: to prevent death, with a long life. There has been for many years a slow but steady rise in the curves of both per capita income and individual life expectancy of the people of the world. There has been, however, a distinct difference, in that these beneficial effects are predominantly seen in the wealthiest parts of the world. It is a sad truism that has been known for centuries, that those who have the most, want more, and get more.[229]

Most of the deaths in the poorer countries are from different causes than those in the countries with the higher GNP, per capita. Infectious diseases (discussed below), nutritional deficiency (starvation: lack of calories and protein, often on a seasonal basis), and exposure to toxic substances (as waste or from products of mining for industrial use in wealthy countries). To solve this, the rich must give to the poor.

The readers of this essay will understand that the causes of death in developed countries are completely different from those mentioned in the rest of the world. For example, in the United States of America in 2017, the ten leading causes of death were heart disease, cancer, accidents, chronic lower respiratory disease, stroke, Alzheimer's disease, diabetes, influenza and pneumonia, kidney diseases, and suicide. Heart disease, cancer, and respiratory diseases now account for about half of the deaths in the United States. These diseases were not mentioned in my medical school course on Preventive Medicine. I suppose this was because there was little that could be done at that time to prevent illness and deaths from these causes. However, during the past sixty years, great strides have been made in research on these issues. Cancer is one example of a disease that has risen to replace the causes of death in previous centuries, and for which much has been accomplished.[230]

Cancer was not considered to be a disease in the early twentieth century, except by the American Cancer Society and a few scientists and physicians who were specialists in the treatment of cancer in Buffalo and New York City. The history of the concept of cancer as one disease that affects different organs in the body, instead of being a group of similar diseases, was discussed in the book by Siddhartha Mukherjee, *The Emperor of All Maladies*. Over the past sixty years, the problem of cancer has been addressed in many ways. The three most important weapons are chemotherapy, radiation therapy, and surgery. Chemotherapy includes treatment with chemical agents, hormones, and immunological methods. Radiation therapy includes external beams and radioisotopes. Studies of the cause of cancer have led to improved methods to prevent the disease. Drugs have been developed that specifically target cancer; radiation therapy has become more powerful and better localized; and surgery has become focused, less destructive to normal tissues, and with an eye toward rehabilitation. The word "cancer" is now accepted by the public, instead of being something that was so dreadful that it could not be spoken. This has allowed physicians and health advisors to speak about the "warning signs of cancer," and to encourage tests that have enabled cancer to be detected in earlier stages of the disease. The practice of medicine at present includes teams of cancer treatment specialists, known as medical oncologists, pediatric oncologists, radiation oncologists, and surgical oncologists, who work with well-trained oncology nurses. The National Cancer Act of 1971, and successive legislative acts, have enabled the National Cancer Institute to provide massive amounts of funding for research into the origin and nature of cancer, of methods to treat the disease, and for education of health professionals and the public. The Surgeon General and the American Cancer Society worked together to show that tobacco smoking was the major cause of lung cancer, and to use this information to restrict the sale and use of cigarettes. As these methods have shown success, other organizations have joined in the work to control cancer, such as the Veterans Administration and the Department of Defense, and new organizations have been formed, such as the Leukemia Society and the Susan G. Komen Breast Cancer Foundation. The American Cancer Society states that the death rate from cancer has decreased by 29 percent since 1991.[231]

Returning to the subject of Public Health, the organization that is now the Commissioned Corps of the United States Public Health Service (USPHS) traces its beginning to an Act of Congress in 1798 to provide care for sailors and immigrants, as the Marine Hospital Service. The USPHS is the tiny seed from which has grown all of the branches of both the U.S. Department of Health and Human Services (DHHS) and the U.S. Department of Education (the ED or DoED). The history of development of these departments and of their many agencies is far beyond the scope of this essay, but a few aspects emphasize the importance of the USPHS. By 1801, government hospitals had been established in several port cities, and by 1871, the Marine Hospital Service had expanded to staff many additional hospitals. The Commissioned Corps of the PHS was created by an Act of Congress in 1889. Most of the older PHS hospitals have vanished, but the flagship institution remains. It is the Clinical Center of National Institutes of Health, where some of the Americans with Ebola were hospitalized in 2018. The PHS staffed the hospital at Carville, Louisiana, which housed patients with leprosy. Uniformed officers of the PHS staff the hospitals of the Indian Health Service and they provide medical care for the Federal prison system. Physicians, nurses, and nine other categories of health care specialists of the PHS serve as the medical department for the U.S. Coast Guard, and they are part of the professional staff of more than twenty government organizations, including the Centers for Disease Control (CDC) and the National Institutes of Health (NIH). As the USPHS was assuming an increasing important role in Public Health, other government organizations were being formed, such as the original National Institute [sic] of Health, formed as the Hygenic Laboratory in 1891, which became the National Institute of Allergy and Infectious Diseases (NIAID), and the National Cancer Institute (NCI). The NCI was created in 1944 and it was established in its current form by the National Cancer Act of 1971. Many of these health-related organizations were brought together in 1953 into the newly formed Department of Health, Education, and Welfare (HEW). This department was divided in 1979 into the two departments shown above: HHS and

DEoD. Several other disease-related institutes have been added to the NIH, such as the National Institute of Heart Disease, National Institute of Neurological Disease and Blindness, and the National Institute of Arthritis and Metabolic Diseases. The NIH conducts intramural research, done by government scientists, and it funds extramural research grants through a highly competitive process. A successful RO1 research grant application from the NIH is the ultimate goal of a university scientist's work. Commissioned Corps officers of the USPHS, led by the Surgeon General, are now grouped with seven other government organizations as the Uniformed Services of the United States government.[232]

A. Infectious Diseases

The discussion of infectious diseases will become increasingly technical, and some readers might skip it, to pick up the thread again with COVID-19. I hope, however, that there will be something of interest in the intervening pages. I would therefore suggest skimming rather than skipping the descriptions of pandemic, parasitology, microbiology, bacteriology, viruses, prions, and so forth. All humans are exposed to at various times to many of these infectious agents, and it behooves everyone to think about them. I have included some comments to entice the reader. Look for them.

From "Plagues" to COVID-19

The word "plague" – has long been a metaphor for an episode of misery, and it is still understood to have that meaning. As a metaphor, "plague" may refer to a single crisis occurring to one person, or to a period of trouble for many people. The word "plague" in science and medicine now refers specifically to illness caused by a bacterium known as the plague bacillus, *Yersinia pestis*.

    In the latter part of the 2nd Millennium BCE, there are accounts of "plagues" in what we now call the Middle East or the Near East. In the Old Testament (Exodus 1-14), Moses asked God to inflict disaster on the Egyptians to induce the Pharaoh to let the Jews return to their Holy Land. The ten plagues of Egypt cannot be identified with certainty. Most of them were probably not infectious diseases, and there is endless speculation about what they may have been. A more convincing case for the existence of the disease now known as bubonic plague is the outbreak of *ophal* (Hebrew), translated as "emerods" (KJV) or "tumors" which afflicted the Israelites and the Philistines, and is described in I Samuel.[233]

    The Trojan War is believed to have taken place at about the same time as the war that is described in the books of Samuel. Troy, in what is now Turkey, is north of Israel on the east coast of the Mediterranean Sea. After the Greeks destroyed the city of Troy, Prince Aeneas led the survivors in a small fleet of ships which sailed west to an uncertain destination. After a sojourn in Carthage, the Trojans eventually arrived in Italy. The journey of Aeneas is described in Virgil's *The Aeneid*, which tells of a disaster known as the plague. Aeneas and his fellow Trojans first landed in Crete, where they hoped to establish a city, to be called Pergamum. They began to have families and to sow crops, and then,

> When, without warning, plague,
> Out of infected air to sap our bodies
> Came on us pitiable to see, and came
> To blight our trees and crops – a year of death.
> People relinquished their sweet lives or dragged
> Their wasted bodies on. …

The Trojans' plantations and grassland withered, and they were starving to death. It is not apparent what their terrible problem was, but the "plague … of infected air" probably meant a hot summer drought.[234]

B. Endemic – Epidemic – Pandemic

Epidemiologists are scientists who study diseases that affect groups of people. Infectious diseases can be classified as endemic, epidemic, and pandemic. Infectious diseases that are present in one part of the world are known as endemic diseases; they are always present, sometimes with alternating periods of resurgence and quiescence. Diseases that occur in episodes in large parts of the world are called epidemic diseases. Pandemic diseases, or simply pandemics, are world-wide variants of epidemic diseases.[235]

Endemic diseases that are always present include infections such as malaria, in tropical areas, and tuberculosis, world-wide; and those that are intermittent, usually in temperate zones, such as seasonal tick diseases, (Lyme disease and spotted fever). Epidemic diseases are episodic waves of resurgence of an endemic disease, such as mosquito-borne yellow fever, or of a disease that previously was unknown in the geographic area, such as cholera in Haiti. The yearly recurring seasonal influenza in the United States are epidemics of an endemic disease, which occur as the result of yearly changes in the genome of H1N1 influenza.[236]

Pandemics of diseases such as cholera, plague and influenza have altered the course of civilizations throughout history. Some of the most famous pandemics are the plague of Athens in 430 BCE, described by Thucydides; the Antonine Plague (also known as the Plague of Galen) in Rome, 165-180; and the Justinian plague in the 6th Century (also known as the Byzantine plague). And then there was the infamous "Black Death" (probably due to the plague bacillus, carried in rats and transmitted by the rat flea) which spread from Asia across Europe in the 14th century, striking Venice in 1630. The recurring episodes of plague killed perhaps one-third of the population of Europe, some 25 million people. Plague continued to ravage Europe. There was the Great Plague or Black Death of London, which spread back across Europe in 1664-66, with additional outbreaks until 1720 in Marseilles, with perhaps 300,000 deaths. A pause, of sorts, and then the Great Influenza of 1918-1919, the so-called "Spanish flu," which was responsible for 50,000,000 deaths from influenza and bacterial pneumonia. In the 20th century, two other pandemics were recognized: the 1957 Asian flu, and the 1968 Hong Kong flu, which caused between one million and four million deaths. More recently, we have had the H1N1 influenza in 2009-2010, which caused more than 14,000 deaths; and the current pandemic, caused by an RNA virus known as severe acute respiratory syndrome coronavirus 2 (abbreviated as SARS-CoV-2). This virus is said to have been accidentally transferred from an animal, perhaps a bat or pangolin, to humans in a food market in Wuhan, China. The pandemic, Coronavirus disease 2019 (abbreviated as COVID-19), caused by the virus SARS-CoV-2, first appeared in Wuhan in December 2019. It spread rapidly to other countries by persons who were infected in China, and who had no symptoms when they traveled throughout the world by air and on large tourist ships. More people in the world have probably been infected in this pandemic than any before, and it is still ongoing at the time of this writing.[237]

C. Biology and Biochemistry – The Chemistry of Life

In order to consider seriously the various little things that prey on human beings, it is necessary to review some aspects of science. Perhaps just enough to bring back memories of high school biology and chemistry. We begin with biology – the study of life – of living things – and biochemistry. Biology is the study of either lower forms (prokaryotes) or complex forms (eukaryotes). In eukaryotes, the genetic material is sequestered in a nucleus and other functions such as respiration are also carried out in distinct subcellular organelles. Prokaryotes perform all the functions of life within a single membranous structure. Many of the chemicals necessary for life contain molecules based on benzene rings that are referred to as organic compounds. Benzene "rings" are composed of six carbon atoms, and the structure of the 6-carbon benzene molecule is actually hexagonal, not a circular ring. In biology, we usually look at the life cycles of photosynthesis and of respiration from the perspective of animal life, in which oxygen is consumed and used for energy, and carbon dioxide (CO_2) is produced as a waste product. From the perspective of green plants, the energy in sunlight is captured by chlorophyll and used to convert carbon dioxide and water to oxygen and sugar. In photosynthesis, carbon dioxide is absorbed and oxygen is released. In the simplest form, six carbon dioxide molecules and six water molecules are converted by light energy into one sugar molecule, such as glucose, and six oxygen molecules. Plants and animals are dependent on each other. Plants cannot live without CO2 and H2O and animals cannot live without oxygen and sugar. A plant's need for water can be seen in the necessity for water to be added on a daily basis to a bowl in which a basil plant is growing in the sun on the kitchen window shelf. The water doesn't evaporate; it is used in photosynthesis. The process is mutually beneficial to animals and plants, because the source of energy is the sun, and it is transferred by photosynthesis from plants to animals. Animals are either protozoan (one-celled organisms, such as amoebas) or metazoan (many cells). Humans are metazoans.

Phototropism (movement toward light) is fascinating to watch in plants, but it usually requires patience to observe it. It can be seen during the day, when a day lily or daffodil opens up its petals. And when a sunflower gradually turns to keep facing the sun throughout the day. The sunflower droops a bit at sunset. Darwin observed phototropism; he called it *The Power of Movement of Plants* (1890). Phototropism is a useful complement for photosynthesis, because without light, plants cannot survive, nor can animals. Sunlight is the source of energy that drives phototropism. Surprisingly, a search for phototropism in *Britannica* is not rewarded. However, with the help of the internet, we can find much about the subject. For instance, there is auxin, the plant hormone that enables plants to face the light. In obscure scientific language, we learn that "Intracellular responses to light cues are processed to regulate cell-to-cell movement of auxin to allow establishment of a trans-organ gradient of the hormone."

Phototropism in animals is seen in many ways, but for different reasons than in plants. In earthworms, slugs, and ticks, negative phototropism is genetically transmitted behavior both for protection and for feeding. In birds, we have the rooster announcing the sunrise, and the sun awakens the robin, because "the early bird gets the worm." The investigator of a crime will ensure that hidden documents "will see the light of day." The phototropism of humans for health – the search for sunlight and warmth – involves many of the components of health, including shelter, communal living, love, lust, money, and also the exceptions. We see "snowbirds" from Canada and New Jersey heading for Florida in winter. From South Dakota to Phoenix, Arizona. In England, to the beach at Brighton; in France, to the Riviera; to the Jersey shore and to the Outer Banks in Delaware. College students search for mates at Spring break in Fort Lauderdale, and when they find each other, it's negative phototropism to cuddle in the darkness. Migrant workers follow the sun to work in cropland and in resorts. For exceptions, we see brilliant sunburns on foolish people who have spent too much time on the beach, and heat exhaustion in Death Valley and the Mohave Desert.[238]

All living things harbor other living things that live inside and outside of them; this is called a symbiotic relationship. Some of these relationships are beneficial to both (mutualism), many are harmful to one or the other (parasitism), and some live together in silent (commensal) harmony. This discussion will focus on parasites of humans. They range in size from intestinal tapeworms, which may be several feet in length; amoebae and bacteria, visible with a standard microscope; viruses, visible with an electron microscope; and abnormally folded proteins known as prions, which cause fatal diseases of the brain.[239]

The chemical composition of humans and their parasites includes mainly compounds of oxygen, carbon, and hydrogen, to which smaller amounts are added of nitrogen, calcium, phosphorus, potassium, sulfur, sodium, chlorine, and magnesium. In humans, oxygen comprises about 65% of the total, followed distantly by carbon (18.5%) and hydrogen (9.5%). The other eight elements are vital to life, but they amount to only 7% of the total. Additional trace elements also occur, amounting to less than 0.1 percent. The elements are combined into groups of compounds, with ratios that vary from person to person; for example, a person might contain water (60%), protein (15%), fat (18%) and bone (7%). The most important chemical compound in living things is deoxyribonucleic acid (DNA). Each species is characterized by the species' DNA; and furthermore, the precise identity of each human being is carried in the DNA of each person. DNA is located in the nucleus of each cell in chromosomes, of which there are 46 (23 pairs) in humans. The circular helix of DNA is composed of two strings of nitrogen base pairs (also known as nucleobases), organized in a spiral structure in which each base pair is linked with its opposite on the other string by a phosphate-ribose backbone. The four nitrogen bases in DNA are adenine, thymine, guanine, and cytosine – ATGC. The functions of DNA are to enable the development, survival, and reproduction of an individual. These functions are performed by enzymes – proteins – which are formed from DNA in a two-step process. In the first step, an enzyme reads the information in DNA and transcribes it into an intermediary molecule known as messenger ribonucleic acid (mRNA). RNA is similar to DNA, except that it has only one string, and uracil is substituted for guanine (ATUC). In the second step, the mRNA molecule is translated into the language of amino acids, from which proteins are constructed. The order of the amino acids determines the unique nature of each protein. Humans have 20 different amino acids, of which 11 can be synthesized and the other nine are "essential," and must be acquired in food.[240]

Humans are mostly composed of water (H_2O), which is the reason that oxygen is the largest component of human body mass. Oxygen has an atomic weight of 16, whereas hydrogen, atomic weight 1, is the lightest element in the universe. The combination of H_2O produces a molecular weight of 16+2= 18; with a ratio of 16/18, 88.8% of the weight of water is oxygen. The other elements that are crucial for humans are carbon (C), of which ribose and other carbohydrates are composed; nitrogen (N), which appears in the nitrogen bases of DNA and RNA and in the amino acids of proteins; phosphorus (P), which is an essential component of the backbone of DNA; and sulfur (S), which is in the essential amino acid, methionine. Calcium (Ca), magnesium (Mg), and other necessary substances are ordinarily consumed in an omnivorous diet. Dietary limitations may produce deficiencies in the requirement for sufficient calories, proteins, and vitamins. A wide variety of insidious diseases may occur, especially in children who live in poverty, but also in vegans who fail to consume the trace substances, and others who have dietary restrictions. However, an ovo-lactovegetarian diet includes eggs and milk, and it will provide all of the vitamins and trace minerals needed.[241]

D. Parasitology and Microbiology

Parasitology

There are five major groups of parasites of humans. Three groups are of very small organisms, which are visible only with a microscope. They include the four species of *Plasmodium*, which cause malaria, causing 400,000 deaths per year in the world; *Leishmania*, which causes leishmaniasis; *Entamoeba* and *Giardia*, which cause intestinal infections; and other unicellular protozoan parasites such as *Trypanosoma cruzi*, which causes Chagas disease. The fourth group, multicellular parasites, consists of small and large parasites that invade the body, including intestinal worms and other large parasites. This group includes such as helminths and arthropods. The fifth group is known as ectoparasites, which live on the exterior of the body. This group includes lice, ticks, and leeches. Examples of the members of each group are in the discussion that follows and in Appendix B, but there are many others that are not mentioned.[242]

Trichinosis is a disease caused by a tiny roundworm known as *Trichinella spiralis*, which is transmitted to humans from poorly cooked meat – usually pork, but occasionally from other omnivorous animals such as bear and dog meat. The worms migrate to internal organs and death may result from invasion of the heart or central nervous system. Trichinosis was probably a factor in the death of three men on a Swedish expedition which attempted to fly over the North Pole in 1897 in a hydrogen balloon. When the balloon failed, they landed on a small island near Svalbard, Norway, and perished within weeks, after shooting a polar bear, presumably for food. At autopsy, the bear had *Trichinella*.[243]

The group of ectoparasites includes lice, fleas, leeches, ticks, and many other small animals that live on the outside of the human body. A few are commensal symbiotics, living contentedly without harm to humans. There are various harmless bugs that exist in dirt and on the skin of an unwashed farmer. One – the bloodsucking leech – has occasionally had a mutualistic relationship with humans, in which both derive benefit. However, most ectoparasites are opportunistic, and the parasite derives benefit from its attachment to humans, without offering anything useful in return. This group includes lice, fleas, ticks, flies, mosquitos, and maggots, some of which are carriers of serious diseases; and many relatively harmless but annoying insects such as bedbugs.[244]

Let us first dispose of the leech. Leeches usually live in the water, but they can be harvested and placed in jars to be admired or to perform needed services. The ancient remedy for many diseases was to withdraw blood from the patient, either with a lancet (to piece a vein, usually the basilic vein at the front of the elbow joint; although occasionally in error, a small artery), or by attaching a leech. Many physicians, especially those who were not skilled in surgery, preferred the leech to the lancet; and so, too, did many patients. Such a physician would be called a "leech," which would not be a pejorative. It does take some courage to handle the slimy little bloodsuckers, but that is what the job calls for. The actual benefit from bloodletting was rare, but if perchance the patient had a condition of excess hemoglobin (known as polycythemia vera) it could be beneficial. In recent years, the leech has returned to the therapeutic armamentarium of surgeons. Leeches are now used to withdraw venous blood from a transplanted organ, such as a finger or leg, which becomes temporarily suffused when the arterial input into the transplant is greater than the venous drainage. After the venous connection is surgically adjusted or the suture line dilates sufficiently, the leech can be removed.[245]

The louse (plural lice) is an obligate parasite, meaning that it cannot live without its host. There are thousands of wingless insects in the order Phthiraptera, but only two are species of lice that affect humans: the pubic louse, *Pthirus pubis*, named for its affection for the nether parts; and the head louse and body louse, which are subspecies of *Pediculus humanus*. The body louse has the smallest genome of any insect. Each louse species is specifically domiciled to the parts of the body on which they live. The eggs of lice are known as nits, as in "nit-picking." Lice feed by chewing or sucking on secretions and debris found on their hosts. When infected by *Rickettsia prowazekii*, the body louse becomes the carrier of typhus, a disease that has recurred in epidemics through many centuries of human history. The Rickettsia are discussed below; they are tiny germs, intermediate in size between bacteria and viruses.[246]

Fleas are small flightless insects that prey on humans and other animals by consuming blood. They are often just pests, causing unpleasant itching, dermatitis, and anti-social behavior. People tend to avoid others who are scratching themselves. However, fleas are also vectors for many diseases. They are responsible for the transmission of two great scourges of humans – typhus and plague – and also for transmitting tapeworms and trypanosome protozoans.[247]

Ticks are members of a large class of invertebrates that are parasites on many animals. Although there are no ticks that are primarily human parasites, ticks carry many serious diseases that attack humans. Most ticks are hard ticks, meaning that they are difficult to squash. They include the common wood tick, which transmits diseases such as typhus and Rocky Mountain spotted fever; and the deer tick, which is responsible for Lyme disease, caused by a bacterial spirochete, *Borrelia burgdorferi*. Other tick-borne diseases include Q fever, tularemia, and various forms of hemorrhagic fever and encephalitis. Ticks are close relatives of mites, which are also transmitters of human diseases.[248]

Mosquitos have a necessary role to play in the ecology of the world, but they are a pest for humans. Some carry and transmit diseases, most notably *Anopheles* and *Aedes* species which infect millions of humans every year with malaria, yellow fever, and dengue. Clouds of mosquitos drove explorers back from northern Canada in the eighteenth century. Mosquitos tend to be larger in the northern latitudes, and the mosquito is said facetiously by some to be the "state bird of Minnesota." Hardly anyone would take a hike in the woods without applying Permethrin or Diamond (N,N-diethyl-meta-toluamide; DEET) to their clothing and exposed skin. The attempts to control mosquitos by spraying with Dichlorodiphenyltrichloroethane (DDT) and other insecticides has produced another series of catastrophes in the ecology of the world, eloquently described by Rachel Carson in *Silent Spring*.[249]

Maggot is the unofficial name for the larvae of flies, usually the common housefly and blowfly. The fly can transmit many diseases in its residue, as it eats its way through feces and foodstuffs and deposits its own fecal matter. The maggot and the fly are ectoparasites; that is to say, they usually are found only on the surface of human beings. Most people find a cluster of maggots to be totally repulsive – a wriggling mass of little wet, wormy things, dead white in color, about a quarter of an inch in length, piled upon each other. However, maggots also have important medical uses. The presence and development of maggots on a corpse, and of flies that develop from these maggots, is used to estimate the time of death. Maggots are also useful medical devices. Live, disinfected maggots are approved by the Food and Drug Administration to be used for debridement of nonhealing wounds.[250]

E. Microbiology

Microbiology is the study of tiny living things using the microscope. The microscope and laboratory techniques involving chemistry were originally used to study bacteria, which can only be seen through the microscope. The field was then called bacteriology. New laboratory methods have since been developed, including tissue culture and the electron microscope, to study smaller microorganisms, such as viruses, and the name of field has therefore been changed to microbiology.[251]

The microbial world consists of prokaryotes and eukaryotes. Prokaryotes are single cells without a membrane-bound nucleus. Eukaryotes include organisms with a membrane-bound nucleus, and all multi-celled organisms, including the largest plants and animals. However, only the smallest of the eukaryotes are considered as microbes. The field of microbiology encompasses the subjects of bacteria, algae, fungi, protozoa, viruses, prions, lichens, and slime molds. The microbiology of humans focuses on bacteria, fungi, viruses, and prions; protozoa were discussed above as parasites, and lichens and slime molds do not ordinarily infect humans.[252]

The field of microbiology began with the development of the microscope in the mid-1670s by Antonie van Leeuwenhoek. His hobby was grinding lenses and making devices to look through them. Leeuwenhoek documented the "animalicules" that he saw with the microscope in letters to the Royal Society, although this seemed initially to have little relevance to scientists at that time. By the 18th century, questions about the origin of life and of disease, spoilage, and fermentation were being studied with the microscope. In the late 1880s, Louis Pasteur, in France, showed that spontaneous generation of bacteria was impossible, and Robert Koch, in Germany, defined the postulates that would prove that a specific organism caused a specific disease. American scientists were slow to accept the microscope and to study microbiology. However, in 1923, in the United States, David Bergey established the modern system for the classification of bacteria, which still remains as the standard system.[253]

Bacteria

Bacteria are categorized in various ways, but for simplicity we will refer to them primarily in relation to the Gram stain. With this staining method, some are gram-positive, and under the microscope they appear to be purple. Others types are gram-negative; they appear to be pink. Some are motile, with one or more flagella. Some produce spores and can live in a dormant stage for many years, while others proliferate rapidly. Some require oxygen; they are called aerobic. Some, known as anaerobes, live without oxygen, and others live best with a reduced amount of oxygen. Some are rod-shaped, some are rounded (cocci), and some have a spiral shape. Some are clustered, while others grow in chains.

Bacteria are also classified on the basis of the medium on which they can be cultured. *Mycobacterium tuberculosis* was difficult to stain for microscopic examination, but this problem was solved with a stain known as "acid fast." *M. tuberculosis* was also difficult to culture in the laboratory, but this problem was solved with a special growth medium and waiting patiently for colonies to appear. It sometimes takes as long as six weeks. *M. tb's* relative, *M. leprae*, cannot be cultured in the laboratory, but it grows in the footpad of the armadillo.

Many diseases of humans are caused by bacteria. Some are causes of death, some cause misery, and others may be causes for concern. On the other hand, many species of commensal bacteria co-exist with humans, and are usually harmless. Some are even necessary for human existence, such as gut commensal bacteria that synthesize and transport some vitamins from foods. Other commensal bacteria are not ordinarily a problem, but in a person whose immune response is compromised, a non-pathogen may suddenly become deadly. Broad spectrum antibiotics upset the normal balance of gut microbes. The ecology of the normal microbiome is of interest to many scientists at this time.[254]

Viruses

Viruses are infectious agents of small size and simple composition that can multiply only in living cells of animals, plants, or bacteria. Viruses can be classified by the type of nucleic acid that they consist of, and which they use in replication. The three viral classes are RNA viruses, DNA viruses, and reverse transcribing viruses, which reverse-transcribe double-stranded DNA and single-stranded RNA viruses. Reverse transcribing RNA viruses includes retroviruses.[255]

Viruses that are transmitted by arthropods are called informally by the term arboviruses (from arthropod borne viruses). Mosquitos and ticks are the arthropods that are most hazardous to humans. The range of mosquitos has enlarged with global warming. Some examples of arboviruses are: Yellow fever, Dengue, Rift Valley (RV) fever, West Nile Virus fever (WNV), Eastern Equine Encephalomyelitis (EEE), Tick-borne encephalitis, and Japanese encephalitis. For more about viruses, see Appendix B.[256]

Some of the important viruses and viral diseases of humans are:
RNA viruses[257]

Rabies, known as hydrophobia, is usually incurable. It is usually transmitted from the bite of a rabid dog or a wild animal such as a bat. The incubation period is usually one to three months, but may be as long as several years. Rabies may be prevented if a vaccine and antiserum are promptly administered, and a vaccine is available for those who are at risk, such as veterinarians.[258]

Measles, also called rubeola, is a highly contagious disease, unique to humans. It is an airborne disease, with an incubation period of 7 to 10 days. It presents with a red flat skin rash, and progresses to pneumonia, diarrhea, and central nervous system infection. Vaccination is an effective preventive.[259]

Dengue fever, or breakbone, is one of several diseases caused by viruses of the *Flavivirus* genus. Dengue is very debilitating, though not usually fatal. It is transmitted by the bite of an *Aedes* mosquito, *A. Aegypti* or *A. albopictus*. Immunity exists after infection, but there are at least four serotypes and infection with each type is required for complete immunity. Epidemics are increasing in frequency.[260]

Yellow fever causes jaundice – yellow skin – as patients die. Epidemics of yellow fever have been some of the most lethal episodes in human history. Dr. Benjamin Rush treated patients in Philadelphia in 1793, when 10% of the population died. The American military physician, Walter Reed, showed in 1900 that yellow fever was transmitted by the bite of an *Aedes* mosquito, and this enabled the Panama Canal to be built. Monkeys are also infected, so the disease can probably never be completely eliminated. A vaccine was perfected in 1937 which conveys lifelong immunity with a single dose.[261]

West Nile fever is caused by another Flavivirus. It is primarily a disease of birds, but it is spread from the avian host to humans by mosquitoes. It is usually a mild infection, with flu-like symptoms, but it can progress to encephalitis and cause death. Formerly limited to Asia and Africa, it has spread to Europe and the Americas in recent years. Zika is another Flavivirus disease, with a similar outcome.[262]

Picornaviruses are the cause of many diseases, most of which are relatively rare or non-specific in nature. Rhinoviruses are in this group of tiny viruses; more than one hundred varieties are the cause of the common cold. Coxsackie A and B viruses cause illnesses that are similar to the common cold, but may progress to involve many organs of the body and can be fatal. Enteroviruses cause diarrhea; hand, foot and mouth disease; myocarditis; encephalitis; and poliomyelitis. Poliomyelitis, also called "polio" or infantile paralysis, is transmitted through the fecal-oral route. The disease probably existed in antiquity; it appears to have been in ancient Egypt, but it became epidemic only in the 18th century. Most infections are not apparent, but muscle weakness develops in a small percentage. Polio causes death in up to 10 percent of these patients, and those who survive may have immediate or late recurring muscle weakness. Vaccines have been developed which may eliminate the disease, but the end is elusive.[263]

Influenza, or "flu" viruses, cause a wide variety of diseases that are spread from person to person through the respiratory tract. The diseases range from minor illnesses, similar to the common cold, to devastating pandemics, such as the so-called Great Influenza or "Spanish flu" of 1918-19 which killed some 25 million people. The Great Influenza was caused by Type A influenza, H1N1, a strain that still exists and which mutates frequently. A variant of H1N1 known as swine flu caused an outbreak in 2009. Other strains of Type A influenza are H2N2, the cause of Asian flu; H3N2, Hong flu; and H5N1, avian (bird) flu. Influenza control requires annual vaccinations and avoiding person-to-person spread.[264]

Corona virus diseases: SARS (Severe Acute Respiratory Syndrome Corona Virus) was first seen in humans in 2002. It probably originated from an animal reservoir, perhaps horseshoe bats or pangolins, with some genetic changes. SARS causes fever, cough, muscle aches, difficulty in breathing, and it may progress to multi-organ failure. MERS (Middle East Respiratory Syndrome) caused by MERS-CoV was first seen in 2012. The present pandemic, COVID-19, is due to a new variant known as SARS-CoV-2.[265]

Hepatitis viruses occur in several strains, labelled as A, B, C, D, E. All affect the liver, hence the name; but many also affect other organs. All are RNA viruses except hepatitis B, which is a DNA virus (see below). The route of transmission and the severity of disease is variable. Hepatitis A is usually spread by the fecal-oral route and patients usually recover without lasting effects. Hepatitis C is also bloodborne and can progress to cirrhosis and death.[266]

Ebola, a virus disease named for the Ebola River, first appeared in 1976 in the northern Congo area. Episodes of Ebola have recurred on several occasions since then, with a 50-90 percent mortality rate. Ebola is a hemorrhagic fever disease, spread by blood and body fluids. Ebola also causes disseminated intravascular coagulation, and patients therefore suffer from both abnormal bleeding and clotting. To date, the epidemics have been contained in Africa. Several strains of the virus have been identified in humans and chimpanzees, but the principal animal reservoir has not yet been found.[267]

DNA viruses[268]

Smallpox (variola major) is one of the most terrifying epidemic diseases in human history. It begins with fever and headache, and an eruption of disfiguring pockmarks, which can be permanent. It appeared in Mesopotamia in the 5th millennium BC, with deaths occurring in 30 percent of patients. Smallpox has no known animal reservoir, and survivors have life-long immunity. Edward Jenner first observed in 1796 that milkmaids who had a similar disease, cowpox (vaccinia), did not develop smallpox. Jenner inoculated cowpox scabs and found that they prevented smallpox; he coined the term, "vaccination." A world-wide program of vaccination led to the elimination of the disease in 1980.[269]

Herpes viruses are classified in three subfamilies: Alpha includes the human herpes simplex viruses and varicella-zoster virus; beta includes cytomegalovirus; and gamma, which includes the Epstein-Barr virus (EBV). Kaposi's sarcoma virus, also known as human herpesvirus 8, has been grouped with the gamma family. Herpes simplex virus, type 1, causes cold sores; type 2 is a cause of genital herpes, which is associated with cancer of the cervix and possibly contributes to Alzheimer's disease. Herpes viruses may be asymptomatic and can be transmitted unknowingly. Cytomegalovirus infection does not usually result in serious illness, although sometimes it is a cause of pneumonia and childhood diseases, and in immunocompromised patients it can be devastating. EBV is the cause of infectious mononucleosis, the so-called "kissing disease" which debilitates students of college age, and it is associated with tumor cells of Burkitt's lymphoma. Human herpesvirus 8 is associated with Kaposi's sarcoma in patients with AIDS (acquired immunodeficiency syndrome) and other sarcomas.[270]

Varicella-zoster virus causes chicken pox (varicella) and herpes zoster (shingles). Chicken pox is a childhood disease that occurs in epidemics, producing itchy papules and fever, but usually without lasting harm. However, in adults and in immunocompromised persons, it can cause fatal pneumonia. Infection produces permanent immunity, but the virus may linger in nerve ganglions and cause painful eruption in the area of a single nerve. An anti-zoster vaccine has been developed.[271]

Adenoviruses are any viruses belonging to the family Adenoviridae. Most of the illnesses caused by more than 40 species of adenovirus are similar in symptoms to those caused by hundreds of slightly different RNA rhinoviruses that cause the common cold.[272]

Enterobacteriophage. Phages are viruses that infect bacteria, some of which in turn are infections for humans. Bacteriophages infect *E. coli*, and have potential for control of coliform diseases.[273]
Reverse Transcribing Viruses and Retroviruses[274]

Hepatitis B is transmitted by blood. A DNA retrovirus, hepatitis B causes chronic hepatitis, and is also an oncovirus (meaning tumor virus). It is a major world-wide cause of cancer of the liver.[275]

HIV-1 and HIV-2 (Human Immunodeficiency Virus 1 and 2) are causes of the acquired immunodeficiency syndrome (AIDS). HIV is a lentivirus, meaning "slow virus," a retrovirus that destroys the body's defense against infection and some forms of cancer by attacking a class of white blood cells known as CD4+ T cells (helper T lymphocytes). AIDS first appeared in 1981 in male homosexuals who had a rare pulmonary infection caused by *Pneumocystis carinii*, and soon after that it was reported in male homosexuals with Kaposi's sarcoma. HIV, the causative agent, was described in 1983. HIV appears to have originated in African apes. AIDS has become a world-wide disease, spread by body fluids, by sexual contacts, and to an unborn child. Behavior modification would reduce the incidence of transmission of HIV, but it has been difficult to effect the needed changes. Antiretroviral therapy and vaccines have reduced somewhat the risk of acquiring HIV and developing AIDS.[276]

Human T-lymphotropic virus (HTLV-1) causes T-cell leukemia in humans.[277]

Human papilloma virus (HPV) is a sexually-transmitted DNA retrovirus. HPV commonly infects most humans, ordinarily with only minor symptoms. Genital warts or laryngeal papillomatosis develop in ten percent of cases, and it is the main cause of cervical cancer. A preventive vaccine is available.[278]

F. COVID-19

The COVID-19 pandemic is the greatest problem of infectious disease in more than a century. COVID-19 is a unique problem in human history, for it has spread quicker and more widely than any previous pandemic. The last pandemic that can be compared with COVID-19 is the Great Influenza of 1918-1919. With no known method of prevention, and no known treatment, the disease caused by the severe acute respiratory syndrome coronavirus 2 (SARS-CoV-2) has infected millions of people in every continent. Many have died, many more have been sickened, and still others have had the disease and are not fully recovered. Many others, unknowingly, have had silent infections. As I began writing this part of the essay on June 29, 2020, I could say that the curve of incidence and deaths is still rising and end of the pandemic is far from sight. By July 6, the U.S. has had 3 million cases diagnosed, with 127,621 deaths. On July 28, 2020, the total had reached 4.3 million in the U.S., with 145,054 deaths. The World Health Organization (WHO) calls it the "most severe" pandemic in history. The reported incidence appeared to level off at about 65,000 new cases per day, although case finding is incomplete and deaths from COVID-19 are probably undercounted. As of May 2021, COVID-19 was still rising in many parts of the world, and on June 16, 2021, the death toll from COVID-19 in the U.S. was estimated to be 600,000.[279]

The actions proposed by public health professionals are (1) mitigation, or (2) containment. Mitigation includes social distancing (separation of people by six feet, whenever possible); wearing face masks; and hand-sanitizing. Containment involves identification of cases, contact tracing, and quarantine. The pandemic has already had enormous consequences, reflected in severe economic distress, disruption of travel, of education, of commerce, and in local and national politics and international relations. Those who already were poor have suffered most. The end is not in sight – not even the beginning of the end.[280]

Howard Bauchner, Editor-in-Chief of *JAMA*, said that 2020 was "a year that will be remembered," along with 1776, 1865, 1941, 1963, and 2001. Bauchner wrote on 21 July 2020 that the "Confluence of events and their immediate consequences during the first half of 2020 have challenged society, government, and medicine in profound and perhaps unprecedented ways."[281]

Responses to COVID-19 are derived from Latin *de*, *disfacere*, meaning negation of *facere* (to do): Denial, Defiance, Despair, Decision, Desert, Defeat, and Death

We now turn to consider the development of human history as it involves all of the components of health that were discussed individually in Part One. In Part Two, we will see how human history moved forward, in sickness and in health, to end with the present Health Care Industry.

Health Matters

Part Two

Health Matters in Human History

Chapter 10

Health and Illness in the History of Medicine, Science, and Technology

This essay proposes that health is the fundamental driving force in human history. *Health Matters* proposes that the search for health involves the knowledge that if you don't prepare for the future, something bad will surely happen, and that you will have poor health. *Health Matters* argues that the goal of life for humans is to delay the ultimate end point, which is death.

Health Matters argues that the goal of humans is now, and always has been, the search for good health and a long life. History depends on humans' beliefs about health. Humans have always asked how to be healthy. The answer in *Health Matters* is to avoid illness, to treat disease, and thus to delay death.

Part One of this essay discussed the fundamental requirements – the needs, urges, desires, and wants – that humans have, and what they must find and secure in order to be healthy. It also examined the various exceptions that humans have made to these fundamental requirements. Some of the exceptions are beneficial, while other exceptions have been harmful, or accidental, or which sometimes benefited other humans. The most prominent exception to the fundamental requirements, however, is the exception that is created by religion. This is the name we give to the invisible, insatiable desire of many humans: a desire of the mind and spirit, to explain what humans could only imagine, and which would help them to achieve health. The desire to explain the unexplainable, which in this essay is called religion, cannot be quenched. It is a fundamental component of the life of humans as they try to explain the past and as they think of the future.

Part Two of the essay on *Health Matters* examines the scope of human history from the earliest humanoids, who preceded *Homo sapiens*, to the present time, when humans have started to make living genetic copies of themselves, and when they also learned to make mechanical copies of themselves – of robots often known as androids. That is admittedly a large project. The subject of religion appears early in this project, and religion in one form or another has been persistent throughout human history. Part Two considers human history from the earliest times that it can be documented in the archaeological record. It focuses primarily on the history of the Middle East and Europe, because the sequential record is well documented there. The history in Part Two is that of the impact of health on humans, as seen in the development of medicine, science, and technology; and on the various ways that good health or illness and death impacted on individuals or groups of people.[282]

****

Health Matters conceives human history to be the movement through time of the human species, *Homo sapiens* subspecies *sapiens*, including aspects that are not documented in writing. In this view, human history is everything that has happened since humans first appeared on earth. The earliest forms of writing appeared only 5,000 years ago in Babylonia and Egypt, some 300,000 years after humans and their humanoid ancestors first appeared in East Africa. That early period, once called "prehistoric," from 300,000 years BCE until 5,000 BCE, is also part of human history. Even today, much of what should be considered as human history is narrated. It is oral history, and it is not documented in writing. Some of it is not even observed by humans. The search for truth in history is complicated because anecdotes give different stories, and written documents are sometimes in conflict.

The search for human health began in Africa, as the first members of *Homo sapiens* evolved from other species of hominids. Other species of the genus *Homo* were probably evolving in different parts of the world at about the same time, and even later, but *Homo sapiens sapiens*, who interbred in Europe with another subspecies, the Neanderthals, eventually became the dominant hominid. Earlier hominids, such as *Australopithecus*, date to 5.6 million years ago in East Africa. Other species of hominids were found outside of Africa about 1.8 million years ago. The primate ancestors of hominids, such as *Afropithecus*, known as hominoids, date to 24 million years ago. Note the slight difference: hominoid vs. hominid.

Paleoanthropologists now conclude that *Ardipithecus*, a climbing, walking proto-human lived in what is now Ethiopia about 4.4 million years ago. And then 3.3 million years ago, it begat a tool-maker, *Kenyanthropus*. The argument in *Health Matters* is based on what can be surmised about human's search for health over the last 2.5 million years, from the beginning of the Stone Age to the end of the Iron Age, and then what is known thereafter in the written and unwritten record about health and history.[283]

Health Matters does not view the history of humans as progress, in the sense of moving upward, but rather as changes that have occurred sequentially in the lifetimes of humans. Before the invention of cuneiform inscriptions, of hieroglyphics, and of writing, these changes took place in different parts of the world, when little interaction was possible between groups of people. The nearly simultaneous development of some aspects of human life is both interesting and relevant, because humans in widely different locations discovered the use of fire, of fishing, and of agriculture. The changes in human history are usually grouped into categories, such as medicine, science, technology, religion, law, the arts and the humanities. However, the many interactions between these fields suggest that another approach is needed. This essay continues by showing some of the ways that each of these categories has influenced the others. The discussion must be anecdotal, for there is neither time nor space to do justice to the entire subject of human history as a single movement of people and things, flowing through space and time.[284]

The view of human history in *Health Matters* is of a much longer period of time than that of some historians, who even now regard history only as that which is documented; or grudgingly and dismissively regard unwritten history as historical supposition, based on published reports of anthropological and archaeological discoveries or oral history. *Health Matters* goes beyond the published reports to speculate on what is likely to have happened in the past, step by step, throughout human history, in the quest for health. This is not the first essay to have proposed connections between some of these fields, but it takes a bolder step than has previously been taken. Other historians have proposed that human social groups have had, since earliest times, a person with an ability to treat illness, using methods that included forms of medicine, of primitive surgery, and ceremonies. These methods are still in use by indigenous people who live in remote areas such as the Kalahari in East Africa, the Amazon jungle, and in the canyons of Papua New Guinea. The priest-healers or, if you wish, the healer-priests, of pre-recorded history and those in the modern jungle or desert have been called "medicine men" or "sorcerers" or "witch doctors" or "shamans" by anthropologists and historians. In the person of a healer-priest, medicine and religion began simultaneously. Others have traced the development of science, technology, and art from this primitive form of medicine; and modern forms of religion must also have evolved from the priest-healers. *Health Matters*, however, asks the reader to accept a novel proposal, which has not previously been suggested. It is that medicine is the mother of science and technology. It is not an orphan, nor a step-child. *Health Matters* argues that the search for health is the primary goal of humans, and the field of medicine was present at the time that humans began that search.[285]

Health Matters also takes an unusual approach to the fields of medicine, science, technology, and the arts, as I suggest that the boundaries between these fields are porous. *Health Matters* suggests that the history of each of these fields cannot be fully separated from the others. Religion is also involved with each of these fields, when they began, and to the present time. A few examples illustrate the shifting boundaries and overlapping histories of medicine, science, technology and the various art forms, which include theatre and dance, visual arts – painting, drawing, and photography – and also literature and poetry, which evolved from the use of language and writing for communication. The study of history – of historiography – is overarching and does not easily fall into any of these categories. History must be viewed with the eye of a scientist and written with the narrative art of a novelist.

Health Matters emphasizes the need to practice whatever has been chosen as a field in which to work. For example, we describe the physician's work as the "practice of medicine," and that a lawyer "practices" his profession. We are reassured that the best outcome for an actor will result from practicing in endless rehearsals. The word "practice" describes the sketches that an artist or composer makes and then revises before completing a final painting or a published work of music. Practice makes perfect, as the saying goes.

There is often overlap between these fields. Some physicians, such as Hector Berlioz, have also been gifted composers of music, and some of the most prolific technologists have also made important contributions to science. For instance, Thomas Edison, America's most famous inventor, also described the "Edison effect" of electric current. Edison was a technologist and also a scientist. Technology is vital in the study of science. Most of the new developments in science have been the result of new tools that are used by experimenters, such as Galileo's telescope, Leeuwenhoek's microscope, the development of tissue culture, and the recent discovery of CRISPR DNA sequences, just to mention a few examples.[286]

A. Human History from the Perspective of Health

In this section of *Health Matters*, the history of human health is examined from two points of view. The first point of view is topical, and the second is chronological. The reader will see the relationship of health to history as it repeats many times in the next few pages. Illness and death and the matters of health are companions in the development of human history.

The previous chapters outlined the components of human health, including what humans need for health, what humans should avoid to be healthy, and what they should use in moderation. Some beliefs about health were also examined as examples of influences on health behavior, as they appeared to groups of people in different parts of the world, over the course of many centuries. The previous chapters showed the many ways in which health is diminished, and how life comes to an end.

All humans have been interested in health, either consciously or subconsciously. The profession of medicine has always been the leading agent for human health. In this section we see that medicine also acted in concert in many ways with science and technology. Additionally, it will show that health and medicine developed concurrently with other aspects of history, such as political history, the history of the arts and humanities, and religion. These other aspects of history include the history of societies and the law, of warfare and conquest, of intellectual history; and also, history examined from various perspectives, such as women's history, and history "from the bottom up." Finally, there will be examples of the various ways that health and medicine have played roles in human history, as individuals and populations either had good health or ill health at crucial moments in time.[287]

The beginning of human history in respect to *Health Matters* is when our species first began to use weapons to project power, and when we first began to use fire. There is no written record that tells when these two events occurred in different parts of the world, and the archaeological record is incomplete. Nevertheless, we can move forward from this uncertain point in time to recognize the development of the various components of health that were mentioned in the previous section. Some of these contributions to human health were discovered and assimilated by many peoples, at unknown points in time. The pace gradually quickened, and in the past few centuries, discoveries can be credited to specific individuals. A few illustrative examples will be given of important moments in the history of human health, though the list must be incomplete.[288]

The idea expressed in *Health Matters* began to germinate many years ago in the course of preparing to give lectures on the subject of history and human health. However, the idea began to coalesce in 1997 with Roy Porter's book *The Greatest Benefit to Mankind*. Porter said that his subtitle, *A Medical History of Mankind,* meant that "My focus could have been on disease and its bearing on human history," which is the heart of my argument in *Health Matters*. Porter continued: "Historians at large, who until recently tended to chronicle world history in blithe ignorance or of or indifference to disease, now recognize the difference made by plague, cholera and other pandemics." However, Porter was not satisfied simply to call attention to this deficiency in historians; he wanted to place "the history of *medical* thinking and *medical* practice at stage center," by concentrating on "medical ideas about disease, medical teachings about healthy and unhealthy bodies, and medical models of life and death." Porter believed that "medicine has played a major and growing role in human societies and for that reason its history needs to be explored so that its place and powers can be understood." He said that writing his book "brought home the collective and largely irremediable ignorance of historians about the medical history of mankind."

Porter observed that "all societies possess medical beliefs: ideas of life and death, disease and cure, and systems of healing." He said that "In Europe from Graeco-Roman antiquity onwards, and also among the great Asian civilizations, the medical profession systematically replaced transcendental explanations by positing a natural basis for disease and healing." He stated that "modern westerners" want "their flesh to last as long as possible." Nevertheless, "Eschewing anachronism, judgmentalism and history by hindsight," and recognizing the "continued phenomenal progress of capital-intensive and specialized medicine," Porter wrote that, "one can study winners without siding with them." *Health Matters* goes beyond what Porter thought about human history. *Health Matters* proposes that the principal theme in human history has been about health. All of the branches of history have been influenced by health beliefs, health practices, and health outcomes.[289]

For purposes of this discussion, *Health Matters* focuses on the history of Western civilization, as it arose in the Fertile Crescent, east of the Mediterranean Sea, and in Egypt. Much of human history occurred before that time, and elsewhere in the world – in central, eastern and southern Asia, in the Americas, and also on many islands, the largest being Australia. The argument regarding the subject of health in human history (including its reciprocal, illness and death) would not be confounded by including what is known or has been reported about history in other parts of the world. However, limits on space and time allow me to include but a few examples from these geographic areas and cultures in this essay.

The subject of health and history begins with archeological evidence and anonymous or pseudonymous stories that precede the earliest written records. The earliest forms of writing in the Western world may be cuneiform inscriptions of financial transactions in what is now Iraq. Or perhaps they were hieroglyphs inscribed in ink on papyrus or carved into stones in Egypt. However, long before there were great cities in the Middle East, such as Babylon, and great civilizations developed along the Nile in Egypt, humans appeared as hunter-gatherers. Many generations later, some hunter-gatherers became the first fishermen, and then some became farmers, and later they became the first to dwell in small cities. Archaeologists have helped us to understand this sequential development of human civilization.

After the last Ice Age began to recede, and the Middle East gradually became warmer, humans began to cluster in small groups to search for food around the waters' edges, and hunter-gatherers became fishermen. Some satisfied their hunger with salt water fish and crustaceans from the Mediterranean Sea, while others found fresh water fish and other edible animals in the Baltic Sea. Still others settled near rivers, pulling up fish and eels by hand or with simple tools, which were forerunners of hooks, lines, and nets. The first villages were formed by these small groups of human families. Some of the coastal villages enlarged, as families clustered into clans of distant cousins. At about the same time, some members of the villages began to study the vegetation near their waterside homes. In this way, hunter-gatherers became the first agriculturalists as they explored ways to convert naturally growing edible plants into annual and perennial crops of vegetables and fruits. The farmers were able to move their families further from the water, and they gradually developed independence from the predominantly meat diet of hunter-gatherers and fishermen. Fruits and vegetable products could be preserved for use in winter, and they allowed for protection against a shortfall in daily needs.

The first inland towns, or small cities, developed at that time – perhaps 10,000 years ago – in the Middle East. Jericho, of Biblical fame, in Jordan, is said to have been one of the first settlements that can be called a city. Specialization in work became possible in cities, and thus new occupations flourished as individuals found that they had useful skills. In addition to the earliest occupation, that of the priest-healer (or medicine man), the handicrafts of weaving and pottery-making soon appeared. Basic weaving with sticks and vines had been known by hunter-gatherers, but the craft of intricate weaving with fibers flourished with specialization and domestication of plants, especially grass. Physicians and potters were the first to experiment with chemicals, including those that produced color – which was used creatively by those gifted with the art of painting. The use of fire and earth in making pottery led to the discovery of how to make glass with sand and fire. This led to making tinted glass and works of art from glazed pottery and glass, such as mosaics. Pottery making, using fire and earth, also led to the understanding of forging metals – first of bronze and later of iron – and then to the methods of making steel for weapons.

Ways were soon discovered to create bricks from earth that was baked in the sun or heated with fire, and homes were constructed in the cities from these bricks. All of these developments, from hunter-gatherers to fishermen and farmers, and then to city dwellers with specialization of forms of work, were the result of a relentless search by humans for health, in all of its components.

The skills of fishermen were enhanced when boats were created to allow them to go far from shore. At first, there would only have been simple rafts, assembled from logs that were tied together with vines, and later tied together with ropes made from stout grasses. Other forms of watercraft included hollowed out logs, and also boats that were made from skins or bark or which were assembled from tightly fitted staves of wood. The first boats were propelled with paddles, but gradually nautical architecture developed and early modern watercraft emerged, using oars and sails of leather and cloth. Some sailors had the gift of navigation, and were able to return to home when it was out of sight, guided by the position of the sun, moon, and stars. They utilized the knowledge that both the sun and moon appeared on one side of the earth in the morning, and both sun and moon disappeared on the other horizon in the evening. This enabled the early navigators to know the directions that we call east and west. The sun at midday was high in the sky, but it was not directly overhead; north of what we call the Equator, it was in the part of the sky that we call south. Some clever observers (also north of the Equator) noticed that at night there was a star that was always seen in the part of the sky that was opposite to where the sun had been at mid-day; we call that direction north, and the star is Polaris.

The sun and moon had different cycles as the year progressed, and the cycles returned each year. The sun had daily cycles and also a yearly cycle. The moon, on the other hand, had cycles that lasted 28 days. These observations led to speculation about the purpose of the cycles. They believed there was meaning to the cycles. The behavior of sun, moon, and stars (some of which we now call planets) were explained by the priest-healer. There could be no doubt at that time that the earth was the center of everything, and that the sun, moon, and stars revolved around Earth. And it was stated in Genesis, and it became a matter of faith. "Flat earth" was not a matter of faith at that time, however, for some people probably assumed that the earth was round. This would be the only way to understand the disappearance of a person as he grew smaller as he walked away, but did not disappear completely as he began to pass beyond the horizon. Also, it was the only way to explain how the sun was higher in the sky at mid-day as they moved in one direction (south) and the sun was lower in the sky at mid-day when they traveled in the other direction (north). But the idea of a "flat earth" was of little interest at that time, and "flat earth" was not then a religious belief. This was unlike the notion of a geocentric universe, in which the Earth was obviously in the center of it all. The geocentric universe was God's creation, as described in Genesis.

Mathematics gradually developed, as humans began to count and to observe the geometry of the world. Humans had four fingers, or five if the thumb is counted, and ten if both hands are counted, and twenty if the hands and feet are counted. These counts would be useful. And although it is said that "nature abhors a straight line," they saw straight lines when objects cast shadows. A straight line was the shortest route for a walk to the well for water and back, so "straight" became the favorite street in the early cities. Early humans were familiar with the circle, because round or circular objects could be seen in nature, such as the circular trunks of trees, and the orb of the moon, when it was full, and the eggs of birds. One of the most important round objects was the wheel. The wheel appears independently in both east and west Asia. Strangely, in eastern Asia, such as Nepal, the wheel is used for conveying prayers, rather than for locomotion or for moving water. There may have been a religious significance for not using the wheel for locomotion. In western Asia, the wheel was used for the many purposes with which we are familiar, including wheeled carts, the water wheel for power and irrigation, and the potter's wheel.

Builders of houses were the earliest architects. They needed to assemble bricks in level courses, and to lay each course on the previous one without vertical variance. Water was used as to mark the level of each course, and a straight side of the building could be assured with a plumb line that measured the vertical exterior. The purpose of architecture was to build a safe structure; beauty of the structure was important, but it was secondary to health and safety.

Domestication of plants and animals proceeded as humans continued to improve their ability to farm and also to dwell in cities. Of the vegetables, the most important was grass, which was bred into strains that were edible (especially wheat, used in the traditional Asian flatbread) and useable fibers (such as flax, jute, and hemp, from which both rope and drugs, such as cannabis, are made). Of fruits, the most important were the grape and plum, because dried, they become durable raisins and prunes; apples, too, were a favorite, because they are long-lasting in storage. Animals that were domesticated early were the dog, horse, fowl (especially chickens), and camel, and there were also opportunistic domesticates such as sparrows and rodents. Some animals were seen as being potentially dangerous for food, such as shell fish and hogs, and consumption of them was regulated by the priest-healers. Domesticated animals introduced many of the ecto- and endo-parasites that have long bedeviled humans, such as fleas, flies, and microbes.

The role of gender in the early cities probably perpetuated what had already been a division of labor in hunter-gatherers and fisher folk. Women were cloistered – sheltered at home – and after puberty they would be covered, or at least their hair would be hidden. A woman was then, as a woman still was in Puritan New England, a *femme covert* (covered woman). During the menstrual period, women would have privacy, but otherwise they were at the mercy of their husbands. Children's lives changed at puberty. Ceremonies were held for boys and girls that announced to them and to their families that they had entered young adulthood. New names, often secret, were given to them in the rites of passage. The hierarchy of men was established in a way that ensured peace in the community. The men would sit for long periods to discuss social problems – to resolve civil disputes without bloodshed, and to determine punishment for crimes. The gathering of tribal elders known as the *loya jirga* persists to this day in Afghanistan. Other gatherings of elders under the baobab trees still make decisions in East Africa. Laws were unwritten at that time, but the principle of *stare decisis* (the precedent stands) provided guidance.

The hunter-gatherers had priest-healers, sometimes known as medicine-men. Often one person would play both roles, but gradually differences appeared that distinguished the priest, whose realm was the unseen or imagined world, from the person who was concerned with the tangible, visible world. The visible world is now known as science and technology, but in the early city, it was ordinary daily life. The early physician was somewhere between these two worlds, sometimes using technology to treat illness and cure disease, and at other times, using incantation and the power of suggestion as an important part of the art of healing. A wise physician always listens to his patients, to ensure that the treatment he or she recommends is consistent with what the patient believes is reasonable. What we call "culture" plays a significant role in this relationship between patient and physician.[290]

B. Developments in Human Health
Topical Viewpoint

Part One explored many aspects of human life, death, religion, and the exceptions. This was a brief trip through human history. We have seen that in connection with life, some of the topics covered were agriculture, anatomy, anthropology, antibiotics, astronomy, archaeology, avocations, biology, the brain, chemistry, clothing, the city, community, dogs and other domesticates, the environment, embryology, exercise, fire, food, law, light, love, mathematics, money, philosophy, physics, shelter, sleep, sex, and water. In connection with death, we considered the arts, bacteria and other microorganisms, catastrophes, cemeteries, execution, immortality, literature, museums, memorials, murders, music, plagues and pandemics, poisons, radiation, suicide, theatre, war, and weapons. Within the subject of religion, the topics included altruism, buildings, dance and performing arts, the healer-priest, religious symbols, self-sacrifice, and religious texts. In addition to religion, other exceptions examined the topics of adventure, birth defects, choices, heroism, irrational behavior, neuropsychiatric problems, and risk. Some of these topics deserve further consideration at this time.

Rituals play an important role in human life, as humans are forced to recognize their mortality. The rituals that are associated with death are especially poignant, and they have long deserved patient attention. Rituals are also associated with other events, such as birth, marriage, or especially good fortune. Praise or thanks is often given in rituals to unseen forces, such as spirits or gods or fire.

Physicians have learned to participate in these rituals as part of their opportunity to assist patients. The Egyptian physician Imhotep, who designed the Step Pyramid, was considered to be a god after he died. The Greeks and Romans also had gods of health and medicine – Hygeia, Aesculapius, and Panacea.

By the time the early cities had been settled, physicians had found many things that could be used to treat patients, including fruits, vegetables and herbs; animal products; substances derived from the earth, and items used in incantations. No account is now available of any medicine man – a physician – in one of those early cities, nor have I read any speculation of what the practice of medicine would have consisted of in those days. However, there are written records of medical advice in ancient Egypt, and statements of what was expected of a physician in the Golden Age of Greece, and later in the Roman empire. They are similar in many ways to what is expected of a physician today. A physician at the present time can see many similarities with the behavior and practice of those who practiced medicine in those early cities. As physicians, they had much in common with the physicians who came later in Egypt, Greece, and Rome, in the Islamic territory surrounding the Mediterranean. In a small community, there would have been only one or perhaps two physicians. They would usually have been competitive, not cooperative. Or perhaps there would be a hierarchy, in which one was regarded as the elder. The physician would have had a certain *gravitas* of manner, which was called "Aequanimitas" by Sir William Osler in 1889 – an appearance of imperturbability, coolness and presence of mind. The early physician would then have been able to suture wounds, to reduce fractures, to lance boils, and to offer sage advice about diet, activities, and bathing. They would have had a large number of substances at hand to offer for complaints that ranged from fever and headaches, to constipation or diarrhea, or anxiety and sexual disfunction, and whatever else may be a worry to the patient. The substances would be secret mixtures, compounded from animal parts and from odd plants, especially odoriferous and bitter herbs. Most importantly, he or she would be able to prognosticate accurately. For thousands of years, the failure of a physician to cure a patient was considered to be a flaw, and it could be considered as a fatal flaw if the patient died. A wise physician would therefore never treat a disease that was surely incurable, or attempt to cure a disease which was inevitably fatal. Prediction of the outcome would enhance the physician's reputation, especially if he chose to treat the patient's illness and the patient recovered.

Some procedures used by physicians were rituals, based on the premise that bad things could be extracted from sick people. Bleeding, using an incision in a vein in the arm or with attachment of a leech, has long been a way to attempt to help a patient in this way. Bleeding was done by physicians for many hundreds of years. After glass was formulated and formed into cups, it was discovered that a heated glass cup could be affixed to the skin of a patient, and as it cooled, the body surface – skin and subcutaneous tissues – would rise slightly into the cup; and "cupping" thus became another way to remove potentially noxious substances from the patient. Astrology has had a long association with health and medicine, and even now, in many cultures, astrology plays an important role in making predictions and in decision-making. Astrology was inseparable from astronomy for centuries. Astrology is based on the belief that the future can be predicted from astronomical events, such as the position of the sun and moon and planets and stars, and the dates and times that alignments of these celestial objects occurred. This seems to be illogical, yet many people with high intelligence listen carefully to astrological predictions.

Plants were the most common source of specific remedies for early physicians. The effects would be found by careful examination, using principally the senses of taste and smell – licking and sniffing. If a plant seemed interesting, and it passed the initial tests, a small amount might be ingested, to see what would happen. For instance, tales would have been told of strange things that happened to some people who tried mushrooms. Some died and others had weird experiences. However, others ate mushrooms that appeared to be similar and were good food when cooked. These simple experiments led to the discovery of the effects of an enormous range of plants. We would now call them dose-related, because the desired effect might be seen with a small amount, while a larger amount is dangerous or deadly. I will mention a few of these herbal medicines to show how they may have been discovered, and a brief list of others which show the breadth of this subject.

An example of the dose-related effect is the leaf of *Digitalis purpurea*, the purple foxglove. When the leaves are dried and formulated into pills, digitalis is known pharmaceutically as digitalis folia (leaf). Foxglove leaf was long known amongst herbalists in England for its beneficial effects in some patients who were fatigued and had "dropsy" – the layman's term to describe the accumulation of fluids in the lower legs and ankles. The active principle in foxglove is digitalis, which acts by strengthening cardiac muscle and slowing the heart rate. If "dropsy" was the result of renal failure, foxglove leaf would have no benefit, and if doses were increased in an attempt to secure an effect in these patients, it would be poisonous. Medical students were once taught to instruct patients that toxic levels of digitalis leaf could be recognized if they began to see strange yellow "spots" (called scotomas). The early warning sign of yellow scotomas did not occur when purified preparations of digitalis, known as digoxin, were used. All of the parts of the woolly foxglove, *Digitalis lanata*, are considered to be poisonous. Surreptitious administration of digitalis has been one of the poisons used in television mysteries such as "Rosemary and Thyme."[291]

Nightshade, from mandragora, is another herb which famously has either beneficial effects (in low doses) or dangerous, poisonous effects (in high doses). The effects are due to the plant's chemicals, atropine and scopolamine, which act on the central nervous system. For centuries, women took the herb with the intent to have beautiful eyes: "belladonna" (Latin = beautiful woman) describes pupillary dilatation caused by nightshade. But the word nightshade, which implies death, is accurate, too: belladonna is a poison in higher doses, and it was also one of the mysterious agents deployed in "Rosemary and Thyme." Atropine and digitalis were formerly mainstays of cardiology through their action on the vagus, the tenth cranial nerve: digitalis would slow the heart rate by stimulation of the vagus nerve, whereas atropine would block the effect of the vagus nerve and thus increase the heart rate. Atropine is important as an adjunct in anesthesia, because it also inhibits secretions in the airways. It is used as an antidote to the poisonous nerve agent, sarin. Scopolamine has effects that are similar to atropine, but its most interesting effect is to produce temporary amnesia; a side effect is disorientation. It was formerly used to accompany anesthesia for childbirth. Obstetrical wards were then easily identified by the sounds of screams from delirious women, who needed little anesthesia because after they delivered their babies, they couldn't remember what had happened. Scopolamine, also known as hyoscine, is used therapeutically to prevent motion sickness with "patches" behind the ear, and it has been used for centuries in Colombia as a dangerous hallucinatory agent called *burundanga*.[292]

Willow bark or leaves of the willow tree (*Salix*) have been used throughout the world for fever and/or pain. More than 400 species of *Salix* exist in nature. The precise nature of the mechanism of action of willow bark and leaves for fever and pain is still a mystery. The effective principle is the chemical salicylate, marketed in 1899 as acetyl salicylic acid (ASA), with the brand name of Aspirin® by the Bayer Company in Germany. In low doses, willow bark and leaves have little likelihood of being toxic. The purified form of ASA has a wide range of effects, some of which are useful while others are dangerous and can be fatal. Aspirin in low doses is an anticoagulant and it has been shown to extend the life of some patients with gastrointestinal cancer. Higher doses of aspirin can cause fatal bleeding, ulcerations of the stomach, and a devastating illness in some children known as Reye's syndrome.[293]

Laurel (*Lauris nobilis*) contains eucalyptol, and its leaves, called bay leaves, have been popular spices since the days of the Roman empire – and probably earlier than that. Other trees known as "laurels" that are not of the genus *Lauris* are toxic. Mountain laurel (*Kalmia latifolia*) and cherry laurel (*Prunus laurocerasus*) contain hydrogen cyanide (yes, cyanide) and all parts of these plants are deadly.[294]

Some of the other ancient remedies for various problems with the gastrointestinal tract are emetics (a medical term, meaning to induce vomiting), such as syrup of ipecac, which contains emetine and cephaline. You don't have to remember the names; they just show that the chemicals have been identified. Diarrhea, euphemistically called "flux" in the eighteenth century, was treated supportively with oral fluids and by removing "roughage" (fiber) from the diet. Good advice then would be what is now called BRAT: bananas, rice, applesauce, and toast. When opium poppies made their way from Asia to Europe, it was possible to treat diarrhea with powerful substances that impair the motion of the intestines; modern derivatives of opium include oral medications such as paregoric and codeine. Oral fluids and opium derivatives were usually insufficient to save patients with profuse diarrhea, such as that caused by dysentery or cholera. Constipation was easier to treat: licorice, or prunes and a high-fiber diet, similar to today's breakfast cereals, such as Kellogg's "All Bran" and "Raisin Bran."

Metals: Diuretics, to stimulate the output of urine, were formulated by Arabic physicians during the European Middle Ages from substances that we know now contained mercury. Mercurial diuretics were prescribed well into the twentieth century. They were useful treatments, though dangerous, because of the toxicity of mercury. Mercury was also formulated into medicine for treatment of the "great pox" (syphilis). It was difficult to abandon mercury. It was fascinating to look at droplets of it rolling around on a plate, separating and then quickly coalescing again into a large drop of silvery, slithery liquid. Few people now have any recollection of seeing liquid mercury. However, mercury was once common in dentist's offices, where it was used in formulating mixtures with silver or gold, known as amalgams, for filling cavities in teeth. Mercury was also used in thermometers, and in the felting process for making hats. Chronic exposure to mercury is toxic to the brain, and in the hat industry, it produced workers who were famously known as "mad hatters."[295]

Other metals were used as medicines for many centuries after they were obtained in relatively pure amounts. Gold and silver, for instance, were expensive and therefore were thought to be especially valuable. Medical students in the 1950s read that gold was sometimes a useful treatment for arthritis, and that it was also the "age old remedy for the itching palm." Silver has anti-bacterial uses, though it is rarely used for that purpose now – it is hard to keep it from disappearing. It was used for many years by placing very thin sheets of sterling silver on nasty looking wounds, which then began to heal nicely. Neither gold or silver has toxic effects on the biology of humans, notwithstanding their troublesome effects on the human mind. And temptation leads to sticky fingers. Other metals have had less benign effects when administered to humans. For instance, in addition to the toxic effect of mercury, described in the preceding paragraph, the danger of lead is well known, yet it is still misused and abused. Lead is malleable and easy to work with. From ancient Rome to modern Mexico, lead has been incorporated in paint and into glaze for pottery. Lead plus white pigment makes beautiful, durable, white paint. In lead pipes, it still leaches into drinking water. Children with lead poisoning are stumbling, and fall far behind their classmates in school. In leaded gasoline for automobile engines, lead prevented "knocking," but at a terrible price to human health. And as other metals were isolated, they, too were tried, often with disastrous results – copper, which becomes poisonous when compounded with sulfur (blue copper sulfate is "vitriol"), and zinc sulfate, too, is vitriolic. Arsenic is perhaps the most famous elemental poison of all. Iron has a double standard. Incorporated into red blood cells for use in transporting oxygen, it is necessary for human health; yet excessive amounts of iron can be fatal, causing a disease known as hemochromatosis. Uranium and radium were considered to be powerful adjuncts for health in the early decades of the twentieth century, to the detriment of many who were exposed to these substances. X-rays were used in stores to show how nicely shoes fitted on children's feet, and dental x-rays were given without protection of the rest of the body of the patient, or for the dentist. All of misguided methods of treatment and diagnosis added up to a massive exposure of humans to ionizing radiation.[296]

Beverages were given for many purposes – as stimulants, relaxants, or simply for enjoyment. Early humans soon discovered that many forms of semi-solid and liquid foods, when left standing for several hours, changed through a process that we call fermentation. Retaining some of their original taste, but with a sparkle or acidic addition, these beverages had a variety of effects: some people became happy, others became wild and unreasonable, and all fell asleep when they were satiated. In some parts of the world, such as in Nepal, the desired quality in fermented beverages was found to be enhanced with a simple form of distillation, which produced a higher concentration of alcohol. Ethyl alcohol became one of the earliest chemicals used in formulating pharmaceutical preparations. "Tincture of iodine" meant that iodine was dissolved in alcohol. The word "tonic" on a druggist's bottle in the nineteenth century also meant that the drug was dissolved in alcohol, and whatever the effect of the drug might be, the tonic would certainly be enjoyed because of the alcohol in the bottle. A teetotaler could accept a tonic that was prescribed by a physician. If enough alcohol was given, the sense of pain would be diminished, surgery could be performed, and the patient would sleep through it. It was soon learned that the useful form of alcohol is that which is obtained from certain plants, but not from fermented or distilled from wood. We now understand that from vegetables and fruits, the fermented product is ethyl alcohol; from wood, it is methyl alcohol. A small difference, two carbon atoms in ethanol versus only one in methanol, but the difference is between happiness and blindness.[297]

For many centuries, mood alteration has been the desired effect of many other medicinal products that have been tried, used, and abused throughout the world. Although alcoholic beverages have always topped the list, four others rank only slightly below it: opium, tobacco, cannabis and cocaine. Opiates, cannabis, and cocaine have important medicinal uses, although the amounts used of each must be carefully regulated. Tobacco leaf was originally smoked in ceremonies by indigenous peoples in North America, and used in that way, tobacco had a beneficial calming effect. There is no longer any redeeming factor in the production, distribution, or use of tobacco, and the cultivation, marketing, and consumption of tobacco is the epitome of pharmaceutical disaster of humans. The earth in which tobacco grows is promptly depleted of nutrients and the nicotine in tobacco is highly addictive, and the chemicals in the leaf and those that are added to it in preparation for market cause many types of cancer. The cultivation of tobacco was an early cause of the societal disruption in America, because it required an enormous amount of enslaved labor, and it still is a socially disruptive force throughout the world. Extracts of hemp produce hashish (meaning "grass" in Arabic), also known as marijuana or "pot," a hallucinogenic agent that is mildly addictive when burned and the smoke is inhaled. Hashish was made famous by the wild behavior of some warriors, known as assassins (from the word hashish), in Asia Minor in the late medieval period. Smokers of marijuana ("potheads") are more likely to drift off into sleep than to become belligerent. Nevertheless, tobacco and marijuana (hashish) have stubborn advocates. They are also gateway agents to other addictive products such as opioids, cocaine, and nitrous oxide. Substances made from hallucinogenic mushrooms, cactus plants (peyote), and other forms of vegetation are less commonly abused. However, societal challenges in the late twentieth century led to use of larger amounts of all of these natural hallucinogens, and this was followed by the discovery of methods to synthesize, produce, and distribute many other deadly addictive chemicals. Most famous of these synthetics were LSD (lysergic acid diethylamide, nicknamed "acid") and PCP (phencyclidine, or "angel dust"), and more recently methamphetamine and fentanyl.[298]

Addictive substances: Opium and cocaine have a similar and often depressing history, from their origins as useful treatments to their present abuse as addictive substances. Opium and its derivatives have been enormously important as pain-relieving agents. The opium poppy has been grown for centuries in the highlands of central Asia, in valleys of the Hindu Kush Mountains, in the western Himalayas, in the country now known as Afghanistan. Extracts from these poppies were carried to Turkey on the Spice Road (now known as the Silk Road), and they appeared as heroin in Europe at the end of the medieval period. Legend has it that opium was secreted in hollowed-out walking sticks. Carried into India on the southern branch of the Spice Road, opium was identified as a valuable trading substance by the British, who transported it north to China. Addiction to opium fueled the desire to continue the use of this substance, enriching British and American traders, but to the detriment of many in the Far East, especially the people of China. Pharmaceutically, heroin became the mainstay of pain relievers, formulated as morphine solutions, usually injected, but also available in solution, and in tablets of codeine meperidine (Demerol), and oxycodone (Percocet). A long-lasting form of oxycodone (Oxycontin) was developed in the 1990s and marketed for control of chronic pain, such as that caused by cancer and rheumatoid arthritis. However, through unwitting overprescribing by some physicians, and illegal prescribing by others, and with complicit distributors, Oxycontin became a lethal addiction that has killed hundreds of thousands of people. Other narcotics such as heroin and fentanyl add to the total, and those who use one of these drugs often take other drugs, especially methamphetamine, that lead to incapacitation or death. The effects of opiates on society are shown in the movie, *The Man with the Golden Arm* (1955).[299]

Addiction to drugs such as those listed above takes many forms, and withdrawal from addictive substances causes a variety of effects. Cigarette smokers usually develop an intense craving which can lead to foolish or even fatal behavior: going out in a snowstorm to buy a package of cigarettes, or careless driving to light a cigarette while driving. There is no physical symptom or sign from withdrawal, but the psychological effect can be strong, as any smoker knows when smelling a whiff of tobacco smoke, many years later. Opiates, however, cause profound changes as addiction develops, and these are only slowly reversed during detoxification. And the changes vary from one person to another. A person with pain can safely take much larger doses of morphine than a person who is taking morphine as an intentionally addictive agent. Also, rising tolerance is seen with increasing doses of morphine and other opiates; a dose which would be fatal as the initial dose is insufficient to relieve pain at a later time. The poorly understood variance in tolerance to opioids is the cause of many fatal mistakes. Sudden cessation – withdrawal – from opioids results in unpredictable behavior and physical effects. Agitation, delirium, sweating, and vomiting are commonly seen. An intravenous injection of heroin typically causes relief of pain, swooning, sleep, and gradual depression of respiration. If an antidote (Narcan) is not administered promptly, breathing may cease, and death will occur. The effects of cocaine are similar in some ways, but profoundly different in others. Cocaine, derived from the leaf of the coca plant, was originally used as a stimulant which enabled miners and farmers to work at much higher altitudes in the Andes than would ordinarily have been tolerated. Chewing coca leaves, they could toil all day, hard at work at more than 15,000 feet above sea level in Colombia, Peru, Ecuador, and Bolivia. Coca leaf tea is a mild stimulant, somewhat like coffee or tea, and coca, like opiates, also relieves pain. Cocaine was used successfully as a topical (surface) anesthetic in surgery for many decades. Cocaine taken illicitly by combustion and inhalation through the nose may result in immediate pleasure but with danger from burning and hyperactivity. In contrast to heroin, cocaine administration produces excitement, and also in contrast with opiates, withdrawal from the use of cocaine does not ordinarily cause untoward effects.

Addiction to alcoholic beverages leads to disability and early death from various causes. Some of these diseases are directly due to intoxication from ethanol and additives in alcoholic beverages, while other effects are secondary. Repeated consumption of beer, wine, and distilled spirits leads to tolerance and the ability to consume ever increasing amounts. The effects initially vary from person to person; after a few drinks, some people become humorous, while others are sad. Eventually, all lose control and fall asleep. They are said to be "dead drunk." Chronic effects include loss of useful work, financial distress, and separation from family and society. Medical consequences include fatal diseases such as cirrhosis of the liver, cancer of the pancreas, accidental deaths from drunk driving and hypothermia, and various forms of malnutrition. And because most alcoholics are heavy smokers, one can add the list of illnesses that are caused by addiction to tobacco. Withdrawal of alcoholic beverages from a serious drinker can also be difficult, because sudden cessation may result in delirium tremens (known colloquially as the "DTs"), as shown in the movie *The Lost Weekend* (1944).[300]

In contrast to the complex mixture of benefits and harms that are present in the history of alcoholic beverages, of opiates, and of cocaine, one natural product, quinine, is purely of benefit to humans. Quinine is derived from *Cinchona*, the "fever bark tree" of South America. Quinine appeared in the Old World after 1492. It is amazing that quinine has never been abused as a product for distribution or consumption, and that it is still useful in the treatment of malaria, which is one of the deadliest diseases in the world. The world-wide deaths from malaria are estimated to be about 1 million each year. Many additional drugs were synthesized for treatment of malaria in the twentieth century, and another drug, artemisinin, long used in China, was recently discovered by Western medicine. Quinine is still the drug of choice for many patients who are in the greatest immediate danger with *falciparum* malaria. Quinine must be used carefully, for it can produce devastating side effects, including deafness, and it is now usually prescribed in combination with other drugs. The precise mechanism of action of quinine is still a puzzle, which if solved could guide the synthesis of new drugs against malaria.[301]

Another tree that has had important medical uses in the past century is the rubber tree, *Hevea brasiliensis*. Drips from a cut on the bark of this tree yield about 30% latex. Cuts on many other plants, such as *Ficus* (the fig tree) and the goldenrod, also produce a similar thick white liquid, but the best producer of latex for rubber is one species: *H. brasiliensis*. It is nearly impossible to enumerate all of the uses of rubber in medical equipment, but to mention a few: gaskets in pump-oxygenators, dialysis machines, and syringes; rubber gloves for surgery, patient care, and handling of dangerous substances; and incorporated into carbon-based plastics for all of the many uses of plastics in medicine.[302]

Returning to vegetable substances that are consumed in medicine: think of sugar, which is perhaps the one that is most important and most widely used. However, like many of the substances listed above, sugar has had a variety of consequential effects on humans in the past few centuries. Many of these effects have been useful, some have been harmful, and others have been deadly. Sugar has been vital as a source of life-sustaining calories in food, and incorporated into syrups, sugar has been "the sweet that makes the bitter pill easier to swallow." Sugar was the source of the healing power of honey on wounds, and a sweet poultice was once a useful prescription for an unhealed sore. Sugar comes in many forms; the sweetest is sucrose, but there are other forms such as glucose (which is also known as dextrose), lactose, fructose, maltose, and more. All of them are carbohydrates – of various combinations of carbon, hydrogen, and oxygen – in combinations that are described in Part One of this essay.[303]

One effect of sugar on humans was unintended. It is a complicated story. The disease known as diabetes (actually, diabetes mellitus), is caused by insufficient production of insulin, which is a hormone produced by the pancreas. Insulin is necessary for the metabolism of sugar. Diabetes can be a life-endangering disease. The discovery of insulin, and of how to produce it as a drug, was an immediate success. However, it has been a mixed blessing. The use of insulin for the treatment of diabetes has enabled patients with this disease to live longer, to become useful citizens, and to reproduce. And as a result, the incidence of men and women and children with diabetes in the population has increased, and the medical and financial burden produced by diabetes has become a major problem, with no end in sight. Add to this, the bleak history of sugar plantations in the Caribbean and the enslaved Africans who were worked to death there. These unfortunate people enriched European and American planters and swelled the economy of England, France, the Netherlands, and their colonies. The sugar industry, known as "Big Sugar," has had enormous political influence in the United States for more than a century. The possibility of having sugar plantations was a force that enabled the invasion of Cuba by the United States during the Spanish-American War in 1898, and ownership of sugar plantations continued to play a role in Cuban and American politics during and after the Cuban Revolution in 1960. "Big Sugar" lobbies on behalf of the sugar industry in the U.S. Congress and in U.S. Departments, such as Agriculture and Commerce. The sugar industry lobbies to ensure tolerance for sugar-containing beverages, in spite of their many harmful effects. A "sweet tooth" for candy, sucrose-flavored chewing gum, and sugared soft drinks are major contributors to cavities in teeth – dental caries – which leads to destruction of teeth and the many economic and social effects of toothlessness (edentualism).[304]

Random thoughts of ancient remedies bring to mind many other vegetable, animal, and mineral substances, some of which were combined in ways that were intended to be both mysterious and useful. Some still are used. The details of some of the concoctions were secret and have, thankfully, been lost. Many others have surely been forgotten. Let us remember coffee and tea, notably used as stimulants and effective in social gatherings – in coffee houses from London to Starbucks, and in the elaborate tea ceremonies in Japan. And there were, and still are, salves for skin with oily substances, especially butter and lard; talc and saltwort, for drying of skin and wounds; and moldy bread poultice, for infections of skin (we now know that this contains penicillin). There were questionable remedies, too, known as polypharmacy, with theriac and mithridates; and useless methods, calling for eye of newt, wing of bat, and dried excrement of various animals, combined with a bit of hocus pocus and waving of hands. Many of the ancient remedies used spices and chemicals that are still used today in the preparation of food, be it to preserve food or to enhance the taste. Salt preserves and enhances and pepper adds to the flavor. Derived from tasty leaves and vegetable powders, the origin and use of these interesting vegetables can be traced to the human urges for food + fire. In the kitchen closet, there may be jars of allspice from Jamaica, almond extract, Angostura bitters, asafetida, basil, bay leaves, cayenne pepper, chile pepper, chipotle (jalapeño) pepper, chives, chocolate, cinnamon, cloves, cocoa, cocoanut, coriander, cumin, curry, fennel, garlic powder, herbs from Provence, honey, horseradish, Italian seasoning, lemon extract, licorice, maple sugar, mustard, nutmeg, onion powder, oregano, paprika, parsley flakes, pepper (ground, black, red), poppyseed, saffron, sea salt, starch, soy sauce, sugar, cream of tartar, Tabasco, tamarind, tarragon, thyme, tomato sauce, turmeric, and vanilla extract, and Worcestershire sauce. Most of these herbs and spices have been used medicinally for centuries, for purposes ranging from aphrodisiacs to diuretics.

Some can be dangerous, such as black licorice, which can cause abnormal heart rhythm and death if consumed daily in amounts that seem innocuous. Some remedies that were useful for hundreds of years have faded away; for example, oil of turpentine.[305]

Many **other methods** were used by early physicians and surgeons, most of which were known in Egyptian, Greek and Arabic medicine, and also known to a variable extent by physicians in Northern Europe. These included, most importantly, prognostication, to take credit or deflect blame for the outcome of an illness; examination of the surface of the skin, thoughtfully touching and taking the pulse at the wrist, and studious examination of the urine. A simple diet was usually advised, especially for a sore big toe, which for some strange reason is a sign of gout. Patients were advised to avoid intoxication, but that injunction was all too often disregarded. Bacchus, the god of drink, would usually win the game against Apollo, the god of physicians. Hippocrates emphasized the proper use of either cold or hot baths, exercise, massage, and personal hygiene. And above all, the physician was advised to "first do no harm." His other aphorisms are still remembered. Rendered into modern English, Hippocrates sagely observed that "Life is short, but the Art is long. Experiment is perilous, and Decision is difficult."[306]

Surgery has been practiced by those who had the gift to perform operations on people from time immemorial to the present. Surgery requires the use of tools, and this is where I would place it in the early history of humans: Tools and tool-making skills developed from the human urges for personal protection and shelter, plus the ability to use fire. The first tools were probably stone knives and primitive swords fashioned from sticks. With the discovery of smelting of metal, bronze and then iron were used to form sharper instruments. Surgeons also needed to use the skills of weaving, because thread and cloth are employed in surgery. Hippocrates advised that a patient must be properly positioned, with good lighting, assistants should be ready, with instruments selected and laid out for immediate use. A pre-operative check list was suggested by Hippocrates, and a version of the check list was recently recreated.[307]

Surgical treatments initially involved reduction and bandaging of fractures; cautery was employed by the physicians of Cordoba in the 10th century; ligature (tying a bleeding vessel with thread) was described in *On Surgical Conditions* by Albucasis of Cordoba (b. 936); styptics were employed for minor bleeding; sutures, using needle and thread, were used to stop bleeding and to sew up wounds; forceps and retractors were employed to aid in surgery; cataracts were removed with a knife, also known as the lancet, which was also used for venesection (bleeding) and to lance abscesses. Many other surgical techniques were re-discovered in Europe after the Renaissance. Barbers, familiar with razors and scissors, became adept at surgery, and the Royal College of Surgeons of England thus descends from barber-surgeons. The Royal College of Physicians, in contrast, has its origin with the "leeches" of the Middle Ages. The "Physician's Tale" of Chaucer in the 14th century is related by a proud and haughty physician, a gentleman, not a barber surgeon of a lower class.[308]

Psychiatry and supportive care have long utilized supportive methods, in addition to trials of various herbs and mineral substances. Psychic methods have been used for anxiety, depression, phobias, and psychoses. Psychics are implored to treat impotence if capsaicin (the "Spanish fly") fails, and for help in cases of female problems, such as menorrhagia, pain, and unwanted pregnancies. Visions of the night sky have been important, but it has been difficult to distinguish between what is observed in the sky (astronomy) and what it is supposed to mean (astrology). Even now, an element of superstition persists regarding the planets and stars; many daily newspapers print the latest information to stargazers.[309]

The physicians of the Arabic world and Persia in the Golden Age of Arabic civilization (750-850) – many of whom were Muslim, some were Christian, and others were Jews – knew of methods to concentrate drugs with distillation, sublimation, and filtration. They also knew of drugs such as senna, camphor, cloves, mercury; solvents such as alcohol, syrups, and aldehydes; and anesthetics such as cannabis and hyoscyamus (nightshade). The physicians of the Middle East and Mediterranean in what was the Medieval Period in northern Europe employed many other substances as drugs but which we now believe were useless or harmful. They persisted in the study of alchemy, the ultimate goal of which was to turn other substances into gold.

Doctors Afield

The contributions of many individual physicians to the history of medicine and of science are mentioned in Part One of this essay. Physicians have also played important roles in human history in other ways than through the practice of medicine.[310]

Physicians are granted a special place in society. Although the ratios vary from one country to another, and also within countries, say from one in two hundred, to one among thousands. The manner in which a physician is addressed is variable, but there is no doubt that to be called "doctor" is a title of wisdom and respectability. The word doctor is derived from *docco* (to teach) in Latin. A physician may be asked to serve on a community's school board, or to be a leader in the Boy Scouts or Girl Scouts, or to serve on the governing body of a church. The physician's obligations also include financial contributions to charitable organizations, because the physician's income is greater than most of the others. Physicians have an income that is in the top five or ten percent of the community, and it is appropriate to return some of this to those who are less fortunate. For hundreds of thousands of physicians, this is what they have done in their capacity as "Doctors Afield."

Some of the physicians who made contributions in other fields surely remembered that they had subscribed to the Oath of Hippocrates, and that in some way this Oath would continue to be a guide in all of their later work. No matter what else a physician may do, he or she is still a physician. A healer. This section of the essay on *Health Matters* recalls the series of biographical sketches of physicians that were composed or edited by Benjamin Castleman, M.D. (1906-1982), and published in the years from 1952 until 1969 in the *New England Journal of Medicine*. He was a pathologist at the Massachusetts General Hospital, and Professor of Pathology at Harvard Medical School. Dr. Castleman memorialized these physicians by calling them "Doctors Afield." Twenty additional biographies were published in a book published by Yale University Press entitled *Doctors Afield* in 1999. The editors credited the name of their book to the series published in the *New England Journal of Medicine*.[311]

Collectively, the non-medical work that physicians have done in their communities and in the larger components of society probably consists of millions of encounters. The impact of this unheralded extra-curricular work by physicians upon human history is enormous yet incalculable. "Medicine has become such a consuming enterprise that a doctor's identity often becomes inseparable from his or her role as a healer."[312]

Please see Appendix C for a list of the physicians and their accomplishments who were profiled by Castleman in his series of articles and in the book, *Doctors Afield*. Brief accounts of additional "Doctors Afield" are also shown in Appendix C. They are grouped in categories listed alphabetically from Actors to Politics. Only a few can be mentioned of the many others and the various fields outside of medicine in which they became famous, so a few examples must suffice. Many additional physicians who are still alive have made contributions to other fields than medicine, especially literature and politics. "Doctors Afield" concludes with the man who I believe was the most famous physician of all, though he is not usually remembered as a doctor. He is Saint Luke, the Evangelist.[313]

A Meditation on Saint Luke
The Most Famous Physician in History

It seemed good to me also, having had perfect understanding of all things
from the very first, to write unto thee in order, most excellent Theophilus.
–Luke, 1:3

The former treatise have I made, O Theophilus, of all that Jesus began both
to do and teach. –Acts, 1:1

This meditation is about Saint Luke, the Evangelist, a doctor, writer, and historian who lived in the 1st century A.D. Much has been written about him, yet little about him is known with certainty. He has been remembered for two thousand years because his name is recorded as the author of one of the Gospels in the New Testament. The "Gospel according to Luke" is the third book in the Christian portion of the Holy Bible, which is the most widely read book in the world. The third sentence of Luke's Gospel, quoted above, shows that he placed it into the hands of a man named Theophilus, about whom we know nothing more. A historian ensures that every document is properly archived. The provenance is established with the chain of custody, and in this case, it began was with Luke's transmission of the document to Theophilus. The documentary evidence provided by Luke enhances the other two Synoptic Gospels, which are those of Mark and Matthew. Without the first three Gospels, the fourth – the book of John – would stand alone, and we would lack many of the interesting stories that bring life to the New Testament. Luke repeated the process when he transmitted another document to Theophilus, which is now known as the Acts of the Apostles.[314]

Luke addresses Theophilus with a title of respect. Perhaps coincidentally, the name Theophilus means "friend of God," which implies that he would be especially interested in what Luke has written. Luke's Gospel is typical of a historian, in that it moves forward in time, with a lengthy side-bar genealogy of the father-in-law of Jesus (i.e., of Mary's line). It is similar to the genealogy of Joseph in Matthew 1:1-16. Taken together, they show that Mary, the mother of Jesus, and his nominal father or step-father, Joseph, were both descendants of King David. Jesus is thus proven to be the "Son of David," and by Jewish law, as the heir of Joseph, he is able to inherit the throne of David. The genealogy is boring to many readers, but historians love this type of documentation. The genealogy would probably be placed in a lengthy Endnote or in the Appendix of a modern work.[315]

E. Earle Ellis, who wrote the article about Saint Luke in *Britannica,* is complimentary about Luke as a scholar and writer. Ellis said, "Luke had a cultivated literary background and wrote in good idiomatic Greek." Ellis also believed that Luke's work in the early Christian church "was no small achievement, and through the centuries it has served the church well." However, Ellis dismisses Luke's professional qualifications, concluding that he was an "otherwise insignificant physician." This meditation disputes the final dismissive comment by Ellis.[316]

The name of Luke, in different translations, has been repeated millions of times, as a given name, a baptismal name, and in nicknames; as a family name, in the names of buildings and cities, and in the names of other saints, noblemen, and royalty. To mention but a few: The English name Luke becomes, in different languages, Lewis, Louis, Louisa, Loúka, Loukas, Luc, Luca, Lucas, Lucia, Lucius, Luigi, Luis, Ludwig, and Lyuk; the nicknames Lee, Lew, Lou, or Louie; and Saint Louis, Missouri. The origin of the name is unclear. Some say it is derived from Greek, meaning "man from Lucania." Others say it is shortened from Lucius (Latin = "born at dawn"), derived from *lux* = light. Luke may be remembered as one of the Gospel writers, but it is rare that anyone will mention that he was a physician. His background as a doctor is either neglected completely or treated dismissively in theological discussions about his life, his work as an early Christian disciple, in the interpretation of his writings, and in the arguments about fact vs. legend in later accounts of his life. Luke only mentioned briefly in the histories of medicine that I have cited for this essay, *Health Matters*. This meditation is intended to show that Luke's career as a physician was a crucial aspect of his life, and also of his contribution to Christianity. It is unlikely that Luke would ever have stopped practicing medicine and surgery.[317]

Saint Luke is the patron saint of physicians and surgeons, and others – artists, students, bachelors and butchers. Many of his likenesses, dating to the 8th century and continuing in the medieval period, show him as an artist, as the first icon painter. We can appreciate these images, although there is nothing in the Bible that would suggest that he was a painter. In the Renaissance, he is often shown accompanied by a bull, for reasons that are obscure. Some say that Luke was Greek, and that he was a Hellenic Jew; others argue that he was a gentile.[318]

A man named Luke was surely a disciple of Paul, although some now doubt that he was the same person as Luke, the author of the third Gospel. The skepticism is puzzling, because Theophilus, mentioned above, is named as the recipient of both the Gospel and the Acts. As the author of one Gospel and also of the book of the Acts, Luke is responsible for about more than one-fourth of the New Testament. However, Luke is mentioned specifically by name only a few times in the New Testament: In the Epistle to Philemon, in Colossians 4:10-11, 14; in 2 Timothy 4:11, and in Acts, 28:16. In Colossians 4:14, Paul says, "Luke, the beloved physician, and Demas, greet you." That's a specific reference to Luke's being a doctor of medicine. The word "doctor" is properly used elsewhere in the Luke's Gospel to refer to a teacher in one place and in another place to a doctor of law. But here, the man named Luke, who was Paul's companion as he traveled in Asia Minor, Greece, and Rome, is a "beloved physician." In his letter to Timothy, Paul says that "Only Luke is with me" in Rome. That's not much, but we know from that comment that Paul and Luke were still in Rome. Luke is mentioned in religious texts which have been dated to the 2d to 4th centuries, although there is little to connect these texts to the actual person named Luke in the 1st century. By tradition, the end of Luke's life came at age 84 in Boeotia, which is a regional unit in central Greece. This tradition states that his tomb was in Thebes, the largest city in Boeotia, and that his relics were transferred to Constantinople.[319]

Luke was a member of the medical profession in Greece and/or Asia Minor when Greek medicine was dominant in that part of the Western world, including Rome. In Ralph Major's history of medicine, we learn although many of the documents that showed the work of individual physicians at that time have been lost, some have remained, and others have been recovered. Major's lengthy chapter on "Medicine in the Roman Empire" is instructive, for it allows us to imagine the life and practice of a Greek physician in the 1st century A.D. A well-educated Greek man, such as Luke, would have entered the profession as an apprentice, whose way would be paved by his family connections. He therefore was probably a gentile. At some point early in his training, Luke would have sworn to the Oath of Hippocrates (c.460 B.C–c.370 B.C.). It begins as follows: "I will impart a knowledge of this art to my own sons, and those of my teachers," and the medical profession continued for the next two millennia to be one of entitlement. A physician in that part of the world was unique, in that he could relocate and earn a living in a new location if he chose to do so. In the Hippocratic tradition, a physician also treated wounds and lanced boils, although some aspects of surgery, such as "cutting for the stone," were limited to those who had special training. It was important to be skillful and lucky, to be of good repute, and to be bold or careful or humble, as the occasion warranted. Luke's skills could have provided the financial means for Paul and his small entourage to travel between cities in Asia Minor and Greece as missionaries. He would have been welcomed by the poor, who never had a doctor, and if his skills in some fields exceeded those of the local physicians, he would be asked by them to be a consultant to the rich. All of these aspects of the practice of medicine were described by Hippocrates, and they are still present today. Physicians in the organization known as Doctors without Borders (*Médecins Sans Frontières*) are but one example of thousands who have been peripatetic doctors. Luke may have accompanied Paul for as long as thirty years, or he may have traveled with Paul intermittently during Paul's years as a missionary. By the time Luke came to Italy with Paul in say 60 A.D., citizenship had been granted to all physicians practicing in Rome. This act by Julius Caesar (100 B.C.–44 B.C.) placed him on a par with Paul, who had become a Roman citizen while working for the government in Judea.[320]

Returning again to the assertion in *Britannica* that Luke the Evangelist was an "otherwise insignificant physician," we now know that Luke, as a Greek physician in the 1st Century A.D., was surely trained in the school of Hippocrates; that he was therefore expert in both medicine and some aspects of surgery; that he could practice anywhere in Asia Minor, Greece, and Rome; that as a physician he was in a position to provide crucial financial support for the missionary work of Saint Paul; that he understood and could interpret the miracles and healing that accompanied Paul's mission; and that he was a physician and citizen in Rome when Paul was nearing the end of his life. Luke may not have added anything new to the history of medicine, but he surely was not an "insignificant physician."[321]

In the academic world, it always has been "publish or perish." But even if a scholar follows the rules, publications are sometimes lost, destroyed, misplaced, or not indexed properly. And even if we do our best, our fate is to "fade away" and to "pass and be forgotten, like the rest." There must be more to the life of Saint Luke, Evangelist and physician, but we are not likely to know the rest of his story.[322]

C. Developments in Human Health - Chronological Viewpoint

The civilization in the West began with the creation of cities in the so-called Fertile Crescent, in the lands to the east of the Mediterranean Sea. Other cities and other civilizations were established at about the same time, or earlier, in China and southeast Asia, in India, and in North and South America. The dates of the development of cities in those parts of the world are less well known, but archeologists are certain that they are also ancient. However, *Health Matters* focuses on the civilization of the West that developed into what, for better and for worse, determines what humans are today.[323]

The Fertile Crescent, where Western civilization began, is similar in shape and appearance to that of a waning moon, which is seen in the eastern sky for a few days before a new moon cycle begins. The waning moon is present shortly before sunrise, with its horns tilted to the southeast. The lower border of the Fertile Crescent of the Near East began at Ur on the Euphrates River, near the Persian Gulf; then west to Jericho, near the Dead Sea. The lower border then crossed the Sinai Desert and Suez and went west and south to Memphis and Thebes on the Nile River. The upper border of the Fertile Crescent extended from Ur in a broad curve into Anatolia, to the island of Cyprus in the northwest. Luxor, Cairo, and Alexandria were later built on the Nile, as was Jerusalem, to the north-east. The four great rivers of the Fertile Crescent were the Tigris and Euphrates, which bordered the east and west sides of Mesopotamia, now known as Iraq; the Jordan, which flowed into the Dead Sea near Jericho; and the Nile.[324]

Sometime before 4000 BCE, the city of Ur had been settled on the Euphrates River. The ruins of the ancient city of Ur were discovered in 1854 underneath a great mound known as the Tell al Muqayyar. It had been an enormous city, with large houses and palaces. The tower known as the Ziggurat of Ur had been built by King Ur-Nammu, ruler of Ur of the Chaldees. Excavations of Ur in the nineteenth century revealed business transactions within the temple precincts that were recorded on clay tablets – the first tax receipts ever issued. The cuneiform inscriptions on the little clay tablets show trading by barter of cereals, fruit, clothing and cattle.[325]

Abraham, the Patriarch of the Jews, is said to have left Ur with his family to find a new home further to the west, near the Mediterranean Sea. Abraham was only a subsistence farmer and herdsman, and the undocumented story of his migration and of what happened to his descendants would be of little interest, except for the momentous impact that Abraham's descendants – the Jews and the Arabs – have had on history. Furthermore, the story of Abraham and his descendants, as told in the Hebrew Bible and also in the version known by Christians as the Old Testament, is the best text that has been recovered to show the many ways that people of the Middle East at that time viewed the subjects of life, of death, of illness, and of health. The first book of the Bible, Genesis (12:1), says that Abraham's wife Sarah grew old without having a child, but with Sarah's permission, Abraham took as a second wife, Sarah's maid-servant, Hagar "the Egyptian," who bore his first son, Ishmael. Then God miraculously allowed Sarah to become pregnant, and Abraham, at the age of 100, had a second son, named Isaac. The teenaged Ismael mocked his little brother, angering Sarah. To solve the family crisis, Abraham gave Hagar some bread and water and sent her and Ismael out into the wilderness. The water was soon gone, and they were close to death, but an angel showed the location of a well to Hagar. They both survived, and Ishmael became the legendary father of the "great nation" of the Arabs (Genesis 21:18). Isaac also survived a close call. Abraham believed that God directed him to build an altar and sacrifice Isaac on it. It was supposedly a test of his faith. Human sacrifice was not uncommon in those days, and Abraham started to do as he believed was God's will. He bound Isaac and drew his knife to finish the deed, but an angel suddenly appeared (presumably directed from God) and told Abraham to sacrifice a goat that was stuck nearby in the bushes. Both Ismael and Isaac were saved and they had long and successful lives. In the stories of both of these children, we see that history is explained by choices that enabled health to occur, rather than by choices or circumstances that would have led to death.[326]

Early deaths or unexpected survivals played roles in many occasions in Biblical history. Some of these are surely fictional and allegorical, but they reflect beliefs about health and illness that were prevalent at that time and are therefore instructive. We read that Cain survived as the first murderer after killing his brother Abel; that Lot survived Sodom (eponym of sodomy) and bred more children (incestuously), though his salty wife did not; that Jacob escaped from his angry father-in-law with the family treasure and two wives; and that proud Joseph barely escaped death at the hands of his brothers. Joseph, it may be recalled, later repaid his brothers' actions with charity, and thus saved the founders of the twelve Hebrew tribes from starvation. Joseph's actions as vizier of Egypt cannot be documented in history, but the poignant tale has never been forgotten.

In about **4000 BCE, Ur was abandoned a result of a flood**. Perhaps it was the Great Flood described in the fantastic Biblical story, which Noah rode out, accompanied by a male and female of all of the animals of the world, in the great Ark that is mentioned in Genesis. Mount Ararat, where Noah is said to have landed, and where he saw the rainbow which signified God's promise not to do this again, is at the northern edge of the Fertile Crescent.

Also, perhaps before 4000 BCE, but probably after the city of Ur was built, the first farmers were settling along the Nile in Egypt. The population is estimated to have reached 1 to 1.5 million in the 3rd millennium BCE. Most people lived in houses built of mud brick in villages and small towns, raising grain crops, fruit and vegetables, irrigated with simple canals, using the annual Nile flood. Papyrus grew wild and was also domesticated and cultivated to use as a food crop, and to make rope and sandals, and later to use as writing material. Many animals were domesticated, including cattle, sheep, and pigs, which were eaten; and cats, dogs, and donkeys.[327]

In about 3000 BCE, the fortress of Mycenae in Crete was built by the Minoan kings, the Bronze Age had just begun in the Balkans, and the last manifestation of the Stone Age was seen in "vast stone tombs" in Sardinia and western France.[328]

In say 3000-2500 BCE, the Ebers and Smith Papyruses were probably originally written. They described the techniques of medicine and surgery at that time in Egypt. The papyruses, which were purchased in Egypt in the mid-nineteenth century, date from 1600 BCE, but they are said to be "compilations" by the writer of one of the papyruses. They were written in hieroglyphics and were translated using the code on the Rosetta Stone, which was discovered in 1799. The inscriptions on the stone were written in three languages: hieroglyphic characters, Demotic script, and Greek. The Ebers Papyrus is a compilation of treatments using incantations and herbal substances, many of which can only be tentatively identified. The Smith Papyrus is a surgical treatise, describing many methods which are still in use today. The era known as the Old Kingdom of Egypt is also known as the Age of the Pyramid Builders. The first great pyramid was designed and built in the Third Dynasty, in about 2630 BCE, under supervision by Imhotep, a physician, priest, and architect, who was the grand vizier for King Djoser. The operation of circumcision is shown on the wall of a tomb at Sakkara, dated c.2400 BC, with a legend in hieroglyphics reading: "The operator says to the man who is standing behind the boy, holding him by the wrists, 'Hang on to him. Don't let him faint.'" The Egyptian physicians of that period were highly specialized in their practices. They were familiar with contraceptives, and in subjects as varied as dentistry, ophthalmology, and proctology.[329]

In about 2900 BCE, Ur was resettled, and in the 25th century, Ur was the capital of southern Mesopotamia. King Hammurabi (2123-2081 BCE) drew up elaborate laws, including laws for those who practiced surgery. By 2000 BCE, when Stonehenge was being built in Britain, and Germans were still using the wooden plow, Babylonians had already developed a high degree of skill in agriculture, commerce, art, science, medicine, mathematics, astronomy, and archeology; and in philosophy, grammar, and literature. The Babylonians made accurate records of the rising and setting of the planet Venus, and of the orbits of the sun and moon and their eclipses; they distinguished between planets and stars; and they divided the day into 24 parts (hours) of 60 minutes and the minutes into 60 seconds, using their inventions of a water clock and sun dial. In 1846, George Rawlinson translated a transcription that was carved on a rock in Persia in three languages – Persian, Elamitic, and Babylonian – which enabled other cuneiform inscriptions to be read. Babylonia would be destroyed and rebuilt several times over the next two millennia.[330]

The Code of Hammurabi is the first known codification of laws. It includes the word "physician" (*asu* = healer), with a section on surgical fees and penalties for surgical failures. For a broken bone, the payment would be three shekels if the patient was a freeman, but if a slave, the owner would pay only two shekels to the physician. If the physician operated on a freeman and caused his death, his fingers would be cut off, but if it was a slave, he would simply restore to the owner a slave of equal value. There was a distinction between physicians (who belonged to the priestly class, which also included judges and lawyers) and surgeons; there were also veterinarians. Law, medicine, and theology were considered to be of divine origin. The "Assyrian Herbal" listed 250 vegetable substances and 120 minerals, most of which can be identified and many of which are still in use today. A eunuch was displayed on a tablet in Babylon, identifiable as being obese and beardless. The close association between medicine and astrology in Babylon persisted for some 3,500 years, lasting into the Middle Ages in Europe.[331]

In 1960 BCE, a nomadic people known as Amorites from the Arabian desert destroyed the empires of Sumer and Akkad in Mesopotamia. They founded Babylon; the center of its power was 1830-1530 BCE; its sixth king was Hammurabi. The most famous kings of Babylon were Gilgamesh, who wrote a now-famous Epic that told of a great flood; and Nebuchadnezzar, who ruled from 605-562 BCE.

In 2000 BCE, Amenemhet I was on the throne of Egypt. The years 1333-1323 encompassed the reign of Tutankhamun, "King Tut," in Egypt. Sophisticated embalming techniques and a profound knowledge of anatomy can be recognized in the Egyptian mummies, such as King Tut, who were carefully prepared for life in the invisible world that they would enter after death.[332]

A decade-long battle between the Greeks and those who lived in a small seaport city on the east side of the Strait of the Dardanelles, now in Asian Turkey, began in about 1260 BCE. It is known in history as the Trojan War. "Based on the evidence of imported Mycenaean pottery, the end of Troy VIIa can be dated to between 1260 and 1240 BCE… Troy VIIa was very likely the capital of King Priam of Homer's *Iliad*, which was destroyed by the Greek armies of Agamemnon." Following the battles described in the *Iliad*, Homer wrote the *Odyssey*. Both of Homer's works are in poetry, originally in Greek. The *Odyssey* told of the long and wandering journey back to Greece by Ulysses, one of the most illustrious victors at Troy. Ulysses finally arrived home alone, and the *Odyssey* is filled with the accounts of starvation, illness and deaths of his crew, and also of Ulysses' slaughter of his wife's suitors when he returned. There is no doubt that health (and ill health) mattered on that long voyage, and at the end of it. According to the legend of the *Aeneid*, written in Latin by Virgil, a few of the Trojan survivors also sailed west, looking for a new place to live. After harrowing adventures in Carthage, they landed in Italy, defeated the native Etruscans, and are now known as the Romans. Many medical issues and surgical problems are described by Homer in the *Iliad* and the *Odyssey*, and by Virgil in the *Aeneid*. We see plagues and starvation, strange herbs and medicines, and gruesome wounds. The Achilles tendon first appears in the story of the Trojan War, when Achilles is killed by a spear that hit behind his ankle. It is the only place where he is vulnerable. His mother had attempted to secure his safety by holding him by the foot while she dipped him in the River Styx. As a chance result of his mother's mistake, the mythical power of the water of the river Styx, which separates Earth from Hades, never touched Achilles' ankle.[333]

Jericho's city walls were destroyed in 1250-1200 BCE, perhaps by an earthquake. Or, as it is said in the Bible, by the Jews who had wandered in the wilderness of the Sinai Peninsula for forty years. Ralph Major estimates that it was in about 1200 BCE when Joshua led the Israelites into the Promised Land. The inhabitants of Jericho were slaughtered except for the family of Rahab, a prostitute, who helped the Israelites. "They burned the whole city and everything in it." The destruction of Jericho was the ultimate sign of ill health. If this was indeed the time that the Jews returned from Egypt to their Promised Land, their journey began with another unexpected bit of good health. As the story goes – and it is only an undocumented story – they were brought to the brink of the ridge overlooking Jericho by Moses, who had led them out of Egypt. As a baby, Moses was carefully placed by his mother in a small basket in the river, where he was found, as intended, by a daughter of the Pharaoh. That his parents were Jewish was unknown, and the orphan was adopted and grew to maturity as an Egyptian. But when he killed an Egyptian who was beating a Hebrew, he was forced to flee for his life. When he learned that he was Jewish, he made arrangements for their departure from Egypt. During the next forty years, Moses was miraculously enabled to save his people from thirst, starvation, and death in the Sinai Desert.[334]

It may have been in about 1000 BCE that David, a shepherd, poet, and warrior, was king of Israel, although the archeological evidence for a precise date is still lacking. David's survival is another success story of good health overcoming death – in this case, it was David's gigantic opponent Goliath that died. But David's good luck story doesn't end there. There are hundreds of commandments and laws in the Torah and at least 13 that are theoretically punishable by death. David certainly violated one of the capital crimes (adultery), and arguably violated another one (murder), but he escaped punishment on both counts. David is said to have lusted after Bathsheba, who he saw bathing, and arranged for her husband, Uriah, to be killed. Sometime after 1000 BCE, his son by Bathsheba, Solomon, became the wise and wealthy king of Israel. The copper industry flourished in his land, with the assistance of the Queen of Sheba, who ruled the area to the south that is now known as Yemen.[335]

The great Nebuchadnezzar II (605-562) was King of Babylon. He built the beautiful Hanging Gardens, and like other rulers at that time he appears to have been a remorseless tyrant. He is said to be the greatest king of Babylon, and he lived in splendor while his people lived in poverty. He conquered Jerusalem, destroyed the Temple, and took its treasures and most of its citizens to Babylon, including the prophets Daniel and Jeremiah. The Jews were held captive in Babylon for seventy years, until he was persuaded by a series of miracles to release them. The Biblical story is of one of harsh confinement by a corrupt ruler, who relents after seeing miracles, such as that of three men (Shadrach, Meshach, and Abednego) who were cast into a fiery furnace but survived; none were burned.[336]

Sometime in the 8th or 7th Centuries BCE, or perhaps earlier in c. 1102, Homer wrote the *Iliad* and *Odyssey* about the Trojan War, mentioned above, which took place in about 1260 BCE. At a date that is unknown, probably sometime between the 6th and 4th Centuries BCE, Buddha Gautama, also known as Siddhartha Gautama, the "Enlightened One," was born in Nepal and died in India. He was a Hindu of high caste, but those who follow his teachings and meditations, and are known as Buddhists, are not accepted as Hindus. Buddha's search for The Way included asceticism, peaceful behavior, and rejection of animal slaughter. Buddhism spread throughout Asia, and it has developed in several different forms of worship. Tibetan Buddhists were formerly the aristocratic rulers of central Asia, north of the Himalayas. Tibetans were notably cruel and fanatic warriors, led by those chosen in sequence to be either the Panchen Lama or the Dalai Lama. The present Dalai Lama, however, is an advocate for peace, and Sherpas in Nepal, who are Tibetan Buddhists, follow his precepts. The Mongolian tribesmen who invaded Europe in the late 11th century were animistic and had no sacred texts, but by the 14th century, Tibetan Buddhism had been accepted in Mongolia. Most Mongolians now are Muslim. Buddhists in Myanmar (formerly known as Burma) have recently used violence to drive out or exterminate a Muslim minority group known as Rohingya. Buddhists control Thailand and are major subpopulations in other countries of southeast Asia, notably Vietnam and Singapore, where they eschew the concept of non-violence that was once espoused by Lord Buddha. The Shinto religion of Japan is considered to be of ancient origin but which later became syncretic with Buddhism.[337]

The Golden Age of Greece, also known as the Classical Period, was in the 5th and 4th Centuries BCE. The majestic white marble building known as the Parthenon was constructed in Athens in 447-432 BCE. A few of the many memorable individuals who lived during that period should be mentioned.

In about 484 BCE, Herodotus, "The Father of History," was born; he died in 425 BCE. Socrates, an important Greek philosopher, was born c. 470 BCE; died 399 BCE, after being convicted of impiety and was forced to drink a poison, probably hemlock. He was famous for his Socratic method of teaching by the use of rhetorical questions, rather than providing direct statements. This method, exasperating to many students, may have been the irritant that led to his trial. The *Argument of Socrates*, written by his student Plato, does not say what Socrates actually spoke to the court, so we do not know what his "impiety" actually was. In about 460 BCE, Thucydides, notable Greek general and historian, was born; he died after 404 BCE. Thucydides wrote *History of the Peloponnesian War* against Sparta. He contracted the pestilence of 430-429 which was known as the "Plague of Athens," but he had the good luck to survive it. We do not know the cause of this "pestilence, but it was sufficient to cause Athens to lose the war." The greatest physician of the Golden Age of Greece, and one of the greatest of all times, Hippocrates, was born on the island of Cos in about 460 BCE; he died in about 375 BCE in Thessaly.[338]

Plato (c.428-c.348 BCE), a philosopher, was the most famous student of Socrates and he was the tutor of Aristotle. He is remembered for his eponymic Platonic lifestyle. However, some aspects of his personal life would now be thought of as scandalous, although sex with men and boys and slaves was commonplace in those days. Aristotle (384-322 BCE) was from the northern part of Greece known as Macedonia. He is arguably the principal philosopher of the Golden Age of Greece. He was also an amazingly thoughtful scientist who is especially remembered for his contributions to biology. He was the teacher of Alexander III of Macedonia, who is remembered as Alexander the Great. Aristotle accompanied Alexander and his army in Central Asia, India, and Egypt.[339]

Alexander the Great (Alexander III, aka Alexander of Macedonia) was born in Macedonia in 356 BCE; he **died at Babylon, 13 June 323**, of a "fever" of unknown cause – or perhaps he was poisoned. He became king after his father, Philip II, was assassinated. His mother, Olympias, was killed in 316 by relatives of those that she had killed. Alexander was unusually lucky in his early life, surviving many dangerous encounters as he led his army into western Asia, and then south across the land now known as Afghanistan into India. He reached the Indian Ocean, but by then, his troops had had enough. Sick and tired, they persuaded his generals to retrace the journey and go home. Alexander's luck ran out; good health suddenly turned to poor health. He died in Babylon, and the lands that he had conquered were divided into three parts. One of his generals, Ptolemy I Soter, born about 367 BCE, took control of the southwestern part of Alexander's empire. Ptolemy ruled Egypt and lands adjacent to it from 323-285. He founded the Ptolemaic dynasty, which lasted until the death of Cleopatra in 30 AD.[340]

Meanwhile, the Golden Age of Greece was fading as Rome was now a rising power in the Mediterranean. Euclid, the most prominent mathematician of ancient Greece and Rome, was born in Greece in 300 BCE. His *Elements* are the source for the theory of mathematics and plane and solid geometry, and the theory of numbers, beginning with five postulates – which are now called axioms – and five common notions. Ptolemy I Soter is said to have asked Euclid if there was not a shorter road to geometry than through his *Elements*, and Euclid replied that there is "no royal road to geometry."[341]

Cleopatra VII, who is usually known simply as Cleopatra, was born in 70/69 BCE. She was the last ruler of the Ptolemaic dynasty and one of the most powerful women in history. Cleopatra was the essence of the *femme fatal*, the lover of Julius Caesar and later of Mark Antony. After the Roman army of Octavian (later known as the emperor Augustus) conquered Egypt in 30 AD (also known as the Common Era, CE), she and Mark Antony committed suicide. Mark Antony fell on his sword, and legend has it that she allowed herself to be bitten by an asp, a poisonous snake; they were buried together.[342]

The Emperor Julius Caesar was assassinated in Rome on March 15, 44 BCE. He was born on 12 July 100 BCE in Rome. Caesar was one of the most successful generals and rulers of all time. *Caesar's Commentaries*, written about his campaigns in France, are still read as classics. Students in Latin translate his words, "All Gaul is divided into three parts," although they rarely ask what those areas of Europe are now called. Caesar's name became the eponym for emperor in Rome and he is still remembered in translation as Kaiser, Czar, and in the words of New Jersey (*Nova Caesarea*). Much of Caesar's life connects with health, illness, and medicine. He is said to have been the product of a difficult labor, which was solved when an incision was made in his mother's abdomen; his was the first "Caesarian birth." He probably suffered from epilepsy. He bathed daily in the icy Rhine River when he was on maneuvers in northern Europe. "Caesar' wife" is model of a perfectly faithful (or at least circumspect) spouse, yet Caesar notoriously dallied with Cleopatra in Egypt and may have fathered one of her children. To Shakespeare, we are indebted for knowing of the danger of the "Ides of March" and of Caesar's unforgettable cry, "*Et tu, Brutus*? (You too, Brutus?)" The moment was when Brutus, supposedly his best friend, stabbed him in the back at the behest of Cassius – he of the "mean and hungry look."[343]

About forty years after the death of Julius Caesar, in the reign of Caesar Augustus, a census was ordered to be taken throughout the Roman territories in Asia. Roman censuses had previously been taken at intervals of fourteen years, and this one has been calculated probably to have been done in about 7

BCE. It was in the reign of Herod, who was appointed as king of Judea by the Romans. Herod (known as "the Great") died in 4 BCE. Christians believe that Jesus, known as the Christ, was born in Bethlehem during this census, because his parents traveled from Nazareth to Bethlehem at that time so that his father, Joseph, would be registered in the city of his birth. Jesus' mother Mary was engaged to be married to Joseph, and she had her baby in Bethlehem. The Christian calendar counts the years since Jesus' birth as 1, 2, 3, and so forth, in the Year of God (Anno Domini, or AD); and the years before that were Before Christ (BC). The Christian calendar got off to a rocky start, however, because Roman numerals lacked a zero, and their calendar went directly from BC to AD. without allowing for a birth year. And because Joseph, Mary, and Jesus were of no particular importance at that time, no record exists of Jesus's birth or of his birth year. It would have been counted in the years of the reign of Caesar Augustus, because there was no sequential calendar in use at that time in the western world. Herod's many activities regarding the reported birth of a competitor for his throne are recorded in the Christian Gospels, so he presumably was alive at the time of Jesus' birth. As a result of the Bible's records of Herod's activities and of the probable year of the census, some theologians place Jesus' birth even a few years earlier, in say 7 BCE.

The birth of Jesus is now celebrated on the night of December 24-25 as Christmas (Christ's Mass). The date was chosen to coincide approximately with the winter solstice, because after that, the days would then gradually begin to lengthen. It was a date that was known and could be predicted by men of wisdom. Jesus's arrival would always be associated with this good fortune of Nature. Many historians now prefer to use non-theological abbreviations for years. BC therefore becomes BCE (Before the Common Era) and AD becomes CE (Common Era) or the years just stand alone; 1066 A.D. is now 1066 and AD or CE is understood. Herod the Great, King of Judea from 37 to 4 BCE, was born in 73 BCE, of Arabic parents. He was considered to be a Jew, however, as a result of his upbringing. He was notably cruel and immensely wealthy, and he was also a builder of palaces, temples, and fortresses. The cause of his slow, lingering death has been the subject of speculation; it is sometimes referred to as "Herod's evil." Some say it was arteriosclerosis, but there was also preceding mental instability.[344]

Jesus died in Jerusalem in 30 AD. He is said to have been a carpenter, as was his father, but he displayed a talent for healing in his later years. There is no contemporaneous record of his years of preaching – estimated to be one and half to three years – or of the end of it by his trial and execution. The Gospels say that he was crucified during the reign of Pontius Pilate, who ruled as prefect from AD 26-36; and that it was at the end of the week of Passover in the spring of the year that he was executed. Nothing was recorded at that time, but only a few years after he died, his followers began to write down what they remembered and told to others about what he said and did. Jesus was a charismatic recruiter, a brilliant teacher, and a spiritualist. He had a gift for speaking in parables, which in many cases he then patiently explained. However, he sometimes deliberately avoided explanation of a parable, or of a question that he posed, and that has allowed no end of speculation about the meaning of it. His ability to draw crowds and preach to them was often enhanced by dramatic demonstrations of his gift as a healer. Some of the patients who were brought to him had terrible physical problems, while others were mentally disturbed. He linked their cure to "belief." Without "belief," there could be no cure; with "belief," nothing would be impossible. Jesus recreated the priest-healers' ancient link between spiritual faith and physical action, and which is still employed by some physicians and many ministers. With his healing touch, Jesus was able to cure a woman who had vaginal bleeding for many years, and as a result had been a social outcast. He is said to have restored sight to the blind, to make a paralyzed man walk again, to drive out devils that had inhabited the mind of a person, and to raise again to life a dead man who had begun to putrefy. One of the four Gospels that tell of his life was written by Luke, who is believed to have been a physician. Luke's story includes many details that show Jesus's healing ability as well as his concern for health. One example: "And Jesus asked the lawyers and Pharisees, 'Is it lawful to cure people on the sabbath, or not?' But they were silent. So Jesus took him and healed him, and sent him away."[345]

Jesus and Buddha demonstrated poverty and sharing and non-violence from a theistic point of view. In Jesus's case, he demonstrated non-violence and sharing with others, and said that was what God required. Jesus made his words thought provoking, by speaking in parables that have led to endless interpretations. At various times, Jesus implied that he was God, but that he also was human, and that he was the Son of God. That is certainly mysterious. There is additional mystery in Christianity, especially with the many miracles described in the Gospels, the Book of Acts, and in the Book of Revelation. Buddha is regarded as the Supreme Being by Buddhists. In Buddhism, the theistic connection is more mystical, with opaque sayings such as *Om Mani Padme Um* (Hail to the jewel in the lotus), and that ultimate purpose of life is a search for The Way. In the 19th century, Karl Marx and Friedrich Engels also spoke of sharing, but their communist movement was not theistic, and it was not a non-violent program. Communism and Socialism have had mixed meanings, but they are both based on the notion of sharing with others, especially with those in need.

Most of the early followers of Jesus were Jews, and many – but not all – of these early Jewish Christians did not welcome non-Jews (known as gentiles) into their homes, or into their small communal gathering places, which they called churches. The early conflict between Christian Jews and Christian gentiles was soon resolved, however, and then all who believed in the teachings of Christ were welcomed to be baptized and to become members of the church. The early disciples traveled throughout the known world, even to Spain and India, and the Christian church grew steadily in membership. The early members were often persecuted for their beliefs, tortured, and killed, but they were not dissuaded. The Christian practice of sharing resources was appealing to the underclass, to the enslaved, and to women, who were welcomed by a Church that attracted people who had previously been outcasts in society in that part of the world.

In about 70-72 AD or CE, if you will, a massive building known as the Colosseum was built on the grounds of the former emperor Nero's Golden House. Seating 50,000 spectators who could sit under a retractable awning, it was the scene of contests between men who were gladiators and between men and animals. Some were said to have been Christians who were put to death in that way, although records to prove that are scanty at best. In about the year 100 CE, another man named Ptolemy, Claudius Ptolemaeus, was born in Egypt. Like those named Ptolemy who preceded him, he was of Greek (Macedonian) descent. A notable astronomer, mathematician, and geographer, Ptolemy died in about 170 CE. He was the author of the geocentric model of the universe known as the Ptolemaic system, which described in detail the solar system as it was described in general terms in the Bible. It was a geocentric universe, with the earth at the center, surrounded in circling orbits by the sun, the moon, and the planets, and outside of that, the stars. The notion of a geocentric universe appeared to be correct, for it was not just stated in the Bible, it appears to be what we see in the sky above us. The geocentric model was accepted without serious objections for nearly 1500 years. Ptolemy constructed maps which showed a round earth, with curved lines of longitude and latitude, and he correctly computed the circumference of the earth. His works on geography were rediscovered by European translators in the 14th century.

Less than a half century after Ptolemy died, a man was born in Anatolia, now Turkey, who became the most important physician of the Roman period. Galen of Pergamum, a Greek, was born in 129 CE; he died in Rome in about 216 CE. He became a wealthy man and was physician to Marcus Aurelius and other emperors. His writings dominated medical practice in Europe, Byzantium, and the Muslim Middle East from the Middle Ages until the mid-17th century – a period of some 1500 years. His multi-volume works, written in Greek, were translated into Latin, and later into French and German. Some, but not all, have been translated into English. They are useful records because they show the breadth of medical and surgical practice at that time, although they broke no new ground from the perspective of medical science. Galen became famous for his demonstrations of anatomy. Public dissections were as popular as contests between gladiators. They were dissections of animals, because dissection of deceased humans was illegal at that time. Galen's anatomical texts, based on the anatomy of animals, include errors that persisted for centuries.

In about the year 280 a Roman nobleman was born who rose to become Constantine the Great, the first Roman emperor to profess to be a Christian. He became the sole emperor of East and West in 324; he died in 337 AD. Christianity was given a tremendous boost by the conversion of Constantine, and tolerance of the faith extended throughout the Roman empire. No longer would it be an immediate hazard to health to be revealed to a Christian. The empire was divided, however, and its power was waning. The Sack of Rome that was accomplished by the Visigoths on 24 August 410 was but one of many occasions known as the Sack of Rome. Within a generation after the Visigoths hit Rome, Atilla the Hun crossed from Asia into Europe and crossed the Rhine into France, in territory that had previously been subject to Rome. The Huns were driven back, but their bloody depredations are still remembered. Health suffered in Europe. Atilla's Hunnic empire is dated 434 – 453. The Fall of Rome is usually said to have been in 455, but Rome had been slipping for some time before that.[346]

Clovis I, King of the Franks and founder of the Merovingian Dynasty, was born in 466. His dynasty survived for 200+ years, and was succeeded by the Carolingians. He died in Paris in 511. The dynasty is named for his grandfather, Merovech (Merovee), who is said to have governed the Salic Franks from 448-457. Merovee is supposed to have defeated Attila the Hun in 451.[347]

Muhammad, The Prophet, was born in Mecca, now in Saudi Arabia, in 570; he died nearby in Medina in 632. He founded the religion of Islam, and he is accepted by Muslims as the last of the Prophets. The *Qur'an* (Koran) is believed by Muslims to be the word of God, transmitted to Muhammad (who was illiterate) and transcribed by his followers; his own sayings are transcribed as the *Hadith*. Muhammad's ancestry is said by his followers to trace to Ismail (Ishmael) and thus to Abraham, as was mentioned above. His influence on the history of the world is incalculable. Many of the teachings recorded in the *Qur'an* and the *Hadith* are concerned with the preservation of health and prevention of illness, and are relevant to the subject of *Health Matters*. Three of the five Pillars of Islam, obeyed by the faithful, have potential, though probably unintended, benefits for health: the dietary restrictions (no alcoholic beverages, and no consumption of pork or shellfish); ablutions (washing hands five times every day before prayers); and the giving of alms (a social need, for the poor). Some of the traditions of Islam also have health benefits: the left hand (which is used for the toilet) is considered to be unclean; and the sole of the foot or of the shoe (which may have traveled through manure) is considered to be foul.

Europe was in what in retrospect is called the Dark Ages. But there were glimpses of grandeur for those who were in power, and who had accumulated wealth. Most of the people of northern Europe at that time were agriculturalists, living on their own small farms; or serfs, who were little better than slaves. In about 747, into the ruling family of France, was born a man who would be called Charlemagne – Charles the Great. He became King of the Franks (in 768) and Emperor of Rome (in 800), and he died 28 January 814, in Aachen, now Germany. He founded the eponymic Carolingian Dynasty. Like many other rulers, he was said to be illiterate, but that term does not properly distinguish between those who could read, but who did not write, and those who could neither read nor write.

The early followers of Muhammad were amazingly skillful and ruthless warriors. Before Muhammad died in 632, they had conquered the Saudi peninsula, to control the entire area between the Red Sea and the Persian Gulf. They rapidly spread the religion and customs of Islam throughout western Asia into Mesopotamia, to Syria, Lebanon, and Anatolia, and across the western and southern borders of the Mediterranean Sea to the Atlantic Ocean. By 661, Muslim rule extended from Persia to Egypt and Libya, and by 750, it would extend across the Straits of Gibraltar to encompass all of Iberia – modern Spain and Portugal – and the part of France known as Languedoc – and into Central Asia, including modern Afghanistan, Pakistan, part of India, and to areas north of the Amur Darya River to include the peoples, known as "stans," from Kazakhstan and Uzbekistan to Turkmenistan. Islam would later extend far to the east, into Mongolia and western China, across India to the East Indies, and across the Sahara Desert to sub-Saharan Africa, from the Indian Ocean to the Atlantic. After each territorial conquest, the rulers would usually be disposed of. However, if the people accepted the terms of the new rulers, they ordinarily would be allowed to practice their own form of religion. In countries ruled by Islam in its early years, religious ceremonies were conducted by Christians, Jews, and Zoroastrians, and they were allowed to do their usual business operations, although they were not considered to have the rights of citizens. Over the next five centuries, scholars of every faith were able to retrieve and translate ancient Greek and Roman documents into Arabic. These documents were carefully studied and were used as the basis for further development in the all of the scholarly fields: of science, medicine, technology, philosophy, mathematics, the narrative arts, and the fine arts. After the Muslim conquest, the territory controlled by Islam became a world at peace. It was the sequel to Pax Romana – the peace that was imposed by the Roman empire. In the major cities, the sick and wounded were cared for in buildings set aside for that purpose, and *madrassas* were developed for study of religious texts. These were the predecessors of hospitals and universities. All of this began to change when Europe emerged from the Medieval Period.

In 825, Muhammad ibn Musa al-Khwarizmi wrote a treatise on mathematics, translated into Latin as *Algebra e Almucabai*, from which the word algebra is derived. Arabic mathematicians introduced the zero and numerical fractions, and numbers begin to be useful in business. One of the important early physicians of the Golden Age of the Arabic world was Abu Bakr Muhammad ibn Zakariya al Razi (c. 841-926), born near Tehran, and known in the West as Rhazes. He first distinguished between the diseases of smallpox and measles. Ibn Sina (980-1037), known in the West as Avicenna, also of Persia, was the perhaps the greatest of all, but his knowledge and contributions to medicine were unknown at that time in England. Avicenna described the use of forceps in obstetrics for "difficult delivery." His work has been called "the most famous medical textbook ever written," and it is still read by students who study the Arabic language. The multivolume text of Galen was at least as famous, and translations of Galen's work into modern languages are still in print. The Arabs described laryngotomy, the use of silk ligatures, catherization of the bladder, and many other operations. In the western Mediterranean, Arabic physicians flourished. The greatest surgeon in the Western Caliphate was Abu'l-Qasim, known in Latin Europe as Albucasis (born in 936 near Cordoba, Spain), who is remembered not only for his original surgical techniques but also as the author of some 30 books. The notion of "publish or perish" could have originated with him. In the 10th century, Cordoba was the most civilized city in Europe, with a population of more than one million, and 50 hospitals. Medical education must have been rigorous in Cordoba and elsewhere in cities in the Arab world, although sad to say, we know nothing much about the details. The largest library in Cordoba had some 225,000 volumes.[348]

In northern Europe, there was nothing like this. **The high point of the Middle Ages was the 11th century** and the largest city in England was London, with a population of less than 20,000. The year 1066, which is arguably the most famous year in English history, shows the importance in human affairs of health and injury, and death or survival. It was the year in which England had four kings. The historical record shows that the first one died; the second was killed; the third wisely resigned and fled; and one conquered, was crowned, and survived. In the same generation, in Scotland, one king was killed; his successor was also killed; and the man who avenged the first killing was also killed. The saintly wife of the third man survived. And legend has it that another man was blinded for lechery. The usual diseases presumably took their toll, but the events resulting from lust are those that are remembered.[349]

The most famous Arab physician is said to have been Ibn Ruischd (1126-1198), known in Europe as Averroës, who also had the gift of writing. He made the useful observation that a person would not contract smallpox again after recovering from the first infection. His most famous pupil was a Jew, Musa ibn Mainun, called Maimonides (1135-1208), who became the physician to Saladin, the Sultan of Egypt, Palestine, and Syria. Maimonides is regarded in the Jewish world today as one of their greatest teachers. His medical practice was lucrative and successful, but he is remembered mainly for his philosophical writings. His patient, Saladin, founded the Ayyubid dynasty. He drove the Christians out of Jerusalem in 1187. Saladin is regarded as unusually benign, because he spared the lives of the defeated soldiers instead of ordering them all to be slaughtered, as was typical in those days.

Hospitals were in common use in the Arab world in the 8th to the 11th centuries, although not in northern France or England until after the 11th century. Many medical schools existed throughout the Arab world, but the first European medical school was established at Salerno in 1080. The pendulum of civilization swung north into Italy and then into the rest of northern Europe. Medical education led the path to the development of universities in Europe, which also included faculties of philosophy and law, and then the other branches of science, the humanities, and the arts. The earliest universities were sponsored by the Church, so Christian theology was a key to their existence and it usually was a required component of student education. For the next millennium, health care was rendered and controlled by a triad of institutions – physicians, hospitals, and universities. The triad was initially dominated by the physicians and surgeons, with tacit consent given to herbalists, midwives, and faith healers. Later, we will see the development of professional pharmacists, known in England as chemists, and of nursing.[350]

The diseases of women, and of their proper treatment, is usually traced to Hildegard of Bingen (1098-1179). The first of the great cathedrals of Europe were the Romanesque cathedrals which were erected in the 11th century. The architectural style known as Gothic began to be employed in the 12th century. Ken Follett, in *The Pillars of the Earth* (1989), set in the 12th century, gave vivid descriptions of health and of the practice of medicine (including home remedies, sorcery, and witchcraft) in that period. Some cathedrals took hundreds of years to complete, because of labor shortages resulting from the Black Death. And their design often changed as they rose. The architects were cautious, but they learned by experience. Many of these enormous, graceful stone structures were erected and stood until they were destroyed by aerial bombs in World War II. Architecture has been a vital component in the history of health care, in the design and construction of hospitals and universities, and of scientific laboratories.[351]

After several additional Crusades failed in the 13th century, Europe finally ceded victory to the Muslims in Jerusalem. The Crusaders turned instead to conquer, in an unimaginably brutal manner, the Christian city of Constantinople, and the schism between the eastern and western branches of Christianity thus became complete. A little village in northern Europe was settled that eventually became the city of Amsterdam, and King John of England was forced to sign the document known as the Magna Carta. Avignon, in France, concerned for cleanliness, decreed that streets should be widened, and that people must not discard bath water or "human filth" into the streets. Genghis Khan expanded the Mongol empire, invaded Russia, and then fell from his horse and died. His son Ogedei continued to expand the Mongol empire into Europe, but was turned back at Vienna. The rats that came with the Mongols were pleased to remain. Genghis' grandson Kublai Khan conquered China, and Marco Polo returned to Venice from China telling stories about Chinese civilization that were almost unbelievable. The bloody institution known as the Inquisition began during the papacy of Gregory IX. The climate gradually cooled near the end of the century, as the Little Ice Age began; it lasted for 400 years, producing a shorter growing season and declining yield of crops. This was a difficult time for health. The two most important figures in medicine in the 13th century were Bartholomaeus Anglicus, an English Franciscan, who composed *De Propretatibus Rerum* (Concerning the Properties of things), an encyclopedia which included 70 chapters on medicine (c. 1250); and Roger Bacon, also a Franciscan, who was called *doctor mirabilis* by his successors. He is said to have known all about everything.[352]

The 14th century got off to a poor start when Pope Benedict X died in Rome, supposedly after eating poisoned figs, and William Wallace, the Scottish hero, was captured and tried for treason in England. He was hanged, drawn, and quartered, an unintended public anatomical demonstration. The first public human dissection was performed in 1315 in Bologna, Italy, by Mondino d'Liuzzi, who also wrote a book about anatomy. Timur, also known as Tamerlane, was born in what is now Uzbekistan; by the time he died, he had become one of the world's leading lethal conquerors, though he is still greatly revered in Samarkand. His empire was greater than that of Alexander of Macedon, who is also called "the Great" in Samarkand. In Europe, war broke out between England and France in 1337, which would continue until 1453. By that time, England would lose most of its possessions in France, and the conflict would be remembered as the Hundred Years War. Shortly after that long war broke out, a devastating disease appeared in Europe. It was known as the Black Death, which probably came with traders along the Silk Road from Central Asia in 1343. Nearly half of Europe died within three years. The Black Death is sometimes said to have arisen in Tashkent, which is now in Uzbekistan, or perhaps it started in China. Waves of plague followed in successive centuries in Europe, and its complex cause and mode of transmission were not understood. There were three forms of the disease: Bubonic plague, with terrible lumps from festering lymph nodes; pneumonic plague, which causes coughing, shortness of breath, and death; and septicemic plague. Plague is caused by a bacterium, spread by the bite of a flea. Rats, which traveled as unwanted companions with traders and conquerors from Asia into Europe, have fleas which were long thought to have transmitted plague. Recent archaeological evidence suggests that the fleas infected with plague may have instead carried the disease directly from person to person. Another disease appeared in Europe in about 1374; it was known as the Dancing Mania or the dance of St. Vitus. The cause of the affliction is unknown, and it gradually disappeared. The 13th century was a problem for health, with climate change, wars, and epidemics of diseases. It was a difficult time for science, too, because astrology was considered to be as important as medicine and it was on a par with law and theology in universities. The end of the 14th century was marked by the death of Geoffrey Chaucer (c.1342-1400), "the outstanding English poet before Shakespeare." Chaucer's prose work, *The Canterbury Tales*, written in the 1390s, provides many examples of health beliefs and practices in England at that time. The cover of a recent edition of *Canterbury Tales* shows a proud gentleman in glorious academic robes, mounted on horseback. His "Physician's Tale" is told in the book.[353]

In retrospect, the Middle Ages in Europe ended during the 15th century. It was the century of the Renaissance, and for many historians, it was also the beginning of the Modern World. There are many other definitions for the Modern World, including that of the Museum of Modern Art (in the late 19th century), and also "Modernity" and "Post Modern" (the late 20th century). The turning point in history in the 15th century is sometimes defined as occurring with the Fall of Constantinople in 1453, when Christians were defeated by Muslims, who called it Istanbul, meaning "to the city" in Arabic. Or perhaps it was Gutenberg's discovery of printing with movable type. The Gutenberg Bible (1455) was the result. Both of these events relate to religion, which was shown in Part One to have originated as an aspect of humans' search for health. Many other events happened which together account for the end of the Dark Ages and a Renaissance ("rebirth") in western civilization. It was an uneven development, with greater changes seen in southern Europe than in the north; and more changes in the cities than in villages and on farms. The brutality that characterized the Middle Ages persisted in many ways. When Timur (Tamerlane) defeated the Christians at Smyrna, Turkey, the inhabitants were all killed. A Czech, Jan Hus, traveled to the Council of Constance to propose reforms, but was burned at the stake. Jews continue to be marginalized, ordered into ghettos, burned at the stake in Poland, and expelled from Sicily, Nuremberg, and Bavaria. Joan of Arc was burned at the stake; said then to be a witch, later discovered to be a saint (except by the English). The Ottoman Turks conquered Athens and moved on into the Balkans, and they defeated Venice to control the Adriatic Sea. Leonardo da Vinci demonstrated his brilliance as an engineer, anatomist, and painter. He also invented the parachute, although it had no useful purpose at that time. Ferdinand and Isabella, as joint monarchs of Spain, drove back Islam by annexing Granada, and they expelled all Jews who refused to become *conversos* to Christianity.

Most people continued to rely on traditional methods to protect their health and to treat disease and injuries. Health was their primary concern. For all of the components of health that were mentioned in Part One, from water, food, and shelter, to communal living in houses, with needs for firewood and sex. Mothers took care of their children's health, grandmothers advised them, and for difficult problems, the local healer was consulted. It was the system of health care that had existed for thousands of years in rural communities. In the few cities that existed in northern Europe, physicians emerged who passed their knowledge and skills from one generation to the next. We know little about them. Most were probably men, although even that is just supposition. The methods that they used were traditional, based on common sense and experience, rather than scholarship. One thing that they all had in common was the "gift" of healing, and the ability to perform simple surgery; without that, they would not be accepted in their community. In the cities, physicians were also appearing who had been trained in a formal manner in medical schools. All of them were men. There was an uneasy relationship between those trained as apprentices, who might be called "doctor," and those who had a university degree: Bachelor of Medicine, or Doctor of Medicine. The academic degrees were written in abbreviations which varied from one country to another, such as B.M, Dr.Med., M.D., and so forth. The duality of apprentice-trained and university-trained physicians would persist for a long time. It continued in the United States until the early 20th century. The impact of the Renaissance on medicine was principally the result of discovery of ancient texts written in Greek and Latin. These writings were preserved with their translations into Arabic, and they were returned to use as scholars in Europe worked with all of these languages.[354]

The 15th century was momentous for other reasons, too. The year 1450 has been called the beginning of the Age of Exploration or the Age of Discovery. Stimulated by Prince Henry "the Navigator," Bartolomeu Dias rounded Cape Horn in 1488 and Vasco de Gama sailed from Portugal to India in 1498. Ominously, the first enslaved people were transported from Africa to Europe in 1441 by the Portuguese. Christopher Columbus reached the West Indies in 1492, and Amerigo Vespucci, John

Cabot, and Nunez de Balboa soon discovered other parts of the New World. A profound impact on human health occurred in the **16th Century, as a result of the so-called Columbian Exchange** in 1492. The roundtrip voyage of Columbus to the New World was the moment when diseases began to spread reciprocally between the continents of America and the Old World. The impact on Native Americans was enormous and their deaths from measles, small pox and other European infectious diseases facilitated the European invasion. As many as 90 percent of the people present when the Europeans arrived were soon dead. Many Indigenous men, women, and children died without realizing what had caused the problem, because they died as diseases spread into towns and villages ahead of the invaders. Smallpox was still killing Native Americans some 250 years later. Arthur Crosby was one of the first to call attention to this problem in 1967. He called it the Columbian Exchange. For decades, school children were taught that the Europeans defeated the Native Americans because they wore armor, had firearms, and rode on horses. The implication was that the Indians were puzzled and afraid of these strange creatures. The Mandan tribe became extinct as the result of measles just before Lewis and Clark came through what is now South Dakota. That was taken to mean that the Mandan people were unusually frail.[355]

In Europe, syphilis, known as the "Great Pox," appeared after 1492, presumably transported by accident from the New World, where it may have been just a troublesome minor disease. Syphilis was usually spread by sexual encounters, hence the lascivious association with the disease, although other modes of transmission are available to the bacterium – a spirochete known as *Treponema pallidum.* Dreadful cases of congenital syphilis occur when syphilitic mothers pass the disease to their babies at birth. Syphilis was initially treated with compounds of mercury, the dangers of which we read about previously. In the 16th and 17th centuries, syphilis was considered to be worse than small pox, and it was probably true at that time. Measles was also more deadly at that time than small pox.[356]

Paracelsus (1493-1541) is emblematic of the 16th century in medicine and science. A genius, he was the son of a Swiss physician. His full name was Theophrastus Phillippus Aureolus Bombastus von Hohenheim. He chose the pseudonym Paracelsus to be remembered as "greater than Celsus" – a Roman author who wrote a compendium of medicine. He repeatedly stated his belief in "first principles," meaning discovery by people of the modern world, such as he was. He denigrated Hippocrates and he publicly burned one of Galen's books. Paracelsus loved his laboratory, and he used it to isolate and purify many substances, such as arsenic and mercury, which he used in medicine. He never succeeded in the goal of alchemists: to transform lesser metals into gold. Nevertheless, his notion of "specifics" was on the path to the present. Although many historians now believe he was overrated, it can be said that he made some important observations. For instance, he saw the relationship between cretinism and endemic goiter, he prepared laudanum (from the opium poppy), and he used in medicines not only mercury and arsenic, but also dangerous amounts of lead and copper sulfate, and potentially useful sulfur and iron. And he observed, amazingly, on chickens, the anesthetic action of sulfuric ether; this effect of sulfuric ether was independently rediscovered 400 years later by a dentist, William T. G. Morton. Some of the contributions of Paracelsus may be controversial or useless, but he can be credited with transforming the way that medicine was taught and the way that textbooks were written. Paracelsus spoke German in his lectures instead of Latin, and his enduring work, *Grosse Wundartzney* is also in German.[357]

Nicholas Copernicus (1473-1543) is credited with imagining and then developing proof that the sun is the center of the solar system, and that the earth and the other planets revolve around it. This conclusion is not an obvious one, for it appears to defy both commonsense observation and the Bible. Copernicus rightly anticipated that it would be controversial and probably heretical. Although he wrote a short unpublished manuscript about his theory in 1514, he delayed publication of the book until he was near death. In 1542, he finalized the book, *De revolutionibus orbium coelestium libri vi* ("Six Books Concerning the Revolutions of the Heavenly Orbs") and gave it to a friend to publish. Recognizing the dangerous ideas in this revolutionary theory, his friend wrote an Introduction suggesting that Copernicus was merely proposing an unproven argument. The idea of a heliocentric universe was gradually accepted over the next century. It now seems obvious – that the earth revolves around the sun, instead of the sun revolving around the earth – but it was controversial for a long time. Two great astronomers followed Copernicus, and who made important contributions to science, although one failed to accept the theory of a heliocentric solar system. They were Tycho Brahe (1546-1601), who accepted Copernicus' conclusion that the universe was very large and could be changing, but he never accepted Copernicus' model of the sun at the center of things; and Brahe's assistant, Johannes Kepler (1571-1630), who developed the concepts known as Kepler's Laws. His first two laws showed that the notion of perfect circular motion in the heavens was wrong, and the third law enabled calculation of the distances of planets from the sun.[358]

Everywhere in Europe, Jews continued to have serious undesired health problems, as they were expelled from cities and countries, and slaughtered. One example: in 1506, Christians killed some 4,000 Jews in Lisbon, Portugal. It is hard to grasp such a number. Meanwhile, in Rome, Michelangelo (1475-1564) worked in the Vatican. In 1512 he finished painting the Sistine Chapel with the beautiful images that have persisted to this day. On the ceiling of the chapel, the finger of God touches the hand of man. Niccolò Machiavelli (1469-1527) published *The Prince* in 1532, which has since been the classic text to measure a politician for his cleverness and ruthlessness, rather than for his courage and morality.[359]

On October 31, 1517, Martin Luther (1483-1546) submitted his academic disputation, *Ninety-five Theses*, to the Archbishop of Mainz. An oft repeated legend says that he may have posted them on the doors of churches in Wittenberg, Germany. The *Theses* stimulated the break in the Catholic Church known as the Reformation. It soon led to more than a century of religious wars in Europe, and to the killing of thousands of Catholics by Protestants, and vice versa. Although most people now are surprised that an ordinary priest would have such a profound effect on history, Luther was actually already a well-known figure at that time because of his prolific writing. He made good use of the printing press. And he also composed, in the vernacular, one of the most famous hymns of all time: "*Ein feste burg is unser Gott*" (A mighty castle is our God). Luther despised the Jews. Luther showed a vicious streak of anti-Semitism in his writings, an aspect of his life that has often been neglected in telling of his work to reform the Christian church.[360]

In 1529, Süleyman I, Sultan of the Ottoman Empire, reached the city walls of Vienna, but he failed to enter the city and retreated back to the Balkans. It was the last Muslim attempt to invade western Europe. King Henry VIII (1491-1547) declared independence from Rome in 1535, and he assumed control of the Church in England. The next year he ordered the beheading of his second wife, Ann Boleyn. He married four more times before he died. Ann's daughter, Elizabeth, nevertheless became Queen in 1558. A physician, Andreas Vesalius (1514-1564), wrote *De humani corporis fabrica*, which was published in 1543. The *Fabrica* is said to be "one of the great books of all time: a combination of art, anatomy and printing." It was "the first medical book in which the illustrations are more important than the text." Ambroise Paré (1510-1590), a brilliant surgeon in France, created artificial limbs in 1550. It was the first step in fashioning the bionic men and women of the late 20th century.[361]

The divisions in the Christian church were profound. On August 24, 1572, St. Bartholomew's Day, and on the following days, more than 20,000 Protestant Huguenots were hunted down and executed by Roman Catholics. A terrible slaughter. Ten years later, in the Catholic parts of Europe, the Gregorian calendar, named for Pope Gregory, replaced the Julian calendar, named for Julius Caesar. The Gregorian calendar was an improvement over the Julian, but its use was long resisted by Protestant rulers.[362]

Galileo Galilei (1564-1642), known to posterity simply as Galileo, was the probably the greatest scientist of the 16th and 17th centuries. In 1593 he invented the thermometer, which eventually enabled a third vital sign to be added to the rates of respiration and pulse that long been recognized by physicians. Galileo is more likely to be remembered for other contributions, such as his invention of the telescope, and his observation of falling bodies. Galileo's *Two New Sciences* (1638) is one of the founding documents of modern physics. Galileo believed that Copernicus was right about the theory of the heliocentric universe, but his sponsorship of this belief led him into trouble with the Catholic church. Near the end of his life, he barely escaped execution by pleading that it was all a mistake. He was then watched carefully, but was allowed to live in peace until the end.[363]

Meanwhile, in England, William Shakespeare (1564-1616), the greatest of all English writers, had published his first play, *Love's Labour's Lost*, in 1588-97. He would compose no less than 37 plays before he died, as well as beautiful poetry. Several have been mentioned previously in this essay, including *Julius Caesar* and *Anthony and Cleopatra*. His *Hamlet* should be included because of the central character's profound meditations on death. Shakespeare's last play was written in 1613, but his last well-known one was *The Tempest*, which was written in 1611.

Francis Bacon (1561-1626) was one of the leading figures in the history of science, noted for his statement that "Knowledge is power," and for encouraging the formation of scientific societies. Like most of the successful early savants, he had acquired money and power – he was Lord Chancellor of England and a Member of Parliament. He enjoyed performing experiments with chemistry, and he recorded his observations about plants and animals. His most important achievement was to inspire the foundation of the Royal Society. The Journal of the Royal Society continues to be a vital source of information about discoveries in science and medicine.[364]

William Harvey (1578-1657), who later became physician to King Charles I and President of the Royal College of Physicians, puzzled about the heart and wondered how it could pump so much blood. Where does all of this blood come from? He has an inspired thought. In *De Motu Cordis* (1628), Harvey proposed that the blood circulates, going out from the left ventricle of the heart in the aorta and returning through the vena cava to the right auricle of the heart. This theory upended thousands of years of teaching. His theory was based in part on the observation that the valves in the veins ensure that the blood will return to the heart by the veins, although no clear connection could yet be seen between the smallest arteries and the smallest veins; nor was there an obvious way for the venous blood to get through the lungs and return as bright red blood to the heart. He performed experiments in dogs, which buttressed his theory of the circulation of the blood; the capillaries in the periphery of the body and in the lungs would soon be seen with the microscope.[365]

An English physician who made no notable contribution to medical history or to science, yet who is important in this essay on health, is Sir Thomas Browne (1605-1682). Browne's portrait and a passing reference to his signature work, *Religio Medici* (1643), is in Ralph Major's *History of Medicine*. In order to assess Browne, one must turn to non-scientific sources. Browne received his M.D. at Oxford in 1634. He was a prolific writer. His reflections on *Religio Medici,* "the religion of a physician," was intended to be as "a private exercise directed to myself." It was circulated among friends and then published in 1643. It was an immediate success and it has influenced the thinking of many thoughtful physicians for the past four centuries. Browne was knighted by King Charles II. For many years, Browne's *Religio Medici* was an important companion for Sir William Osler (1849-1919), who was one of the most notable physicians of the early twentieth century. Osler carried a copy of the *Book of Common Prayer* in his doctor's bag, and he was always prepared to pray with a patient, if asked to do so.[366]

René Descartes (1596-1650) is best known as a philosopher, but he was a practicing scientist who was familiar with the telescope and microscope. He studied Harvey's theory of the circulation of the blood, and he believed it was correct. Descartes also decided that Copernicus was correct, but as a devout Catholic, he was careful not to offend Church authorities by saying much about it. Descartes doubted everything, and took nothing for granted. His most famous saying was *Cogito ergo sum* ("I think, therefore I am"). It was the summation of the Enlightenment. Descartes introduced the letters "x, y, and z" into algebra, to indicate the unknown. Descartes died of some type of infection shortly before his fifty-fourth birthday. Once again, ill health in the form of death trumps life, and a promising future was lost.[367]

King James VI of Scotland became James I, King of England in 1603. He was the eldest son of Mary, Queen of Scots, who was beheaded by order of her cousin, Queen Elizabeth of England. Once again, life and death played a significant role in history. Elizabeth died childless, and James was able to claim the throne of England. The crowning of James VI of Scotland as James I of England produced a personal merger of the two countries. This was formalized in 1707 to form the United Kingdom. Ireland joined the Union in 1801. The U.K. has survived for more than four centuries, but it has been a bit shaky in recent years. Sixteen of the 22 counties of Ireland became independent in 1922, when the Irish Free State was formed; the remaining six were in the northern province of Ulster. Rumblings have occurred recently in Scotland. Some wonder if Cornwall and Wales would follow, if Scotland leaves the U.K. King James somewhat reluctantly authorized the translation and printing of the Bible in English, but it has since borne his name: The *King James Version* of the Holy Bible (1611). For vivid descriptions of health and illness at this time, and what might be done to delay death, novelist Ken Follett continues his story of people in a fictional town in England. His earlier novel in this series, *The Pillars of the Earth* (1989), was set in the period of cathedral building in the 12th century. *A Column of Fire* (2017) is set in the late 16th and early 17th centuries.[368]

English adventurers successfully created a colony in North America in 1607, after several previous attempts failed; the most recent failure is still remembered as the Lost Colony of Roanoke. The successful settlement was known as Jamestown, in Virginia. The first enslaved people were brought there from Africa 1619. The first barrels of tobacco were shipped to England in 1614, soon to be followed by tons of tobacco annually, to the dismay of King James. He wrote a treatise in opposition to "this filthie noveltie." Intense cultivation of tobacco expended the nitrogenous nutrients in the soil, leaving the colonists at risk of starvation. They were also more interested in looking for gold than in growing crops for food, which supposedly led Captain John Smith to say, "He who does not work, does not eat." Ill health played a significant role in the history of the colonies of Virginia, Maryland, and the Carolinas. Early English settlers in Virginia and along the southern part of the Chesapeake Bay had a high mortality rate from tropical diseases and poor sanitation. These settlements survived only because of continued importation of men to replace those who died. Population in this part of North America began to increase only after new settlements were built in upland areas that were less prone to disease, and after women arrived and families developed.[369]

In 1608, the French built a small settlement at Quebec, which barely survived its first winter. In 1609, Henry Hudson traded with the Dutch at Manhattan Island and sailed up the Hudson River, looking for a passage to the Far East. The Dutch bought Manhattan from the Wappinger Confederacy in 1626. The Dutch East India Company built a factory in India in 1611 to make gunpowder, which was invented in China in the Tang Dynasty in about 850-900 CE. A simple formula was known to amateur chemists many centuries later: charcoal, sulfur, and potassium nitrate. The chemicals were included in the popular Gilbert Chemistry sets that were sold in the 1940s, and the recipe for making the explosive was in the *Americana Encyclopedia*. Gunpowder, and its derivatives of guncotton, nitrocellulose, nitroglycerine and dynamite, have caused countless deaths over the past several centuries. It is ironic that Alfred Nobel (1833-1896), who invented dynamite, is now famous for the prizes that are awarded annually in his name, including the Peace Prize and the Prize for Physiology or Medicine.[370]

The *Mayflower* landed in Massachusetts in November 1620, bringing religious separatists from England known as Pilgrims. They created the Plymouth Colony. The ship was sailing for Virginia and it was said to have been blown off course and landed far to the north, although some are skeptical about the excuse. The 102 Pilgrims who landed at Plymouth in late autumn had a terrible first winter. About half of them died, including most of the women, of starvation and hypothermia. One probably died of suicide. They also had to contend with skeptical tribes of Native Americans, which threatened their continued existence. They had but one physician, Samuel Fuller, who did not have a degree of M.D., but was simply called "doctor"; his wife was the colony's midwife. *Mourt's Relation* (1622) was the first publication to tell of life in the Plymouth Colony. The text was written by Governor William Bradford and others in the new colony. It was intended to please investors in England and to encourage others to emigrate to the colony in America. The editor and publisher, known only as "Mourt," is believed to be George Morton. *Mourt's Relation* is not wholly objective, but it gives a glimpse of what life was like in the early 17th century in America, including some things about health and illness. We now know that the mortality of the Pilgrims during that first winter in Plymouth was actually horrendous. Bradford's *History of Plymouth Plantation, 1620–47* was written as a manuscript and it was left in Boston's Old South Meeting House. It was discovered in 1844, and it was first published as *Of Plymouth Plantation* in 1856. It tells a redacted story of life in the colony. In spite of the rosy pictures that they paint, these two books are better primary sources than any others for early English colonies in America.[371]

A large fleet of ships arrived in Boston harbor in 1630, under the leadership of John Winthrop. The flagship of the Winthrop Fleet was the *Arbella*, named for Lady Arbella, daughter of the Earl of Lincoln, who arrived on the ship with her husband. These English were well-heeled and most were well-born. They were known as Puritans, disenchanted with the rituals of the Anglican Church, who wanted to "purify" the church. During the course of 1630, the Great Migration sponsored by John Winthrop brought between 700 and 1000 new settlers to New England. Nary a one of them was a physician, so they had to rely on the usual home remedies: women took care of the sick and delivered babies, and men treated those who were wounded in accidents and in conflicts. They founded the Massachusetts Bay Colony, which soon absorbed several smaller settlements on the coast in Massachusetts. The Pilgrims of Plymouth were even more radical than the Puritans; they were separatists, who had left the Anglican Church. The Plymouth group refused to join the Bay Colony at first. However, after the Pequot Indians raided the English colonies in 1638, Boston and Plymouth began to work together. Dr. Samuel Fuller and his nephew, Dr. Matthew Fuller, became physicians and surgeons for both Boston and Plymouth. The Wampanoag Indians, led by their chief, Metacom, called "King Philip," attacked the settlements of the English in 1676, but the Indians were defeated. King Philip's War ended with Metacom being cut into quarters and his head was mounted on a pike at the entrance to Fort Plymouth. The wife and children of the Wampanoag chief were shipped enslaved to Bermuda.[372]

The English colonists on the coast of Massachusetts gradually spread outward, and they established new settlements in what is now Maine, New Hampshire, Rhode Island, and Connecticut. There were very few doctors among them. They continued to use the same methods that had served in families and small communities for thousands of years: Men took care of injuries with needle, thread, knives and splints. Women prepared herbs and potions from powders of leaves, bark, roots, and beer; cleansing soap made from ashes and pork fat; and soothing salves made from butter and sour cream. The health of New England colonists was dramatically better than those in the southern colonies. The agonies of childbirth were unrelieved, but women usually bore children every two years until menopause, and most of the children survived. Families were very large. Tombstones on Nantucket Island show that in the seventeenth century there were many men and women who lived into their late nineties.[373]

Disease was rampant in Europe in the 17th century. In 1631, the bubonic plague killed about 500,000 people in Venice, which accelerated the decline of that Republic. In 1648, the Peace of Westphalia ended the 80 Years War between the Hapsburgs and the Dutch, and Spain recognized Dutch independence. In 1649, King Charles I was defeated by the Puritan Oliver Cromwell and he was beheaded. Parliament ordered Cromwell to subdue Ireland, and he carried out notorious massacres of Catholics there. Cromwell died in 1658. After this brief period known as the Commonwealth, England returned to rule by hereditary monarchs. King Charles II, son of the beheaded Charles I, was crowned in 1660. Five years later, the Black Plague (the Black Death) struck London, killing about 70,000 in one week. In the following year, 1666, the Great London Fire destroyed much of the city, and it was rebuilt with stronger materials – brick and stone, instead of wood and thatch. The 1660s were bad years for health in England. The last plague in Europe ended in 1679, and in thanks, many Plague Monuments were created. The most elaborate is probably the Baroque Pestsäule (Pest Column) in Vienna.[374]

Thomas Sydenham (1624-1689) was the most respected English physician of the 17th century. He is said to be the founder of clinical medicine in England. His fame rests on many publications, originally in Latin, but which were later translated into English and other European languages. He described St. Vitus' dance (Sydenham's chorea) and he commented on hysteria and hypochondria. He is sometimes attributed with the aphorism *primum non nocere* (first, do no harm), although variations on that famous phrase can be traced back to Hippocrates. He realized that Peruvian bark (quinine) was useful for some fevers (i.e., malaria), and he began to search for other specifics. He dedicated his great work on fevers, *Methodus Curandi Febres* (1666) to his contemporary, the chemist, Robert Boyle. One of his close friends was another physician, John Locke (1632-1704), better known as a philosopher. Locke published his own *Observationes medicae* (1699), but his great contribution is *Essay concerning Human Understanding* (1690). In his publications, Sydenham did not mention William Harvey or Harvey's theory of the circulation of the blood, which shows that this new theory had little immediate impact on the practice of medicine. It is similar in many ways to the slow acceptance by astronomers of the theory of the heliocentric universe of Copernicus.[375]

Robert Boyle (1627-1691) and his assistant Robert Hooke (1635-1702) were instrumental in the progress of chemistry. Boyle should be remembered as the man who developed litmus paper. Every high school student knows from his chemistry class that a strip of litmus paper turns red when it is dipped in vinegar (acidic) and it turns blue in bleach (alkaline). From his experiments, Boyle concluded that the ancient theory of the four elements – earth, air, fire, and water – was incorrect. And so, too, would be the mixture of these elements that had long been thought to be the human body: yellow bile, black bile, blood, and phlegm. Boyle thus set chemistry on a path to discover what the elements might be.[376]

Antonie van Leeuwenhoek (1632-1723), a skilled crafter of lenses in Amsterdam, began in 1674 to peer through a combination of lenses at tiny things that could not be seen, unaided, without this device. It was the first microscope. Leeuwenhoek carefully drew pictures of what he saw. Others later found that he had discovered many forms of bacteria. He also discovered motile sperm, which did not appear spontaneously under his lenses. He was probably curious about how copulation led to pregnancy.[377]

Isaac Newton (1642-1727) presented his *Principia* to the Royal Society in 1686. He explained gravity, inertia, and other laws of nature. Two years later, King James II was deposed in the Glorious Revolution, and William of Orange was invited by Parliament to rule in England. His wife, Mary, a distant descendant of the English Royal family, was intended to give legitimacy to the revolution, and they ruled together as King and Queen. In retrospect, the 16th and 17th centuries are sometimes called the period of the Scientific Revolution. These centuries also included the end of the Renaissance and the beginning of the Reformation, which had little to do with science, although the intellectual ferment in these centuries had an impact on science. By this reckoning, Newton and his theories are usually considered to have been the climax of the Scientific Revolution. Science continued to advance in the 18th century, but this period is usually termed the period of the Enlightenment.[378]

William Penn (1644-1718) was the privileged son of an immensely wealthy and well-connected Englishman, Admiral Sir William Penn. After toying with the idea of becoming a warrior himself, and dallying as only a playboy can do, Penn was attracted to the novel ideas of the Quakers – known as the Society of Friends – and he became a Quaker in about 1667. It was dangerous to be a Quaker, for the radical activities of this sect were considered to be treasonous. Quakers recognized only their personal beliefs, whatever they might be, and they would not swear allegiance to the Crown. The men would not even bow or doff their hats. In Protestant England it was more likely that a Quaker would be tortured and executed than would a Roman Catholic. One of the ways that England had dealt with the problem of radicals, such as Separatists and Puritans early in the century, and now Quakers, was to allow them to go to America. Admiral Penn died in 1670, and the large debt that King Charles II owed to the admiral was paid to the son by granting him an enormous province in America. The boundaries were ill defined in the grant, but Pennsylvania would be located between New York (on the north) and Virginia (on the south), and from the Delaware River (on the east) to as far west as could be imagined. A few months later, his friend, the Duke of York (who later became King James II), granted him the three counties that are now Delaware. William Penn was a shrewd businessman as well as being a devout Quaker. He sold large parcels of his land along the Delaware River to Quakers in England and in the valley of the Rhine in what is now Germany. The new owners bought their thousand-acre properties without seeing them. They knew that they would have to find the boundaries after they arrived in America, and then purchase the land again from any Swedes or Indians who might already be settled there. The owners of Penn's grants would also be awarded five acres of land where the small Schuylkill River enters the Delaware River. This became the city of Philadelphia, which within a century would become, next to London, the greatest city in the lands ruled by the United Kingdom. William Penn sailed to America and arrived at the site of his new city in the ship *Welcome*, in October 1692. Twenty-one more ships came to Pennsylvania in 1692, some before, some with, and some that followed Penn. Collectively, the passengers on these ships, perhaps as many as 355, arrived in what is called the Welcome Fleet. It was a dangerous voyage. Many died during the passage and were buried at sea, and those who arrived late in the year had a difficult time getting though their first winter. Many barely existed in dugouts in the hillsides.[379]

Pennsylvania was the only one of the original thirteen colonies that welcomed all Christians, Quakers, Baptists, Catholics, Jews, and non-believers. Pennsylvania thus contrasted with the rigorous puritan Protestant beliefs in much of New England, the high church Anglican Protestants of Virginia and the Carolinas, and the Roman Catholics of Delaware. The fortuitous combination of a sheltered deep port in Philadelphia and the Quaker principles of fair dealing in business, led to the development of several institutions in Philadelphia that positively affected the health and welfare in Pennsylvania and in the other colonies. During the century after the Welcome Fleet arrived, the first hospital in the thirteen English colonies in North America would be established in Philadelphia, and also the first medical school.[380]

Only ten years after the Quakers arrived in Pennsylvania to create a province that is famous for religious tolerance, in Salem, Massachusetts, Puritans hanged nineteen men and women as witches. The infamous episode of Salem's "witch hunting" would become forever known as a symbol of intolerance. One man was pressed to death; countless others were accused and were jailed in Essex County, Massachusetts; some children were tortured to give evidence against their parents; and many died as they languished in prison during that year of terror. Various aspects of the episode of the witch trials have been examined previously in this essay. I will only repeat here that the events in Salem in 1692 have aspects that demonstrate relationships between all of the subjects discussed in this essay: these events involved individuals, families, and communities; of aspects of physical and mental health; of sickness and death; and of religion, medicine, and politics. Health mattered in both Philadelphia and Salem, but it had a positive effect in the City of Brotherly Love, and it was negative in Salem.

Rev. Dr. Cotton Mather, FRS (1663-1728), a Puritan minister in Massachusetts, would appear to be an odd candidate to introduce into the history of medicine. He provided the theological support needed for conviction with "spectral evidence" of the accused witches at Salem in 1692. However, Mather can be credited for providing leadership for the successful introduction of inoculation to prevent smallpox in Boston. "Inoculation" was the method used before the discovery of vaccination by William Jenner in 1798. Inoculation (also known as variolation) utilized implantation of small amounts from pustules of patients with mild cases of smallpox. The medical establishment in Boston opposed the use of inoculation, but in 1721, Mather backed the use of it by a physician named Zebadiel Boylston, who did not have a doctoral degree. Mather published statistical evidence which showed that inoculation reduced the mortality from smallpox in those who received the inoculation to 2% compared to 14% in those who were not inoculated. Inoculation/variolation was not without risks, and it was difficult for parents to make the decision to ask for it to be given to their children. Benjamin Franklin failed to do this, and he deeply regretted his indecision when one of his sons, Francis Folger Franklin, died of "natural" smallpox at age four in 1736. John Adams, who became the second president of the United States, was in Philadelphia in July 1776 when his wife Abigail decided to do it. She took their four children from their farm in Braintree to Boston to be inoculated by Dr. Thomas Bullfinch, one month after Boston suspended its prohibition of the procedure. Abigail and all of the Adams children, including John Quincy, age 4 – who became the sixth U.S. president – had the treatment, and all eventually recovered. But it was a hard business. Three had to be inoculated a second time, because the first attempt to produce smallpox failed, and one needed three tries before it was successful. The children's illnesses ranged from mild to severe – "puking" and "sick with fevers, terrible body aches, and erupting pustules" – before Abigail could write to John that it was finally over.[381]

In retrospect, the **18th Century was an auspicious time for medicine**. Dr. Herman Boerhaave (1668-1738), is said to have tipped his hat to Sydenham. As we have seen on many occasions with previous notable physicians, Boerhaave's reputation persists because of his books. He wrote two, which are usually printed in many volumes: *Institutiones medicae* (Medical Institutions, 1708) and *Aphorisimi de cognoscedisi de et curandis morbis* (Aphorisms, 1709). Copies of these two works, in English translation, extend most of the way across a 3-foot-wide bookshelf. The *Aphorisms* went through 10 Latin editions and it was translated into English and French. The *Institutions* went through 15 Latin editions and it, too, was translated into modern languages. He was undoubtedly a fine physician, and a very busy one, but his books set him apart from all of his contemporaries. Boerhaave made no important discoveries, but his books were used to teach many generations of physicians.[382]

One of the important figures in the history of science would be a surprise to most readers in the 21st century. Benjamin Franklin (1706-1790) is best remembered as a long-lived politician who lived in Philadelphia at the time of the American Revolutionary War. Some might recall that he spent most of the Revolutionary War in France, working on behalf of the new United States, and that he was involved in some way with the Continental Congress, the Declaration of Independence, and the Constitution. A few might remember various disconnected stories about Franklin, such as that he was the author of *Poor Richard's Almanac*, and that he flew a kite in the rain to show something about electricity. In fact, he did all of these things, and more. Franklin was a brilliant man, an autodidact, and he had just the right charisma to succeed in the quiet, staid, Quaker land of Philadelphia. He was not a Quaker, but he appreciated their beliefs, and he persuaded the leaders of Philadelphia to create the first hospital in the English colonies of North America (the Pennsylvania Hospital); and the first American medical school, at the University of Pennsylvania; and the first insurance company; and the first lending library; and more. Many of these activities were stimulated by Franklin, who came from Boston to Philadelphia as a young man. *The Autobiography of Benjamin Franklin* is based on notes that he wrote. It is incomplete, but it is a window into the first century of the city of Philadelphia.[383]

Franklin achieved success in many business enterprises, and he became one of the wealthiest men in the British Empire. His restless mind also led him to solve his personal health problems: he invented bifocals, to improve his reading ability; and the flexible rubber catheter to by-pass urinary obstruction from his bladder stones. But to make a pun, it was in the field of electricity that his light really shined. Franklin imagined that lightning had some similarity to the electricity in the Leyden jar, with its "positive" and "negative" poles. He proved the connection with his experiment in a rainstorm, flying a kite with its attached metal key. He protected himself with a wax handle to hold the kite string, and he "grounded" himself with a wire that he attached to himself and to the ground beneath him. He made the first battery (a word which he coined) by placing a piece of glass between the two strips of lead in a Leyden jar; and he created the world's first lightning rod, which he placed on the peak of his own house. Thomas Alva Edison (1847-1931), who was the Great Electrician of the 19th and 20th centuries, was, like Benjamin Franklin, largely self-educated, and restlessly curious. Edison's creative work began with batteries which produced low voltage direct current, which was a connection, so to speak, with Franklin. Benjamin Franklin has an incomparable role in the history of health. It includes not only technology – his medical inventions – and his leadership in the establishing the first hospital and medical school in America, but also for his discoveries in the science of electricity, which drives most of the devices used in medicine and health care in the 21st century.[384]

Carl Linnaeus (1707-1778) was a physician in Sweden, although he is remembered for his work in botany and biology. His great goal, which he finally completed, was to work out a way to classify all of the plants and animals. He assigned the name of the genus and species, *Homo sapiens*, to us.[385]

The prevention of the disease known as scurvy, which we now know is due to deficiency of Vitamin C, was discovered at this time by a British Navy surgeon, James Lind (1716-1794). It was a clever piece of work, which was the fore-runner for controlled trials in medicine. Others had previously proposed that citrus fruit would prevent scurvy, so Lind's treatment was not an original idea. His contribution was to study the effects of various treatments on 12 sailors who were developing scurvy on a long voyage in 1747. He divided them into six groups, which he treated with different supplements. One pair received two oranges and a lemon, and they were the only ones that were improved. Lind believed that administering citrus fruit for scurvy was something akin to using Peruvian bark for malaria. It was not realized that scurvy was a disease caused by deficiency of Vitamin C (ascorbic acid) until 1932. British sailors later received dietary supplements of limes, hence their nickname "limeys."[386]

Joseph-Ignace Guillotin (1738-1814) was a prominent physician in Paris. He was elected to the National Assembly in 1789, where he was instrumental in having a law passed requiring all sentences of death to be carried out by "means of a machine." A decapitation "machine" was constructed in 1792 by a man named Antoine Louis and first used in that year. Guillotin was later imprisoned during the Reign of Terror, but he survived to practice medicine again, and was a supporter of Jenner's technique of vaccination to prevent smallpox. He died of a carbuncle, which is an infection caused by *Staphylococcus aureus*. By coincidence, a physician of Lyon named J. M. V. Guillotin, apparently unrelated to Joseph-Ignace Guillotin, was put to death by the guillotine.[387]

William Withering (1741-1799) was a graduate from Edinburgh and he practiced medicine in Birmingham. He had a large practice, and he traveled widely about the countryside to see patients. He was an ardent student of botany and in 1766 he published a major work on the "all the vegetables" of

Great Britain. Withering heard that an old woman in Shropshire had a secret remedy for dropsy, and he obtained the recipe for the concoction. He realized that the active principle in the thirty ingredients was the leaf of the foxglove plant, and he thus introduced digitalis into the list of useful pharmaceuticals. Withering published *An Account of the Foxglove and Some of its Medical Uses* (1785), and digitalis became the mainstay of treatment for heart disease for the next two centuries.[388]

One of the most significant events of the late 18th century in Europe and America is known as the Revolutionary War, or the War for American Independence – depending on which side the conflict is viewed from. In the thirteen colonies that became the United States, those who won the war are called Patriots, while those who wished to remain in the Empire were called Tories. In Canada, the Tories were known as Loyalists, and their descendants still refer to their opponents as Rebels. I will not argue that question, but instead I will attempt to discuss the impact of the new nation upon the history of the world. I will instead give a few examples to show how health and illness played a significant role in the outcome of the war. The war was fought for "life, liberty, and the pursuit of happiness" and the slogan of the Patriots of New Hampshire is now the motto of the state: "live free or die." These are frank statements about the purpose of the war; it was all about health. We can also look at the Revolutionary War from the perspective of individual participants. For instance, George Washington (1732-1799) was able to play his crucial role as general and later as president only because he escaped death on many occasions when his life was in danger. Washington contracted smallpox as a young man, but survived it; he survived his early service in the French and Indian War, when his commanding officer was killed; and he personally led his troops into battle at Trenton, Princeton, Monmouth, and Yorktown, when many around him were killed. He knew that he would be a target, for he was a tall man, in a glorious uniform, riding on a distinctive white horse. Washington's genius as a military leader has often been unappreciated. He won only a few battles, yet in the end, he won the war against the British by his strategy of attack and retreat. It was a strategic method that was unknown in Europe, and would largely be forgotten until it was used successfully by Ho Chi Minh in Vietnam in the 20th century. At the end of the war, Washington changed the course of history: he surprised the world by resigning his commission instead of becoming king of this new country. And then he established a precedent for American presidents that lasted for more than 150 years when he declined election to a third term in office. None of these events would have been possible if Washington had not survived all of his close encounters with death.[389]

Benjamin Rush (1745-1813) was the most famous American physician of the late 18th century, and he was arguably the most important of all of the physicians in colonial America. He was a careful observer, uniquely thoughtful of patients with mental illness, and he had a large and successful practice. He has been criticized for his use of bleeding in treatment, although that was commonplace at that time. He was a Signer of the Declaration of Independence, and he often demonstrated personal bravery as a surgeon during the Revolutionary War. Under a flag of truce, he traveled across enemy lines to see if he could help the fatally wounded General Hugh Mercer in Princeton, New Jersey, in January 1777.[390]

The storied lives of three other physicians of the 18th century must suffice to show something of the ways that medicine advanced in England during that interesting period. These physicians are Sir Percival Pott, John Hunter, and William Jenner.

Sir Percival Pott (1714-1788), who described tuberculosis of the spine (known as Pott's disease). In 1775, Pott was the first person to describe a form of cancer that was the result of something in the environment – a carcinogen in soot which produced squamous cell cancer of the scrotum in chimney sweeps. It is known as Pott's cancer. After young boys were not sent to clean chimneys, this disease disappeared. However, the chemicals in soot that caused Pott's cancer are similar to the carcinogens in tobacco smoke, which has caused millions of deaths. John Hunter (1728-1793) was a surgeon, born in Scotland, who followed his older brother, William, to London, to practice at St. George's Hospital. William rose to become a prominent obstetrician and anatomist; he delivered the boy who later became George IV. John was somewhat of a rougher cut. He left Oxford after two months and assisted his older brother in the dissecting room while becoming a surgeon's pupil at St. George's, and then house surgeon. He joined the army and served in battle, where he learned much about wounds and their treatment. On his return to London, he embarked on a successful career in surgery, while at the same time teaching, dissecting, collecting anatomical specimens, experimenting (including self-experimentation), and writing on medical and surgical topics. Astonishingly, he inoculated himself with pus from a patient with gonorrhea, to see if the disease was the same as syphilis. He developed both gonorrhea and a chancre, but he failed to recognize that the two diseases were different. When he realized that he had acquired syphilis in the experiment, he took mercury for three years. He later developed angina pectoris, probably caused by tertiary syphilis. Hunter had a ferocious temper, and he sometimes pushed the boundaries of decency. But he should best be remembered for his statement, "Why think – why not try the experiment?" His students are said to have loved him, calling him "the dear man." Several of them became famous, such as Philip Syng Physick (1768-1837), known as the "Father of American Surgery"; Sir Astley Paston Cooper, a brilliant but "sadistic" surgeon; and William Jenner, who discovered vaccination.[391]

William Jenner (1749-1823) was the son of the vicar of Berkeley, Gloucestershire, on the Little Avon River, about 100 miles west of London. At the age of 13, he decided to become a physician and he apprenticed for six years with a surgeon near Bristol. He then went to London to study with John Hunter, and he lived in Hunter's home for two years. In Bristol, Jenner had seen a young woman who said that because she had had cowpox, she couldn't get smallpox. Jenner is said to have discussed this with Hunter, and it continued to be a source of wonder and curiosity to Jenner. He returned to Berkeley to practice medicine, but he also did experiments on animals. He reported his observations to the Royal Society in London and was elected as a Fellow. Like many physicians at that time, he performed inoculation (variolation) to prevent smallpox. In 1796, he saw a case of cowpox in a milkmaid. He obtained pus from the sore on her hand and injected it into the arm of a boy. The boy developed a small pustule, followed by a scab and scar. Six weeks later, Jenner inoculated the boy in the usual manner with smallpox, but no smallpox developed. He repeated the procedure on three more patients, with similar effects. He prepared a paper for the Royal Society about the four cases, but it was rejected. Jenner therefore published it privately in 1798, entitled *Inquiry into the Causes and Effects of the Variolae Vaccine*. Vaccination, as Jenner called it, was controversial in England at first, but it was soon accepted by physicians in America, France, Germany, and Italy. After English physicians accepted the procedure, Jenner was honored in his own country. In 1802, Jenner received thanks from Parliament, and the first of two grants of money, totaling 30,000 pounds. Jenner lived in London after he received the first grant, but he chose to return to work as a family doctor in Berkeley. Ralph Major says appreciatively that, "Jenner's discovery ranks among the greatest discoveries in medicine."[392]

William Bynum says that there were two important characteristics of medicine in the 18th century, especially in France: "Health mattered, and people were prepared to pay for it." It was a time of "busy optimism. ... The idea of progress, including medical progress, was taken for granted [and] medically oriented philanthropy was common." We now know, however, that medical progress has not been entirely free of negative consequences. Thomas Robert Malthus recognized the problem that presses upon us today. In 1798, he published *An Essay on the Principle of Population as It Affects the Future Improvement of Society*, in which he argued that population will always tend to outrun the growth of production. And if unchecked, population will expand to the limit of subsistence and will be held there by famine, war, and ill health. Malthus may or may not be correct; we do not know what the future holds. But he predicted that demography would show that health matters in human history.[393]

One of the most influential physicians of France in the **19th Century, when Paris was the "Mecca of the medical world"** was René T. H. Laennec (1781-1826). His contribution will serve as a model for many others who, like him, made the rigorous, complete physical examination of each patient a mainstay of diagnosis and treatment. Laennec is credited with introducing the stethoscope, which he also named. It was originally just a piece of heavy paper, rolled into a tube. In 1816, Laennec placed one ear on the outer end of the tube, while he placed the other end against the patient's chest. He made this device to avoid placing his ear against the chest (i.e., the breast) of a young woman, in what was the usual, though embarrassing, way to listen to the heart and lungs. This form of auscultation, as it was called, was surprisingly effective. Laennec promptly converted the stethoscope to a hollow wooden tube. It was soon modified to be a metal horn, with a narrow earpiece and a wider endpiece that was placed against the chest. It was again modified to have two earpieces that were connected by two rubber tubes to a large endpiece with a diaphragm that was placed against the chest or abdomen. In the late 1950s it became the modern 'scope with a small endpiece and diaphragm, and one tube connected to two earpieces. It dangles symbolically around the necks of millions of doctors, medical students, nurses and first responders. Since the time of Laennec, the physical examination of the chest (including the heart and lungs) has included the Paris doctors' group of four tests: inspection (looking), palpation (touching), percussion (tapping), and auscultation (listening). As a specialist in pulmonary diseases, Laennec treated many patients with tuberculosis, and like many of his contemporaries, he died of this disease.[394]

While Laennec and other physicians were at work in Paris, a vastly different form of the practice of medicine was taking place across the Atlantic. A midwife on the frontier in Maine, Martha Ballard, was keeping a diary that told of her daily struggles to reach mothers in time to deliver their babies. Ballard also worked with local physicians, and she recorded what they thought and did in their practices. Her diary was thoughtfully edited by Laurel Thatcher Ulrich, *A Midwife's Tale: The Life of Martha Ballard* (1990), for which Ulrich was awarded the Pulitzer Prize. Ballard (1735-1812) was the aunt of Clara Barton (1821-1912), who founded the Red Cross movement after serving as a volunteer nurse with the Union Army during the Civil War. Barton was motivated by the hundreds of patients that she treated with war wounds and illnesses in the camps. The observations that moved Barton were similar to those seen by Walt Whitman (1819-1892), who served as a volunteer nurse's aide in Union Army hospitals in Washington, D.C. Whitman's poetry about sorrow and death in hospitals reached an even more profound depth as he composed *Oh Captain, My Captain* (1865) about the death of Abraham Lincoln.[395]

For medicine and surgery at sea in the early 19th century, a fine account is given in the novels written by Patrick O'Brian, CBE (1914-2000). At that time, there were great ships that moved only from wind in their sails. His books feature the competition and cooperation between two fictional characters: a warship's commander, Captain Jack Aubrey, and a ship's surgeon named Stephen Maturin, who also happens to be a spy. The British honorific for a surgeon was then and still is "Mr." Maturin is familiar with all of the latest treatments in medicine and surgery at that time, and they are described in perfect detail by the author. Two of the books, *Master and Commander* and *The Far Side of the World*, were combined in the script of a movie (2003), with the former title, in which the action was changed from combat at sea between Britain and the U.S. in the War of 1812, to conflict with a French ship, sailing for Napoleon, near the Galapagos Islands.[396]

The Lewis and Clark Expedition (1804-1806) was sent to explore the new American territory known as the Louisiana Purchase. This Corps of Discovery was led by Meriwether Lewis (1774-1809) and William Clark (1770-1838), who were dispatched under orders from President Thomas Jefferson. They had incredible success without loss of life after they left the Missouri River. Following military rules, careful preparation, good luck, and good health allowed the expedition to succeed. There was a downside to the expedition, however, that is rarely discussed. Upon their return, William Clark did not free his enslaved servant, known only as York; and Meriwether Lewis died three years later, apparently a suicide, after suffering from bouts of depression.[397]

The Industrial Revolution was well underway in England in the mid-18th Century and it was over in Europe by the 1840s. It was named for the technological revolution that was more clearly demarcated than the so-called Scientific Revolution which preceded it. The histories of science and technology were always intertwined, and neither field was independent of the other. Both were based on a search for health, as I have defined it, and both had enormous impacts on human health. Some of the outcomes were sought for and have been helpful to humans, some were incidental and questionable, and some were terrible and their bad results have persisted. The Industrial Revolution is said to have begun in Europe in 1760, as the world of individual farms with workers centered around small towns, was replaced by a new world of industry, with large numbers of men, women, and children, who toiled in cities with machine manufacturing. This period of revolution ended in Europe in about 1840, by which time it had become the normal economy. Advances in science of course continued. John Dalton (1766-1844) is credited with introducing the atomic theory into chemistry; he also studied colorblindness, which as a result is called "Daltonism." And Michael Faraday (1791-1867) discovered many of the important principles of electricity. Faraday also discovered benzene, the key molecule in organic chemistry – the chemistry of life. The Industrial Revolution began a generation later in the United States, because the large labor force that was needed to work in mills and factories was not immediately available. Immigrants streamed into America from Europe, but they could not be induced to work for long in mills and factories. Land vacated by or taken forcibly from Native Americans, which was available for individual family farms, beckoned irresistibly in the North, and the pioneers spread west across the land that was north of the Ohio River. In the Southern states, the workforce consisted largely of enslaved people of color, living on large plantations, or stubborn descendants of Scots-Irish highlanders, content with their contrariness, who lived in small clearings in the Appalachian mountain forests, and were unwilling to toil in factories.[398]

The Industrial Revolution had enormous and persistent effects on the health of humans, in addition to its effects on the ecology and health of the planet. To mention but a few: the mining of coal and its conversion to steel, in industries that employed thousands of men; the invention of the steam engine, which became a source of energy, replacing wind and water mills; invention of the spinning jenny and power loom, on which workers toiled endlessly in factories, with children running underneath to do dangerous jobs that only they could do; and all of the secondary effects on agriculture. Machines enabled farms to become larger and more productive, with simultaneous destruction of forests and industrial contamination of surface water. Social divisions in the population became pronounced, as the owners learned to live uphill and upstream from their factories and the factory workers. By the mid-19th century, the grumbling workforce in continental Europe began to think of revolutions in politics. Karl Marx (1818-1883) conceived of the *Communist Manifesto*, which was published in 1848, co-authored by Friedrich Engels (1820-1895). Engels had previously described the negative impact of industries in England. The first volume of Marx's *Das Kapital* was published 1867; the second and third volumes were published posthumously, edited by Engels. Marx's vision of Communism was set in motion in Russia by Vladimir Lenin (1870-1924), whose legacy persists to the present time. The goal of humans was still the same as it ever had been: to live as long and healthy a life as possible. However, during the 19th century, this goal continued to be elusive for most people. Only the rich and powerful had a chance to have good health. Even those with privilege and wealth continued to be struck with untreatable diseases of mysterious origins. Nevertheless, the Industrial Revolution offered a measure of hope, because in the 19th century, there were also significant advances in science and medicine.[399]

Before examining the discoveries related to health in the 19th century, we must confront a paradox. What is considered to be a healthy goal for one person, or one population, is considered by another person or another country to be the antithesis of good health. This is the paradox of war and of deadly conflicts. The 19th century was the period in which ships transitioned from power by sails to steam engines; the period in which rifles, pistols, and larger guns changed from firing with single shots to rapid fire; when black powder was replaced by dynamite; when ships of wood became ironclads and then ships of steel; and when wars, both large and small, became commonplace and continuous. Most wars and most deadly individual conflicts are based on false beliefs. The beliefs usually include the notion that the conflict is inevitable, that the outcome will be victory, and that it is necessary or even good to get on with it. And thus, the world saw the great conflicts known as the Napoleonic Wars, with tragedies including the march to Moscow, Trafalgar, and finally Waterloo; the Crimean War, with more than 700,000 casualties, and with the outcome an unchanged stalemate; the American Civil War, fought for reasons that are still not agreed upon; and Theodore Roosevelt's "splendid little war" that ended with the transfer of the Empire of Spain to the unnamed empire of the United States. The Spanish-American War was preceded by brief hostilities in which the Hawaiian monarchy was deposed and the islands became available for transfer to the United States; and it was followed by more war with the Indigenous people of the Philippines. Add to that, innumerable other wars: The War of 1812 between Britain and the U.S.; the Franco-Prussian War of 1870, which was the first of several conflicts over the bilingual province of Alsace-Lorraine; the British wars in Afghanistan, India, and Africa, all to enlarge or protect their Empire; the undeclared wars of the Germans, French, Belgians, and Portuguese against African tribes to subjugate and divide that continent into their colonial empires; and by the British, French, Dutch, and Portuguese in south and east Asia. By the end of the 19th century, control of most of the land on earth had been divided between the Great Powers in Europe and the United States. The U.S. occupied Cuba, and it acquired

Puerto Rico, Hawaii, and the Philippines. The U.S. used the threat of the Monroe Doctrine to keep the European countries out of Latin America. The exceptions to Euro-American control included only Japan, China, Korea, and some of the Muslim areas in Asia, but even in those areas, the economies of Europe and America were in play. Many humanitarian excuses have been given for the development of these Euro-American empires, but the true reason for these adventures was the search for power.[400]

One of the incidental benefits to the health of humans that arose from these conflicts was the development and rise of the profession of nursing, and of the treatment of prisoners of war. The nursing profession traces its modern role to the leadership of Florence Nightingale, OM (1820-1910), who was in charge of treating the sick and wounded of the Crimean war in hospitals in Istanbul. Known as "the Lady with a Lamp," Nightingale was a powerful voice for nursing after she returned to England, and the profession benefited from her long life. Nightingale's work was similar, in a way, to the development of the International Society of the Red Cross and Red Crescent, which arose from the work of her contemporary, Clara Barton, who volunteered to work as a nurse in the American Civil War. Barton founded the American Red Cross, which became the International Committee of the Red Cross. The ICRC later incorporated the symbol of the Crescent of Islam and is now known as the International Red Cross and Red Crescent Movement (IFRC). As it evolved, the ICRC deserves credit for stimulating many humanitarian activities which include the Geneva Conventions for treatment of prisoners of war, and of the sick and wounded; for outlawing of some weapons, such as land mines, that are considered to be inhumane; for the trials of German and Japanese war criminals after World War II; and for creation of the World Health Organization by the League of Nations and continuing under the United Nations.[401]

Cholera arrived in Britain in 1831. Some, who were known as "miasmatists," believed that it was spread through the air, while "contagionists" thought it was spread from person to person by humans, especially by poor, filthy, unwashed people. Enter Edwin Chadwick (1800-1890), a lawyer, who had been secretary to the reformer Jeremy Bentham (1748-1832). Bentham coined the phrase, "the greatest good for the greatest number," which has come to exemplify the concept of public health. Chadwick became Secretary of the Poor Law Commission, which was created to investigate the conditions of the poor, and to make recommendations to improve them. Cholera returned to London in 1854, and the question was: what to do about it? Chadwick believed that the lower classes lived in filth; this was true, because they had no easy way to have water, especially clean water. They could dip it out of the Thames, which was a tidal cesspool. A physician of London, John Snow (1813-1858) studied the problem and worked out a solution. Snow found a way to prove that cholera was a water borne disease, and that some areas of the city had clusters of it. He removed the handle from the pump on Broad Street which was at the center of a group of houses with cholera patients, with the effect of halting the small outbreak in that neighborhood. Snow became prominent, and he later administered anesthesia to Queen Victoria when she delivered her eighth child. She was happy with the outcome. But Snow's evidence for the mode of transmission of cholera was not enough to convince everyone. In retrospect it seems obvious, but science, including medicine, does not always work in straightforward ways. The problem of finding and reporting cases of specific infectious diseases, tracing for contacts of the cases, and quarantining all of them, is still a contentious issue. It has been called "the enforcement of health."[402]

Two major developments occurred during the 19th century which changed forever the practice of surgery. The first was anesthesia, and the second was asepsis, which I will mention later. The first use of ether for relief of pain during surgery was dramatically demonstrated in Boston on October 16, 1846, at the Massachusetts General Hospital. The most respected surgeon in Boston at that time was Dr. John Collins Warren (1778-1856), who at age 68 was at the height of his career. He had been Dean of the Harvard Medical School, of which one of the founders was his father, Dr. John Warren (1753-1815). His uncle, Dr. Joseph Warren (1741-1775) was killed at the Battle of Bunker Hill in the Revolutionary War. A young dentist, William T. G. Morton (1819-1868), proposed to administer a gas which would make a patient insensible to pain, and he said that he had used it successfully to extract a tooth without pain. Dr. Warren agreed to let Morton use his method on a patient who was scheduled to be operated on for a tumor of the face. The operation was concluded successfully. The patient did not exhibit the screams and movements that were expected from an incision that was several inches long, accompanied by a deep dissection to ligate the tumor. Warren turned to the surrounding physicians and medical students and exclaimed, "Gentlemen, this is no humbug." The amphitheater in which the operation was performed has been preserved as a memorial known as the "Ether Dome."[403]

Morton called his gas "Letheon," but it was soon revealed to be sulfuric ether, also known as diethyl ether. It has since been known simply as "ether." Ether is difficult to work with, for it is highly explosive and it is easily ignited when it is near an open flame. The search for pain relief during surgery had been something like the alchemist's search for transmuting other elements into gold. Many clues had been missed before Morton and Warren demonstrated that ether would be successful. Surgeons had previously learned to prepare their patients with alcohol and opium, and to operate very quickly. It was never easy for either surgeon or patient. Recently, nitrous oxide, a non-explosive gas formulated by Sir Humphrey Davy, had been shown to have a useful effect, though not as dramatic as ether. Nitrous oxide, with a chemical formula of NO_2, known as "laughing gas," had been inhaled at parties, and after the effect of ether was demonstrated, NO_2 was also found to have a role in surgery, especially as an adjunct or for short procedures. In contrast to nitrous oxide, ether produces profound insensibility. Another gas, chloroform, was soon discovered in England to be an excellent anesthetic agent. Chloroform had the advantage of being non-explosive, although in rare cases, some patients developed liver failure after exposure to it. Although there was resistance from some surgeons and others, ether, chloroform, and nitrous oxide soon became accepted, both for surgery and for obstetrical delivery. By the end of the century, a role was also found for cocaine, a topical anesthetic agent derived from leaves of the South American coca plant. Cocaine had long been used by Native Americans in the Andean region, but it had not been appreciated by Western medicine. The demonstration of "painless surgery" in 1846 stimulated the search for all of these discoveries, and more, which have continued into the 21st century.[404]

While we are thinking of surgery and anesthesia in the United States, it is appropriate to consider of one of the most important political figures of the 19th century, who was born in America midway between John Collins Warren and William T. G. Morton. It was Abraham Lincoln (1809-1865), known as the Great Emancipator, who was President of the United States during the Civil War. Lincoln's health and his impact on the health of others is an important example of the many ways in which health matters to us all. We will examine some aspects of Lincoln's own health, the health and illness of his family, and his many escapes from death. We must first discuss the many ways in which Lincoln mattered to enslaved people, all of whom at that time were Black. They were simply chattel (moveable) property, an important part of their equity, and permanently embedded in a web of trans-generational owners. They could be bought and sold like other property, including real estate, crops, and farm animals. Most owners considered the health of their enslaved people in a way that was similar to their farm animals[405]

Lincoln's election in November 1860 was the proximate cause of the American Civil War. It was known in the South as the War Between the States, or the War of Northern Aggression. Most people believed, correctly, that as President, Lincoln would oppose the continuation of slavery. The issue of slavery was crucial to the South, because it was then the basis for southern economy, which was primarily based on agriculture. Slaves also amounted to a large portion of equity in the South. Slavery was also considered in the South to be a State's right, guaranteed by the Constitution, and which only a State could modify or abolish. Lincoln had campaigned on the Republican Party's platform of abolition of slavery, in opposition to candidates from three other parties. Lincoln won a plurality of votes, and because votes were split between the other candidates, he received a clear majority of votes in the Electoral College. The Southern States began to prepare to leave the Union, to secede, in the event that Lincoln won, and as soon as the result of the election became clear, the States in the south immediately declared their independence. Armed conflict began on April 12, 1861, when Fort Sumter in the harbor of Charleston, S.C., was fired upon by Confederate soldiers. The Constitution did not explicitly address the issue of whether or not secession was permissible, but Lincoln was determined to preserve the Union by force of arms. And he did. War was never formally declared between the United States and the Confederate States, and no peace treaty ever signed to conclude it. The end became clear began in April 9, 1865, at Appomattox Courthouse, Virginia, with the surrender of the Army of Northern Virginia, commanded by Robert E. Lee, to the Union Army of the Potomac. Lee's surrender was accepted by Ulysses S. Grant,

Commanding General of the United States. This event was followed over the next several months by desultory fighting throughout the south, which ended with the surrender or drifting away of other Confederate Armies and of individual soldiers. The last enslaved people were notified of their freedom on June 19, 1865 in Galveston, Texas. The date has been celebrated since then as "Juneteenth." In the meantime, on April 15, only six days after Lee's surrender, Lincoln died in Washington, D.C., having been shot in the head the previous evening by John Wilkes Booth. And that changed history.[406]

Lincoln was succeeded as President by Vice President Andrew Johnson, a Democrat from Tennessee. The details of Lincoln's plans for Reconstruction, which included reconciliation of the States and bringing previously enslaved people into the social fabric of America, are unknown. Success in Reconstruction would have required Lincoln's determination and his ability to make political compromises. Reconstruction was despised by the white leaders of the former Confederate states, so it continued only with armed force during the eight years when Ulysses S. Grant was President. Reconstruction ended with the installation of Rutherford B. Hayes as President in March 1877.

Reconstruction, from 1865-1877, was regarded for decades as a time in which the South was ruled by opportunists from the North acting illegally in concert with newly empowered, uneducated Blacks from the South. It was said that these two groups deprived the majority white population of property and other Constitutional rights. This version of history was taught in America for almost a century. It was written by the leading historians in America during the late 19th and early 20th centuries, who were mostly Southern in ancestry. The opprobrium of "Reconstruction" also derived from the fact that there were few people in the North who wanted to have anything to do with people of color. Many would not have fought for abolition, which was considered to be a radical solution to a problem that should have been settled peacefully. The notion of the Lost Cause of the South, and the bravery of soldiers on both sides, became the predominant view of the Civil War. The Ku Klux Klan was regarded in the North as an organization of former Confederate Soldiers similar to the North's Grand Army of the Republic. Both organizations were perpetuated by the inclusion of children and male relatives of the soldiers. The misbehavior of some elements of the Klan was rarely mentioned, and it was thought not to be typical of the entire organization. Chapters of the KKK were also formed throughout the North, to discourage Black migration to farming country in the Mid-West. Lynching was rarely mentioned in the North. It was assumed that Blacks had no difficulty in their Southern communities, and that they would gradually become educated there and would work their way up to success. They should stay there.[407]

Abraham Lincoln's personal health and health issues involving his family played a significant role in his life before and during his years as the country's chief executive. He was born in a log cabin in rural Kentucky. His mother was "stoop-shouldered, thin-breasted, sad." The family was desperately poor, and she died when he was nine years old. However, his father married again to a widow with three children, and she raised both sets of her husband's children as if she had borne them all. Lincoln said she was his "angel mother." Abraham was a healthy, vigorous man who was self-educated, with the help of his step-mother. He was known as the "rail splitter" because of his skill with an axe in building fences. He taught himself law, and he served as a volunteer captain in the Black Hawk War of 1832. No one who has not been in service can appreciate what it is like to be elected captain of a company in wartime, even if no battles occurred. The respect of a hundred men, all of whom know and look up to you, is special. He wooed Mary Todd, who belonged to the social aristocracy of Springfield, Illinois. Her family looked down on him; he broke their engagement, but they reconciled and were married. They had four children, although only one survived to adulthood. Robert Todd, "Tad," was born with a cleft palate and a lisp, and he outlived his father. Mary Todd Lincoln developed fits of anger, and she became increasingly a burden to him when he was President. In 1875 she was officially declared to be insane. With apparent calm, Lincoln traveled to Washington to be inaugurated in 1862. He passed through hostile Baltimore under the protection of armed guards. During the Civil War he repeatedly visited the line of battle, consulting with officers in tents. Lincoln became ill on the train as he returned from giving his famous address in Gettysburg, Pennsylvania. It is now believed that he had smallpox, and that he barely survived it. He traveled to Richmond, Virginia, shortly after the Confederate capital had been captured by the Union Army, and walked calmly through the streets without any special protection. He was unprotected when he was shot by John Wilkes Booth on April 14, 1865. His Emancipation Proclamation, which was issued in September 1862 and became final on January 1, 1863, freed only slaves that were under Confederate control, but the symbolic effect was great. It may have been unconstitutional, but it was ratified after his death with the 13th Amendment, which was proclaimed as being in effect on December 18, 1865.[408]

We now return to England, where a contemporary of Abraham Lincoln was born in very different circumstances, and whose life altered health matters and world history in an entirely different way. He was Charles Robert Darwin (1809-1882), who was born in Shrewsbury, England, the son of a society doctor, Robert Darwin, whose father was Erasmus Darwin, a noted physician and author. His mother was the daughter of the industrialist and pottery maker Josiah Wedgwood. Darwin grew up in a life of privilege, and he was buried in Westminster Abbey. After traveling on a Royal Navy ship that was dispatched from London to explore areas in South America and the Pacific, and many years of worrisome thoughts about what he had seen, Darwin published his theory of *The Origin of Species* in 1859. The book was a best seller. It was the most important non-fiction book published in the 19th century, and it is still in print. Darwin's work was immediately, and correctly, regarded as a direct challenge to the Biblical account of the origin of the world, its plants and animals, and of humans. Darwin's theory of evolution is still regarded by some as unbelievable. Even now, although students are required to know and repeat on tests what they read in science textbooks about the origin of the universe and the earth, and of the evolution of plants and animals, they cannot be compelled to believe it.[409]

Darwin's theory of evolution by natural selection, which was soon called "survival of the fittest," was preceded by the theory of inherited characteristics, which was proposed by Jean Baptiste Lamarck (1744-1829). Lamarck said that a useful quality, such as the long neck of a giraffe, would be derived from stretching upward by giraffes over many generations. Lamarck and Darwin were actually not far apart, but Lamarck's reputation has suffered as a result of the perversion of science in the Soviet Union by a neo-Lamarckian, Trofim Lysenko (1898-1976), when Josef Stalin ruled the USSR, and Mao Tse-tung (Zedong) was in power in China during the Great Leap Forward. Lysenkoism, as it was called, was the official policy of biology and agriculture in the Communist world. It is estimated that it was the cause of crop failures which led to the death of millions of people, and dissent from Lysenkoism doomed thousands of scientists over a period of more than forty years.[410]

Darwin's theory of evolution was difficult to prove, but it received a boost with the work of a Moravian monk, Gregor Mendel (1822-1884). Mendel studied the breeding of peas with different colors (yellow and green) and variations in skin of peas (smooth or wrinkled) and he enumerated the results of his experiments. Mendel published his studies in an obscure journal in the 1860s, but it was re-discovered in 1900. Mendelian inheritance is the foundation for the field of genetics. Mendel's work led to a search for the molecular key to inheritance, known as the gene. The search lasted more than fifty years. The puzzle was solved in 1953 with the discovery of DNA. The impact on human health from the work of Darwin, Mendel, and others who followed them in the field of genetics is incalculable.[411]

Sir Francis Galton (1822-1911), Darwin's cousin, and a physician, was also studying inheritance. He was interested in whether development of individuals was due to "nature or nurture," and he coined the word "eugenics." His book, *Hereditary Genius* (1869), showed that the most highly educated people had the most successful children. Eugenics soon became the darling of the upper class in England. Eugenics has spawned problems that have adversely affected the health of millions of people, and problems related to the idea of eugenics exist today. To add to the problem, the human genome can be edited to eliminate potential defects but this activity raises major moral questions. Should we do this?[412]

Also, in England at that time, Henry Bence Jones, FRS (1813-1873) became the first person to describe a biochemical abnormality that was specific for cancer. In 1845 he showed that an unusual protein occurred in the urine in patients with a disease that was then called mollities ossium (meaning soft bone). We now call it multiple myeloma. The Bence Jones protein, as it is called, is diagnostic of that disease. Meanwhile, in Budapest, Hungary, Ignaz Semmelweis (1818-1865), an obstetrician, was desperately concerned about puerperal (post childbirth) sepsis in his hospital. He noticed that the mortality rate was much higher on the ward where medical students worked than on an adjacent ward where midwives were being trained. He surmised that it might be the result of "cadaverous material" carried by medical students from the autopsy room to the delivery room. The student midwives did not conduct autopsies on their patients. In 1847, Semmelweis proposed hand-washing using a solution of calcium hypochlorite, because it was used to remove the smell of the dead tissues in the autopsy room. Hand washing produced an immediate reduction in mortality on his ward. Semmelweis' proposal was, however, met with derision by physicians, and he died in an insane asylum. Semmelweis' proposal was shown to be correct a decade later by Louis Pasteur, who showed that invisible germs caused disease.[413]

The cell theory, as it became known, began with Johannes Müller (1801-58), who studied microscopy and decided that all tumors were composed of cells. He was the teacher of Mathias Schleiden (1804-81), a botanist, who reported in 1838 that cells are the building blocks of plants; and of Theodor Schwann (1810-82), who reported in the following year that animal cells arose in tissues from a substance that he called "blastema." Rudolph Virchow (1821-1902), a physician and pathologist, decided from his study of microscopic tissues that Schwann was correct in his belief that all animal tissues are composed of cells, but Virchow added that every cell arises from an existing cell. In Latin, that is *Omnis cellula e cellula*." It was similar to Pasteur's later conclusion, based on laboratory research, that there is no spontaneous generation of germs; that every microorganism is derived from an existing microorganism.[414]

Louis Pasteur (1822-1895) was a French biologist, not a physician. During the course of his career, he followed the hunches of his "prepared mind" with experiments in the laboratory and in the field to show that he was on the right path. He learned to court the press, and by doing so, he antagonized many of the leaders of the medical profession. Pasteur solved important questions in the fields of agriculture and medicine, but his most memorable demonstration was to show that there was no such thing as "spontaneous generation." This concept was transforming, and it was utilized in the development of new methods in surgery and new developments in microbiology. Some of Pasteur's guesses were amazing, and his luck was astounding. He never failed. His string of successes included the way to prevent the spoilage of milk, with a special technique of heating, known as "pasteurization"; of correct methods to ferment wine and beer, by adjusting the necessary yeasts; of his method of vaccination to prevent anthrax, a devastating disease of both sheep and humans; and of his spectacular prevention of the disease of rabies after a person has been bitten by a rabid animal. There are still puzzles regarding anthrax and rabies, yet Pasteur solved the necessary problems correctly with both diseases.[415]

A somewhat older Parisian physician, Claude Bernard (1813-78), was a leader in the medical profession in France at the time when Pasteur burst onto the scene with spectacular public demonstrations of the effects of what he called microorganisms, that could not be seen with the naked eye. Bernard was a man with many talents, including that of a playwright, surgeon, and author of a pioneering textbook of surgery. But the most important aspect of Bernard's work in the history of health is his successful research in the field of physiology. One of his many discoveries was a carbohydrate known as glycogen, found in the liver. By a serendipitous accident, he found that it was a polymer of glucose, also known as dextrose – the sugar needed for energy. On a signal received by the liver, glycogen is broken into molecules of glucose, which is secreted into the blood and provides a stable source of energy. Claude Bernard recognized the existence of a *milieu interieur* – the internal environment of the body. The concept of the *milieu interieur* was accepted in America by Walter Bradford Cannon (1871-1945), who called it "homeostasis." It is the principle of what Cannon called the "wisdom of the body." Bernard also experimented with unanesthetized animals, and his work with animals, known as vivisection, was considered abhorrent in England. Bernard's book, *An Introduction to the Study of Experimental Medicine* (1865), is the foundation for research using large animals. Without animals, it would not have been possible to develop many of the areas of medicine in the next century. For instance, experiments using animals were the basis for organ transplantation, which has saved the lives of tens of thousands of men, women, and children; cardiac surgery, with development of the pump-oxygenator, to enable the heart to be stilled and carefully repaired. And for vascular surgery, with replacement of blood vessels and heart valves with those made from plastic or from animals; and much of the research in the fields of cancer, immunology, and infectious diseases, with development and testing of new drugs and vaccines.[416]

A significant consequence of Pasteur's work in France took place in Britain. It was "antisepsis," which was the second great advance in surgery in the 19th century. The first important advance in surgery in this century was anesthesia, in 1846, which was mentioned above. Joseph Lister, later 1st Baron Lister (1827-1912), was well known as a surgeon and scholar, and he was experimenting with ways to improve his results. Lister studied reports of Pasteur's work and he considered how they might be applied to surgery. He thought of using a known disinfectant – carbolic acid, the chemical known as phenol – to cleanse the skin before incising it. Lister and Pasteur corresponded cordially and Lister had visited Pasteur in Paris. In 1865, Lister was confronted with a boy who had an open fracture of the thigh bone – the femur – in a street accident. The usual treatment in this case would be to amputate at the level of the thigh, because to reduce the fracture and return the broken bone into the thigh usually led to death from infection. A fatal infection known as "gas gangrene" was likely to develop. Lister decided to try carbolic acid to clean the ends the broken femur, and then to replace the bone into the thigh. Lister and his patient were lucky; the patient survived without an infection, and Lister continued to use carbolic acid as a spray or wipe to prepare the skin before surgery. His method was rapidly accepted by German surgeons, and it slowly gained acceptance in France and England, but "antisepsis" was resisted by many older surgeons, and it gained little favor in the United States. Antisepsis was soon replaced by the concept of asepsis, with complete sterilization of the operating field, the patient's skin, the instruments, and the personnel involved. Antisepsis, which led to asepsis, was the basis for modern surgery."[417]

The most prominent leader in the next generation of microbiologists was Robert Koch (1843-1910), in Germany. The political turmoil in Europe affected the relationships between French and German scientists, and so it also was with Pasteur and Koch. However, with his superb powers of observation and relentless determination, Koch was able to succeed in some areas that had eluded Pasteur. Koch discovered the peculiar spiral shaped organism that was the cause of cholera, no mean feat, for it was one of countless bacteria that infested sewage; and he also found and successfully cultured the organism that cause tuberculosis – which was then the most common cause of death in Europe and North America. Koch is credited with both the identification, by a special stain of his own design, known as the "acid-fast stain," and for the technique of culturing the bacillus, which required special media and a long waiting period. Koch named Four Postulates which were needed to prove that a bacterium was the cause of a disease. Another German academician, Carl Ludwig (1816-95), invented the kymograph, which enabled the fourth vital sign of blood pressure to be recorded. You may recall that previously, the three vital signs had been respiration, the pulse, and temperature.[418]

It is strange to add to the history of health in the 19th century the name of Thomas Alva Edison (1847-1931). But add him I must, in spite of the fact that Edison does not appear in any of the histories of science and medicine that I have cited as references for this essay. This is appropriate, for Edison stands apart from all others in the history of technology, which overshadows his important contributions to medicine and science. For his many inventions and for his influence on world history, Edison was named by *Life* magazine at the Man of the Millennium. Edison is also an appropriate person to consider in this essay, for in his personal life, he is yet another example of a person whose life and work was significantly impacted by illness. His biographer believed that "Edison's deafness strongly influenced his behaviour and career, providing the motivation for many of his inventions." He narrowly escaped death on several occasions, and because he lived so long, he had time to accomplish much – both for good and otherwise. Edison's life bridged two centuries. In the 19th century, Edison obtained the first of his 1,093 patents. Most were in the field of electricity, and in the sub-fields of telegraphy, direct cell batteries, the telephone, and magnets. In 1877, Edison invented the phonograph (which was considered to be a form of telegraphy at that time) and in 1879, the first incandescent electric light. Four years later, he observed the unusual glow in a light bulb which is known as the "Edison effect." It became the basis of the electron tube and the electronics industry. With his success in electricity, Edison became involved with making movies, using images that were portrayed on film, with projectors driven by electricity, and lighting that only he could arrange. He was a pioneer of in the film industry. He was also working with chemicals in the production of his batteries and phonograph records. He developed new phenol-formaldehyde plastic polymers which were produced with great heat and pressure. He founded the Edison General Electric Corporation, now known simply as *GE*. In the early 20th century, his interests shifted to magnetic separation for iron mining, and then to the use of mining equipment and chemical separation to produce high quality cement. His discoveries were often not patented, but were instead regarded as industrial secrets. All of these interests coalesced into the Edison Company.[419]

Thomas Edison's impact on health can be measured in many ways. The incredibly important fluoroscope was his invention, although he never patented it. He also invented a battery-powered miner's safety head lamp and the free-standing warning light for safety at railroad crossings. In the 20th century, he created the lithium battery, which is used in many medical devices such as cardiac pacemakers and hearing aids. On the other hand, Edison's factories were dangerous places for workers and they were destructive to the environment. His factories used and released large amounts of toxic products that included mercury, lead, chromium, and phenol. He neglected his responsibility for the health of other people, and he was often cruel to animals. He obfuscated, dissembled, feigned forgetfulness, blamed his poor hearing, and simply lied at times about all of these issues. Edison employed thousands of people in his factories, which extended across eight counties in northern New Jersey, from the Hudson River to the Delaware. His orders and his shabby workplaces resulted in countless injuries and deaths in his factories, and in the permanent pollution of thousands of acres of land and of rivers and underground water in New Jersey. The Great Inventor understood how to manipulate the media, and he lived a charmed life. Long after he died, the facts of his complex life story slowly emerged. One New Jersey governor later said that he wasn't respected in his own town, and another governor said, "He wasn't a nice man, either."[420]

The great classical composers, from Vivaldi to Mendelssohn, include Bach, Handel, Haydn, Mozart, Beethoven, and Brahms. In their lifetimes, death was considered to be inevitable, unpredictable, and largely unpreventable. They therefore celebrated life, sometimes with quiet thanks and sometimes with grand music, because death had been temporarily held in abeyance. The epitome was Beethoven's Ninth Symphony, with its "Ode to Joy." The classicists were especially good at composing farewells to life, as in "Missa Solemnis" by Mozart. Death was sometimes sudden, from "fever" of unknown cause, or from a "wasting disease" which was probably tuberculosis. Death was nevertheless feared, and those whose death was slow and lingering were sometimes shunned or even loathed. The dead were mourned, however, and their passing was memorialized in ceremonies, poetry, tombstones, and statuary. Religion played a much larger role at those times as humans dealt with dying and death; medicine rarely played anything but a watchful part, but physicians would claim credit if the patient survived.[421]

Repeated episodes of illness also impacted on the life and work of two other classical composers. Franz Peter Schubert (1797-1828) was a Viennese composer whose work bridged Classical and Romantic types of music. He was noted for his *lieder* (songs), his great *Symphony in C Major* and the unfinished *Symphony in B Minor*. His work was influenced by feelings of rejection, instability, and finally exhaustion. He had a serious venereal disease in 1823 (probably syphilis) and he died of typhoid fever. Robert Schumann (1810-1856) was a German composer, born in Saxony. He is considered to have been in the "front rank of German Romantic musical figures." His work was influenced by Franz Shubert. He had a "very strong and painful" undiagnosed ear malady, which I think must have been *tic douloureux*. He was also "mentally unstable" and he attempted suicide on several occasions. His wife Clara was a musical prodigy, who overshadowed her husband at times, but whose professional life was truncated by what she believed were her family responsibilities.[422]

Development of the first gasoline powered motor cars and the first attempts in the field of aviation began at the end of the 19th century. The automobile was the first: Karl Benz, in Manheim, Germany, and Gottlieb Daimler, in Stuttgart, independently produced gasoline-engine automobiles in Germany in 1885 and 1886, respectively. The companies they founded were merged in 1926 and became Mercedes-Benz Company of the 21st century. Men had attempted to glide or fly for many centuries, and many types of mechanical gliders were built and tested during the 19th century. These were forerunners of the first successful powered flights, which were made in 1903 by Wilbur and Orville Wright, in Kitty Hawk, N.C. The Wright brothers' design was a bi-plane with a small internal combustion engine. The upside and downside of automobiles and airplanes might be imagined, but it could not be predicted. Automobiles soon enabled cities to become remarkably cleaner, when automobiles, trucks, and street cars replaced horses, and the streets were free of manure. The automobile has also been the cause of death and injury of millions of people. "Unsafe at any speed," was the slogan of Ralph Nader, and it led to improvements in the design and construction of automobiles and regulations, such as seat belts and air bags, that improved the safety of riders. The public, loving speed and the *frisson* of danger, has been resistant to accept what might be better, and bystanders, pedestrians and bicyclists are still at risk; they always lose when hit by a car. The movement of both people and products has been immensely enhanced by airplanes, large passenger liners, and container transport ships. Our earth has become what Wendell Willkie called "One World," when COVID-19 loosens its grip. Business and tourism flourished before the pandemic, and travel has been increased, to flee for fear, or for immigration, or from war. Exotic pests and diseases can now spread to distant places within hours. Toxic industrial products produced in developed countries are now easily transported to the third world, to be dumped and out of sight.[423]

War is one of the most prominent sources of bad health. If health really matters, war should be avoided at all costs. However, one side or the other usually thinks it will win, and the contest begins. I will mention two individuals in the 19th century who serve as examples of wartime leaders. They represent countless other leaders of people who went enthusiastically to war. The 19th century had more than enough like these two to prove that point, if it needed proving. My examples are Otto von Bismarck and Queen Victoria. Bismarck (1815-1898) was prime minister of Prussia and Founder and first chancellor (1871-90) of the German Empire. He unified Germany by force and he provoked the Franco-Prussian War. It ended in a humiliating defeat for the French and by the annexation by Germany of most of the bilingual province of Alsace-Lorraine. It set the stage for the bitter ending of World War I, when Germany was forced to yield the province back to France. Germany did not for long accept this loss, and it rearmed. War resumed in just over twenty years, as the disputed province again became a battleground and World War II began. Alexandrina Victoria (1819-1901), Queen of the United Kingdom (1837-1901) and Empress of India (1876-1901), was the eponymic ruler of the Victorian Age. In her personal life she exemplified the pomposity and falsehoods that marked that period in British history. Her grandchildren led the countries of Britain, Germany, and Russia that stumbled into war in Europe in 1914, and which evolved into World War I. After an Armistice in 1918, war began again in 1939. It was World War II, which lasted until 1945. Long life and good health for Bismarck and Victoria, as leaders, concurrently resulted in ill health for hundreds of thousands, perhaps many millions, of other people.[424]

Much of the world was becoming urbanized in the 19th century, but farming was still a vital occupation. Farm workers followed patterns that were established centuries earlier. In Europe, most farmers lived in small towns and walked back and forth during the day from their homes to their farms. Most American farmers owned and lived on their farms, and they only went to town to buy or sell or socialize. In some parts of Europe, farmers owned their own small plots of land, but in other countries, most of the land was possessed by absentee owners, who rarely visited their property. Some of the farmers share-cropped with the owners, and others had long rentals – up to 99 years.

Towns and cities were situated for different reasons in different parts of the Western world. Initially, a waterfront location was desired. A favored place was a sheltered harbor on the ocean, especially with a river running into the harbor at that point. The river would allow goods to be exchanged between those who lived inland and those who lived in the city on the waterfront. Boston and New Haven are good examples of a good harbor and a slow-running river. New York's harbor is difficult, but the Hudson River is magnificent. Philadelphia is upstream on the Delaware, but the river is navigable, the port is perfect, the Schuylkill River is a good feeder stream for it, and first falls on the river are upstream at Trenton. The cities of Europe follow similar guidelines, but they were formed at a time when strategic location was a principal concern. Other choices included attractions such as the natural hot water in Bath, England, which became a city in Roman times, or Marienbad (German: Mary's Bath), Czechoslovakia, now the Czech Republic. In America, railroads became the principal reason for situating a new town, or to enlarge a village into a city. Towns would be built at exact intervals, depending on where the train crews would change places; they were called "divisions" or "sections." The location where two railroads crossed would be best of all: Atlanta, Georgia, was a crossing point; so, too, was Elizabeth, New Jersey.

The 19th century was a time of tremendous change in agriculture. Cyrus McCormick (1809-1884) invented the mechanical reaper at age 22, in 1831. Wheat and oats then lay on the ground and were raked by hand into rows or piles to be beat with flails. Then a machine was invented to do the job. The threshing machine is a stationary machine to separate the seeds from the stems (aka stalks) and husks of grain. The threshing machine beats the plants after they have been cut (with a reaper), winnowed (raked into rows), gathered up, and fed into it. *Britannica* says the first one was patented in 1837. A mechanical rake was invented in 1871, known as a dump rake, drawn by horses. It enabled farmers to gather the harvested plants into windrows. The windrows of grain plants were scooped up and laid out in rows with a threshing machine. The "combine" was then developed. It is a moveable threshing machine which combines the functions of reaping, threshing, and winnowing (leaving the stalks and husks in rows). All of these machines have helped farmers do more with less expenditure of energy. They required farmers to become capitalists – more than subsistence farmers, who had to buy and sell their products and have a bit left over. The products for sale were usually meat animals, wool sheared from sheep or goats, and extra amounts of hay, grains, eggs, and butter.[425]

Bridge building was the premier accomplishment of architects in the 19th century, and the greatest of these was the Brooklyn Bridge. The bridge spanned the East River, which is actually a branch of Long Island Sound. It was built to connect Brooklyn, on Long Island, with the island of Manhattan. John Roebling (1806-1869), designed the Brooklyn Bridge and he personally directed the beginning of its construction. His foot was crushed and it was partially amputated. He refused to accept his physician's recommendation for post-operative care. He treated himself, and he died of tetanus. Work on the bridge was continued by his son Washington (1837-1926) and it was then finished under the direction of his wife Emily Roebling, after Washington Roebling was disabled from a disease now known as caisson sickness. Washington Roebling's mysterious illness led to the beginning of the understanding of how to work at depths under water, to avoid nitrogen accumulation in the blood (the "bends").

Large open fireplaces, fires, and candles were major causes of injury and death in Colonial America, especially of children, who played in the fireplaces, and with long hair and skirts that easily caught fire. To wit: Fanny Appleton, second wife of the poet Henry Wadsworth Longfellow (1807-1822).

The idea of sanitation in cities was developed during the 19th century. Old ways still persisted in isolated homes, on farms, and in small towns. Water was carried by hand from dug wells, and slop jars and outhouses were still in use in houses and hotels. But in many cities, fresh water was channeled through iron pipes from intakes upstream or from reservoirs at higher elevations. Natural pressure allowed water to exit, but not to enter, at joints or breaks in the pipes, so clear water flowed from taps. Chlorination and fluoridation were unknown then, and methods of water purification and treatment would come later. Toilet water and industrial waste was channeled downstream by sanitary sewers, connected into a sewer system. Individual septic tanks were yet to come. New York City was famous for its reservoirs, and Paris for its sewers. Baltimore, Maryland, had a unique opportunity for its sanitary and septic system. There were rapidly running rivers on the high ground above Baltimore to provide fresh water, and a huge tidal estuary, Chesapeake Bay, to dump what remained. The Bay would gradually become polluted, but that was far in the future. The estuary of New York harbor also became polluted, and wells drilled around the city were contaminated. As the water levels fell with inadequate replenishment from rain, they became the source of typhoid. Then they dried up. In the end, sanitation did more for health than all that medicine could do. However, lead pipes, or iron pipes that were plumbed together, using lead at the joints, leaked lead into the water. Thousands of children have been brain-damaged from lead in their drinking water. One example was Flint, Michigan, revealed in 2014.[426]

In the last decade of the 19th century, the Western world was optimistic. Health wasn't perfect, but there were reasons to be hopeful. The germ theory had taken hold in science, and there were vaccines for smallpox, rabies, and anthrax. More would surely come. Surgery could now be painless, and women could have anesthesia for delivery. Cancer was understood to be a disease of cells, and there were glimpses of its causes. The night was lighted with natural gas conveyed through copper pipes, instead of candles and kerosene lamps, and then arc lights and incandescent lamps which used electricity. The city streets thus became safer, and work could continue through the night. Buildings were rising with steel above ground and with caissons under water. Railroads and ships were powered with coal and steam, connecting people and markets.

The change in attitude near the end of the century was recognized in music composed and enjoyed at that time. In Russia, there were the beautiful symphonies and the heroic *War of 1812* overture of Pyotr Ilyich Tchaikovsky (1840-1893) and *Pictures at an Exhibition* by Modest Mussorgsky (1839-1881). In Bohemia, there were the reminiscences of "Going Home" in the Largo of Symphony No. 9, *From the New World*, of Antonín Dvořák (1841-1904); the comic operas of W. S. Gilbert (1836-1911) and Sir Arthur Sullivan (1842-1900) in England (remember *Pirates of Penzance*, and more), and in 1901, the triumphant *Pomp and Circumstance March* by Sir Arthur Elgar (1857-1934), with the words "Land of Hope and Glory" that were later added and were sung by millions in the 20th century; and Claude Debussy, *Prelude to the Afternoon of a Faun*, in France. The warfare between science and religion receded by the end of the 19th century, because of the obvious benefits that were seen from science, technology, and medicine, which did not seem to be based on religion. There was still a theoretical conflict between science and religion, but for most people in Europe and America, religion had its proper place, and so, too, did everything else. A person could read the Bible, go to church on Sunday, behave like a Christian should do during the rest of the week; and also go to work, raise a family, and enjoy the benefits of modernity. Some people even shrugged off the Christian religion: a few were atheists, others were agnostic, and there were also Unitarians and Quakers who denied the divinity of Christ. Deism, which accepted the idea of a supreme deity, but which avoided the issue of the divinity of Christ, persisted behind closed doors in Masonic temples. England was mostly Anglican, and the monarch was the Head of the Church, but church attendance was no longer required. France was nominally Roman Catholic, but after the French Revolution, France was Catholic in name only. Germans were allowed to choose between Catholicism and Lutheran Church, or neither. Most Jews in Germany chose to be assimilated into the mainstream as Lutherans, or silently avoided religious practices. In Europe and America, religion was no longer the driver of health. Instead, as the story is told in *Health Matters*, health was in the late 19th century was based on science, technology, and medicine.[427]

When the 19th century passed into the **20th century, it was the *fin de siècle*** (end of the century), and it was emblematically marked with the architecture and décor of Art Nouveaux.

Theodore Roosevelt (1858-1919) was the 26th President of the United States. During his eventful life, he achieved greatness in many areas that are too numerous to mention in detail in this brief sketch. Suffice it to say that he is the only person ever to have won both the U.S. Medal of Honor and the Nobel Peace Prize. Roosevelt expanded the area of control of the United States to rival that of the British Empire at its height. With his grasp of the role of sea power in history, his charisma, good luck, and political savvy, he made an empire for America that succeeded that of Spain. Health and illness each were important in his life and career. Teddy, or TR, as he was often called, was a nearsighted sickly youth, who suffered from asthma. By sheer determination, he rose above those health problems, only to see both his mother and wife die on the same day from typhoid fever. He was devastated at that time, but as a widower with one daughter, he married again and had five more children. He dared death on many occasions: as a volunteer Rough Rider in the Spanish-American War, on safari in Africa, and in exploring the interior of the Amazon rain forest. His death at age 60 was probably hastened by an unknown tropical infectious disease. He died when he was the odds-on favorite to be the Republican candidate for election in 1920 against Woodrow Wilson. Two of his sons also dared greatly. Quentin, an aviator, was killed in Europe in World War I. Brigadier General Theodore Roosevelt, Jr., died in Normandy in 1944, soon after D-Day in World War II; he received the Medal of Honor posthumously.[428]

The 28th U.S. President, Woodrow Wilson (1856-1924) made significant contributions to history in spite of his duplicity and his personal health problems. He introduced racism in U.S. government employees, and he persisted in negotiations for the Treaty of Versailles without considering the political consequences of not including the opposite party (Republicans) which controlled the Senate. He was also ill with influenza in 1919, and perhaps overly confident as a result of his sudden celebrity in Europe. He failed to honor his declaration of national choice, except in Europe. People of color, in Africa and Asia, continued to be in colonies ruled by England, France, the Netherlands and Belgium. German colonies in Africa were divided between England and France, and in the Pacific, they were transferred to control of

Japan (which had been on the side of the Allies in World War I). Wilson had a series of disabling strokes before ending his second term in office.[429]

Herbert Hoover (1874-1964) was basically a good man. The 31st President was a Quaker, born in a tiny farmhouse in Iowa, and he performed heroic humanitarian service as the head of the world's food relief organization in Europe after World War I. But he failed as President.[430]

Winston Churchill (1874-1965), later Sir Winston, had a long string of post-nominals that began with KG (Knight of the Garter) and OM (Order of Merit). He was arguably the most important person in English history after William, Duke of Normandy, who successfully conquered England in 1066. Churchill had noble ancestors, and perhaps the Conqueror was one of them. By his unquenchable determination, his domestic political savvy, and by his gift of speech, Churchill mobilized the querulous people of England to mobilize and to defend their island in the "Battle of Britain" against Hitler in 1939. Churchill had a long life after that. But what interests us here is his early life, in which he experienced the thrill of combat in the Boer War, and in the battles against the Pathan tribesmen along the North-West Frontier of India (now the Afghan-Pakistan border). He wrote in his first book about the thrill of hearing a bullet pass "without effect" in Malakand, at that time. He later fumbled in World War I in his distant leadership of the British Empire's failed invasion at Gallipoli, in Turkey. He then reclaimed his honor by serving as a battalion commander in the trenches in France. He somehow escaped the many causes of death in World War I: by gunshot, artillery, bombs, land mines, or disease. There was no guarantee that he would survive the war, but he did, unscathed. And he was ready to fight again.[431]

Joseph Stalin (1879-1953), born in Gori, Georgia, in the Russian Empire, was secretary-general of the Communist Party of the USSR (1922-1953) and premier of the Soviet State (1941-53). His biographer in *Britannica* sums it up by saying that he "probably exercised greater political power than any other figure in history." By 1920, he held two ministerial posts in the Bolshevik government. He defeated Leon Trotsky (b. 1879) and became the successor to Vladimir Lenin (b. 1870), who died in 1924. He arranged for Trotsky to be assassinated in Mexico in 1940. Stalin's devastating impact on the health of others in the Soviet Union and elsewhere in the world is vast but impossible to enumerate. It was made possible by his personal good health, which was apparently phenomenal. At the time of the crucial Tehran Conferences in World War II, Stalin took charge, when Churchill was suffering from a near-fatal case of pneumonia, and Franklin Roosevelt, while not well himself, was attempting to mediate between the two of them. Stalin created a system of infamous prison camps, the *Gulag Archipelago*, and he systematically starved millions of Ukrainians. He helped to defeat Germany in World War II by his wiliness to sacrifice thousands of Soviet troops. Stalin's legendary mendacity did not prevent him from creating a "mighty military industrial complex" which "led the Soviet Union into the nuclear age." Stalin's USSR and its allies opposed the Western Powers in the Cold War that followed the conclusion of World War II, in battlegrounds throughout the world – most notably in the Korean and Vietnam Wars, but in smaller conflicts elsewhere in Asia, South America, and Africa – and the tense stand-off at the Iron Curtain in Europe. A succession of leaders of the USSR followed Stalin until 1989, when the USSR began to implode after it withdrew from Afghanistan. The eight leader, Mikhail Gorbachev (b. 1931), dissolved the USSR in 1991 and the Cold War came to an end. The world had sat on that "powder keg" since the end of World War II. Gorbachev is honored in the West for his personal bravery, although he is said to have few supporters in Russia. He deservedly received the Nobel Peace Prize and for his concepts of *glasnost* and *perestroika* (openness and restructuring). After more periods of unrest, Russia has again returned to dictatorship with Vladimir Putin as leader with the title of President.[432]

Franklin Delano Roosevelt (1882-1945), known as FDR, the 32nd U.S. President, followed Herbert Hoover. He was the fifth cousin of Theodore Roosevelt, but he was a generation younger in age. He looked on Theodore as a role model, and followed many of the older man's steps to success in politics. He married Theodore Roosevelt's niece, Eleanor, in 1905. Unlike Theodore, he did not court danger, nor did he boast about his bravery, but he sailed to Europe through submarine infested waters in WWI as Assistant Secretary of the Navy and took an extended tour of the battlefront. He recovered from an attack of typhoid fever in 1912. Remember: typhoid was the infection that killed both Theodore's mother and his first child. Franklin's recovery from typhoid made the rest of his eventful life possible.

He contracted poliomyelitis in 1921, and although he recovered, he was unable to walk without support. He hid his infirmity as well as he could, and there are few photos of him in a wheelchair. A gregarious politician, he waved jauntily from the back of an open car, and enjoyed stirring martinis for others. His other health problems were numerous. They probably weakened his decision-making and clouded his judgment, especially at the Tehran Conference. He had heart disease and hypertension, which probably led to his death from a stroke. He is also suspected of having a metastatic melanoma, which arose at the left eyebrow, and some say it may have been the cause of his terminal cerebral hemorrhage.[433]

FDR had a long sexual affair with his wife's secretary, Lucy Mercer, which began in 1916. It led his wife to distance herself from him, though they never divorced. They had six children, all of who became famous and two were decorated for bravery, but they had little direct guidance from either parent. Eleanor Roosevelt (1884-1962) came into her own after FDR died. By 1932, she had a romantic relationship (hidden from the public at that time) with a well-known journalist, Lorena "Hick" Hickok. In later years, Eleanor was an active force in the Democratic Party. Eleanor's good health led to a long life. As Ambassador to the United Nations, she is rightly regarded as being a distinguished humanitarian. Eleanor Roosevelt authored the UN Resolution on human rights, which set an example for conduct of nations that has been difficult to follow but which has nevertheless endured.[434]

Adolph Hitler (1889-1945) led Germany and the Axis powers to disaster and defeat in World War II. His name is synonymous with death; of the Nazi movement and the swastika; and of the death's head insignia of the dreaded SS (*Schutzstaffel*). He organized the killing of six million Jews in what has become known as the Holocaust. Hitler was born in Austria. His father was a customs worker, and Hitler's education did not extend beyond secondary school. He volunteered for service in the German army in World War I, and rose to the rank of corporal. He spent most of the war on the front lines; he was wounded in 1916, gassed in 1918, and twice decorated with the Iron Cross. He was still hospitalized at the end of the war. Like many others, he was bitter about the defeat. In 1920, he joined the German Workers' Party which was renamed in that year as the National Socialist Party (Nazi). He conceived of a movement to unite the German-speaking people on the basis of national identity. His autobiography, *Mein Kampf* (1925; German for "My Fight"), became the inspiration for the Nazi movement. Hitler's uncanny ability to speak for many hours to adoring audiences resulted in his subsequent successes. He became Chancellor of the Republic of Germany and then the undisputed Führer of the Third Reich – the father of the long-awaited new Empire of Germany. His diet was mysterious. Sometimes it was said that he was a vegetarian and that he abstained from alcoholic beverages, but that may have been propaganda. What is certain is that he had megalomania, a psychiatric condition, which led to world-wide devastation and countless deaths. His physical and mental health deteriorated as the German army retreated from its high points of victory in World War II. He survived an attempted assassination with a bomb that was left in a briefcase in his conference room, which killed and wounded others who were near him. He committed suicide in Berlin as the Russian army was approaching the city.[435]

The Nazi movement resonated with similar nativist sentiments in other countries in Europe, in which black-uniformed German soldiers were welcomed. The word Nazi and the swastika logo have become symbols, along with the Confederate battle flag, of the unorganized but politically powerful movement of white nationalist supremacists in the United States. Hitler is an example of the importance of health in history: for survival after his injuries in war, for his personal health problems as he saw the end approaching, and for his enormous impact on the health of the world.[436]

Two examples from show business will illustrate the various ways that health can play a significant role in the performing arts. Hedy Lamarr (1913-2000) was said at one time to be the most beautiful woman in the world. She was enormously famous in her time as a film star, but she is now perhaps even more famous for another aspect of her life: Hedy was an incredibly gifted worker in a laboratory that she created in her home. She invented a method to scramble and unscramble radio waves that was used in World War II. Her invention, patented under the name of Hedy Markey when she was married to her second husband, movie producer [later Rear Admiral] Gene Markey, is still in use today. Sad to say, late in life, she suffered from dementia, and in the end, she did not have a dignified death. Cole Porter (1891-1964) was also a gifted celebrity in his lifetime. He enjoyed the good life. "I get my kicks from cocaine" was written into lyrics for one of his songs. At the height of his career, he was paralyzed in an accident while riding a horse, and he spent the rest of his life in misery and pain.[437]

Many important discoveries were made in science and technology in the 19th century by men and women who lived into the 20th century. These discoveries and inventions had enormous impacts on health, usually for better but sometimes otherwise. Three of them, the Curies, also had significant personal health problems. A sample would include Albert Einstein (1879-1955), Nikola Tesla (1856-1943), and Guglielmo Marconi (1874-1937). The Curies were Pierre Curie (1859-1906) and Marie Sklodowska-Curie (1867-1934), husband and wife, and their daughter Irène Joliot-Curie (1897-1956).[438]

A few of the physicians and scientists who made important contributions in the history of medicine in the period from 1800 to 1920 includes the following:

Sir William Osler (1849-1919) was notable for his thoughtful teaching and writing. Osler was the model of a kind and caring physician, who advised students to steel themselves for the tragedies that they would encounter in their career. He was the author of *The Principles and Practice of Medicine* (1892) and the essay *Aequanimitas* (1889). He was devasted by the death of his son Revere as a soldier in World War I. Osler slowly died of complications of pneumonia near the end of the Great Influenza pandemic.[439]

William Stewart Halsted (1852-1922) was a brilliant surgeon, both bold and precise, whose techniques have since been followed by thousands of surgeons. He founded modern American surgical training as the first Professor of Surgery at Johns Hopkins University's School of Medicine. Halsted became addicted to morphine and perhaps also to cocaine as the result of experiments with methods to produce anesthesia. It was a secret known only to a few of his friends. Halstead often spent months away from sight, in places unknown, and then would return to function normally again.[440]

Paul Ehrlich (1854-1915) developed the first chemical that was synthesized to treat an infectious disease – syphilis. On his 606th attempt, he succeeded with a drug known as Salvarsan. Although it contained a large amount of arsenic, it was not toxic, and it opened the field of chemotherapy. Ehrlich had previously participated in the development of a vaccine against diphtheria.[441]

Dr. Sigmund Freud (1856-1939), an Austrian neurologist, created the field of psychoanalysis, "and the seeming inexhaustibility of the intellectual legacy he left behind." His daughter Anna, who died in 1982, founded the field of child psychoanalysis.[442]

Walter Bradford Cannon (1871-1945), mentioned previously, developed the concept of homeostasis. Alexis Carrell (1873-1944) won the Nobel Prize for developing a technique to suture blood vessels. During World War I, Carrell worked with Henry Drysdale Dakin (1880-1952) to develop a successful combination of chemicals to irrigate wounds: the Carrell-Dakin solution. Carrell later worked at the Rockefeller Institute in New York City with the famed aviator, Charles Lindbergh, to cultivate cells, tissues, and organs *in vitro*. Insulin was discovered by the brilliant combination of serendipity and hard work in the summer of 1921 by Dr. Frederick Banting (1891-1941) – later Sir Frederic Banting, MC, KBE – and his assistant, a medical student, Charles Best (1899-1978). Banting was wounded while working as a surgeon in the Canadian Army in World War I.[443]

At this point, I interrupt the historical sequence of physicians and scientists, to mention a few leaders in this period in the fields of fine arts and literature, whose lives show examples of the ways that health matters in human life. Two painters show the difference between a life of ill health and a life of good health: Vincent Van Gogh (1853-1890) and Pablo Picasso (1881-1973). Each has a prominent place in art history. Yet they are very different. Van Gogh never sold a painting during his lifetime. He was schizophrenic and self-mutilating, desperately unhappy, and he died at the age of 37. Picasso, on the other hand, had a long life and was recognized in his own lifetime as a genius. He had many sexual affairs, and he died as a wealthy man, with enough left to fought over by those who claimed to be heirs.[444]

Harvey Cushing (1869-1939) was the founder of neurosurgery in America, and in his day, he was possibly the most famous physician in America. He received the Distinguished Service Medal for work on the front lines in World War I, and he won the Pulitzer Prize for his biography of Sir William Osler. His name is remembered today for describing a rare tumor of the pituitary gland, now known as Cushing's disease, and for the associated Cushing's syndrome (due to a specific type of adrenal tumor or, more commonly, from long-term administration of cortisone or its derivatives). His collection of rare books in the history of medicine is now at Yale University, where he received his undergraduate education. He left only a 3-foot shelf of books at Harvard Medical School, where he spent most of his career. His ego was enormous, and it is said that his fellow faculty members were glad to see him go back to Yale when he retired from Harvard.[445]

Other physicians who were famous in their day for their discoveries or for their contributions to public health, are, in roughly chronological order: Ivan Pavlov (1849-1936), who documented many of the ways that mind and body interact (the dog salivates when it hears the dinner bell); the Mayo brothers, William J. Mayo (1861-1939) and Charles Mayo (1865-1939), of the Mayo Clinic in Rochester, Minn.; and George Crile (1864-1943), a brilliant surgeon who created the Cleveland (Ohio) Clinic.[446]

Most of the prominent military leaders in World War II had served previously in World War I. I will mention a few, with comments on health crises in their lives, to suggest that history would have been altered, to some extent, if they hadn't survived. Douglas MacArthur (1880-1964) was wounded by a German bullet as he stood calmly on the top of the trenches as deputy commander of the 42nd division. He was dramatically carrying only a riding crop, although he was qualified as an expert with the service rifle. George C. Marshall (1880-1959) suffered a near fatal wound in an accident when he was a cadet at the Virginia Military Institute; Dwight D. Eisenhower (1890-1969) had a knee injury while playing football at the U.S. Military Academy, followed by troubles with the knee for the rest of his life. He had a very close call as a result of this in France in World War II. Eisenhower and his pilot, in a single engine plane, were forced to land on a beach near enemy lines, and he had to limp back in the sand to safe territory. Eisenhower had additional health problems when he was president, including intestinal obstruction from regional enteritis, which required emergency surgery, and later, a heart attack. Eisenhower was elected as the 34th President of the United States, and he served from 1953-1961.[447]

In other countries, there is Lord Mountbatten (1900-1979), a second cousin, once removed, of the present Queen Elizabeth II, and uncle of her husband, Prince Philip. He had many heroic adventures as an officer in the Royal Navy in combat in World War I, and again in World War II. He was later in India in World War II as Commander of the South-East Asia Command (SEAC); he was assassinated by Irish Republican Army terrorists. In Germany, the example is General Erwin Rommel (1891-1944), the brave and initially successful commander of the Afrika Corps. He then commanded the German Army's defense against an expected invasion of France in June 1944. Rommel was accused by Hitler of being a participant in the assassination plot in 1944, and was coerced to commit suicide to save his family from imprisonment or death. In Japan, there is Admiral Isoroku Yamamoto (1884-1943), head of the Japanese Navy in World War II. He had been wounded during the Russo-Japanese War in 1904-5. He was sent to Harvard to study from 1919-21, and he served twice as Naval attaché in the Japanese Embassy in Washington. He was ordered to plan an attack on America. Yamamoto understood the ways that Americans thought and planned. His suggested a surprise attack at Pearl Harbor, while the U.S. was expecting it in the Far East. He believed that the initial attack would be successful, as it was, and he also believed that the U.S. would rise "like a sleeping giant" and would defeat Japan. He was unable to convince the others in the wartime cabinet of the fallacy in their thinking. Yamamoto died when his airplane, flying alone, was shot down. It had been identified as a target by U.S. Navy code-breakers.[448]

Two others, who were neither generals or admirals, but who were both, in very different ways, involved in World War I, and later in World War II: Harry S Truman and Charles Lindbergh.

Harry S Truman (1884-1972), who became the 33rd U.S. President, was an Army artillery captain in Europe in World War I. He was in great danger at that time, but no one who has not been in combat would realize it. Artillery is a high priority for attacks by airplanes, other artillery, and infantry. Truman learned to make quick and decisive decisions, as he showed when FDR suddenly died. As Vice President, he suddenly was in charge of finishing the war for the Allies. He faced off successfully with Stalin at the Potsdam Conference at the time when his principal ally, Churchill, was weakened politically. He then authorized the drops of atom bombs on Hiroshima and Nagasaki, without regret. He broadcast the unforgettable Sunday message of V-J Day in his Mid-Western twang. It can still be heard on the National Archives website. "The Buck Stops Here" was the motto on his desk. Truman's untroubled health made his work achievable.[449]

Charles Lindbergh (1902-1974) graduated from high school on June 5, 1918. Some of his contemporaries had left high school to join the Army, and many others enlisted or were drafted that summer. Why Lindbergh did not enter service is unknown, but what is known is that his father was one of the few U.S. Congressmen to vote to oppose war against Germany in 1917. Lindbergh's father left office shortly before the Declaration of War was voted upon. By June 1918, the U.S. had a large American Expeditionary Force in France, consisting of Army and Marine Corps troops, supported with Naval forces in the Atlantic. Lindbergh became famous in 1927 as the first to fly alone, in a single-engine monoplane, from New York to Paris. His fame was instant and it continued for the rest of his life. His relationship to this essay is in connection with his personal life and his work in science: After he flew across the Atlantic, Lindbergh worked with Alexis Carrell (1873-1944) at the Rockefeller Institute in the development of tissue and organ culture, which led eventually to be useful for many other techniques in medicine. In the 1930s, Lindbergh was feted and decorated by Hitler, and he then followed his father's path in respect to the U.S. and Germany. He became a leader of the "America First" movement which opposed joining the Allies in World War II. He resigned his commission in the Air Corps, although he flew 50 missions in the Pacific as a civilian consultant during the war, and shot down a Japanese plane. Lindbergh married Ann Morrow, daughter of the wealthy U.S. ambassador to Mexico, and they had six children. Their oldest son, Charles Lindbergh, Jr., was kidnapped and killed at the age of two in what was said to be the "Crime of the Century." Lindbergh also had a secret life, which involved having seven children with three other women in Germany. Lust is an aspect of health, and he surely had it.[450]

World War I and World War II are now merged into one World War in the minds of many American school children. They can't remember which side Italy and Japan were on. That's understandable, because those countries switched sides after World War I, and then Italy switched sides a second time in World War II!! And anyway, wasn't it just one long 30+ year war that lasted from 1914-1945, with an Armistice that allowed for a pause of 20 years from 1918-1939? Especially because Winston Churchill called it a Thirty Years War, and he should know, shouldn't he? He was in it from start to finish.

Speaking of lust, no less than three U.S. presidents had illegitimate children: Thomas Jefferson is now known to have had several children by his deceased wife's enslaved servant. Grover Cleveland had at least one ("Ma, Ma, Where's my pa? / Gone to the White House, Ha, Ha, Ha"). Cleveland also had a secret operation for a malignant tumor of the palate. The operation was performed on a yacht in 1893, shortly after began his second term in office. He was under general anesthesia for one and one-half hours, supplemented with topical cocaine. A major piece of his palate was removed, which affected his speech. The operation was said at that time to have been a dental procedure; the truth was revealed in 1917. He never completely recovered from the operation and his term in office was adversely affected by it. Warren G. Harding, who had at least two extramarital affairs, had a daughter borne by one of these mistresses.[451]

Insurance became a vital part of medical care in the 20th century. The insurance industry has an ancient beginning with "bottomry contracts" for shipping, in which the risk was shared between the owner of a ship and those who invested in hopes of its safe return. These contracts date back to 4000-3000 BCE in Babylon, and with similar contracts in ancient Greece and Rome. The industry expanded when Lloyd's of London was formed in 1688; Lloyd's would insure almost any risk. In America, the first insurance company was the Philadelphia Contributionship, founded in 1752 by Benjamin Franklin. It was one of the many organizations created by that brilliant polymath. And then there were many others, including both specialized and general insurance companies: Prudential in Newark, N.J., Aetna, Blue Cross/Blue Shield, Kaiser-Permanente, Hospital Corporation of America (HCA), and the later New Jersey behemoth, Saint Barnabas Health Care System – Robert Wood Johnson (SBHCS/RWJ). Some of these are publicly owned, some are privately owned, and some are categorized as not-for-profit. Competition between them is fierce. Public opinion about health insurance is divided. Some want free health care for all; that government (i.e., taxes) should pay for it; and that there should be no limit on what "health care" should mean for a person who desires a service or product that he/she (or a health care provider) believes is needed for health. On the other end of the spectrum, there are those who believe that health care is an individual responsibility; if you can't afford it, that's just too bad. In the middle are those with low income who are covered by Medicaid (which varies from state to state), or who by virtue of reaching 65 years of age (or who are eligible because of disability) are insured by Medicare with a paid or earned supplement; or partially covered by the Affordable Care Act (ACA, also known as "Obamacare"). The American elections in 2020 heard many candidates proposing "Medicare for all" or "Health care for all," and some said that "Health care is a basic human right." The election of Joe Biden as President in November 2020, and with a thin majority in both houses of Congress, meant that the ACA would likely continue for at least another two years. Most Americans now want some form of health insurance, and the ACA is supported by a majority of voters. However, a determined minority continues to press for its overthrow in Congress and in lawsuits.[452]

Lobbyists for various groups compete to enable their members to obtain government insurance benefits through Medicare or military Tri-Care (for those on active duty, and their dependents), and insurance coverage is now an important part of labor negotiations. About 4 million retired military veterans have thus achieved a higher level of coverage known as Tri-Care for Life, which is Medicare Plus, without co-pay. Health care "providers," such as various specialties of physicians, chiropractors, and independent nurse practitioners, have lobbied to have Congress set aside benefits on behalf of their specific professions. The final details are delegated to the powerful Center for Medicare and Medicaid Services (CMS), where the lobbying continues. The cost of pharmaceuticals is an interesting issue. If a drug or other product is on the shelf in a pharmacy, and can be bought without a prescription, it is usually not covered by insurance. If a prescription is required, the cost to the patient varies greatly, depending on who is paying. Full price, without insurance, could be $100; with some insurance, it might be $10, or with another policy, it might be free. (These are estimates, not specific examples.) The computer tells the pharmacist what to charge. Dental care lags seriously behind in benefits, and there are few benefits for those who have problems with vision or hearing. The discrepancies are partly the result of ineffective lobbying by dentists, optometrists, and audiologists, and also because the cost of coverage of these problems would be very high.

A line of thought can be traced for leaders who espoused non-violent behavior and thus changed human history, at the cost of their own lives. Henry David Thoreau (1817-1862), who went to jail to protest taxation to fund the U.S. war with Mexico in 1846. Thoreau saw this war correctly as a land grab by English-speaking Americans that would also enable slavery to move further west on the North American continent. Non-violence was successfully employed against British imperialism by Mahatma Gandhi [Mohandas Karamchand] (1869-1948), who wore a dhoti as a symbol of unity with disadvantaged people of India. He was assassinated. Non-violence was later used successfully by the Rev. Dr. Martin Luther King, Jr., who also was assassinated. He gave his life in the cause of freedom for Blacks in America. Non-violence was espoused by Congressman John L. Lewis, who followed King's precepts.[453]

Fiction often provides vivid descriptions of the ways that human history is affected by health. Works of fiction that show the importance of health in human affairs is endless. However, any selection could begin with the classic series of *Sherlock Holmes* mysteries, in part because they were written by a physician: Sir Arthur Conan Doyle (1859-1930). The brilliant diagnostics of Sherlock Holmes were humanized by his partner, Dr. Watson, to whom he carefully explained his solutions. The fictional Watson served in the 2d Afghan War; Doyle himself served in the Boer War. Both of them knew much about illness and death.[454]

Other distinguished 19th century authors whose writings show the role of health in human affairs are: Harriett Beecher Stowe (1811-1896), whose novel, *Uncle Tom's Cabin* (1852), captured the imagination of the public in the North regarding the need for abolition of slavery in America. The novels of Charles Dickens (1812-1870), *Oliver Twist* and *A Christmas Carol*, among many others, show the widespread existence of poverty in the midst of wealth in London, and of what it was to be poor in the city at that time. And Émile Zola (1840-1902), whose many novels emphasized with the downtrodden in France. He wrote *J'Accuse* (1896) about the conviction and false imprisonment of Captain Alfred Dreyfuss, and for this, he was forced to flee to England to escape punishment himself.[455]

A list of some of the most popular writers of the 19th and early 20th centuries, whose works can be read from the perspective of the components of health – including shelter, lust, illness, and death – are shown here in the chronological order of their births: Herman Melville (1819-1891), *Moby Dick* and *Billy Budd*; Fyodor Dostoyevsky (1821-1881), for *The Brothers Karamazov* and *Crime and Punishment*; Leo Tolstoy (1828-1910), for *War and Peace*; Thomas Hardy (1840-1928), *Far from the Madding Crowd*; Joseph Conrad (1857-1924), *Heart of Darkness*; Willa Cather (1873-1947), *My Ántonia* (1918); James Joyce (1882-1941), *Ulysses*; Franz Kafka (1883-1924), *Der Prozess* (1925; *The Trial*) and *Das Schloss* (1926; *The Castle*); Aldous Huxley (1894-1963) *Brave New World* (1932); F. Scott Fitzgerald (1896-1940), *The Great Gatsby* (1925); Ernest Hemingway (1899-1961), *A Farewell to Arms* (1929); and George Orwell (1903-1950), *Animal Farm* (1945) and *Nineteen Eighty-four* (1949).[456]

The hazards to health of country life, especially on the frontier, are sometimes easier to perceive when they are told in well-written novels than in biographies and period histories. As adventurers and explorers proceeded across the United States, they were followed by farmers and ranchers. Usually men on horseback at first, and then entire families in covered wagons. Early settlements were founded, consisting of only a few houses and a store and a saloon with rooms for rent on the second floor. The small town might grow by attracting more businesses, especially if a railroad was laid down through it. The frontier moved West from New York state to the Mid-West, and then to the Rockies, to the Pacific Coast and to the Last Frontier, Alaska. The adventures and mishaps of men, women, and children in these distant, isolated places included illnesses, wounds, and deaths. The causes included combat with guns between those of English descent and between whites and people of color – Mexicans and Native Americans – using bullets and arrows. Both in the novels and in local histories there are examples of loss of life from exposure to the elements, with hypothermia or heat prostration, and deaths from starvation, thirst, drowning, falls from heights, fire, lead poisoning and infections from gunshot wounds, mysterious fevers, insanity, suicide, cannibalism, accidents with livestock (thrown from a saddle horse, attacked by a bull, trampled by a runaway team of work horses), and attacks by wild animals (especially grizzly [brown] bears, an angry moose, or a mountain lion). The possibility of a wolf pack attack was probably overrated, but it is legendary. The saddest stories are those that tell, as in real life, of death or permanent disability, when a wrong turn is taken at a fork in the road; or from potentially treatable injuries that were, due to circumstances, untreatable at the time that they occurred.

Some of the great story tellers and novelists of the frontier whose characters were concerned about health are: Washington Irving (1783-1859), for what was then the frontier, in the Catskills, west of the Hudson River, for "The Legend of Sleepy Hollow" and "Rip Van Winkle"; LeGrand Cannon, Jr. (1899-1979), for *Look to the Mountain* (1942), a novel of the Revolutionary War era when the frontier was in northern New Hampshire; and Mark Twain (pseudonym of Samuel Clemens) (1835-1910), for *Huckleberry Finn*, on the Mississippi River before the Civil War, and after that war, *The Celebrated Jumping Frog of Calaveras County and Other Sketches* (1867), in the Rocky Mountains and the Far West. Twain had many experiences as he was growing up with illnesses, violence, and deaths. There is also Owen Wister (1860-1938), *The Virginian* (1902), on the Western frontier; classic cowboy stories by Bret Harte (1836-1902) and Louis L'Amour (1908-1988), and Alaskan frontier stories by Jack London (1876-1916), such as "To Build a Fire" (the 1908 version) and *White Fang* (1906).[457]

Many movies focus on health and illness, recovery or death. For instance, *Gaslight, Rebecca, Pasteur, Magnificent Obsession, Bataan,* and *La Strada*. A vivid depiction of the Salem Witch Trials in 1692 is recreated in *Three Sovereigns for Sarah* (1985) with Vanessa Redgrave and Kim Hunter. More recently there are genres that include murder, torture, and various methods of violence and death. These are seen in unrealistic action movies, murder mysteries, true crime stories, fantasy and science fiction, and in biopic films with dialogue and characters and scenes that are said to be "based on" actual events, but are actually fictionalized.

Grand opera is the ultimate combination of all of the arts: vocal music (in all of its ranges), instrumental music (in all of its forms), visual arts (in all media, on all textures), and performance art: theater, drama, text, and occasionally spoken. Opera usually tells a story that is based on history or legend. Operatic themes include the full range of human problems and emotions, especially those that are related to illness: torture, homicide, tuberculosis, valiant death, prostitution, poverty & hunger, tragic accidental death, and insanity. One example of opera and the subject of health is the second opera of Giuseppe Verdi (1813-1901). It was *Nabuccco* (1842), written soon after his wife and small children had died. *Nabucco* (Italian, for Nebuchadnezzar) was about the Jewish period of Captivity in Babylon. They cried "Va, Pensiero" (Italian, for Go, Thought) as they begged to return to Jerusalem. This haunting aria was the song that became the unofficial anthem of Italy. In Larry McMurtry's novel, *Dead Man's Walk*, the aria appears in connection with leprosy, as it saved the last few survivors of the legendary Jornada del Muerto (Spanish, Dead Man's Walk) in the desert. The fictional character of "Lady Lucinda Carey" sings the aria from *Nabucco*, while riding slowly, bareback and completely nude, with blotches of leprosy on her skin. She rides alone, apparently without fear, in view of the awestruck Comanches who were poised to annihilate the white men. The doomed Texans are allowed to pass because they accompany this ghostly figure. Many other operas could be cited as examples of illness and death in their plots. For instance, *Aida* with its star-crossed lovers, who commit suicide; and *Romeo and Juliet*.[458]

****

Historians sometimes say that it is not appropriate for a historian to discuss current events, and that historians should never make predictions about the future. Nevertheless, historians certainly think about the future. In order to do that, let us think of the recent past. Perhaps we can regard the first twenty years of the 20th century as if it were the end of the 19th century. The *Fin de siècle* or the Period of Art Nouveau in Europe was also known as the Gilded Age in America. The last decade was known in America as the "Gay Nineties." In this way, for *Health Matters*, the 19th century is the period from 1800 to 1920. Strictly speaking, in chronology, the 20th century began in the year 1900, so there is a bit of overlap in the history of the 19th and 20th centuries.[459]

The 20th century was a dramatic period without precedent in human history. There is no simple term that defines the last century in the second millennium of the Common Era. It was marked by a period of explosive growth of the human race, and of the unparalleled impact of humans on the planet that they call Earth. It could be called the Atomic Age or the Nuclear Age, because during this century, scientists split the atom and made it possible to develop previously unimaginable amounts of energy. The twentieth century could also be called the Space Age. It was when humans landed on the moon and sent spacecrafts on missions to the other planets, and then two Voyagers that left the solar system and drifted into deep space in the universe, sending back radio signals that indicated how far they had gone. Voyager 1 and Voyager 2 still communicate with Earth via the Deep Space Network from a distance of 23 billion miles. The radio telescope at Arecibo, Puerto Rico, fascinated both scientists and laypeople until it collapsed from storms and old age in 2020. The Hubble telescope, launched from a satellite that was built by humans, sends back images from within the Milky Way. The Space Station, a cooperative international venture, continues in operation.[460]

Surgery in the late 20th Century

The pioneering work of surgeons in the early 20th century was the background for other surgeons' successes in the second half of the century. Three major areas are seen: organ transplantation, cardiac surgery, and replacement of body parts with prosthetics. Each of these three areas were developed as the result of three aspects of research: from experiments that explored bold new surgical techniques; by discoveries in basic science and in pharmacology involving the hematologic system; and from technology, which developed machines that incorporated metal and plastics, and then by miniaturizing and computerizing the new devices.

Research on organ transplantation had its first great success in 1954 with the transplantation of a kidney from one identical twin to his brother, who was suffering from renal failure. The surgical technique required months of experiments on dogs, using techniques to join blood vessels and ureters (urinary tubes) that had been developed by others. A new machine known as an "artificial kidney" was also a necessary part of the treatment of the patient, who was kept alive by this extra-corporeal device long enough to receive the transplanted organ. The next piece of the puzzle of transplantation was solved when drugs were developed to manipulate the immune system. These drugs permitted transplantation of organs between unrelated individuals. Other contributions to the field of organ transplantation were made by Christian Barnard (1922-2001), who first transplanted a human heart in 1967, and Thomas E. Starzl (1926-2017), who did it with the liver. The Nobel Prize was awarded in 1990 to Joseph E. Murray (1919-2012), who led the team that performed the kidney transplant in 1954. Murray was a surgeon at the Peter Bent Brigham Hospital (now Brigham and Women's Hospital). The surgical techniques were developed in his laboratory at Harvard Medical School. Alexis Carrell had been awarded the Nobel Prize in 1912 for developing the technique of blood vessel anastomosis that made Murray's work possible.

The dramatic use of a heart lung machine, which allowed surgeons to operate on a beating heart, was another development of the second half of the century. This work was preceded by many previous operations on the heart and blood vessels, involving surgery to remove bullets and shrapnel from the heart, from preliminary experiments that included a flexible cup that was sewn to the heart, and with the successful use of blood vessels that had been obtained from cadavers. Two surgeons at the Harvard Medical School, Robert E. Gross (1906-1988) and Dwight E. Harken (1910-1993), were pioneers in these operations. Bio-medical engineers worked with surgeons in the development of machines and plastic tubing that allowed the heart to be emptied and operated upon. All of the blood in the body was pumped out to the cardio-pulmonary bypass machine which performed the function of the lungs, oxygenating it, and returning it to the patient. Several types of these "heart-lung" machines were developed, beginning with the one created at the University of Pennsylvania by Dr. John Gibbon (1903-1973), with the assistance of engineers from IBM. None of this could have been possible except for the previous discovery of the anticoagulant effect of heparin; of human blood groups, which made it possible to use transfusions of blood obtained from other people; and of the use of plastics, made from carbon-phenol polymers, which were needed for the tubes, machines, and storage of blood. The machine used for extra-corporeal circulation of the blood was a direct predecessor of the extra-corporeal membrane oxygenator (ECMO), developed by Robert Bartlett (b. 1939), also at Harvard and later at the University of Michigan, which has saved many lives during the COVID-19 pandemic.

The third field which was developed by surgeons in the twentieth century is the use of implantable prosthetics and associated new technologies. This field is similar to the developments in organ transplantation and cardiac surgery, in that it was based on many years of attempts, failures, and successes. The field blossomed when engineers introduced new metals and plastics, and the ability to create ever smaller and more delicate bionic parts. To mention but a few: Microscopic surgery, using magnifying lenses that enable threads that are almost invisible to be used in surgery on the eyes. Laparoscopic surgery, using flexible tubing with lights and small telescopes that enable surgeons to operate through small holes, called "ports," made in the skin, instead of through grand incisions. Robotic surgery, in which the surgeon operates with a laparoscope, but is not necessarily in the operating room with the patient. He may view the operative field indirectly, on a television screen. This technique can be used to perform surgery on a someone who is under anesthesia a thousand miles away, if another surgeon is standing by the patient, prepared to operate in case a problem arises. And bionic replacement of limbs and internal organs, of which perhaps the most dramatic was the artificial heart. The first mechanical heart, the Jarvik-7, named for inventor Robert Jarvik, M.D., was implanted in Barney Clark, age 62, by William DeVries, M.D., at the University of Utah in 1982. Clark lived for 112 days after the operation.[461]

Chapter 11

The Health Care Industry

A. Health Care at Home

Most of health matters has always depended on the best practices that had evolved in each society. The practical aspects of health matters have always been at home. Physicians were rarely involved. "An ounce of prevention is worth a pound of cure," as the saying went. Prevention of illness was based on a healthy life style, safe behavior, and good luck. Mothers began the search for good health, without calling it "prevention," by serving food that they had learned to prepare. Food would be economical, available, and sufficient. Mothers also taught about safety inside the house. From Mother, children learned potty training and how to blow their noses; the dangers of fire, sharp tools, and heights; about loving others and peaceful behavior; and girls had "the talk" from their mothers. From Father, children learned about safety outdoors and in more distant locations – on the farm or in a factory, and while hunting – and to be wary of strangers. Sometimes boys had "the talk," but usually not from Dad. It was older boys who told younger boys the fibs, fables, opportunities, and of interesting things that could happen by playing with girls.[462]

In 1940, a typical breakfast in the American Midwest would be cereal with milk and sugar (oatmeal in the winter and dry cereal in the summer – Wheaties for boys, and Rice Krispies for girls). Milk would be from a bottle delivered by a local dairy, with a layer of sweet cream at the top. Brown sugar would be a treat, or even better: wild honey or black sorghum molasses. Breakfast would usually start with a teaspoon of cod liver oil. It was a hateful thing, although it was full of vitamins, so it was supposed to be "good for you." There might be another hateful teaspoon of castor oil if the child didn't report having a "B.M." yesterday. Older children would have scrambled eggs, bacon, and toast with home-made churned butter (making it would be a tedious chore for children) and apple butter. And sometimes pancakes, made with white wheat or brown buckwheat flour. For lunch (it was called "dinner" in farm country), a bread and cheese sandwich, with horseradish mustard. Older folks would have a "beef sandwich," which consisted of several thin slices of roasted beef between two slices of pieces of white bread, served on one plate with a mound of mashed potatoes and gravy. White bread would otherwise be a rare treat. Or a wiener with mustard on a hotdog bun, home-made sweet pickle relish, and sauerkraut on the side. There would be Jello or a piece of home-grown fruit for dessert. "An apple a day keeps the doctor away." Sometimes pears or grapes instead. A very special treat would be home-made ice cream. It often had a tasty bit of rock salt that slipped in from the churn, where it was packed into the water around the side to lower the freezing point. For supper, there would usually be another piece of meat, probably hamburger with ketchup, or a tough piece of pork; on occasion, it would be beef. The President promised that there would be "chicken every Sunday." There would be vegetables on the side. A white vegetable, such as potatoes – mashed or boiled. Maybe some cabbage, boiled, or as sauerkraut. And a green vegetable, such as gas-producing green beans (Grandma called them "light ammunition") or brown beans ("heavy ammunition"). It was said that "The more you eat, the more you toot." And sometimes carrots (good vitamins for the eyes) or celery, peas, lima beans and big onions; sometimes shallots. Corn, always on the cob, was the favorite, starting in mid-summer. Corn was expected to be "knee high by the Fourth of July." There was always gravy for meat and it was slathered over the potatoes, too. Beef gravy was best; or chicken gravy, if chicken was being served. There was no store-bought cooking oil. It was called "shortening" and it came from a can beside the stove where fat was collected after cooking bacon. Lard was plentiful and it was much used, but it was gradually replaced by Crisco. There were lettuce and radishes, but only in the spring, because those plants were early to rise and early to die. Tomatoes were rare. Mushrooms were eaten only in a few houses, and they were not sold in grocery stores. It took a daring person to eat wild mushrooms because everyone knew they were usually poisonous.

Families rarely ate in other families' houses, except at harvest time and on very special occasions. Families usually only with other families at church, especially after funerals. "Funeral food" was a casserole, also called a "hot pot." A family meal was served at noontime every day, with father at the head of the table and mother at the foot. Only the hired man or a cousin might be seated with the family. There never was garlic in most houses; that would only be eaten by immigrants, such as Bohemian or Polish families or gypsies. Perennials were harvested, too: the stalks of asparagus (never mind the smelly urine) and the beloved red-streaked stalks of rhubarb. Every housewife learned how to "can" properly to prevent botulism (meaning to boil vegetables and fruit and put them into Mason or "Ball" brand jars with screw-top lids and red rubber gaskets) and to make "preserves" (using vinegar or sugar to bottle slices of boiled cucumbers or fruit). Women learned to cook and bake with on a kitchen stove, fired with coal or split wood or dried corn cobs. They could bake deep dish pies, layer cakes, sugar cookies, and wheat bread and corn bread. Desserts were scrumptious. No coffee or tea for children, and rarely for adults. And no alcohol – or perhaps just a cordial now and then – but certainly no low-class wine or beer. And no cigarettes, although men might have a pipe of tobacco after a meal, or a chew on occasion, if there was a spittoon nearby. The hired man might roll a cigarette from a pack of "Bull Durham" tobacco. People were guided by idioms of the farmland: "Hold your horses"; "Make hay while the sun shines"; "Don't count your chickens before they're hatched"; and "Don't cry over spilled milk."

Grandmas taught the mothers about the ways to make lye soap, cottage cheese, and other aspects of the home economy. Soap was made from ashes and pig fat. The ashes, from each cleaning of the kitchen stove, were saved in a pile near the back door. They would be combined with rancid fat scraped from pork, which had been preserved in a wooden tub. When enough of the ingredients had accumulated, a fire would be built in the back yard, and the tub of fat would be suspended over it. Ashes and water would be added, and this alkaline brew would be stirred with a long wooden ladle while it bubbled and boiled. Gradually, the mixture would condense into a cake of grey soap, which would be cut into pieces. "Cleanliness is next to Godliness," so this soap would be used to wash hands before every meal, and also to scrub out the dirt from wounds. Manure was everywhere in those days and lockjaw (tetanus) was always a threat. A small bottle of acetone, and a box of powerful powder known as twenty-mule team "Boraxo" were sure ways to achieve cleanliness. Grandma made cottage cheese in a two-gallon porcelain jar with a tightly fitted lid. Unpasteurized milk was added from time to time to the "starter" mixture which always remained in the jar. Milk wasn't pasteurized in most dairies at that time, and unpasteurized milk was always available anyway. Adults loved the sour curds, but children held their noses when the lid to the jar was lifted.

Many homes did not have indoor plumbing, and each bedroom had a set of bowls: a large bowl for washing, one or two small pitchers containing fresh water, and a slop jar on the floor for waste water. If there was a bathroom in the house, that is where the home medicine cabinet would be located; otherwise, it was in the kitchen. Every kitchen cabinet contained aspirin, used for headaches and fever; and then assorted pills and bottles of whatever Mother and Father believed would be important. A jar of Vaseline was the universal home remedy for most skin problems; it would be tried first for redness and itchy rashes. The home pharmacy would usually include a styptic pencil, to staunch minor bleeding from a razor; Campho-Phenique, for pimples and other minor skin infections; a little bottle of tincture of iodine for a more serious infection; possibly gentian violet for skin abrasions; a tube of soothing zinc oxide for sunburn; Listerine, for a sore throat; and perhaps Carter's Little Liver Pills and Lydia Pinkham's universal remedy (which contained a generous supply of ethyl alcohol). There would be a box of cough drops, a small bottle of Mentholatum to rub onto a wheezing chest, and a jar of honey ("a teaspoon of honey helps the medicine to go down"). For severe coughing, elixir of terpen hydrate with codeine, though ETH with codeine is no longer available without a prescription. A tablespoon of Pepto-Bismol would be tried for loose stools, but if that didn't work, a teaspoon of paregoric (which contained codeine) would stop the flood. Paregoric would also induce sleep, which would be welcomed by both Mother and child. It, too, is no longer available as an over-the-counter product at pharmacies. There would be oil of cloves, to apply to a sore tooth; and a thick creamy white liquid, lard or Neutragena, to sooth an itchy skin. Women kept sanitary napkins (Kotex) out of sight.[463]

A large clean bandana was always available; it could be folded once to make a triangular bandage to use as a sling, or it could be folded twice to make a compress to place over a laceration. It was known as "first aid," until the doctor could look at it. Mothers taught their children how to tie the corners of a triangular bandage with a secure square knot, and also how to tie a slightly modified "granny" knot that was easier to untie. The kitchen cabinet would also include a few tools: a sturdy needle that would be used to pry out a splinter, after the tip was sterilized with a burning match; a safety razor blade; a small set of tweezers; a box of Band-Aids; Q-tips; and a small pair of scissors. Lifebouy and Ivory soap would be there; Lifebuoy supposedly was medicinal, whereas Ivory offered purity. A pitcher or syringe to wash out an eye if something nasty was spilled into it. Men would always be prepared mentally and physically to deal with bad injuries, and women would be prepared to help them. Most men in small towns and on farms throughout the Mid-West would encounter in their lifetime many of these injuries, and a country doctor would have seen them all: gunshot wounds, either from accidents or hostile intent; amputations (usually fingers or forearms; rarely a leg); dislocations (most commonly of the shoulder, but also of the hip, wrist, knee or ankle); fractures (of arm or leg, or worse – the back or neck); deep lacerations with exsanguinating bleeding (put a hand deep into the wound to grasp the blood vessel); evisceration (a slash in the abdomen, and the bowels spill out; they are replaced and held there with a tight wrap until the doctor comes); impalement (falling onto an upright pole; for instance, sliding from a haystack onto the handle of a pitchfork; bad news indeed if the handle goes up in the body between the legs). If the victim is obviously dead, he or she would be laid out respectfully and a cloth would be gently placed over the face. If the victim was unconscious and appeared unlikely to live, an expectant watch would be kept until a doctor could decide what to do. The dangers of country life were always there: machines with moving parts and belt drives, sharp tools, open fires, boiling water, guns, roofs of tall barns and houses. And animals: a horse's hooves and teeth, a kicking milk cow, a bull's horns, an angry sow's crushing weight. Hornets, bees, and rabid animals added to the list of worries that every parent had for their children.

For a sick child, there would be a bowl of hot milk toast, buttered and with salt. (This would also be a Sunday-evening dish, presumably to ensure good health.) If the child was seriously constipated, there would be a spoonful of castor oil. Fever would be treated expectantly, with foreheads gently wiped, pajamas changed, and blankets and sheets adjusted tenderly. A hot water bottle would relieve a chill. Every child was expected to endure all of the usual childhood diseases (UCD's they were called). The order varied, and hopefully they would come separately: measles (the most dangerous), German measles (rubella), whooping cough (the most worrisome); mumps (the most painful, for boys); and chicken pox. All parents knew that it was best to for the kids to have them all. Scarlet fever was dangerous (the only one that was quarantined); and God forbid if anyone got strep (a worse form of streptococcus than scarlet fever), or meningitis or [Rocky mountain] spotted fever (both of which would be, sadly, fatal). Polio, called "infantile paralysis," was the most feared of all, because it could cause permanent paralysis and wipe out a family's finances. Most of these measures did not require a doctor's attention. If the patient was really sick, a doctor would be asked to make a house call. Nurses only worked in hospitals, and they never made home visits. Doc would give an injection of something that was supposed to help. It didn't make any difference, but it seemed to everyone that it was the right thing to do. If the patient was elderly, it would be a medical gesture that usually preceded the preacher's last visit. Then each person would quietly step into the room, to say Good bye. The Bible says that miracles do happen, and we can pray. Maybe that's what happened to tuberculosis and diphtheria and tetanus, which used to be so common. Almost all of health matters were taken care of at home, but when necessary, it was good to have a family doctor. He could write a prescription, and there was a pharmacist in every town who could fill it.

Sulfa drugs became available in the late 1930s, and they were the first "wonder drugs." Patients sometimes had terrible allergic rashes from sulfanilamide, and after a slow recovery, it was, for them, "back to the good old days." Never again would they dare to take sulfa. Doc could set a broken bone without an x-ray and then put on a cast made of plaster of Paris. Doc could stich up a deep wound and deliver a baby. A family doctor would not usually perform surgery, if anesthesia was required, but he could assist another general practitioner and the two of them would get the job done. The patient might be told to lie down on the kitchen table. Then someone else, perhaps one of the women in the family, would be instructed how to drip ether from a can onto a gauze that was wrapped over a screen that fitted close to the patient's face. The instruments would be boiled up, and after the procedure – it might be an appendectomy, or repair of a rupture (hernia), or a difficult delivery, or a scraping out huge carbuncle – the instruments would be washed in the kitchen sink, and everything would be tidy again. Say a prayer.

B. The Health Care Industry

1945-1975   Seventy-Five Years

The twentieth century was a time when more people were born than ever before, and also when more people than ever were killed by other people. It was a time of paradoxes: It was a time of increased human life expectancy from disease control, yet it also was a time when billions of people died prematurely from disease. In the field of health care, the triad of physicians-hospitals-universities expanded to a pentad, with two additional components: government and industry. And now hidden behind the five components of this new Health Care Industry were the fields of science and economics.

For many centuries, health matters had primarily consisted of:
Medicine & Science & Technology
and
Religion

In the 20th Century in Developed countries, health matters became the Health Care Industry:
Physicians & Hospitals & Universities
And then, with the addition of Governments and Industry, the Health Care Industry became:
Physicians & Hospitals & Universities & Government & Industry
and
Science & Economics

There also has been a role for the legal profession, for doctors of the law, throughout the history of health since the end of the Middle Ages. Lawyers have a special place in *Health Matters*, but this essay has skipped from the earliest days of the hunter-gathers to the present time. The deficit will now be rectified, as the subject of the legal profession is re-introduced in connection with its involvement in health care.

Lawyers

Lawyers are needed in every part of the modern Health Care Industry. The profession of law, and its practitioners, namely lawyers and judges, can trace the origin of the profession to the earliest settlements of communities of humans. Communities needed ways to ensure that disagreements would be settled amicably, and to set punishments for outliers, and thus to set examples for others who would disrupt the peace of the community. Originally meeting as elders to make these decisions, the specialty of lawyers developed the profession on its own path. In this essay on health care, the legal profession has up to this point had little attention. However now, at this point, it is appropriate to show the ways that law and lawyers are involved in health, as part of the Health Care Industry.

The twin professions, law and medicine, have developed in different paths. Medicine, being primarily a branch that is scientific and seeks one truth, though it accepts the fact that there are several versions of truth. Physicians may debate, but they agree that there is preferably one best solution to every medical question. Law, on the other hand, is combative. Lawyers are taught to argue a point, and to debate it effectively from either one side or the other. The combat may be settled with a compromise, but the goal is to secure the best position at the end. To a lawyer, winning is everything. There is, however, a specialty in law for negotiators, and they are interesting to observe. The case may be a dispute in a contract, a claim of tort, or of a crime. A defense lawyer may recommend that the client plead guilty to a lesser charge. Many criminal cases are now settled in this way, although many of the accused fail thereby to have a fair trial. Wise lawyers and physicians have learned to appreciate each professions' ways, and to accept them. With that preamble, let us look at the ways that lawyers are now involved in the Health Care Industry. It is not a small part. Although no estimates are available, perhaps not less than ten percent of the time and money spent on health in the United States can be allocated to legal costs. Perhaps more, but surely not less than that. Legal costs are an appropriate part of every budget in the Health Care Industry. It is an appropriate cost of doing business, known in the financial world by the acronym CODB.[464]

Lawyers have been chief executive officers of many hospitals and physicians' organizations. Two lawyers in succession have been CEOs of the Medical Society of New Jersey for more than forty years. Lawyers have argued cases both for the "right to live" and the "right to die." They have assisted in developing contracts, Non-disclosure Agreements (NDAs), and compliance with the Sarbanes-Oxley Act, which includes whistle-blower protection and retention of records. Lawyers have taught physicians how to bill for time spent in conversation with patients, as lawyers do. They take depositions and argue on behalf of physicians charged with malpractice (and they also argue on behalf of the plaintiff), and they ensure that group billing is properly done so that it does not appear as fee-splitting. They advise physicians not to attempt to retaliate against a patient who loses a case charging malpractice, because in the United States (in contrast to Britain) it is difficult to win a judgment by charging that the original suit was frivolous. They advise physicians about compliance with the difficult requirements of the Health Insurance Portability and Accountability Act (HIPPA). Lawyers and physicians are often collegial friends.

Since the end of World War II, the human search for health has become the business of the Health Care Industry. A brief summary of this health care-industrial complex is now in order. The focus in this essay will be on the United States, but similar trends have taken place throughout the world. Many of the details are available in Paul Starr's book, *The Social Transformation of American Medicine* (1984) and in Roy Porter, *The Greatest Benefit to Mankind* (1999). The trends that Starr and Porter observed have accelerated. Health care now represents almost one-fifth of the United States economy, and the end of this growth is not yet in sight. And as much as one-quarter of the spending on health is wasted. There was a bump in the road in 2020-2021, but on the whole, the Health Care Industry has sailed along nicely. The industry profits most when people are sick, and there has been much sickness with COVID-19.[465]

In the United States the death toll from COVID reached 500,000 in February 2021, and COVID has become the nation's leading cause of death. Hospitals are full, and many others are out of sight in nursing homes. Predictions vary widely; some say that "herd immunity" will be reached in the summer of 2021, while other experts expect that masks and social distancing will be needed until Christmas. Several mutations of the SARS-CoV-2 virus have developed, which lends a new air of uncertainty.

The five principal components of the Health Care Industry were shown on the outline on the previous page: Physicians, hospitals, universities, government, and industry. They have each changed dramatically in the past seventy-five years. These components are overlapping in their corporate relationships. The search for health, money, power, and fame are threads that binds them together. Many components have joined into conglomerates that incorporate people and industry in all five areas. Some individual leaders in the health industry – CEOs – are reported to have achieved immense incomes, with little concern for conflict-of-interest. Science is involved; patentable discoveries yield new ways to provide health care, and profit for the discoverer. Economics is also involved; when a new product or service is developed and marketed, the income statement shows a profit, and Wall Street is bullish.

Physicians are still at the center of the health professions. Although rural areas are still served by generalists, the increasing urbanization of America has enabled physicians to specialize and practice in groups. What was formerly "general surgery" (all of surgery), is now divided into specialists who limit their practice to specific parts of the body. The brain, spinal cord, heart, lungs, trachea, abdomen, breast, and so forth. They do it well, by repeating the same operation day after day. A trauma surgeon is an exception; he or she must be able to handle anything. Physicians now lead teams that include nurses, paramedics, social workers, and medical students. They work in shifts. The laparoscope, the flexible endoscope, robotic surgery, and outpatient surgery have transformed American surgery. Organ transplantation and replacement of body parts with bionic substitutes have let people live longer than ever. The broad reach of organizations such as the American Medical Association and state medical societies have gradually diminished, as specialty organizations have developed. The American College of Surgeons is still a power to be reckoned with, but so, too, are specialty organizations such as the American Society of Clinical Oncology and the Society of Surgical Oncology. Other health professions' organizations, such as the Oncology Nursing Society, have also developed scholarly and political activities that have extended their role in patient care and partnership with each other health care workers.

Hospitals have also undergone dramatic changes in the past seventy-five years. Public charitable hospitals, organized by cities and counties, have largely disappeared. Most free-standing psychiatric and tuberculosis hospitals have been closed and abandoned. Psychiatric patients now often wander in the streets, homeless, with inadequate supervision. Sometimes on drugs, but often forgotten. Tuberculosis is still a threat, with drug-resistant TB now rising in incidence again. Small rural hospitals have closed. The remaining hospitals are now enormous, gleaming, brilliant complexes with impressive office suites for the administrators and heads of medical staff services. These medical centers have become efficient machines to move patients from the emergency room to the CT scan, to a treatment room, to the recovery room, and out the door as soon as possible. All is usually done within a day or two, because the cost is calculated by the hour. Hospitals now employ physicians: hospitalists, who work through the night, and specialists whose offices are in adjacent buildings. Patient care not as personal as it used to be, but it is extremely efficient and the result in most cases is excellent. It is, however, very expensive.[466]

The universities continue to be one of the pillars of the Health Care Industry. Medical schools have bonded with other schools and departments of the universities to develop new methods for patient care and for profit. A typical medical school's health care complex may include physicians (some full-time, others part-time), a university hospital, and science laboratories which are working to develop new treatment methods. The university will have medical students and graduate students. In contrast to the situation seventy-five years ago, about half of the medical students are now women. There is a gradually increasing percentage who are from minority groups in the population. Efforts are being made to train all students to work with cultural differences, although this seems to be an uphill battle at times. Science laboratories are funded by government grants, pharmaceutical industry grants, and private philanthropy. The university's administration and the laboratory scientists are always looking for a patentable product, and for ways to share the profits if it is successful.

The U.S. government is a major funding source for universities through research and teaching grants. Some of these grants are intensely competitive, whereas others are negotiated quietly behind doors. The RO1 grants from National Institutes of Health (NIH) are the ones most desired. An RO1 grant is the route to academic success in many medical schools in America. It is often required for tenure. The NIH grant program has enabled American medicine to be the world's leader in discovery and development of new ideas and treatments. The U.S. government also is a major funder of patient care, and in this way, it supports universities, hospitals and physicians.

"Industry" is now the fifth component of the field of health care, of the complex that is involved with people and health. The pharmaceutical industry and the insurance industry are the principal groups, but "industry" also includes many other individuals, companies, and organizations. Some are for-profit, such as food service companies, trash collectors, office supply stores, and HVAC corporations that provide electrical/plumbing/air conditioning service. Some are not-for-profit, such as the American Red Cross and the American Cancer Society. Nursing homes may be either for-profit businesses, such as Marriott's chain of Brighton Gardens, or operated as not-for-profit charitable organizations by churches.

The complex relationships between the various individuals, groups, and businesses involved in health care appear in their internet addresses. The "dot coms" in the field of health care include .com (business), .gov (government), .org (charitable organization), and .edu (not-for-profit education). The latter two organizations are exempt from federal taxes by 501(c)(3) and its associated regulations. They may have offices or buildings adjacent to each other, and they can be either competitive or cooperative. Their administrators must have superb business skills, and they may have backgrounds in medicine, nursing, laboratory science, or other professions related to health. Physicians are, however, the key to success. The epitome of the Health Care Industry at this time is a 2.1 square mile medical district in Houston, Texas, which is known as the Texas Medical Center Corporation (TMC). The TMC traces its start to a donation in 1945 that created the M.D. Anderson Cancer Center, in cooperation with the state of Texas. The TMC has become the largest medical complex in the world. The area known as the TMC now includes more than sixty medical organizations, including Baylor St. Luke's Medical Center, Houston Methodist Hospital, the Texas Heart Institute, Memorial Hermann medical office building, Shriners Hospital, DeBakey Veterans Affairs Medical Center, and the TMC Library. More than 100,000 people work on the TMC campus, and some 10 million patient encounters take place there each year. The annual gross revenue is a staggering $25 billion. The TMC is considered to be a not-for-profit educational institution, with a website of www.tmc.edu.

    The Health Care Industry is now composed of many uncoordinated and highly competitive components which are subject to regulations and oversight by government agencies. The system, as it may be called, is imperfect. However, in the past seventy-five years, it has achieved remarkable results.

****

History is continuous. The 20th century passed into the 21st century, and thus into the Third Millennium, without a pause. There was a slight hiccup at the moment when midnight occurred at 00:00 hours, because all of the computers in the world needed to reset. But a Millennial catastrophe, that some predicted, such as the End of the World, did not occur. It is now 120 years since the end of the 19th century. In contrast to the previous narrative for each century in this part of *Health Matters*, there will not be a review of the last one and one-fifth centuries. Some readers may be disappointed in this decision, but most will probably be satisfied, or even grateful. There are already many examples of important events of this period of 120 years in previous sections of this essay, and they should be sufficient to show the influence of this period upon health. To repeat them would be a tiresome exercise, and to add more would be superfluous. A brief paragraph will suffice to show a few of the ways that health matters impacted upon the last eleven presidents of the United States. These are the presidents who followed Dwight D. Eisenhower, who was mentioned above.[467]

    From the 34th President (John F. Kennedy) to the 45th (Donald J. Trump), the following medical conditions have been reported: adrenal insufficiency (Addison's disease); chronic pain following spinal surgery, requiring treatment with corticosteroids and injections; addiction to extra-marital sexual activity (three presidents), one of which impacted on governance and one on national security; megalomania and the appearance of paranoid behavior; exhibitionism (perhaps a usual phenomenon for presidents); hyperthyroidism; cardiac disorders; excessive sweating (hyperhidrosis); excessive risk-taking (gambling addiction), a condition common to presidents; insomnia; excessive alcohol consumption (at least one, while in office, or possibly more); near-asphyxiation from aspiration of a potato chip; a torn quadriceps tendon at the knee; a bone spur of the ankle (sufficient for deferment from military service); smoking of marijuana (two presidents); previous history of alcoholism (followed by abstinence); colonic cancer; and three assassination attempts with guns (a rifle, successful; a pistol, nearly fatal; and a pistol, deflected, without injury). Positive effects on the health of others includes sponsoring legislation that enacted Medicare (which greatly reduced the cost of treatment for those who are eligible for Social Security), new controls on marketing of tobacco products; the National Cancer Act (which provided an enormous increase in federal funding for cancer research); and funding for medical problems in African countries.

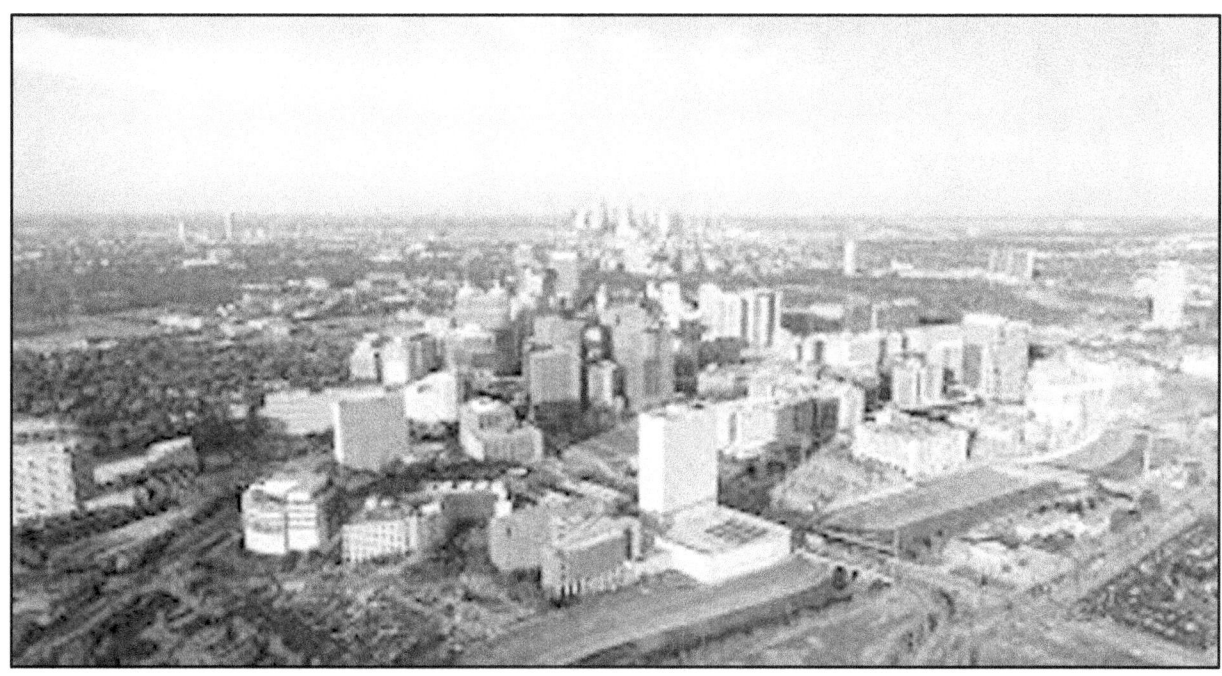

"Texas Medical Center" aerial view from www.tmc.edu.

Texas Medical Center
Houston, Texas
The Largest Medical Complex in the World – 2.1 Square Miles

Health Matters

Part Three

Discussion and Conclusion

Chapter 12

Historiography

A. Three Other Books

Warfare Between Science and Theology

Is It Irrelevant Now?

Religion appeared in the first part of this essay, but it has rarely appeared later until now. There were about 150 references to religion in Part One. Most of them were in connection with the urges and the exceptions in the search for health, including sacrifice and self-sacrifice. In Part Two, which focused on the role of medicine in history, there were less than 20 references to religion. It is now appropriate in conclusion to re-examine the role of religion in health. The reader may recall the thesis in *Health Matters* that religion and medicine were inseparable in the earliest days of our species. This was not an original thought; it was first stimulated for me when by James George Frazer's *The Golden Bough*. It has been reinforced over the past sixty years in studies of history and medicine. *Britannica*, in its essay on Anthropology, says that Frazer "posited a progressive and universal progress from faith in magic through to belief in religion and, finally, to the understanding of science."[468]

The primal needs and urges of *Homo sapiens* for health led to the identification of men and women who had the gift of healing. In *The Greatest Benefit to Mankind*, Roy Porter observed that "medical expertise became the *métier* of particular individuals" known as the "medicine-man or healer-priest," who provided for health care in early societies. They have sometimes been called "witch doctors" or "shamans," both of which have pejorative connotations. The existence of the healer-priest has been recognized by anthropologists in some cultures that are currently in existence in remote areas, such as Africa, South America, and Papua New Guinea. Two branches can be traced from the healer-priest. One is to medicine, and the other to religion. Relationships between these two great components of human life still exist. Several connections between medicine and religion have been described in this essay, such as one by Sir Thomas Browne, *Religio Medici*. However, each of these fields of endeavor has mainly developed, or evolved, in different directions. In medicine, we now have medical practitioners (such as physicians and nurses), and developments from medicine into the related fields of science and technology. In religion, we now have designated leaders (such as priests, nuns, rabbis and imams) and development into the fields of the arts and law (including theatre and politics). Another example of the connections between these two tracks is the alphabet – which originated in technology – and which is important for both religion and medicine. Mathematics, a scientific discovery, is used in law and government. Architecture, a branch of technology, owes its existence to both science and art. Architecture has been crucial to the building of edifices of worship – churches, cathedrals, mosques, synagogues, and temples. Structure and form are both important in architecture; the structure must be scientifically perfect, but the product must be pleasing to the eye. And above all, architecture is based on safety. The architect's plan must pass the test for safety beyond normal conditions, to withstand fire, flood, and earthquake; the quality of the building materials must be examined as they are inserted; and the final construction must satisfy the inspector. Philosophy and epistemology – the study of knowledge, existence, and truth – can be said to encompass both science and religion.[469]

A three-day conference on the "so-called warfare thesis" was held in 2015, sponsored by the Issachar Fund and the Department of Zoology, University of Wisconsin-Madison. Some of the papers presented at the conference became the basis for a book by Jeff Hardin and others, *The Warfare between Science & Religion: The Idea That Wouldn't Die*. The book which stimulated interest in the "warfare thesis" was of course a major topic at the conference. A full citation was not given in the publication by Hardin, et al. It is: Andrew Dickson White's 1896 work in two volumes, *A History of the Warfare of Science with Theology in Christendom*. There is no bibliography in Hardin's book, and the full title only appears in the Index and in the essay by Lawrence M. Principe, "The Warfare Thesis."[470]

The principal puzzles with which each Christian must wrestle include three Stories and two Questions. The three Stories are (1) Is the Bible literally true? (e.g., the Creation story); (2) the Nativity story; and (3) the Resurrection story. The Questions are: (1) Is there Intelligent Design, a Prime Mover in the Universe? [called God by some, or YHWH, or Allah] And (2) Is there is a Heaven and Hell?

By "literally true," is meant that some Protestants believe that every word written in the King James Version of the Bible is true. The term "Evangelical Christians" is a pejorative expression that is applied to those who accept the King James Version as truth. Many college-educated Christians believe that all three of these Stories are myths. They cannot be reconciled with science. Many of them enjoy reading the King James Version, and comparing it with other translations, but they do not believe that it is literally the "word of God." The KJV can be inspiring, and it is also challenging to read and to understand. The two Questions posed above cannot be answered by science. Perhaps the answer is Yes. Or Maybe. It's comforting to imagine that they are, but what is done in daily work, today, is what is important. Most of the members of the health professions and scientists do their jobs without wrestling with these two Questions. Many of them go to church or synagogue or temple occasionally, or once a week, celebrate religious holidays, and never think about a conflict between science and religion.[471]

The Creation myth has two components that are especially troublesome to scientists. One is the short period of time from the First Day in Genesis to the present moment, which some Creationists believe to be about 4,004 BCE; and the other is the implication that the earth is the center of the universe, and that revolving around earth are the moon, the sun, the planets and stars. There are additional stories about Creation in the book of Genesis, such as the story of Adam and Eve, their expulsion from Eden, and so forth. These could be thought of as metaphorical. The geocentric universe was a fundamental belief of Christians for many centuries, as it had been for the Hebrews. Both Copernicus and Galileo hesitated to suggest that it might be wrong. Nicolaus Copernicus (1473-1543) developed a theory that placed the sun at the center of the solar system, with planets such as Earth and the other planets circling the sun, each in a separate orbit, and with the moon circling Earth. Copernicus' theory was based on his observations and calculations. He proposed that the starry sky was a universe that extended far beyond the solar system; and that it was the earth that moved, giving the appearance of motion of the stars. (We now believe that the stars are also moving, away from us, but that is a later story.) Copernicus realized that his theory would upset the leaders of the Church in Rome, and he withheld publication of it until the year he died.[472]

Galilee Galileo (1564-1642), after inventing the telescope, was able to confirm the existence of many additional stars, previously unknown, and other findings which convinced him that Copernicus' theory was correct. Galileo attempted to advance the ideas of Copernicus by suggesting that it was just a debatable question. However, the papal authorities recognized what Galileo was trying to do, and he was forced – at the peril of his life – to recant. Tycho Brahe (1546-1601), a prominent astronomer, never accepted Copernicus's theory of the heliocentric solar system. Others, too, are said to have been reluctant. Brahe's assistant, Johannes Kepler (1571-1630) accepted it, but perhaps more because of his "sun worship" than because of scientific evidence. As a result, it took about 100 years to become accepted by science. A heliocentric solar system is, in fact, contrary to our common observation. The appearance of a geocentric universe is what we see every day. The sun rises in the east in morning it sets in the west in the evening, and the moon follows the same pattern at night, rising in the east and setting in the west. And the starry heaven appears to rotate around the earth. Copernicus' universe is still not accepted as truth by many Evangelical Christians, who must learn it to pass exams in school, but who believe the true account is told in Genesis.[473]

We now return to the collection of the essays that were written after the conference in 2015, and edited by Hardin, et al, on the "warfare thesis ... the belief that an inevitable and irreconcilable conflict exists between science and religion." For anyone interested in this question, this book is important for its discussion of the origins of the conflict, and for recent comments on it by scholars in various fields. The conflict reached its climax with two books that were published in the 19th century. In his chapter, "The Warfare Thesis," Lawrence M. Principe says that these were the "chief vectors of the conflict thesis": William Draper, *History of the Conflict between Religion and Science* (1874); and Andrew Dickson White, *A History of the Warfare of Science with Theology in Christendom* (1896). The personalities of Draper and White, and their backgrounds, play significant roles in development of their ideas. Principe says that "Draper's thought can be characterized as an obsession with law" and that he "promotes a religion of his own devising, a theology opposed to Christianity – and to Roman Catholic Christianity in particular." Draper, according to Principe, says that Islam introduces monotheism in opposition to Christianity, which is polytheistic. White's "ponderous" two volume work was published later than Draper's but his "opening volley" was fired in 1869, and his "attacks" on religion continued for a longer period of time than Draper's. Principe: "Modern historians have regularly seen the *Warfare* as a response to critic from clergy and denominational colleges aimed at White during his work to found Cornell University as a nonsectarian institution." Principe says he ended his first lecture on this subject "with a rather peevish allusion to these events."[474]

The attacks on the "conflict model of science-religion interactions" continues throughout this book. As an example, in his Chapter "Social Scientists," Thomas H. Aechtner writes that "adherence to the conflict model still persists within anthropology and sociology [and] the conflict model narrative perseveres as a conspicuous historical narrative in modern university-level pedagogical materials." But as I mentioned above, the "conflict model" does not appear in the teaching materials of several universities. It may be there, but it is certainly not prominent. However, Aechtner doesn't mince words in offering his opinions. He refers to Draper's *History* as a "notorious text" with its "infamous contentions." Aechtner's view of the profession of anthropology is sadly truncated: he does not refer to Frazer or to *The Golden Bough* in his description of the origin of anthropology. John H. Evans, in "The View on the Street," takes the position that "conflicts in the public are typically not ultimately about epistemology. Rather the conflict is often over issues like whether religion or science will have more social authority." And he is certainly correct in saying that "a conservative Protestant may completely accept the mainstream scientific account of human origins but still be opposed to the social/moral influence of scientists' account of human origins." Many chapters in this book are written in the language of the elite or those who do crossword puzzles. It is wise to have a dictionary at hand, for few people ordinarily use words like these: Humean empiricist, hermeneutics, semiotics, polygenism, theophanic, epistemic and otiose (which means "serving no useful purpose").[475]

One chapter, "Neo-Harmonists," by Peter Harrison, aligns with these thoughts. Harrison's latest book is on *Territories of Science and Religion*, and he writes on both subjects. He speaks of the "false historical claim that since antiquity 'science' and 'religion' in the West have been engaged in a perpetual warfare." Harrison approves the views of Rodney Stark, a sociologist of religion, who wrote that "religion and science are compatible, and that the *origins* of science lay in theology" [emphasis in original]. This was the argument that appears in Frazer's *Golden Bough*. However, Harrison does not give Stark an easy pass, saying that "he is right for all the wrong reasons ... owing to [his] unfamiliarity with relevant primary sources and lack of knowledge of the specific detail of much recent work in the history of science." In conclusion, Harrison profiles the life, faith, and work of Francis Collins, director of the National Institutes of Health. Harrison says that as an "advocate of harmony," Collins espouses the "venerable seventeenth-century idea that the formal study of nature is a form of religious worship."[476]

It is admittedly a difficult issue to summarize the thoughts and beliefs of Christians in the United States, in order to draw conclusions regarding their attitudes regarding science and religion. We will return to that in a minute, but it should be said that there is a profound difference between those who understand science and those who do not. Just as there are some for whom mathematics is easy, while others struggle with numbers. Some people enjoy reading the Science pages in the newspaper; others read the Business section or Sports. For those who are not interested in science, or for whom it is a difficult subject, there are two choices: to ask for, and to accept, the observations and conclusions of scientists; or otherwise, to reject science. The plot thickens when scientists disagree, and that does happen. And when a majority of scientists agree on something, it still may be wrong. A good scientist knows that there is often some uncertainty in what is reported, and it is necessary to keep an open mind. A thoughtful non-scientist appreciates the fact that scientific opinion may change. This is especially important in the time of COVID-19. For instance, the original recommendation for mitigation included (1) hand sanitation, (2) wearing masks, and (3) social distancing. Nine months into the pandemic, it now appears that the SARS-CoV-2 virus is usually transmitted by airborne aerosols. Contaminated surfaces are now considered to be a minor vector for transmission. Hand sanitation/washing is still recommended, but the emphasis is now on masks, to reduce viral transmission in both directions. The recommendation for social distancing is unchanged (6 feet apart), but for young children a shorter distance appears to be satisfactory. The changes in recommendations should not be taken as evidence that science is faulty.[477]

There are five major groups of Christian denominations in the United States at this time. All of them believe in the divine nature of Jesus Christ; i.e., that he was (and still is) both man and God: Roman Catholics; mainstream Protestants; non-liturgical Protestants; the Church of Jesus Christ of Latter Day Saints (also known as LDS, or Mormons); and others. The Roman Catholic Church includes both faithful and nominal members, most of whom are birthright Catholics, but rarely attend church. The Catholic Church differs from the Protestant in two principal ways: Catholics believe in the supreme authority of the Pope, who has the final word on all matters of faith; and they elevate Mary, the mother of Christ, to a high level of devotion: "Ave Maria" (Hail Mary). Faithful Catholics attend Mass regularly, and although some may waver in respect to birth control, they usually follow doctrine in opposing abortion. For many years, Catholics were not encouraged to read the Bible, and the Bible still does not play as important role in Catholic services as in Protestant worship.

Mainstream Protestants include Methodists, Presbyterian Church USA, Lutherans, Episcopalians, and smaller groups that include Church of Christ (formerly known as Congregational) and Reformed Churches (Dutch or German). Protestants are encouraged to study the Bible, and many develop their own notions about the meaning of Biblical texts. Community pressure, rather than the hierarchy of the church, prevents Bible-readers from straying too far from conventional beliefs. In the 19th century, the Methodist Church was the largest denomination in the United States. The largest is now the Catholic Church, as the result of immigration from Ireland and decreasing birth rate among congregants of mainstream churches. The non-liturgical Protestants include several groups of Baptist churches, all of which have in common their belief in adult baptism: that faith requires a personal commitment, rather than infant baptism, in which adults agree to raise the child as a good Christian. Most of the other non-liturgical Protestants are grouped together as Evangelicals. Their worship services are generally informal, conversational, and family-oriented. The preacher reads one or more passages from the King James Version of the Bible, and these are discussed – witnessed – with affirmation by the congregation. No one questions the text, regardless of internal conflicts that exist within the Bible, or with history or science. Evangelicals believe the Creation Story, the Ten Commandments, the Nativity Story, and the Resurrection Story, including the hope of the Second Coming. Most of the Evangelical congregations can repeat these stories, using the exact words of the KJV. The LDS Church also requires "belief in the Bible as the word of God" and belief in the Book of Mormon, which was written on "golden plates," unearthed by Joseph Smith in the late 1820s, along with the Urim and Thummim, a "translating contrivance" that allowed Smith to read the engravings on the plates. The Eighth Commandment, "Thou shalt not kill," said to have been given by God to Moses, and which is believed by millions of Christians, is a powerful weapon against abortion.[478]

Many other groups gather for worship in the United States. Some of them originated within the Protestant Christian Church, and they retained belief in the divinity of Jesus, although they have differing views about what "divine" means. Others regard Jesus as one of the important figures in history, and that his sayings should be studied, along with others; but that Jesus was not divine. The other religious or meditation groups range from those who believe in the literal truth of the Bible, to those who regard the Bible as just one of many important sources to consider for inspiration. Some of them are communal and pacifistic and some have specific dietary beliefs. They include large groups such as the Seventh-Day Adventists, the Society of Friends (Quakers), Eastern Orthodox Churches (Greek, Coptic), Christian Scientists, and Unitarian-Universalists; and smaller organizations, including Amish, Mennonites, Jehovah's Witnesses, the Amana Colony in Iowa, Hutterites, Swedenborgians, and the Ethical Society, which includes people of different faiths. There are also many Black Church groups; the largest is the African Methodist Episcopal Church. And there are the Mega churches, which seat thousands inside their buildings and hundreds of thousands observing, worshiping, on television. There are also Wiccans, who believe in witches; and voodoo, from Africa via Haiti. And of course, there are Jews, Muslims, Hindus, Buddhists, Zoroastrians, and Native American religions. All of them theoretically have Freedom of Religion, guaranteed by the Bill of Rights, in the First Amendment to the Constitution.[479]

Religion also appears in the background of many other organizations. There is a belief in Divine governance in various Masonic orders, which date back to the late Middle Ages. They are secret, and the details are not available to outsiders. It is public knowledge that some of the Masonic groups in America are the Masonic lodges, marked A.F.&A.M., composed of Third Degree "Blue Lodge" Masons; and the 32nd Degree Masons of the Scottish Rite and Knights Templar, the Shriners, Order of the Eastern Star, DeMolay, and Rainbow Girls. In theory, they welcome anyone who passes the required written and oral tests, but there was, and perhaps still is, racial segregation in Masonic lodges in the southern states. The counterpart for Catholics is the Knights of Columbus. A religious tone was established in the Boy Scouts of America when it was created more than a century ago. Millions of young men and women and adults memorize and recite at the beginning of Scout meetings, and at other times, the Scout Oath and Law. The Oath begins with "On my honor, I will do my duty to God and my country," and the Law begins with "A Scout is," and it ends with the 12th point: "Reverent." Scouts are encouraged to earn religious awards, such as one named "God and Country," for service in their respective churches.[480]

Religion plays an enormous role in the polity of America. Freedom of Religion has allowed for many views to be expressed, and we have overt political maneuvering on behalf of the beliefs of churches. The Methodist Church became the principal organizer of prohibition, through the Women's Christian Temperance Union (WCTU). The Methodists were not opposed to alcohol when the church was founded by John Wesley, an Anglican priest. However, in the mid-19th century, the leaders of the church saw the need to reform society, and church doctrine added prohibitions against alcoholic beverages, tobacco use, dancing, and gambling. This was especially pointed at newly arriving immigrants from Europe, many of whom were Roman Catholics, and who enjoyed these pleasures. It was pure politics: On the side of temperance were Protestants, whose ancestors had arrived in America several generations earlier from the British Isles (although few from southern Ireland) and Germany. They lived in small towns and on farms, and they were staunch Republicans. On the other side were the Democrats. Most of them lived in cities; they had recently arrived in America, did not speak English well, and were Catholic. Republicans sensed an odor of corruption about the Democrats, who seemed to enjoy politics, whereas the Republicans liked to pretend that they were righteously above political maneuvering. But politics in America has always been about money. A surgeon who became a Republican member of the New Jersey Assembly (the lower house) said, "There are three important things in politics. The first is money, the second is money, and I can't remember the third." An obstetrician and a Democrat, who was also very active in New Jersey politics, said the first rule in politics is "Never say no." Without saying so, he implied that it's better to suggest "Maybe," and then to see if any money appears.

The historic conflict between science and religion is similar, in a way, to the conflict between Democrats and Republicans in the twenty-first century. There are about 150 million voters in America, with a wide spectrum of beliefs, so this generalization is fraught. However, Democrats, in general, are now more willing than Republicans to turn to science for answers. Republicans are more likely to turn to religion and to be suspicious of science. The polarization continues into the field of health care. During the runup to the election in November 2020, many differences were seen between the two candidates in several important areas. The differences were summarized as follow: On COVID-19, Donald J. Trump downplayed the severity of the pandemic, whereas Joseph Biden pledged to put scientists and public health leaders "front and center." On the Affordable Care Act (ACA), Trump attempted to overturn the

ACA entirely, whereas Biden proposed to build on the ACA and to increase insurance coverage. Regarding prescription drug prices, Trump emphasized the need to address high drug prices, but did little about it; Biden's plan is to give the federal government the authority to negotiate drug prices for Medicare and other insurers, with a cap on payments. For reproductive health, Trump expanded restrictions on abortion, whereas Biden supported *Roe v Wade* and promised to nominate judges who would uphold abortion rights. Polices on immigration and health care also differ: Trump took many steps to restrict immigration, including building a wall on the U.S-Mexican border; Biden proposes to reverse many of the Trump administration policies on immigration.[481]

The issue of conflict between science and religion has come to the foreground in the United States during the COVID-19 pandemic. The conflict had long been present, but the dispute now has elements that are so violent that warfare may be a more appropriate word to use. The division between believers and deniers of science in America has been present for many decades. However, the division lay beneath the surface of daily life, because there was little reason to argue about science, and anyone could believe what they wanted to about religion. On one hand, scientists might argue with each other, but the technology that was produced from science was confirmed by the marketplace before it was accepted by the public. Children learned to repeat and recite what they were taught in science classes, and anyone was free to believe whatever they wanted to about any subject that was not in the realm of science. The First Amendment prevented discussion in public schools of God, Jesus, Intelligent Design, or anything related to religion. As a result, the study of history, literature, and philosophy was truncated in public schools, because students were unaware of the texts on which these subjects depend. For instance: the Torah and the other books of the Jewish Bible, the New Testament. Shakespeare, Milton, the Religious wars, and plays such as *The Crucible*. What were they all about? There could not be a complete discussion in public schools. In some private schools, students could be assigned to read and discuss these texts. However, many private schools were religiously oriented. In these schools, the perspective was usually one-sided; one side was taught as being correct, and the other side was wrong. Formerly, the disputes about science and religion and between religious groups were non-violent, and did not become a matter of public record. It was this way until the early years of the 21st century.

During the competition for the presidency in America in 2008, a loose coalition formed which opposed the election of Barack Obama as the 44th President of the United States. This movement included White nativists and Christian fundamentalists, who said that Obama was not born in the U.S. (the "birther" theory); that he was not a Christian (because his father was a Muslim, from Kenya); and that he was therefore not a legitimate president. One of the sponsors of the "birther" theory was Donald J. Trump, who had been planning his own campaign for the presidency for many years. Trump's attraction to a large segment of American voters was overlooked by intellectuals and most of the news media. His successful campaign depended on his mastery of communication, and it appealed to a large segment of the American public. His followers were enchanted by his outlandish and repetitive comments in speeches, in public, on television, and on Twitter. He rarely spoke of matters of religion, or of science, and his personal behavior included a profligate life-style of gross indecency. However, it was clear to his supporters that Trump's motto, Make America Great Again (MAGA), and his slogan, "Drain the swamp," as an outsider in politics, would support the goal of White Christian supremacy and Biblical righteousness. Trump anticipated that he would not win the popular vote, but he knew that he could win the Electoral College vote if he focused on winning several states in the Mid-West. These states had large populations of White Evangelical Christians, who were the key to his success. Trump's words and actions satisfied the usual Republican voters in many other states. Hilary Clinton's campaign failed to recognize the strength of Trump's message, and he ultimately prevailed. She won the popular vote, as was expected, but it was mainly in the urban areas. Trump's victory was based his winning the votes in rural and "rust belt" areas, which dominate the American system of the Electoral College. The Electoral College was established to ensure that small states would not suffer from the "tyranny of the majority." The Electoral College is composed of 538 electors, whose members represent the two Senators from each state and all of the state's Representatives in Congress. The U.S. Constitution gives two Senators to rural states such as Wyoming and Alaska, the same number as New York and California.[482]

You may ask, in what way did the presidency of Donald J. Trump relate to the question of science and religion? The answer is two-fold. In the first three years, the issue was simply the antagonism to science by the president and by those who he appointed and his followers. He showed that the power of the presidency extended to areas that had never previously been tested. Scientific advice was marginalized, in respect to climate change, the environment, and research. Religious conservatives were pleased with Trump's appointments to key staff positions and to the federal courts. The possibility of overturning *Roe v Wade* was not without hope, and lower courts approved repeal of many of the opportunities for abortion that had been enacted in the states. And then, in the last year of Trump's presidency, COVID-19 arose to cast a shadow on the health of the world. Trump's dilatory and confusing approach to COVID-19 was criticized by most scientists and physicians. However, his supporters increased in numbers, and they have cheered for him – wearing red MAGA baseball caps, and standing side-by-side, without masks. Many have been quoted as saying that they wouldn't take the COVID-19 vaccine. They pride themselves on their opposition to science. The Evangelical Christians – the so-called "fundamentalists" – represent a major group within the Republican party. It is too soon to unravel the relationship between science and religion in the belief of many who supported Trump. However, the numbers are staggering. Trump received 63.0 million votes in 2016, and that number rose to 74.2 million in 2020.[483]

For an Evangelical Christian, religion is more than theology. It is a way of life. This imaginary passage is intended to capture the beliefs of Evangelicals:

A typical Evangelical Christian family is a man and a woman, dressed appropriately, with both boys and girls. The man wears trousers, and the woman is in a dress, with a skirt; the boys wear blue overhauls and the girls wear dresses, pink preferred. "Boys and girls behave as God intended when they were born"; no wavering about their sex. Marriage is between a man and a woman. Marriage should precede intercourse, although a bit of lusty behavior can be excused. It is in the Bible, from Abraham to David. Not bestiality or sodomy though. Sodom got its bad name when Lot left town. There is nothing in the Bible that would suggest that abortion is proper; but it is killing, and that is prohibited by the Commandments. A woman should be respected when she is in the time of her custom, as was Rachel. You remember that story. Genesis 31:35. Life on a farm is hard, but hard work is expected, and it is the gateway to success. Just as it was for Joseph's father, and for Jesus' father, too. An individual sometimes needs help, but that should come from others, not the gov'ment. They only take taxes from you, like the tax collector that Jesus told about. In farm country, there were no colored people here until the Mexicans arrived. Immigrants. Black folks passed through this country before the Civil War, and that was a good thing. They didn't stay. On the way to Canada, they were. We're glad that Mr. Trump is putting that wall up in Texas. It's the only way to protect our border. My shotgun, my rifle, and my pistol are secure with the Second Amendment, and Mr. Trump is all for that. Our family is safer with those guns. I do go huntin' once in a while, too. We believe those folks from Asia and Africa and Cambodia should stay where they came from. We've got friends who are Catholic – Germans and Czechs – but them Irish and Italians, they are city folks, and they drink beer and wine. They're Democrats, too. We don't drink. Not much, anyway, and only a taste of that hard stuff. We're Republicans, in case you didn't know it. Our family has been Republican since Mr. Lincoln's time. We don't understand why China seems to tell us what to farm and all our clothes are marked Made in China now. Mr. Trump is going to stop China. Socialism is bad. Never mind that our old folks are glad to receive them Social Security checks. Mr. Trump will protect them. He's all for veterans, too. All that talk about him being a draft dodger and stuff is phony. He went to military school, didn't he? Well, it's coming time for church today. Ma will make a casserole, and Daddy will put on a coat and tie. I hope we don't run in to any of those immigrant folks from Somalia or India or wherever before we get back home today. Now, I've got to get to my Bible."[484]

The current dilemma about religion and science is a concern that is not new; it is medieval. This was well stated by Harry Flickinger, who reacted to an article entitled "Pastors struggle to spread the vaccine gospel." He said, "I will not be joining those who are hellbent on holding to the ignorance of the Middle Ages and science skepticism. Given the choice between getting the vaccine and exposing oneself to dying with a tube down your throat gasping for air, I'll take the vaccine."[485]

Health Matters and *The Structure of Scientific Revolutions*

Is *Health Matters* a new paradigm for history? Yes.
But it is not the same as the paradigm in *Structure*. *Health Matters* is about history.

History is both art and science. Thomas Kuhn's use of "paradigm" refers to science, not to art. He discussed the evolution of graphic art from realistic art (scientific) to non-representational art (post-Renaissance, as in "Mannerism"). He does mention "in the eye of the beholder," which could mean that there could be exceptions. But it is clear that Kuhn intends to have his "revolutions" or "paradigm shifts" refer to science itself, rather than to the history of science. At one point, Kuhn mentions both the "history of science" and "science" itself, which might mean that the two are conflated in his book; but usually he speaks of "science" as the way scientists do their work, and how fields of science accept change. I would also say, how they evolve, almost always progressing. He differentiates the world of science from other fields, such as politics and art. He doesn't mention "Whig history," but his view of science is clearly that of Whig history – always progressing forward and upward.

Kuhn's choice of words and his slow progression through *Structure* makes his argument difficult, even tedious, to read. This is perhaps understandable, because every age, or generation, has its own language and its favorite expressions. In the half century since Kuhn wrote *Structure of Scientific Revolutions*, many words have been given new meanings, and many neologisms have been coined. For example, "trope," "meme," "woke," "rap," "twerk," and more. Acronyms have become substitutes for words. Kuhn took a rarely used word (paradigm) and defined or re-defined it, and captured it. The words "paradigm" and "paradigm shift" now have a new life of their own. Ian Hacking wrote in 2012 that it is "pretty hard to escape the damn word, which is why Kuhn wrote even in 1970 that he had lost control of it." Kuhn gave new meaning to other words such as "anomaly" and "revolution." Words that Kuhn used such as "incommensurability" and "exemplar" seem to be intentionally highbrow. Would that Kuhn had been a story-teller, or that he could write in language that is straightforward and explanatory.[486]

Kuhn's examples of scientific revolutions are used and re-used *ad nauseam* throughout *Structure*, but they must be largely unintelligible to anyone who has not studied the fields of science that he used as examples, and then remembered the details. In order to follow his argument, the reader must have retained a good understanding of the history of chemistry, of physics, of astronomy, and mathematics. Otherwise, the reader must unquestionably accept Kuhn's examples. Kuhn makes little effort to explain the examples that he chooses, as in the contributions of John Dalton and Benjamin Franklin, and in the debate between Antoine Lavoisier and Joseph Priestly. What were they? A simple explanation of the geocentric universe of Ptolemy and the heliocentric universe of Nicholas Copernicus, and how they differ, would have been better than simply mentioning them as being different. I suppose I might do this now for Kuhn, but I will forgo that pleasure. Kuhn states that the reason for the difficulty in shifting from the geocentric to heliocentric concept was both religious and scientific. But he failed to give a clear description of the problem that astronomers, such as Johannes Kepler, had with the heliocentric model. The heliocentric "model" became the only way to view the universe until the Big Bang was added, and the universe was then seen as expanding, not static. We now believe that the heliocentric solar system of the sun and its planets is located in an ever-expanding universe.

Ironically, unintentionally (or perhaps from some unstated reason), Kuhn neglected to mention, by comparison with Ptolemy's brilliant though incorrect view of the solar system, Ptolemy's equally brilliant deduction that the Earth was globe of about 25,000 miles in diameter. It has long been forgotten that the idea that the Earth was round was probably made in the ancient world before Ptolemy and by many after him – before Columbus captured the popular imagination. But Ptolemy accurately calculated the circumference of the Earth. He used the Pythagorean theorem, after having measured the distance between two points on the Nile and the length of the shadow cast by a pole at each point at noon.

The writers of the Bible probably knew that the Earth was round. In the first place, none of them said or implied that the world was flat. How else could anyone explain the warmth of the climate and the longer days in summer as one moved from north to south in the lands of the Bible – in what we now call the Middle East? Sailors must also have observed that the sun gradually rose to a higher point in the sky at noon as they sailed south along the coast of Europe, until, while sailing south along the coast of Africa, they reached a point when the sun began to cross the sky in the north at noon. Every ship had a navigator, and this was clearly evidence of a round Earth. The disappearance of the hull of a ship as it sailed away from land was also a puzzle to landlubbers, but not to sailors. Prince Henry of Portugal must have known that his ships were sailing south, across the Equator, along the coast of Africa. Christopher Columbus and his sailors must have known it too, as they sailed west from Europe to find what they believed would be islands off the east coast of Asia. Columbus hoped to find more islands after the Canaries and the Azores, and the islands known to be off of the east coast of Asia. He was right, but they were far apart. Think of Hawaii and Australia. But to Columbus' surprise and pleasure, he found an island, just in time. Though he never saw it, there was a huge land mass there. He thought it was Asia. But it was America.

History also has another dual meaning. History is everything that has happened since time began, and it is also the story of what has happened. There is no longer a "pre-historic" period. History extends from the moment that the universe was born until the moment we call "now." It is everything that has happened from the Big Bang to Modernity. The study of history depends on facts. Facts are the basis for the science of history. History is also the story of what happened, and why it happened. The story of history can be told in many ways; this is the art of history.[487]

Science is the study of things: of "how," not "why." It thus is in contrast to philosophy and religion, both of which ask "why," not "how." The argument in philosophy is rigorous, based on rules; in religion, there are both rules and beliefs. Science, philosophy, and religion are in contrast with art, which asks "what do the senses say?" In judging art, the argument is won by the eye (and ear, and the other senses) of the beholder. Medicine is the science of health. It is also a form of art. Technology is the work of useful science – of making things that can be used.

Health Matters is similar, yet in many ways is different, from the essay by Thomas Kuhn on *The Structure of Scientific Revolutions*. Kuhn's *Structure* was based on a thorough review of the history of mathematics, astronomy and physics, and to a lesser extent on the history of chemistry. Kuhn had little to say about biology, biochemistry, and medicine, but he implied that these fields of science developed in the same way; i.e., with episodic revolutions that were due to "paradigm shifts," after enough evidence accumulated that was incommensurable with an existing theory. In *Health Matters* there are many similarities and also important differences in the history of medicine and biology with respect to Kuhn's model of paradigm shifts in *Structure*. Some of these were mentioned previously in this essay, and a few additional examples will now be added which show similarities and conflicts with Kuhn's model.

There have been two important scientific revolutions in biology in the past two centuries. They are examples of contrasts. One shows the accumulation of incommensurable conflicting evidence and then a paradigm shift such as Kuhn described in *Structure*. The other was different. It was immediately accepted by all biologists, without reservation. The first example is in the mid-19th century, when the revolution known as "Natural Selection" took place. Others had observed some of the changes that Darwin mentioned, but they had explained them in various ways. Darwin challenged these old ways of thinking. The *Origin of Species* by natural selection was promptly accepted by many scientists, reluctantly by some, and not at all by others. Reception by the public was also variable, and often was hostile. Although the details are still being debated, Darwin's *Origin* was the greatest revolution in biology in that century. However, Darwin and the *Origin* appear on only three pages in *Structure*. The first instance is but one long sentence, in which Kuhn quotes *Origin* to show that Darwin realized that he did not "expect to convince experienced naturalists" to accept his views, but instead he looked "with confidence to the future, – to young and rising naturalists … to look at the question with impartiality." A longer discussion in *Structure* deals with the "conflict" issue, of science versus religion, rather than the paradigm shift. Kuhn wrote that "the least palatable of Darwin's suggestions," was that *Origin* "recognized no goal set either by God or nature."[488]

The greatest scientific revolution in biology in the 20th century was immediately accepted. In contrast to the slow, halting, and incomplete acceptance of the Darwinian theory of evolution in the 19th century, the model proposed in 1953 by Watson and Crick of double-stranded DNA was promptly recognized by all of the scientists who were searching for the molecular structure of the gene. The question that James Watson (b. 1928) and Francis Crick (1916-2004) were working on was not of any particular interest to scientists in general. Their solution did not challenge current philosophical or religious beliefs, and the public took little notice of it. Yet their answer spawned a vast new field of research in biology. There is nothing in *Structure* that encompasses both Darwin's revolution and Watson-Crick's revolution in biology. Why did Kuhn not mention this? We'll probably never know. The model structure of DNA as a double helix was published in 1953, nine years before the publication of *Structure*. The enormous impact of DNA upon biological research was well established by 1962. Earlier in 1953, Linus Pauling (1901-1994) announced his theory that DNA was a triple helix, but he immediately accepted the Watson-Crick model of the double helix when their paper was published. Pauling had received the Nobel Prize in chemistry in 1954 for his "for his research into the nature of the chemical bond and its application to the elucidation of the structure of complex substances." Ian Hacking, in the Introduction to the fiftieth-year edition of *Structure*, mentions Watson and Crick as an example to show that by 1992, "biotechnology rules," and "physics is no longer where the action is." However, Hacking did not mention whether or not he thought that the Watson-Crick theory was a "paradigm shift" revolution. Linus Pauling is not mentioned by either Kuhn or Hacking.[489]

There are many revolutions in the history of medicine that show the spectrum that are exemplified by these two examples. Some revolutions in medicine were immediately accepted, some were slowly accepted, some have faded away, and some are still under consideration. The idea of a "paradigm shift" in thinking has not been a major consideration either for physicians or for their patients. The reasons for acceptance of the changes include the obvious benefits of some, the apparent benefits of others, and non-scientific considerations such as deliberate falsification of results, finance, nationalism, ego, politics, and religion. The subject of bloodletting (venesection) is a curious phenomenon. It appears in methods used by tribal physicians. It was used for centuries in the far East, in India, and in the West. But it gradually disappeared. No sudden conflict or debate can be recognized as a paradigm shift in connection with bloodletting. This is a clear exception in the history of medicine to Kuhn's hypothesis of paradigm shift in scientific revolutions. Darwin observed, as quoted above, that young people are more likely to accept change, whereas older men and women are generally more conservative and are less willing to try something new. The spectrum of humans ranges from those who appreciate something that is "bright and shiny" to those who favor a thing that is "tried and true."[490]

Immediate acceptance by the medical profession and the public is a matter of record for the use of chemotherapy for many diseases, beginning with infectious diseases: Salvarsan (called "606"), sulfa drugs, penicillin, and then the full spectrum of antibiotics – one after another. Patients would begin to expect to have a "shot" of something for a sore throat or cough, and physicians would gladly accommodate. There was little concern about other miracle drugs that appeared in the 20th century, because the benefits appeared to outweigh any apparent or possible side effects. Chemotherapy became the treatment of choice for psychiatric disease, for hypertension, arthritis (even though cortisone had its downside), and cancer. There were problems of treating tropical infections, because the drugs were often as challenging as the infections, but patients were advised to take them anyway. Chemotherapy worked miracles for all of these diseases, and complications were simply tolerated. And then there were all of the vaccines – for tetanus, diphtheria, polio, yellow fever, cholera, anthrax, and yearly against influenza – and for diseases of children, too, until the anti-vaccination movement rose as the result of problems with polio vaccine. And then there came a false report about autism associated with vaccination against childhood diseases. Vitamins were safe, and a daily dose of a multi-vitamin became a welcome shift from cod liver oil. When it came to new options for surgery, there was little reason to hesitate: cardiac surgery in all of its forms, organ transplantation, and replacements of body parts with titanium or plastic substitutes prepared from hard or soft polymers of carbon or silica.[491]

There were other new chemicals that appeared to be wonder drugs, but which were found to cause new problems. Elimination of malaria – the world's leading killer – seemed possible, if the many species of the mosquito could be destroyed; and DDT appeared to be that miracle. But DDT has poisoned the well, so to speak, with a *Silent Spring*, and malaria, yellow fever, dengue, and other mosquito-borne diseases are still with us. All of these new drugs were accepted promptly without a paradigm shift, though perhaps a longer period of consideration would have been better.

False reports regarding chemotherapy for cancer with Krebiozen and Laetrile were made by unscrupulous scientists. Discussed previously, these claims for useless chemicals led physicians down wrong paths and led to hopes that were dashed for patients and their families. Disproof was insufficient to cause them to be rejected; it was necessary for the public to tire of hearing of success that was occasionally reported but which could not be confirmed. Laetrile is still a hoax that is perpetrated in a clinic in Tijuana, Mexico, but Krebiozen (Kreb = German, cancer) has vanished. This was a potential paradigm shift that was quietly reversed in the same way that venesection disappeared.[492]

Treatment of suspected myocardial ischemia with oxygen and heparin was displaced by elaborate pharmaceutical methods. The old ways to treat a suspected heart attack with relatively inexpensive methods and drugs have been replaced by expensive drugs. The results of the new methods are probably better than the older ones, but the shift was gradual, and were not subjected to rigorous study. Ethically, this would be difficult, and it would be hard to devise a randomized study protocol that would pass review by an Institutional Review Board. Whether the new methods are better, or not, has not always been tested for other types of heart disease. Relatively inexpensive drugs such as digitalis and quinidine were replaced by expensive beta blockers and other drugs, which let to profit for some physicians and the pharmaceutical industry, without an independent randomized study to prove that the new therapies are better. The same was true with pharmaceutical derivatives of thyroid hormone, but in that case, the whistle was blown: the pharmaceutical manufacturer attempted to suppress the result of trials that questioned the superiority of the new drug, but the truth was finally revealed in *JAMA* and the *Wall Street Journal*. Were these paradigm shifts, or not?[493]

Paradigm shifts could be described for pharmaceutical treatment of hypertension and type 2 diabetes, instead of simpler methods such as reduced dietary salt and reduction in caloric intake, but is the pharmaceutical treatment better, or not? Once again, it would be difficult to plan an ethical randomized trial, and then who would pay for it? The paradigm has shifted, but not as a result of the debate of the type that is described in *Structure*.

Questions of competition between science, public policy, and profit arise in many areas of biology and medicine. For instance, it is clear that there is overuse of antibiotics in the food of domestic animals that are raised for slaughter. This is an almost impossible conundrum, given the fact that animals are allowed to be kept in pens that foster transmission of infectious disease. There has been a serious mix of good intentions, political maneuvering, of profit for some, accidentally harmful intent, and ignorance plus profit in the widespread use of opioids, non-smoking tobacco products, and marijuana. These medical issues have been revolutionary, but they cannot be said to have passed the paradigm test.

Scientific research in bio-medical fields is also complicated with competing values. Paradigm shifts are difficult see in this mixture, in which grants are funded based on the basis of new ideas that are just ahead of the pack, but not too far, and which appear to be likely to succeed. In fact, in many cases, the best applications describe proposals that have already been tested and proved to be correct, using previous grants from less demanding sources, such as funds from faculty practice groups, or uncommitted money known as "overhead funds" that can be allocated by administrators in universities. The top level of NIH research grants, known as RO1 grants, needs to be in the same direction but with new and significant improvements, compared to previous publications. And they need to point to newer possibilities. There is temptation to do research to prove that the proposal will be successful, using other funding, and to pick data from the experiments that fits the expectation. Bio-medical science is troubled with frequent retractions of papers, and by other reports of fraud that are reported but are not retracted.[494]

A major paradigm shift occurred twice during the past three decades in connection with a protein with the innocuous name of "p53." This protein was discovered independently by four groups of investigators, who originally gave it different names. As the research coalesced, and the name p53 was agreed upon, it was designated as one of the so-called oncogenes, meaning genes that cause cancer – and there were many who believed it was the most important of the oncogenes. Additional research over the next few years led to the conclusion that cancers that were thought to be caused by p53 were actually caused by a mutant form of p53; and that normal p53 was, instead, an important protein that stabilized cells. That is to say, p53 was an anti-oncogene. The paradigm thus shifted twice; once to call p53 an oncogene; secondly to call p53 an anti-oncogene. The shift happened quietly, no one was embarrassed, and the earlier conclusion can only be seen by historians who search for the entire record of p53.[495]

There are many theories in medicine which have developed in the same way that Kuhn describes paradigm shifts in *Structure*. That is to say, the theories that are now accepted were initially rejected or were questioned or appeared to have little relevance at the time they were proposed. But as it was with Copernicus' theory of the heliocentric solar system, William Harvey's theory of circulation of the blood initially had many opponents, and it made no difference in the treatment of patients, so it took much longer to become commonly accepted than is now remembered. The same can be said, for various reasons, that the discovery of Galen's errors in some aspects of anatomy; and of the cause and prevention of cholera, the use of anesthesia, the germ theory, of asepsis and antisepsis, the cause of yellow fever, the difference between syphilis and gonorrhea, the cause and prevention of scurvy, and the risks and benefits of vaccination. In addition, we have seen some beliefs fade away without being replaced. The ancient Greek theory of the four elements and the four humors also gradually faded away, leaving only a residue of metaphors, such as "choleric" and "sanguine," but there was no paradigm shift in that instance. The use of animals in experiments is still a contested issue, with the outcome uncertain at this time. The proper use of specimens obtained from humans without specific consent is also questioned. The same is true with the use of embryonic human tissues. These questions cannot be answered simply by science or medicine, because the lay public is involved, too, with interactions of politics, religion, and ethical questions. Kuhn said correctly that a scientific community typically consists of perhaps one hundred members, and that communities of this size make the decisions which he calls paradigm shifts. However, although medical research is conducted in groups of about this size, the revolutionary changes that occur in medicine usually depend on groups that are much larger – and they include oversight by the public.[496]

Advances in medical research continue, in spite of confirmed evidence of fraud, duplicity, greed, plagiarism, guesswork, and personal ethical failures. The list is actually longer. All of these problems, and more, have been repeatedly documented over the past century. Reports of discoveries of problems such as these would embarrass many others, so the incidents are often hidden, and never revealed to the public. The perps are warned but allowed to continue, or to retire quietly, and all is soon forgotten. Papered over, as the saying goes. However, it is of greater interest at this point to emphasize that these human failures have not prevented the vetting of research results by the ultimate test: Does a report of a discovery lead to additional discoveries? If it does, that's good enough. In most instances, no attempt is ever made to repeat the original work. The original report may have been fabricated, or based on carefully selected data that would not stand a statistical review, but if it was a lucky guess, so be it. Science stumbles along successfully in this way.

In the 21st century, one area in biological research stands out thus far as the stellar achievement. It is CRISPR. It is too soon to know if CRISPR will have an effect comparable to the impact of Darwin in the 19th century or Watson-Crick's discovery of DNA in the 20th century. One thing is certain, however: CRISPR is not easy to understand, even by a scientist, without expertise in the same field.[497]

The definitions of the acronyms are:
    CRISPR-Cas   This means a specific DNA and its associated protein
    CRISPR = **C**lustered **R**egularly **I**nterspaced **S**hort **P**alindromic **R**epeats, of DNA
    Cas = **C**RISPR **as**sociated protein. There are several, each with a different number

The Whig Interpretation of History

Is *Health Matters* a Whiggish History?

The answer is probably no. *Health Matters* is not Whiggish history. *Health Matters* encompasses all of human history, from the cave dwellers to the present time. It would be possible to take the position that human history has been a history of progress, as the Whigs in England viewed history in the mid-nineteenth century. However, "Whiggish history" has taken on a series of meanings since it was first coined as a scornful term by Herbert Butterfield (1900-1979) in 1931. The term "Whiggish history" now encompasses much more than what the Whig political party intended in the 19th century, and probably also from what Butterfield meant. We will examine some of the ramifications of this term, as it has evolved into the 21st century. However, "Whiggish history" is a complicated subject, because there is no perfect definition of this term, nor is there anything that would satisfy all who render opinions about it.[498]

The Whigs and Tories were political parties in England from the 17th to the mid-19th century. The Whigs were progressive, and they sought to limit the royal authority and to increase parliamentary power. The term "whiggish" in England was used to express belief in the progress of mankind. Ironically, in contrast, the Whig party in the United States was conservative, and it was dubious about progress. A young British intellectual named Herbert Butterfield took the position in 1931 that the Whig movement, as it applied to history, was incorrect. Butterfield believed that a historian's position in the present can lead that historian to misunderstand, and thus to misrepresent, the past he/she is studying. He stated that a historian's duty is "to evoke a certain sensibility towards the past, the sensibility which studies the past 'for the sake of the past,' which delights in the concrete and the complex, which 'goes out to meet the past,' which searches for 'unlikenesses between past and present'." That is to say, the historian will find in the past what he/she is looking for. Butterfield's thesis has been debated for nearly ninety years. Most historians now decry whiggish history by calling it "presentism" or "present-centeredness." Nevertheless, historians recognize some aspects of history are properly viewed through present eyes. Three examples are the history of slavery, the history of the Holocaust, and the history of non-violence. Historians of slavery can document the movement through the centuries toward the emancipation of enslaved people, even though this is Whig history. The horrors of the Holocaust are now viewed by historians through present eyes, even though millions of people in Germany, Europe, and the United States turned a "blind eye" to what was Hitler's "final solution" in the 1940s. This, too, is Whig history, but it is not debatable. Finally, historians would surely agree that the history of non-violence, of peace between individuals and nations, has been beneficial to humans, and that this history, though Whiggish, is properly recorded through presentist eyes.[499]

Historians of science also waver about "whiggery," because scientific discoveries and theories are built upon prior discoveries. Kuhn's *Structure of Scientific Revolutions* proposes the way that new theories are developed by "paradigm shifts," revolutions in science, which usually result in improvements. The Nobel-prize winning physicist Steven Weinberg stated unequivocally the case for Whig history of science, as follows: "I have come to think that whatever one thinks of whiggery in other sorts of history, it has a rightful place in the history of science." He continued, "It is clearly not possible to speak of right and wrong in the history of art or fashion, nor I think is it possible in the history of religion, and one can argue about whether it is possible in political history, but in scientific history we really can say who was right."[500]

Health Matters concurs with Weinberg's opinion regarding the history of science. This brief summary of the history of science and of medicine is integrated in this section of *Health Matters* into the totality of human history, one century a time, with that in mind. Science and medicine have progressed, sometimes slowly, sometimes erratically, and sometimes with great breakthroughs. There have been blind alleys in medicine, but medicine has usually moved forward. *Health Matters* does not offer an opinion as to whether human civilization has progressed, or not. It simply tries to tell the story of human history from the perspective of health, without implying that it is a triumph.

Leonardo da Vinci's career shows the two sides of historiography: Is Leonardo's life Whig history, or not? Leonardo's imaginative drawings of parachutes, gliders, and anatomy were beautiful. However, they were considered to have no importance in the history of science, because they led nowhere. The machines were never built, tested, and improved by others. And although his famous drawing of a man in a circle with outstretched arms and legs, was accurate, it also did not become a step forward in the depiction of anatomy. Leonardo is supposed not to have had any impact on Vesalius, whose anatomical textbook is regarded as the starting point for realism in anatomy. That is a Whiggish view of Leonardo's work in science and technology. However, from the point of view of history in general, Leonardo's drawings of machines and anatomy are just one part of his oeuvre. He can be appreciated for that. The question begs: why did he not pursue these interests? That would be what Butterfield would be interested in, and that is why he gave the derogatory name, "Whig history," to those who would fail to look for the problems that Leonardo may have contended with in his own lifetime.

The history of civilization, from the hunter-gathers to city dwellers, shows progression from the discovery of fire to the discovery of the neutrino. But civilization may have reached a tipping point. The steady increase in life span has begun to slow, and in some parts of the world, to show regression. One of the goals of health is a long life. A new pandemic arrived in 2019, and it has rapidly spread. The possibility of a long life has now ended for millions of people. The virus causing COVID-19 prospered from the world's large population and from its many connections. We expect more viruses such as this.

B. Telling the Story of History: Several Ways to Do It

Famous People

Should history be told as "The Great Men (and a few Great Women)"? I believe this is an important way, although not the only way, to tell the story of history. History can also be written as a narrative story, in which the events move along like a river, flowing to the sea. The popular series by Will and Ariel Durant in eleven volumes, *The Story of Civilization*, shows that this can be done. Nevertheless, individuals do make important changes in history, as I have shown above. Can anyone deny that these individuals are game-changers, and their roles in history should be studied: Homer, Hippocrates, Euclid, Aristotle, Alexander the Great, Buddha, Julius Caesar, Cleopatra, Jesus, Mohammed, Charlemagne, William the Conqueror, Genghis Khan, Tamerlane, Copernicus, Galileo, Christopher Columbus, Leonardo da Vinci, Shakespeare, William Harvey, Queen Elizabeth I, Martin Luther, Isaac Newton, René Descartes, Napoleon, Beethoven, William Penn, Benjamin Franklin, Louis Pasteur, Otto von Bismarck, Karl Marx, Abraham Lincoln, Washington Roebling, Theodore Roosevelt, Lenin, Stalin, Mussolini, Hitler, Churchill, Franklin Roosevelt, Marie Curie, Werner Heisenberg, and Albert Einstein. I mention Heisenberg and Einstein, not for their scientific contributions, but for introducing, respectively, the concepts of "uncertainty" and "relativity." These philosophical principles altered the ways of thinking in the 20th century from the absolute truths that were the beliefs, or which were sought, in previous centuries.[501]

To illustrate the importance of discovery of a new idea, even if the discoverer is anonymous, remember that in south Asia, wheels were fashioned, and were used for prayers and to lift water. But the wheel was never used as a means of transportation, as it was in western Asia and in the Mediterranean basin. Another example: elaborate mathematical systems were developed sequentially by the Sumerians, Egyptians, Greeks, and Romans, and were used in finance, philosophy, and architecture. It seems strange to us that these great mathematicians never saw the need for a zero, or for fractions, exponents, and negative numbers. Their concept of infinity was very different from ours. The idea that force, mass, acceleration, and velocity are related seems obvious to us. Every high school student now learns that "F=MA" (Force = Mass times Acceleration) for velocity, and "P=MV" (Force = Mass time Velocity) for momentum, although these formulas were unknown until they were described by Isaac Newton in 1686. To Newton that we also owe the description of calculus, with its infinitely beautiful mathematical curves. Einstein gave us the opportunity to ponder the relationship between energy, mass, and the speed of light. The counterintuitive formula "E=MC^2" (Energy = Mass times the square of C, the speed of light) is a clear example of the way science finds the "what" of things, but not the "why." Why should the speed of light have any relationship to energy and mass? Short answer: It is not the job of science to attempt to answer "Why." Another counterintuitive observation was the statement by Copernicus in 1453 that the earth was not the center of the universe. It looks like it is, but things aren't always as they seem to be.[502]

Perhaps someone else would have altered the way that history moved from one century to another. However, it would not be the same as it is now. Someone else could have been the Father of Medicine, but the collection of writings that are attributed to Hippocrates have had a beneficent influence on physicians for centuries. His attributed dictum, "first, do no harm," has been repeated as a word of caution in the lay world, too. Someone else from Europe would surely have sailed west to America, but the voyage of Columbus from Spain in 1492 was the first step in the development of the Spanish and Portuguese Empires in the New World. Four hundred years later, Theodore Roosevelt took the empire away from Spain. Someone else would have been the first human to set foot on the Moon, so although Neil Armstrong's place in history is unique, it was not crucial in the same way as that of Otto von Bismarck, who united most of the German-speaking countries of central Europe. The same might be said of Napoleon, who created an empire for France that was evanescent, but who left the Napoleonic code of laws that rival the other legal codes of the world.[503]

However, great artists are unique: Homer, Leonardo, Shakespeare, and Beethoven are examples to remind us of that. And the great novelists, such as Geoffrey Chaucer, Emile Zola, Charles Dickens, Mark Twain, Franz Kafka, Leo Tolstoy, and Ernest Hemingway, whose writings both shaped history and our understanding of it. The Industrial Revolution might have happened without Isaac Watts and Michael Faraday, but they played key roles in it, and the history of that period is best told by looking at their inventions. Architecture changed forever when Washington Roebling showed how it was possible to build under water, at great depths. Someone else would probably have done it, but the process started at that moment with the Brooklyn Bridge. We can imagine that others might have revolutionized communications throughout the world, but this subject cannot be taught or understood without mentioning the contributions of Samuel F. B. Morse, Alexander Graham Bell, Thomas Edison, and Guglielmo Marconi. The changes in longevity in the 20th century and longevity's impact on population growth in the 21st century cannot be understood without mentioning antibiotics and their discoverers: Gerhard Domagk's sulfa drugs and Alexander Fleming's penicillin. And also, Frederick Banting's insulin, which has enabled millions to live with diabetes. The possibility of non-violence as a possibility for human development owes much to Henry David Thoreau, who influenced both Mahatma Gandhi and Martin Luther King. The names are a matter of record for the inventors and industrialists who have polluted the world, using the work of ordinary people, but for this aspect of history the person who is best to remember is Rachel Carson and her book, *The Silent Spring*. This is "Whiggish history," but I would argue that it is the duty of a historian to report this "presentist" view of the effects of population increase and industrialization. It is also history told through "Great Men and a few Great Women."

Some of the most interesting contributions to history are by people whose names are unknown. Perhaps several collaborated on these things, but they probably did not develop without the input of specific talented thinkers. The architecture of the Mayan, Inca, and Aztec temples, and the perpetual calendar of the Mayans, which rival anything that was developed in Europe or Asia. We can also admire the water storage facilities of the Mayans and the irrigation ditches of the Inca Empire; and of the unique form of communication of the Incas and others in the Andes who used *quipu* (knots) in a coded language. The Incas also developed a fine understanding of astronomy and utilized this knowledge in their religious ceremonies. The leaders of these cultures are known through pictographs, but there is little that connects specific individuals with advancements in science and technology. We should not hesitate to use the word "advancements," although some critics might say it is a whiggish view.

There certainly are other ways to view history and to tell the story of history. The history of the sequence of events featuring "Great Men" looks very different from history as it is seen "from the bottom," who are the nameless and faceless underclass. Emile Zola's stories of French coal miners' families is a window into that side of history. Or historical events as they are seen by women. For instance, when woman is at home with her children, and a man goes off to war. Their perspectives are very different, although the basic event is the same for both. History that is a story of "Great Men" also differs dramatically from history seen from the perspective of children, even though all of us were children at one time.[504]

Making Choices

Is history about making choices? Is that the way history should be taught? A focus on "Choices" in teaching history should also include a discussion of the causes which led to the need to make a choice at that time, and of the consequences that followed the choice that was made. For example, the focus on "Choices," does not encourage discussion of the causes and consequences of the U.S. involvement in these two wars: The war with Mexico in 1846 and the entry of America in World War I in 1917. The initial conflict between the United States and Mexico is oversimplified by recalling the bravery of the Texans at the Alamo. The Mexican War that followed is remembered now for the words, "From the "Halls of Montezuma," in the Marine Corps Hymn. The miseries on both sides of the war have largely been forgotten in the United States. The cause of the war is now believed to have been President Polk's goal to increase the territory available for slavery, and its success became one of the causes of the Civil War. In the case of World War I, the historical record also shows more complexity in the cause of American entry in the war, and of its consequences. An intense spirit of patriotism immediately followed the declaration of war, and the triumphal end of the "war to end all wars" led to Wilson's receiving the Nobel Peace Prize. We now know, however, that President Wilson had long been preparing to enter the war in Europe. Wilson had been elected having promised to keep America out of the war, so when he made the decision to enter the war on the side of the Allies, he knew that he would have to proceed carefully. There were many Americans who were isolationists or pacifists, and also many of German and Irish descent who did not want America to enter the war on the side of Britain.[505]

On the other hand, although many of the important decisions in history are made by small groups of leaders, it is clear that people do make choices, as individuals. Furthermore, most of the people of the world attempt to have as much agency as possible in their own lives, and in the lives of their families. The agency to make decisions also extends to their social groups in ever-widening circles. These decisions involve choices regarding the basic needs, urges, and exceptions that were discussed in Part One of this essay. There is nevertheless a wide spectrum in the ability of individuals to make choices. Agency to make choices is severely restricted in the case of prisoners and very young children. Throughout most of the world, men have more power than women to make choices. The ability to choose is also limited by other conditions, such as geography, financial status, race, education, and health.[506]

A typical example in the life of one hypothetical person will show what is meant by the agency to make decisions. What choices are available? Most of the readers of this essay are likely to be college graduates who understand English. The example is one day that is typical for such a person to face on a daily basis. Most of the actions of this person will be based on habit. This day starts with sleep, something that everyone needs. Hopefully, it will be in a safe, quiet place, to dream, to refresh, and then to awaken spontaneously. Some have more success with this than others. Perhaps a small nightcap of whisky or wine, or a non-prescription sleeping pill. After awakening, habit takes command for the usual routine events, such as toilet, dressing, food, drink, and planning the day's activities. At mid-day, habit often dictates a break, and after several more hours, habit again tells how the day will end. The daily routine may be interrupted by family responsibilities or gifts of time and energy to others – sometimes offered by good will, or under orders, by direct command. Health issues may interrupt the habitual routine. The day may be going well, and then, suddenly: a migraine headache, a broken tooth, chest pain from angina pectoris or a heart attack, or sudden weakness in one arm from a stroke. The vagaries of nature may play a large role in the lives of some people, especially those who work outside. Catastrophic events may necessitate changes: for instance, an accident, a sudden storm, or declaration of an emergency. The individual is likely to be part of a social or religious group, or a member of a workforce. Depending on the position in the group, the individual may be given responsibility to make decisions for the organization. The choices are weighed; sometimes the decision may be made by one person, while in other instances, others may be involved. History is based on the accumulation of daily events such as these, with endless variations, in the lives of billions of humans.[507]

An Argument

What is "history"? The term, "history," has been redefined in the past half-century. To recapitulate, the term "pre-historic" used to mean something without a written record, or which had not been translated. It was a pejorative expression that is now rarely used. "History" is now considered by many to be all that has ever happened; a chronology, as it were, of all of the events since time began. And "History" is also the story of what has happened. It is a narrative story that tells of these events; it is thus both a selection and an interpretation of the events, not a simple chronology. Another way in which human history has been redefined is that it is now said to be based on choice. The singular "great man" approach has been replaced by "choices" made by anonymous groups of people. However, individuals do play a seminal role in history, and history, when it is written, should mention these individuals. That is to say, history is not simply a series of choices made by groups of people; individuals are important, too. There is no need to be embarrassed by mentioning their names, their actions, and the time and place in which they took place. Whether it is in the creation of new ideas, the discovery of new lands, or winning or losing battles and wars, individuals have played a crucial role in history. Seen through the lens of the present period, many of the people (mostly men) of the past have done things that are now considered to be inappropriate, or terrible. Nevertheless, the argument becomes more focused, and more interesting, as we study the ways that health and illness, and the search for health, have played such an important role in human history.

Is history about "what happened in the past," as is taught in many secondary schools and colleges, or is history about an argument? This question was posed in the Introduction to *Health Matters*. Several years ago, a seminar was given by Robert Darnton, Professor of History at Princeton University, who had been President of the American Historical Association. In the discussion period that followed his lecture, he was asked, "What is history?" Professor Darnton immediately replied, "History is informed argument." This essay makes the argument which states, perhaps provocatively, that health matters. Does the reader believe that this argument is informed, and has it succeeded?[508]

C. A Driver of History?

In his book, *The Influence of Sea Power on History*, Alfred Thayer Mahan proposed that the quest for sea power was the driver of history. Edward Gibbon proposed a similar argument in *The Decline and Fall of the Roman Empire*. Gibbon proposed that it was due to the unrestrained excesses of the Roman Catholic Church. *Health Matters* suggests that if there is a driver of human history, that it would be the search for health: it is that health matters.[509]

D. On the Subject of Intellectual History

Health Matters proposes that the search for health has been the driving force in human history. This search has resulted in the development of science, technology, medicine, politics, and religion. And thus, of the development of urban life and all that goes with it, including specialization in the work force, a middle class of urban workers, and of the acquisition of capital. It is not as easy, however, to fit the development (or evolution) of intellectual history and the arts into this new paradigm of human history. Nevertheless, intellectual history can be incorporated into the new paradigm. For example, David Brion Davis wrote, "I have long believed that what most distinguishes us from all other animals is our ability to transcend an illusory sense of now, of an eternal present, and to strive for an understanding of the forces and events that made us what we are." Davis' belief is consistent with my argument, which is that humans understand that life is more than "now" and we must prepare for the "forces and events" that not only "made us what we are," but which still lie ahead.[510]

Archaeology and anthropology have shown that art and music were present before humans began to evolve from hunter-gatherers to become fisherman, farmers, and city dwellers. The genes for artistic expression including drawing and musical instruments must have been present, and favored in selection, for thousands of years – and perhaps even in other species of hominids. The development of a written alphabet occurred independently in several parts of the world, so intellectual history developed at an early time, too. Philosophy and story-telling and writing could have begun with religious beliefs, which can be traced to human's search for health. The humans who were born with the genes for intellectual and artistic skills would have been favored, and propagated successfully, within families, and then in tribes, in clans, and in early settlements.

Chapter 13

Recent History

The Last 120 Years

Should the last 120 years, from 1900 to 2020, be thought of as the Age of Modern Warfare? If instead of the appearance of triumph, as in the Atomic Age or the Space Age, we might look at the history of this period with a cool eye as the Age of Modern Warfare. Or is there another name for the present Age? If so, what should it be called? We remember the Renaissance and the Reformation, the Age of Exploration, the Enlightenment, the Napoleonic Period, and the Victorian Age. In the past 120 years, we have seen two great conflicts which were caused by apparently unresolvable differences. The first was the 31-year period of World Wars from August 1914 until September 1945, with a hiatus from 1918-1939. The World Wars were caused in part by nationalism, to pride in country of origin. It was warfare in the western word, which involved the dominant Christian countries. It included Japan, which was allied with one block of European countries. But it was not a religious war. The second great conflict was a resurgence of the ancient war between Islam in Asia and the Christian countries of European origin. Ominous warnings occurred over a period of years, but this conflict broke into the open with the attacks on the United States in 2001. Two important dates in this Age of Modern Warfare are November 11, 1918 and September 11, 2001. The first date was when an Armistice was signed to end the fighting in World War I. The Armistice of 1918 was followed by the Treaty of Versailles, which imposed the harsh conditions that led to the rise of Adolph Hitler and resumption of war. The second date is remembered as "9/11." On that day, Islamic terrorists, organized by al-Qaeda (Arabic for "the base"), hijacked four commercial airliners and deliberately crashed three of them into buildings when the planes were filled with fuel. The intent was to cause massive numbers of deaths. Two of the planes were crashed into the Twin Towers in New York City, and one was crashed into the Pentagon. Passengers on the fourth plane fought back and forced it to crash into a field in Pennsylvania. Nearly 3,000 people lost their lives on 9/11, and the consequences – with toxins and dust released from the buildings – led to many more deaths over the following years.

    The action by al-Qaeda was a dramatic escalation that followed many years of bombings, shootings, and hijackings by Islamic terrorists. War immediately broke out between the nations of America and Europe on one side, and on the other side, a group of Islamic organizations which operate internationally, without claiming a nation of origin. The most prominent name in this 120-year period of intermittent international warfare is that of Adolph Hitler. In the years to come, this period may be regarded as the Second War of Islam against Christianity. But for now, it could also be considered as the Age of Hitler. His legacy persists in the anti-immigration movements in Europe in the 21st century, and in the nativist "America First" movement that originated with Charles Lindbergh before World War II. That movement receded from view after the war. Americans appeared to accept the role of their country as the leader of the United Nations. Elements of the public simply maintained a quiet watch until they found another isolationist leader. The words "America First" were used again successfully in 2016 by the nationalist MAGA (Make America Great Again) movement of Donald J. Trump. However, it seems doubtful that the present period will be remembered as either the Age of Hitler, or as the Age of Modern Warfare.[511]

    Another way to regard the 20th century is to think of it as the American Age or the American Century, from 1898 to 2001. We can say that the American Age began with the Spanish surrender of its Empire to the U.S. in 1898. The end of the American Age is not yet known, but United States may have reached the zenith, the high point, of its existence in the period between 1898 and 2001. The post-Civil

War "Gilded Age," which some say ended with World War I, was followed by the Roaring Twenties, the Great Depression, and then World War II, and the Cold War. After the Soviet Union began to collapse in 1989 and was dissolved in 1991, America was without doubt the most powerful nation in the world. And it was also arguably the world's most admired country. In 2020, America may still be the most admired (or at least the first choice of immigrants), but for many, it is also the most feared. Its light has dimmed. After nineteen years of an unending and unwinnable war in Afghanistan and Iraq, and with battlegrounds elsewhere in Asia and Africa, America has withdrawn from its leadership role in the world. America is not the healthiest country in the world, although it spends the most, per capita, of any country. It is the most inefficient country in respect to health matters. The American Age may be coming to an end.[512]

The idea that America was a "shining city on the hill" evolved into a belief in American exceptionalism. The expression of "Manifest Destiny" enabled Americans to believe that they had created an example of beneficence that spread around the world. It was rarely said that this version of the American Dream was based on white supremacy, and that it was dominated by Christians – originally only Protestants, but gradually also including Catholics. People of color were marginalized, though they played an important role in the labor force. Blacks continued to have problems with racism, which existed to a greater extent than most white people were willing to admit. Asians were slowly and incompletely accepted into American society. The belief in a goodhearted America was supported by U.S. sponsorship of the United Nations and its agencies, the U.S. Agency for International Development (USAID), the help provided to friendly governments by U.S. military personnel, and American charitable organizations. The role of secret intelligence and of individuals working in deep cover for such organizations as the CIA, NSA, and DIA, was sometimes mentioned, but it was rarely discussed. Some regarded this world-wide spread of influence as an American empire, in fact if not in name, with a person called President at its head, instead of using the title of Emperor. The previous behavior of Presidents of the United States has been revealed since 2016 to have been the result of self-restraint. It now appears that there are very few limits that exist on Presidential power in America.[513]

It seems that we are on a Malthusian search for the end of our species. We are *Homo sapiens,* subspecies *sapiens*. But our subspecies could instead be called *imperfecta.* Our warring is continuous, the population of the world continues to increase, and pestilence has become repetitive and unending. We continue to degrade the earth's natural environment to produce more food, as it is needed for world's growing population. Malthus predicted that war, or pestilence, or starvation would limit an increase in population. If we succeed in making peace, and if we control pestilence, starvation will nevertheless occur because the food supply cannot be limitless; the earth cannot produce an infinite amount of food. As Malthus predicted, all of these functions are in play: war, disease, and food supply; and population growth will be limited by death.

As an aside, but not connected with the Malthusian proposition, it should be added that humans also degrade our environment through careless actions and inactions, such as dumping of plastics in the ocean, toxic chemicals on land, and radioactive wastes that contaminate the earth and the oceans; and we also speed the increase in environmental degradation by global warming. The normal geological cycle of the Pleistocene age is now being accelerated with the "greenhouse effect" of gases such as carbon dioxide and methane. Unless we control these foolish actions, it will not be enough simply to balance the Malthusian prediction. *Homo sapiens imperfecta* will still be doomed.[514]

Humans should be able to control conflict with each other. "First, do not harm," is the maxim of a physician. The same phrase is often referred to in the context of international relations. It could be regarded as the goal of the United Nations and of its agencies, such as the World Bank, the World Court, and the World Health Organization. Cooperation, mutual defense, and peaceful solutions to international problems, rather than offense, is the objective of many multi-lateral organizations. These include the North Atlantic Treaty Organization (NATO), the South-East Asia Treaty Organization (SEATO), Organization of American States (OAS), the African Union, the European Union (EU), the Conference on Security and Cooperation in Europe (CSCE), and the British Commonwealth of Nations. Hopefully, this is also true of the states of the former Soviet Union (USSR), most of which became members of the

Commonwealth of Independent States in 1991 with Russia as its leader. The CIS now includes nine member states and one associate state.

Humans need to discover the correct demographic balance for the population of the world, and some way to achieve it. This is a complex issue, but it must be solved. An increasingly aged population needs a younger working population to support it. And at the same time, children must be born and raised in precisely the same numbers that are needed each year to enter the work force. They must then work long enough both to support those who are children and also those who are aged or disabled. Even if the numbers are calculated that are necessary, there are at least two problems to achieve the goal of a stable population. One problem is that the goal must be achieved within the populations which exist, and which are wildly disparate; the population is very old in Japan, and it is very young in Africa. The other is the difficulty in gaining acceptance of population control. It is resisted by many religious organizations, such as officials of the Roman Catholic Church, Hasidic Jews, many Muslims, and others, including some academicians, and the poor and uneducated, who depend on children in their own families for work. Zero Population Growth (ZPG) was a slogan that never caught the imagination of enough prominent leaders or of the public to be taken seriously, and it appears now to be dead. Demography – the size and age of the population – is a key aspect of health, yet it is difficult to make it interesting enough to matter.[515]

We also may be able to exert better control over infectious disease, but that is going to be difficult. Parasitism is a fact of life. All living things are dependent on others. We are teeming with bacteria, most of them harmless, some are useful, and others are dangerous, just waiting for a chance to advance. We harbor diphtheria and staphylococcus in our noses, our mouths are full of spirochetes, and our intestines are filled with E. coli. All are quiet, unless they find a break in the surface and become invasive. It is unlikely that we will ever achieve total freedom from endemic and pandemic diseases. The diminished natural environment, which is the result of population increase and the need for more farmland, causes humans and wild animals to live near each other. This is thought to be the likely cause of the transmission of SARS-CoV-2 from animals to humans in Wuhan, Hubei Province, on the Yangtze River in China, in December 2019. The likely mode of transmission appears to have been from bats via an intermediate host, perhaps a small mammal known as pangolian, which is eaten as a delicacy – an exotic food – in China. An alternate possibility is that humans decided, foolishly, to buy bats in a "wet market" for food, as they have been doing for many centuries. Or that the virus may have escaped from a research laboratory in Wuhan where it was being studied. Bats are eaten in many countries in Asia. The other problem is the facilitation of the spread of each new infectious disease by international travel. The methods of travel have increased greatly, with large airplanes and enormous tourist ships, and thousands of shipping containers on freighters, traveling throughout the world.

Furthermore, the mosquito is likely always to be with us as a carrier of deadly parasitic diseases. In past centuries, various methods were used to prevent disease and treat infections. Early in the 20th century, scientists synthesized chemicals such as Salvarsan and sulfadiazine that were successful in the treatment of some infectious diseases. These successes were followed with the discovery of antibiotics, starting with penicillin. And many more antibiotics, one after another: the tetracyclines, streptomycin, nitrofurantoin, ciprofloxacin, azithromycin, chloramphenicol, and other second and third generation derivatives of penicillin. Germs have developed resistance to almost all antibiotics that have been developed. War between the pharmaceutical industry and microbes seems likely to continue indefinitely. Unless microbes win this war. Health matters in the crucial war with microbes.

The goal of health should be a long and comfortable life, and to be as useful as possible, with changes required for age, for as long as possible. This goal is achieved for some people, but probably only for a minority. For some, it is instead an issue of finding a balance between achieving a reasonable quality of life versus a desire to have life come to an end. And for others, dementia, early onset Alzheimer's, and other debilitating neuro-muscular diseases make it necessary for others to make decisions as surrogates for the slowly dying patient. These are not easy decisions. Some choose assisted suicide, and in some cases, patients are probably hastened along toward the end without knowing that someone else has decided to do it. Little is known about these instances, because they would be illegal. Nevertheless, in any event, we know that health matters.

Chapter 14

Summary and Conclusion

Final Thoughts

Humans don't always do what is best for their own health and the health of others. But even when humans reject the search for health, it has usually been a conscious decision. Humans are instinctively aware of pain and they recoil from danger, but as sentient beings they can foresee that harm or death may result from choices they make. Adult humans usually anticipate the need for food, water, clothing, and a safe shelter. These are the basic requirements for daily health and well-being. They also look ahead to the next day, and week, and season, and year – planning and building, keeping the future in mind. The thoughts of individuals become the norm for society as well. Our species became organized to ensure that families and clans, and then unrelated persons, gather together to produce safe and long-lasting lives for all. It is remarkable to see the sacrifices that some individuals make on behalf of good for the rest.

Many scholars have previously described the evolution of the healing arts from their earliest beginnings in so-called primitive societies. Frazer, in *The Golden Bough*, described the human concern for both spiritual health and physical health. The term "witch doctor" is often used pejoratively, although Fraser didn't look at it that way. A person with these skills would utilize them in the same way a generalist physician would do today. Or of a family doctor in a small town in a remote area, combining the skills of a psychiatrist, internist, and surgeon. It's a long stretch from this ancient history to the present time. The branches of history that are involved in this are the history of technology, and the history of the city. Anthropology, archaeology, the history of agriculture and architecture are involved, too, and also political and economic history. The development of civilization is now understood to have passed through stages from the hunter-gatherer of the distant past to the city dweller of today. Cities became sites of specialized workers; they were hubs of transportation, and they were walled for safety. Stones and wood for tools were replaced when metals were discovered: copper for bronze, and then iron. Plants were found from which textiles could be made, and cloth replaced animal skins for clothing. The marketplace arose in the cities in which products were exchanged for profit. A stationary population could accumulate foods for future use, and items could be held for personal enjoyment or a hedge against catastrophes. These developments were intended to produce safe, healthy, and happy humans.

How does modern medicine fit into this history of human beings? The answer is that all important events in human history can be directly or indirectly attributed to the loss of health, or concerns about health. This has usually been by illness or injury, or other processes that led to death, disability, or health concerns; and sometimes beliefs about health that profoundly affected polity in other ways. This notion is somewhat analogous to Alfred Thayer Mahan's *The Influence of Sea Power upon History.*" Mahan would say that choices are made by nations on basis of knowledge of the importance of sea power. I would say instead that they are made on the basis of health, illness, and the search for health. Other historians have glimpsed a portion of my argument, but I think that none has ever previously seen the full picture of it. When Kuhn proposed his concept of "paradigms" in *The Structure of Scientific Revolutions*, he didn't include any examples from the history of biology and medicine. A few historians have recognized that infectious diseases have been the underlying cause of many historical events. For example: William McNeill's *Plagues and Peoples* and Alfred Crosby's *Columbian Exchange*. Other scholars and science writers have also written about the impact of infectious disease on history; see Hans Zinsser's *Rats, Lice, and History* and Jared Diamond's *Guns, Germs, and Steel*. Roy Porter showed that our search for health begins with our beliefs about health. This is, in the end, a question that each group of people answers in its own way. Lynn Payer demonstrated this in her book, *Medicine and Culture*. However, it is difficult to engage the interest of most historians in this discussion, and also many others who are well-educated, but who don't have a mind for science. This problem is what C. P. Snow called *The Two Cultures.*

Battles and wars are ultimately won by the superior force, a fleet or an army that has, or is expected, to prevail by capturing or killing the opposition. It's brutal, but that's history. Infectious disease and warfare have affected historical events, but so, too, have other diseases and types of illness. Many events in history have turned on the fortuitous avoidance of death and illness. For example, Alexander III "The Great" dodged death on many occasions as he expanded the Alexandrian Empire throughout Asia. His sudden illness and death in Babylon put an end to that. There are other examples of dodging death, if only temporarily, and death deferred, with history thereby altered. Can anyone doubt that the course of American history would have been very different had Franklin Roosevelt died in his third term, when he would have been succeeded by Henry Wallace, instead of dying two months into his fourth term, when he was succeeded by Harry Truman.

Many diseases have profoundly affected history: starvation, thirst, vitamin deficiency and inherited diseases. To this list, others can be added, such as Mediterranean anemia and sickle cell anemia, which sapped the strength of many Africans and those who lived in the Mediterranean basin; and the growing population of diabetics, which produces a social, economic, and ultimately a moral dilemma. History has also been changed by accidents of nature, or by the unintended consequences of human actions. Volcanic eruptions, tsunamis, typhoons, blizzards, tornadoes, and 'little ice ages' have profoundly affected human history. However, it is not the geological or climatic event itself that changes human history, it is what each event does to humans, and how they respond to it accordance with their health beliefs. In early days, a catastrophic natural event was looked at as something that was as inevitable as it was unpredictable, and it was best to look at it as the will of the gods. In that way, the catastrophe was incorporated into the health belief system, and re-enforced the system.

Not everyone seems to want good health or a risk-free life. From the earliest days, before there was a written record, people have been willing to inflict pain on others and also on themselves, and even death, because they believed that this was the right thing to do. We see it in the pre-Columbian Meso American's carved stones, which show sacrifices they performed, some by drowning, and some by mutilation. It is believed that many of those who were sacrificed knew and accepted what was in store for them. We also read of it in the legend of the death of Jesus, which has been considered remarkable but believable by many millions of his followers. That he would willingly accept this death is considered a cause for piety, not for disbelief. More recently, in World War II, "Banzai" suicide charges were made by Japanese troops and suicidal missions were carried out for the Emperor-God by kamikaze pilots. Their courage was matched by the U.S. Marines who waded ashore at Iwo Jima, not expecting to survive. The motive was different in all of these examples, but the result was the same; they were giving up health, happiness, and well-being for what they considered to be a greater cause.

This issue continues to permeate our lives and our thoughts, without our recognizing it for the historic force it has been. The most difficult domestic issue in the past century has been societal welfare. It is clearly based on what we believe should be the goal for the health of society as a whole. It is a major element in the economy, and in politics. The first major step in the U.S. government's solution for social health was social security, which was enacted as part of the plan to end the Great Depression, during the administration of Franklin D. Roosevelt. The next big step in social health planning was Medicare, enacted during the Lyndon Johnson administration. The next stage was the development of a "health care industry," as Paul Starr has described it in *The Social Transformation of American Medicine*. We are now struggling with this issue again in the Affordable Care Act. This is the most contentious and expensive issue that America now faces in its domestic policy debate.

We are in the midst of a world-wide pandemic, known as COVID-19, caused by a novel coronavirus. We see once again that history is changed by illness and by the responses that are made to the potential of illness and death that are faced by humans everywhere in the world. *Health Matters.*[516]

Acknowledgements

I am indebted to many people for inspiring me to become a physician and a historian. My parents, Essie Mae and Gerald Hill, taught me about my duty in life: to be thoughtful and kind. My mother taught me to read, and my father taught me always to be honest. Mother had been a geologist, and she taught me about geology, which was then called "pre-historic time." Father had been a journalist, and he taught me that every story needs to answer six questions: who, how, what, why, when, where; and as a banker, he added a seventh question: how much. Thirty boys and girls were first cousins in my generation. And many more who were my great-aunts and great-uncles. By studying our family's genealogy, I began to understand that history is based on people and geography.

Miss Betty L. Ralston, Cornell College '45, inspired me. When she was a college senior, she taught American History to my eighth-grade class in Mount Vernon, Iowa, in 1944-45. As a sophomore at Yale, I took my first college course in history. It was Classical Civilization, taught by Mr. Robert Woolsey, who had just received his Ph.D. at Yale. As a junior, I chanced to take a seminar course on Human Populations, which introduced me to the apocalyptic prediction of Thomas Malthus: it was that the growth of population would be limited by starvation, warfare, and/or pestilence. In my senior year, I took Professor Frederick Kilgour's class in the History of Science. I was assigned to write a term paper on the history of cancer research in the mid-19th century. Research for that paper took me to the library at the Yale School of Medicine, where I read some of the books that had been donated to Yale by Dr. Harvey Cushing. I decided to follow Harvey Cushing's footsteps from Yale to the Harvard Medical School. The Harvard Medical School had many faculty members who were interested in the history of medicine. I am especially grateful to Dr. George Ericson, bibliophile and Professor of Anatomy; Dr. Daniel Funkenstein, Professor of Psychiatry, who gave me his neurosurgical instruments; Dr. William B. Castle, Professor of Medicine, who inspired me; Dr. Otto Krayer, Professor of Pharmacology, who interviewed me (partly in German) as a candidate for admission; and Dr. Edward D. Churchill, Professor of Surgery, who complimented me for research on Claude Bernard. I am grateful to Henry R. Viets, M.D., Head of the Boston Science Library, who discussed my paper for the Boylston Medical Society on "Cancer Research in the mid-19th Century"; and to Ralph T. Esterquest, Head of Harvard Medical School's Countway Library, for many kindnesses. My research on the history of cancer research continued under the guidance of Dr. Robert E. Gross, Ladd Professor of Pediatric Surgery.

In 1996, I retired from surgery and began graduate education in history. My application to study for a master's degree included my proposal that human history was based on the search for health. The application was accepted by Jan Ellen Lewis, Ph.D., who was Chairman of the Department of History at Rutgers-Newark. She called me to say that my proposal was interesting, and that she hoped I would pursue it. Dr. Lewis encouraged me to continue to explore it as a "think piece." Others encouraged me to continue to work on this subject, including Dr. Christopher Sellers and Dr. Clement Alexander Price at Rutgers-Newark; Dr. Richard Sher of the New Jersey Institute of Technology, and Dr. Perry Leavell and Dr. Donald Kent at Drew University. I thank the Medical History Society of New Jersey, especially Bob Vietrogoski, Ph.D., Sandra Moss, M.D., M.A., Vincent Cirillo, Ph.D., and Alan Lippman, M.D.

Thanks, too to the reviewers of early drafts of this work and commented on it, especially Captain Peter Pennington, RN. I am grateful to Leslie Wolfinger and Debbie Riley at Heritage Books. The final decision about what to include and how to phrase it is nevertheless my own, and no fault of theirs.

Appendix A

Death

Death from the Perspective of Science

It is worth pondering about the subject of Death, because throughout the centuries that humans have lived on earth, the definition and meaning of Death has changed. *Britannica* says it well:

Death is "the total cessation of life processes that eventually occurs in all living organisms. The state of <u>human</u> death has always been obscured by mystery and superstition, and its precise definition remains controversial, differing according to culture and legal systems."

I will mention but a few of the issues about death that involve science, including biology, medicine, and sociology. Biology is, paradoxically, the "science of life." The primary purpose of medicine is to prolong life, and thus to defeat death, at least for a time. Sociology is the study of groups of humans, and thus to count the living and to subtract the dead. This study includes the percentage of deaths in specific periods (say, annually) and enumeration of deaths from various causes.

We can look at death in humans from the perspective of a cell, an organ, a body, and a population. The simple definition is that for a cell, life depends on the presence of metabolism, and death occurs when metabolism is not present. However, if a cell is properly prepared, it may be frozen or dried, and restored to metabolic activity when thawed or hydrated. The same is true with an organ, such as a heart or kidney, which is being transported from a recently deceased person to a recipient in another city. The organ will be preserved by cooling, and it will not be functional; but it will become functional when it is rewarmed. And this is also true for a person who is deeply hypothermic. Recovered from an under the ice of an avalanche or from an accident on thin ice of a lake, the victim may have no signs of life – not breathing, and no heartbeat. But the rule to remember is that "no one should be declared dead until they are warm and dead." Rewarming restores the heartbeat in many cases, and breathing resumes.

The statistics of deaths of human populations show variations that change with geography and time. The World Health Organization (WHO) keeps a record which shows the principal causes of deaths annually in each of the member countries of the United Nations. The range is great, with some diseases seen as major causes of deaths in developed countries, and a vastly different group of diseases in developing countries. The "natural" causes of death in the United States, for instance, includes diseases of the heart and blood vessels, cancer, pulmonary disease, and diabetes. Accidents (falls and automobile accidents) and gunshots (intentional and unintentional) also appear as causes of death in the U.S. Until the present pandemic began in 2020, infectious disease has not been a prominent cause of death for many years in the U.S. In contrast, countries at the low end of the Gross National Product (GNP) per capita, the prominent causes of death include nutritional deficiency and infectious disease.

Death in Literature and the Arts

Literature: Death is the subject in many forms of literature. One of the earliest works of fiction is *The Satyricon of Petronius the Arbiter*, which follows the vagabond life of several young men in the reign of Nero. There is always a foreboding of death in their careless antics ("That you may'st know that Death is on his way"). In both slang and bawdy literature, "die" is a synonym for orgasm, as in *la mort doucé* (sweet death) or *la petite mort*.[517]

Charles Dickens wrote about death in novels such as *Bleak House* and *A Tale of Two Cities* ("It was the best of times, it was the worst of times") during the French Revolution. Edgar Allen Poe told many macabre short stories about death, including *The Pit and the Pendulum*, *The Masque of the Red Death*, *The Premature Burial*, and *The Murders in the Rue Morgue*. Death is in the background in many other novels, such as Thomas Mann, *Death in Venice* (1912) and *The Magic Mountain* (1924); and Harper Lee, *To Kill a Mockingbird* (1960). And in fictionalized history: Henry Wadsworth Longfellow, *Evangeline* (1847), which ends dramatically with the yellow fever epidemic in Philadelphia in 1793. Sinclair Lewis wrote *Arrowsmith* (1925) about the search for a bacteriophage which will prevent death from bubonic plague. Albert Camus, *The Plague* (1947), is set in the 1940s in Oran, Algeria, in which "plague" is a metaphor. Camus accurately describes bubonic plague, but the novel conflates an epidemic of cholera in Oran, Algeria, in 1849, in which a large portion of the population died, and bubonic plague in 1944, in which only 95 cases were recorded. Novels about death in World War II include the horrors of being a soldier in Norman Mailer, *The Naked and the Dead*, and Kurt Vonnegut, who wrote about deaths in the firebombing in Dresden in *Slaughterhouse Five*.[518]

History: True stories about death were composed in the form of gripping narratives by Truman Capote, *In Cold Blood*, whose initial research was done in company with Harper Lee, author of *To Kill a Mockingbird*; and by Vincent Bugliosi, in *Helter Skelter*, writing about the gruesome murders that were orchestrated by Charles Manson in Los Angeles. Death is described in historical periods, such as the Civil War, by Drew Faust, *This Republic of Suffering* (2009); and in specific locations, by Jessica Mitford, *The American Way of Death*. Berton Rouché wrote many true stories about deadly illnesses for the *New Yorker* magazine. Some were republished in his books, *The Incurable Wound* (rabies) and *Eleven Blue Men* (accidentally poisoned from sodium nitrite).[519]

The true story of the Trojan War and the travails of the survivors will never be known, but Homer's *Iliad* and *Odyssey*, and Virgil's *Aeneid* have survived as both literature and imagined history. These books tell of the epic battle to the death between Achilles and Hector, and of the desecration of Hector's body; of the savage destruction of Troy and most of its people by the Greeks; and of the aftermath of the War, with revenge killings by Ulysses and other returning soldiers, and of disgusting torture by imaginary fiends. The Trojan War began with lust, and it ended with death, in Greece, Asia Minor, Carthage, and Italy. The most notable year in British history was in 1066, when England had four kings. The Stamford River ran "red with blood," Harold died at Hastings, and William the Conqueror marched to London. Millions of deaths accompanied the march across Asia to the Adriatic Sea from Mongolia by Genghis Khan (1162-1227), and by the Uzbeks: Tamerlane (1336-1405), who emulated the great Khan and conquered most of Asia; and Babur (1483-1530), the great Khan's descendant who founded the Mughal dynasty in India. The march of Napoleon's army from Poland to Moscow which began in June 1812 and its retreat during the bitterly cold winter of 1813 is one of the most inglorious failures of any army in any war. More than 412,000 soldiers died. The army began with 422,000 soldiers, and only 10,000 returned. The deaths were largely due to non-battle losses, from starvation, scurvy, pneumonia, hypothermia, drowning, and the usual infectious diseases that accompany an army such as typhus and dysentery. In the twentieth century, William Shirer bookends the deaths caused by the Nazis, beginning with *Berlin Diary* before World War II and ending with *Fall of the Third Reich*. One of the most amazing stories of death is that of the family of the Romanovs by the Soviets, and the recovery and identification of their bodies many years later.[520]

Biography and Diary: Hannah Arendt, *Eichmann in Jerusalem: A Report on the Banality of Evil*; this biography was a window through which millions of deaths in the Holocaust could be viewed. Probably the most famous diary about death is *The Diary of Anne Frank*. The reader knows that the diary ends before Anne died in a concentration camp.[521]

Obituaries: Publication of death notices, paid for by relatives of the deceased, are typically part of the services offered in the United States by a funeral director. The death notices, accompanied by a photograph and often a symbol, such as a Star of David or the emblem of a branch of military service, appear in local newspapers and on the website of the funeral home. If the deceased had been prominent in local affairs or was of interest to history, the newspaper may publish its own summary, known as an obituary. Large daily newspapers maintain a file of draft obituaries that is updated daily, placing clippings or notes into files of people who are expected to be subjects of obituaries. Everyone dies, and the "morgue" (the morbid name for the newspaper's library) then produces the last few sentences, including the date and cause of death, and who reported it. The credibility of the report, and of the reporter, is important, because the paper does not want to publish a false report of death. The most famous instance of an incorrect report was that of Mark Twain, who commented with characteristic wit, "The report of my death was an exaggeration." The praise showered upon people in the death notices is unfortunately unknown to them in their lifetime, unless it is prepared in advance by the author. Many of the on-line searches for the term "false death" now relate to counter-claims of deaths reported from COVID-19.[522]

Histories of Medicine that focus on the cause and prevention of death include Paul de Kruif, *Microbe Hunters* (1926), discussing infectious diseases; and Siddhartha Mukherjee, *The Emperor of All Maladies: A Biography of Cancer* (2010). Six notable books about deaths from infectious diseases in human history use language that is accessible to the educated layperson: *Rats, Lice, and History* (1935), by Hans Zinsser, a scientist; a science writer, Geddes Smith, *Plague on Us*; the historians, Alfred Crosby, *The Columbian Exchange* (1973) and William McNeill, *Plagues and Peoples* (1976); Jared Diamond, who is both a scientist and historian, in *Guns, Germs and Steel* (2003); and Frank Snowden, a retired professor of history and the history of medicine, in *Epidemics and Society* (2019). Many other books tell of the deaths in individual epidemics, but these six books are remarkable insofar as they reveal the enormous scope of deaths from infectious disease in history.[523]

Poetry: Walt Whitman composed *Oh Captain, My Captain*, about the death of Abraham Lincoln, *Leaves of Grass*, and other memorable poems about death. Robert Frost, in *Stopping by Woods on a Snowy Evening*, wrote "I have promises to keep, and miles to go before I sleep," with sleep as a metaphor for death. Henry Wadsworth Longfellow reflected on death in *A Psalm of Life* (1838), saying "departing, leave behind us, footprints on the sands of time." T. S. Eliot thought pessimistically about death in *The Hollow Men*, saying that "[T]he world ends. Not with a bang, but with a whimper."[524]

Many poems about death were written during World War I: Robert Graves, "The Soldier"; John McRae, "In Flanders Fields"; Wilfred Owen, "Anthem for Doomed Youth"; Alan Seeger, "I have a Rendezvous with Death"; and Siegfried Sassoon, "The Kiss." The stalemate of trench warfare of the Great War provided time for contemplation in the midst of danger. When fighting resumed, the war was called World War II. It was a war of action. Soldiers and sailors usually were either in active combat, or far removed from it. As a result of these changing conditions, World War II produced little poetry. Also, in contrast to the sad poetry of World War I, the music and songs that were produced during World War II were mostly upbeat and looked forward to victory, no matter at what price.[525]

Theatre: Arthur Miller's play, *The Crucible* is a story of illicit love, with the hangings in Salem in 1692 in the grim background; and there can be no doubt that death will happen in another memorable play by Miller: *Death of a Salesman*. R. C. Sherriff, *Journey's End* (1929), is a haunting story of trench warfare in World War I in which men exit, one at a time, to die.[526]

Of Shakespeare's tragedies, *Hamlet* is the most memorable, as the Prince in his famous soliloquy, ponders, "…to die, to sleep." Shakespeare's *Macbeth* is the story of murder engineered by a scheming wife (although the true story was fictionalized by the Bard). His other tragedies revolve around deaths: *Romeo and Juliet*, *King Lear*, and *The Merchant of Venice*. T. S. Eliot's *Murder in the Cathedral* is based on the martyrdom of Thomas Becket in the reign of Henry II of England.[527]

Music: Many romantic songs have a wistful or sad ending: *Lili Marlene* was sung by soldiers on both sides in the Great War; the song, *As Time Goes By*, which was sung by Dooley Wilson as "Sam" in the movie *Casablanca* (1942); and American folk ballads, such as *Clementine*: "You are lost and gone forever, Clementine." The bugle sounds *"Taps"* at the burial of an American soldier, and *"Last Post,"* at a British soldier's funeral. The final movement of Gustav Mahler's monumental *Das Lied von der Erde* is about death: *"Der Abschied"* ("The Farewell"). In *Death and Resurrection*, Richard Strauss explores the struggle of a man between life and death. It is a meme for the struggle faced by everyone, although death always wins, as in Johann Sebastian Bach's plaintive organ piece, *"Alle Menschen müssen sterben"* ("All men must die"). The eerie D-minor music of Camille Saint-Saëns, *Danse Macabre* (Dance of Death, 1874) is played as skeletons escort living humans to their graves in a hectic waltz.[528]

Folk songs, spirituals, and hymns: "It takes a wearied man … but I won't be wearied long," "Carry me back to ol' Virginny," "Deep River," "Dem Bones, dem dry bones," and "Crossing over into Jordan." Note the irony: The settlers of Jericho were all killed by Joshua's troops. Spirituals were usually based on Old Testament stories before Emancipation, and thereafter they usually found themes from the New Testament. In spirituals and hymns, "Home" is always a metaphor for Heaven. Dr. Leon Sullivan once said, "We have crossed the river, but the ocean lies ahead." The Other is represented in modern America by African Americans.[529]

Funeral music: Chopin's stirring *Funeral March*, and the haunting violin solo in Saint Saëns, *Tais*. Both are associated with death, though each evokes a different emotion. Funeral hymns are in the section entitled "The Eternal Life" in *The Methodist Hymnal*. Methodists tried to normalize death. They believed that death should not be feared, for Eternal Life is ahead:[530]

Death is mentioned in the title or verses of hymns

"And when my voice is lost in death / Praise shall employ my nobler powers." (Isaac Watts)
"Assured alone that life and death / God's mercy underlies" (John G. Whittier)
"In life, in death, O Lord, abide with me" (Henry F. Lyte)
"Sickness and sorry, pain and death, are felt and feared no more" (Samuel Stennett)
"Not Jordan's steam, nor death's cold flood, should fright us from the shore" (Isaac Watts)
"Where neither death nor sorrow invades their holy home" (Hugh R. Haweis)
"'Tis finished, all is finished, their fight with death and sin" (Henry Alford)

Death is implied in hymns, though not stated explicitly

"'Earth to earth, and dust to dust,' calmly now the words we say" (John Ellerton)
"Thanks be to God that such have been, tho' they are here no more! (melody: Auld Lang Syne)
"The land of rest, the saints' delight, the heaven prepared for me" (Charles Wesley)
"Servant of God, well done! Thy glorious warfare's past" (Charles Wesley)
"When on my day of life, the night is falling" (John G. Whittier)
"Rest comes at length, though life be long and dreary" (Frederik W. Faber)

The "Navy Hymn" is sung at funerals of those who have served in the Navy: It begins with "Eternal Father, Strong to Save," and its first three verses end with the words, "those in peril on the sea." The Navy Hymn was sung at the funeral of Franklin D. Roosevelt, who had served as Assistant Secretary of the Navy, and also when the body of John F. Kennedy was carried up the steps to lie in state in the Capitol. At retirement or death, a sailor or Naval officer is said to have "swallowed the anchor."[531]

Opera: Giuseppe Verdi's *Aida* ends with entombment and suicide of the two lovers, and his *La Traviata* concludes with the death of Violetta, "the fallen woman," from consumption (tuberculosis). At the climax of Verdi's unforgettable *Rigoletto*, Gilda dies, while offstage, the Duke repeats his ironic aria, "La Donna e Mobile" (the woman is fickle). In fact, ironically, it is the Duke who is fickle. Giacomo Puccini's *La Bohème*, also about two young lovers, ends with the death of Mimi from consumption. Mimi's death was seen at that time, by some, as punishment for the lovers' carefree life.[532]

Movies: Death appears or is implied in the titles of many films, such as *Murder for Hire*, and *Dial M for Murder*. The genre of *film noir* includes films that rise to a terrifying climax, accompanied by ominous music and dark lighting. A classic is Alfred Hitchcock's *Rebecca* (1940), which was based on Daphne du Maurier's novel of the same name. Hitchcock produced many other horror movies, such as the unforgettable *Psycho*, and *The Birds*. Agatha Christie, on the other hand, explored death in a genteel, almost bloodless fashion, in a series of delightful movies. Christie's most intriguing one was *Murder on the Orient Express*, in which many people, each with a grudge, participated in knifing the victim. The term "Gaslighting," referring to psychological manipulation, originates with the *film noir* movie *Gaslight* (1944), starring Charles Boyer and Ingrid Bergman. Orson Welles' *Citizen Kane* ends with Kane's death, and then flashes back to explore his life. Death (or the escape from death) is the theme in most of the recent films in the genre of science fiction (*Star Wars* series, 1979ff., and *Gravity*, 2013), and in the genre of fantasy (J. K. Rowling's *Harry Potter* series).[533]

Wars all involve death, and although there is love and humor and irony in war, war movies are mostly about death: Erich Maria Remarque, *All Quiet on the Western Front* (1930), is based on his incredibly grim World War I novel, published in 1929; and *A Farewell to Arms* (1932), from Ernest Hemingway's novel (1929), is about love and death in World War I. The random, almost casual, sacrifice of men in the Great War appears in *Paths of Glory* (1957) about the French army; and in the apparently preventable deaths of many soldiers in the British army in the recent film, *1917*.[534]

More books and movies with death in the background: in the nineteenth century, Wilkie Collins, *The Moonstone* (1868), and Sir Arthur Conan Doyle, the *Sherlock Holmes* series, beginning in 1887. *Love Story, Mrs. Miniver, Casablanca*, and many others like them in the early twentieth century. And in the past half century, there has been an odd surge of interest in murder mysteries. You wouldn't be aware of that from reading the New York Times Book Review, which has only two major sections: Serious non-fiction and serious fiction. Poetry is sometimes featured, but crime fiction is barely mentioned, on one inside page. Nevertheless, the three most popular genre at this time of books and movies are mystery, romance, and fantasy. The underlying fascination in mysteries, romance novels, and fantasies is usually an unsolved murder (or many of them), or the danger of death of one or more of the principal characters.[535]

Violent death is often seen in war movies, and death is always hovering in the background in *They were Expendable* (about PT boats in the Philippines); *The Sands of Iwo Jima* (the heroism and deaths of United States Marines); *Tora Tora Tora* (the attack on Pearl Harbor, seen from the Japanese point of view); *The Best Years of Our Lives* (the challenges faced by returning veterans); *The Longest Day* (D-Day, with the largest war fleet ever assembled); *Saving Private Ryan* (a gripping fictional account of war in Europe); and the British film, *Dunkirk*.[536]

Fairy tales: Death or the fear of death appears in many fairy tales and nursery rhymes, to caution children. The stories by the Grimm brothers, Jakob and Wilhelm, include the fearsome wolf in "Little Red Riding Hood" and the child-eating witch in "Hansel and Gretel." Other stories intended to scare children include many of Hans Christian Andersen's *Fairy Tales*. In one story we read that "Big Claus" went home and "killed his grandmother and put her in the cart," and he offered to sell her for "a bushel of gold." And in "The Story of a Mother, "the old man – he was Death – gave a nod that might mean yes or no." In the anonymous Mother Goose story, "Sleeping Beauty" lies in suspense between life and death. The tale we know as "Cinderella" is based on a legend that can be traced back for thousands of years. Cinderella is consigned to live in a dangerous place by her evil stepmother and stepsisters; "cinders" means death, the residue of fire. Nursery rhymes may have a macabre background: "Ring around the Rosie" in which "all fall down" is thought by some to refer to death from the plague, although this theory has its detractors. *Alice in Wonderland* and *The Wizard of Oz* are exciting because of the frisson of death that is in the background of the little girls' weird adventures. These stories are in vivid contrast with pleasant books for children, such as *Green Gables* and the *Little House* series and – more recently – happy books for children, such as Dr. Seuss's *Cat in the Hat*.[537]

Folk art: Death is seen in the Jack o' Lantern, which is the traditional symbol for Hallowe'en (All Hallows' Evening). This is the night that precedes the Day of the Dead (*Día de los Muertos*, or All Hallows Day). It is celebrated in Latin America with parades in which *calacas* (skulls) are shown on masks or painted faces, and by breaking *calacas piñatas*.[538]

Cartoons: *The Addams Family* in the *New Yorker*, and the movie with the same title (2019), dealt with the subject of ghouls and the supernatural in an amusing way. A recent comic strip, *Non Sequitur*, deals with death in strange images, such as a man holding his own head on a platter, yet speaking; and flashbacks through time, involving humorous views of Heaven and Hell.[539]

News media: Four memorable events will be mentioned to illustrate the coverage of death on television. The first was the "Four Days That Made TV News" when millions watched continuous television coverage of the events following the assassination of President Kennedy on November 22, 1963, until his funeral on November 25. The "Four Days" included the on-camera shooting of his assassin, Lee Harvey Oswald, by Jack Ruby. Ironically, the media's desire to show Oswald being transferred as a prisoner enabled Ruby to get close enough to shoot him.[540]

Two others were sudden, unexpected deaths of beautiful celebrities. Many hours of television coverage, including images and interviews, followed the deaths of Princess Grace and of Princess Diana in automobiles. Princess Grace Rainier (née Kelly) had had a spontaneous cerebral hemorrhage which caused her accident, which occurred in 1982 when she was driving with her daughter near their home in Monaco. Before she married Prince Rainier, Grace Kelly had been one of Hollywood's most famous actresses. By coincidence, Grace Kelly had co-starred in several of the scariest murder mysteries of Alfred Hitchcock.[541]

Princess Diana's limousine crashed in Paris in 1997 while the driver was attempting to evade the *paparazzi* who were following her. Lady Diana Spencer's marriage to Prince Charles in 1981 had been one of the most famous events of that decade. It appeared to be a real-life fairy tale, in which a commoner becomes a Princess. She then has two sons; the elder is next to his father as heir to the throne. Diana's grace and beauty appeared to grow as time passed, and it was hardly diminished when she and the Prince had a messy separation and finally a divorce in 1996.[542]

The terrorist attacks on September 11, 2001, provided both challenges and opportunities for television coverage, especially in New York City and Arlington, Virginia. Coverage of the events in New York began shortly after 8:15 a.m., when the first airplane hit the North Tower in the World Trade Center, and soon all news cameras were focused on the Twin Towers. Eighteen minutes later, a second plane hit the South Tower, and at a distance, viewers watched in horror as the buildings were engulfed in flames and collapsed. Hand-held television cameras in the streets below showed panic-stricken people running away from the buildings, surrounded by smoke and debris and the sounds of shouts and sirens. Some people who worked in the upper floors chose to leap from windows to escape being burned to death. The ghastly sight of bodies dropping from the towers was not clear to most television viewers on 9/11, but recovered footage has shown it. At 9:45, a third hijacked airplane crashed into the Pentagon, and television coverage of that burning building was then split-imaged with sights of the continuing tragedy in New York. A fourth plane was hijacked, but it crashed in Shanksville, Pennsylvania, as the passengers fought to take control away from the terrorists who had seized it. The hijackers apparently had intended to crash the plane in Washington, D.C., into either the White House or the Capitol. The deaths caused by the attacks in America on 9/11 are said to total some 2,996, including the 19 hijackers.[543]

Fantasy: Witches are in the background of *Hansel and Gretel* and *The Wizard of Oz* and *The House of the Seven Gables*. However, witches are in the foreground of the terrifying *Blair Witch Project* and are parodied in *The Witches of Eastwick*. Fiction and fantasy reach new heights in the gruesome *Texas Chain Saw Massacre* and in the series of films about the fictional cannibal Dr. Hannibal Lecter, most notably in *Silence of the Lambs* (1981).[544]

Art and Sculpture: Christ crucified is the most common image of death in art and sculpture in the Western World, with the legend INRI nailed to the cross; it is translated as: "Jesus, King of the Jews" (John 19:3). The terrifying image of Christ on the cross appears above the altar in thousands of churches, often accompanied by the twelve Stations of the Cross that preceded the crucifixion. Absolute terror, in which death can be imagined, appears in the painting, *The Scream* by Edvard Munch; and death by beheading is anticipated by the sorrowful men sculptured by Auguste Rodin in *The Burghers of Calais*.[545]

Science fiction: Much of this genre places death at the center of the action, or as an ever-present foreboding shadow. Robert Heinlein's *The Moon Is a Harsh Mistress* ends with the death of the protagonist, and quotes Robert Louis Stevenson's *Requiem* as an epitaph: "Home is the sailor, home from the sea, / And the hunter home from the hill." The classic science fiction movie, *2001: A Space Odyssey* (1968), featured the apparently soothing but terrifyingly voice of "Hal," the talking computer.[546]

Medicine and Science

Science: Important observations about death have been made in other branches of science: In psychology, five stages of grief were proposed by Elizabeth Kubler Ross and David Kessler in *Grief and Grieving*: Denial, Anger, Bargaining, Depression and Acceptance; a sixth stage, Meaning, was later added by Kessler. The stages of grief that were described by Kubler Ross and Kessler have been disputed, but their concept continues to activate many conversations about grief. The discovery of the tomb and mummy of King Tut in Egypt is one of the high points of the field of archaeology. Tourists will spend hours waiting to see the ancient burial sites in the Valleys of the Kings and other *memento mori* in Luxor and Cairo. Anthropology and archaeology have worked together to identify the bones of those who died in remote locations throughout the world – in the peat bogs of the British Isles, in the lands occupied by indigenous peoples throughout North and South America, in the caves of the Neanderthals in Europe, in burial locations of ancient peoples across central Asia, and in east Africa, where the most ancient bones of the genus *Homo* have been found.[547]

Experiments on humans without their permission: Some were dangerous and some were responsible for deaths; and others were intentionally brutal and lethal: The surgical experiments by Dr. J. Marion Sims to repair vesico-vaginal fistulas (bladder to vagina), without anesthesia. Most were said to be "successful" although we don't know how many died. Death was always a possibility in the U.S. Public Health Service studies of diet and vitamins; the USPHS Tuskegee study in which patients with syphilis were observed without treatment, even after effective treatment was discovered; the experiments conducted by the USPHS in Guatemala, deliberately infecting hundreds of prisoners, psychiatric patients, and soldiers with gonorrhea and syphilis; and the experiments at the National Institutes of Health (NIH) with prisoner "volunteers" to study infections with adenovirus and malaria in the 1960s. Dr. Hubertus Strughold, who was brought to the United States by the secret Operation Paperclip in 1947, was revered for decades as the Father of Space Medicine. However, as a German army colonel (*Oberst*) in World War II, he was intimately connected to infamous Nazi experiments on prisoners at Dachau and elsewhere. There were also unconscionable biological warfare tests by Unit 731 of the Japanese Imperial Army on thousands of subjects, including prisoners of war; and the atrocious experiments by Dr. Josef Mengele, "the Angel of Death," in Nazi concentration camps in World War II.[548]

Religion

Altruism: Altruistic behavior occasionally leads to death. Sometimes it may occur as the result of an act of heroic altruism – to try to help another person. The intent may not be death, but death may happen in the course of the event. Death resulting from a desire to help someone else may be a carefully planned decision, or it may happen at the spur of the moment. The altruistic act may be a spontaneous secular decision; or it may be enhanced and encouraged by religion. The decision to help another person at such a cost would violate the principle that health matters for the individual. It would therefore be an exception to needs and urges in this essay on *Health Matters*.[549]

Selfless behavior, trying to save others, in the face of certain death: Captain Lawrence Oates, on return from the South Pole with Sir Robert Falcon Scott, and suffering from gangrene of the feet, left his companions to go for a walk into the darkness, so his companions would have what little is left of their food. An old Eskimo woman traditionally leaves her family in the igloo and walks down wind until she can't walk any further; if she decided to return, it would be impossible to walk back, with the wind in her face. Her goal was to spare whatever food was left for the younger people.[550]

The Bible: Death is a central theme in the Bible. In the Old Testament, death is seen to be inevitable, after Adam and Eve have made their fatal mistake and have been expelled from the Garden of Eden. But God will decide when and how each person will die. All humans are mortal; to be human is to be subject to death. The word "mortal" is itself derived from *mors, mortalis* (Latin), meaning death. God has the ability to prolong life, as he did with Methuselah, who lived 969 years; or to shorten it – as suddenly, Lot's wife became a pillar of salt. In the first book, Genesis, in the generation that follows Adam and Eve, one son killed the other. God commanded Noah to build the Ark to avoid death. And death reappears in the stories about Abraham and Isaac, of Joseph and his brothers, of Esther, of King David, and more. The ten plagues that Moses asked God to inflict on the Egyptians cannot be identified with certainty, but one or two of them could have been infectious; one was perhaps an infestation of lice (which carry the plague bacillus), although it did not affect the Jews, and another, sometimes translated as "boils" could have been smallpox. Moses dies dramatically, just as he is about to lead the Jews into battle for their Promised Land. In the New Testament, death is still inevitable, but there is the promise of

Resurrection, as it was with Jesus. All of us will die, but God takes some into Heaven. The execution of Jesus by torture and crucifixion was followed by the stoning death of Stephen, the first Saint.[551]

Other religions also had deadly customs. Ritual sacrifices of young people, usually maidens, were performed in Aztec and Mayan temples in Mexico and Central America. The climax of one ritual was when the priest performed a thoracotomy (cutting the chest open) in order to display the still-beating heart to the worshippers. In another ritual, the maiden would be thrown into a cenote – a deep water well. The epitome of death appears as the lord of the Underworld in Genesis 3:1-17 as the serpent, and as the devil in the New Testament (Matthew 4:1-11). He is Hades in the gods of Greece and Pluto in Rome, with many assistants. He is Satan. He is Lucifer in Milton's *Paradise Lost*, banished to Hell, or Tartarus. Death reappears as Lord Voldemort ("mort," from Latin *mortalis*) in J. K. Rowling's *Harry Potter* series; and as Darth Vader (rearranging "Darth" into "Death," with "r" changed to "e") in *Star Wars*.[552]

War

The Civil War: Much has been written about death in the American Civil War, and rightly so, for April 1861 until April 1865 was saddest period of death and dying in the history of the United States. It was a devastating time, with hundreds of thousands of soldiers' deaths in battle and later from wounds, and civilian deaths from many causes. It has been estimated that more than two percent of the population in the United States was killed or died as a result of the Civil War. The deaths in the Civil War were preceded by thousands of deaths of enslaved Africans who were brought to the English colonies and the states of the American republic, beginning in 1619. But the premature deaths of African Americans did not end with the Civil War, because racial profiling has continued to shorten the lives of Black people and other people of color to the present time. The Museum of African American History in Washington, D.C., tells of this tragic history, which has not yet ended.[553]

The Civil War was preceded by an intense period of conflict in the United States, characterized by armed resistance to the Federal Government's struggle to satisfy both slave owners and abolitionists. Many deaths resulted as a result of resistance to the Fugitive Slave Act of 1850, and in actions led by John Brown in "Bleeding Kansas" (1856) and in his attack on Harper's Ferry, Virginia (now West Virginia) in 1859, in which Brown was captured and hanged. Several versions of a popular song, *John Brown's Body*, soon appeared, and the patriotic *Battle Hymn of the Republic*, written by Julia War Howe in 1861, was set to the same familiar music as *John Brown's Body*. Brown has not been forgotten; a poem, *John Brown's Body*, by Stephen Vincent Benet (1928) won the Pulitzer Prize. Other notable works about the period of the Civil War include Harriet Beecher Stowe's novel, *Uncle Tom's Cabin* (1852), Abraham Lincoln's *Gettysburg Address* (1863), the novel by Shelby Foote, *Shiloh* (1952), and the movie *Glory* (1989). Death is an underlying theme in all of these works.[554]

Memorable museums about the Civil War include the Gettysburg, Pennsylvania, museum and mass burial ground, and Ford's Theater in Washington, D.C. The most dramatic incident that ever occurred in any theatre took place at Ford's Theatre in 1865. On April 14, 1865, an actor, John Wilkes Booth, shot President Abraham Lincoln in the head, and he then leaped down onto the stage of the theatre and broke his leg, but escaped. The President died the following morning, and Booth was killed on April 26, shot when a barn in which he was hiding was set ablaze.[555]

The World Wars: What Winston Churchill said was a "thirty years war" began in August 1914 with the assassination of Archduke Ferdinand of Austria and his wife at Sarajevo, in Serbia. The *Guns of August* soon roared as the nations of Europe slid into the first Great War, with the Allied Nations of Britain, France, Italy and Japan against the Central Powers of Germany and the Austrian Empire. The United States joined the war on the side of the Allies in April 1917. An uneasy Armistice was finally agreed upon on November 11, 1918. By that time, seventeen million soldiers and civilians had died. These deaths probably included some of the fifty million – yes, estimated at 50 million – from the Great Influenza pandemic that began in 1918 and continued until 1920. Miseries and deaths continued for several years as Europe slowly recovered. But the angry nations of Europe couldn't agree on enough to keep the peace. The Lost Generation in the U.S. danced its way in the post-war "flapper period." The

U.S entered the Great Depression, and it forgot Europe. The punishment inflicted by France on Germany, and payment of war debts insisted upon by the U.S. and Britain, kept the old international conflict alive. It gradually developed into another World War. Fighting resumed on September 1, 1939, and again the nations of Europe were at war with each other, the Allies against Germany and its so-called Axis. Japan and Italy changed sides, and Japan's Imperial designs came in conflict with America's goals in the Pacific. Tensions rose during 1941. Conflict between the U.S. and Japan was expected, but the initial location was a surprise. On December 7, 1941, Japan attacked America at Pearl Harbor, in Hawaii, and the U.S. immediately declared war on Japan. Germany, as Japan's ally, soon declared war on the U.S., and the conflict then became another World War. After a long and deadly struggle, Germany finally surrendered in May 1945. An estimated sixty million more people died, and after two atomic bombs were dropped by the U.S. on Japan, World War II came to an end in September 1945. The relief was immense, but short lived, for a Cold War soon continued between the Communist world, led by the Soviet Union, and the non-Communist countries, led by the United States. The post-war period has been called Act III of World War II, and some would say that it still isn't over.[556]

Conflicts after World War II have caused many deaths. The Cold War between the United States and its allies, and the Soviet Union and its allies – the Communist bloc – lasted from 1945 until 1989. Atrocities were committed on both sides of this conflict. The U.S. Central Intelligence Agency was deeply involved in destabilizing governments in Central America and Indonesia, and in the failed attempt to overthrow Fidel Castro at the Bay of Pigs in Cuba in 1961. There were many active military conflicts during this period, beginning with the Korean War from 1950-1953, which produced an unresolved armistice; a long period in Vietnam from a small start in 1950 to final failure of the United States in April 1975; and the CIA's coup d'état of the Iranian government in 1953, which was paid back by the Iranians in 1979 with the capture of the American embassy and the establishment of the present Iranian government. Throughout this period, the Soviet government showed no mercy in its fierce determination to defeat America and its allies. The abominable prison system of the Union of Soviet Socialist Republics (USSR) was described in Aleksandr Solzhenitsyn's novel, *A Day in the Life of Ivan Denisovich* (1962), and the Soviet Union continued the antisemitic pogroms that had begun during the reign of the Czars, and with intentional starvation in Ukraine. When the Communist People's Liberation Army (PLA) of Mao Zedong drove Chiang Kai-shek's Nationalist Army to the off-shore island of Taiwan, the People's Republic of China (PRC) took control of a vast area of Asia, from the Great Wall in the north to the Himalayas in the south, and from the Pacific Ocean on the east to the Hindu Kush in the west, including Tibet. China then took The Great Leap Forward, with millions of deaths by starvation and relocation. The PRC continues to brutally suppress minorities: Buddhists in Tibet and Muslim Uyghurs in Xinjiang.[557]

There are authoritarian governments in many other countries in the world, and much of the so-called "democracy" in Africa and Asia is represented by autocratic, hereditary kleptocracies that are savage to many people. Death is often the consequence of being on the wrong side of the government.

Western Expansion of the United States: The terms "Manifest Destiny" and "The Winning of the West" have been retitled appropriately by historians as the "Western Expansion of the United States." The Western Expansion occurred at the expense of indigenous peoples and the destruction of much of the habitat for animals and plants in North America. The first step was the Lewis and Clark Expedition, in which death took a holiday. However, the massacre described in *Bury My Heart at Wounded Knee* in 1890 is the sequel to Custer's Last Stand in 1876. *The Virginian, High Noon* and *The Lone Ranger* told tales of valor, redemption and punishment of white settlers in the West, including combat, survival, and death – in which Native Americans played minor roles, or were non-existent. One of the famous legends of the West was that of the noble Texas Ranger, who worked alone. This was a myth, however, which hid a "history of lynchings, massacres and ruthless white supremacy."[558]

Museums and Cemeteries: Death is shown in many exhibits in the United States Holocaust Museum and the National Museum of African American History and Culture, in Washington, D.C. In New Orleans: The National WWII Museum. In Europe, countless cemeteries honor dead soldiers of both sides in both World Wars. Many U.S. veterans are buried in government cemeteries. Some of the most memorable are at Arlington, Virginia; on Oahu, Hawaii, in the Punch Bowl and in Pearl Harbor, on the U.S.S. *Arizona*; and the Gettysburg National Military Park Museum, and the surrounding battlefield and Gettysburg National Cemetery. Family members in many countries in Europe and America visit cemeteries in towns and on farms to remember their relatives with prayers and flowers. In Latin America, the *Dia de los Muertos* (Day of the Dead) is an occasion to decorate the graves of family members, to spend a bit of time with them, and to reminisce with children about their ancestors.[559]

Monuments and Memorials honoring the dead: In addition to monuments in many U.S. veterans' cemeteries, there are three that are especially moving in Washington, D.C.: the Vietnam Veterans Memorial Wall, designed by Maya Lin, on which more than 58,000 names are inscribed; the adjacent Three Soldiers Memorial and the Vietnam Women's Memorial; and the Korean War Veterans Memorial nearby, with the haunting expressions of nineteen soldiers who are trudging aimlessly, with weapons trailing at their sides. There are many other memorable sites in Washington that honor the dead, notably the Washington Monument, the Lincoln Memorial, the Thomas Jefferson Memorial, the Martin Luther King, Jr., Memorial, and the National World War II Memorial. In London, on Whitehall, near Piccadilly Square, is the United Kingdom's Cenotaph, which honors the dead of both World Wars and British military who died in later wars. A cenotaph is an empty tomb; this one was designed by Sir Edward Luytens. It has been reproduced elsewhere in many of the countries of the Commonwealth.[560]

Memorial days that honor the dead are annual events in many countries. There are many legends about how "Decoration Day" in the United States began, but it probably was a day on which women placed flowers on the graves of Civil War soldiers, and they would also visit graves of other family members. The date of May 30 became the usual date for Decoration Day, and in 1868 the day was designated as Memorial Day. The date was in the spring, when flowers were bursting into bloom. The reason for the name of the day and its date have largely been forgotten. Many people seem to be unaware of the reason for calling it Memorial Day. The day is now a holiday, and it is the opportunity for a three-day weekend of picnics and pleasure at the end of May. Yet the graves in veterans' cemeteries are still decorated with flags, and older members of veterans' organizations still hover near supermarkets, selling poppies to wear in memory of the dead. They return in November to sell poppies for Veterans Day. In England, Canada, Australia, and New Zealand, "Remembrance Poppies" are worn through the month of November, in honor of the dead in World War I. Armistice Day (November 11, 1918) is the annual Remembrance Day in the British Commonwealth Countries. In the last century, children remembered the Armistice by standing silently beside their desks in school on November 11 at 11:11 a.m. In Russia, the annual celebration of Victory Day (VE-Day) is on May 9, because the Great Patriotic War ended at midnight on the Eastern front during the night of May 8-9, 1945. Many other remembrances have been forgotten, as if they were but "footprints on the sands of time." The commemoration was a quiet one for the family from New Zealand who came to the Gallipoli peninsula in Turkey to honor their son, who died as a soldier in the failed amphibious operation of 1915-1916. His parents placed a slate shingle from the roof of their home to mark the land where he died, although his exact burial place is unknown.[561]

Suicide

Depression is probably the most frequent reason that a person takes his or her own life. It may be the result of intractable anxiety or sadness, as it was with the poet, Sylvia Plath. Or it may be an acute overwhelming tragedy; or a situation that seems impossible to deal with; or from a mistake in belief or judgment. Or impetuous anger, thinking "I'll show you!!" Suicide may be an accident; intending to be a gesture, but instead, it succeeds in death. If the victim showed no warning signs, and did not leave a note, it leaves a perpetual wound in the heart and mind of the survivors. In paranoid schizophrenia, the cause of death is delusional, not real.[562]

Other reasons for suicide include a conscious decision: Socrates, who drank a poison made from hemlock at the behest of the state; Field Marshal Erwin Rommel, who committed suicide using a cyanide capsule in October 1944, to spare his family from imprisonment by Adolph Hitler; and then Hitler, who shot himself in the head in April 1945, as the Russian army was entering Berlin – his wife,

Eva Braun, bit a cyanide capsule at time. Suicide may be a duty fulfilled: A spy may carry a cyanide capsule in case he is captured, to prevent disclosure of secrets. General William Donovan, head of OSS, is said to have carried a cyanide capsule in his mouth when he landed in France shortly after D-Day in June 1944, but he wasn't captured, and didn't need to bite into it.[563]

Methods of suicide include an almost endless array of possibilities, ranging from gruesome to bloodless. Hanging, jumping from heights, drowning, exposure to the elements, refusing nourishment, guns, knives, carbon monoxide, barbiturates and other drugs. Brahmans of India formerly tolerated suicide and self-immolation of a widow, called *suttee*, though it is now illegal. In Japan, suicide was once regarded as a noble gesture, as in the traditional suicide of a samurai by disemboweling, known as *seppuku* or *hari-kiri*, and in suicide bombers by *kamikaze* pilots in World War II. This was an eerie precedent for the suicide terrorist bombers on September 11, 2001. "Suicide by cop" is tragedy for two people, the policeman and the victim; it happens when a person intentionally threatens a law enforcement officer, provoking death by shooting.[564]

There is also **assisted suicide**, most commonly with a lethal dose of a drug, usually a barbiturate or a narcotic, with the help of a physician or family member; it may be legal, or not, depending on the law in that locality. Euthanasia, in which the physician actively administers a lethal dose of a drug, was made famous by Dr. Jack Kevorkian, nicknamed "Dr. Death." Euthanasia is an area into which few physicians would venture to go. See Appendix E for the Hippocratic Oath, which physicians usually take at some point in time, either early in medical school, or at the time of graduation.

More Methods of Death

Ionizing radiation: The electromagnetic spectrum ranges from extremely short gamma rays and X-rays, to longer rays, including invisible ultraviolet light (UV C, UV B, and UV A); visible light (which can be refracted into the colors of the rainbow, from the shortest, blue, to the longest, red); invisible infrared light; and radio waves, which are the longest wavelengths in the spectrum. At the short end of the electromagnetic spectrum, X-rays and gamma rays have important effects on the human body, and they also can be deadly. So, too, are the effects of UV C and UV B, but as the wavelengths become longer, their danger decreases. The first scientists to work with these dangerous rays were Wilhelm Roentgen (with X-rays) in 1895, and Pierre and Marie Curie (with radium) in 1898. Marie Curie died of aplastic anemia, which was caused by radiation that she received inadvertently from her work in the laboratory. Soon after Roentgen announced his discovery, Thomas Edison began working with a glass vacuum tube – a cathode ray tube – that would generate X-rays. His device became the fluoroscope, an enormously important medical invention, which he never patented. Edison and his glassblower, Clarence Dally, both developed radiation sickness. Dally stood on the opposite side of the device from Edison, and he thus received a higher dose of X-rays. He died a horrible death from radiation-induced squamous cell carcinoma. Fifty years later, the discoveries of physicists and chemists in this arcane field, led by the theoretical research of Albert Einstein and the technology of the U.S. Manhattan Project, produced the atomic bombs that were dropped on Hiroshima and Nagasaki. Atomic weapons were then followed by nuclear weapons and the standoff of the MAD (Mutual Assured Destruction) Cold War. The Cuban Missile Crisis in October 1962 nearly ended in an unimaginable catastrophe, but by good fortune, the moment passed. It seemed for several years that nuclear power might be the best way to avoid the problems created by burning fossil fuel, but the accidents at Three Mile Island in the U.S., at Chernobyl in what is now Ukraine, and the disaster after the earthquake and tsunami at Fukushima in Japan, have put a pause on that possibility. Deaths of countless humans have been caused by radioactivity. The strange deaths of miners for metal that occurred for several centuries in Schneeberg, Saxony, can now be explained as due to radioactive uranium that was present in the mines. Many other radioactive elements have been identified, some occurring naturally and others produced synthetically; one of them, polonium-210, was used as a poison to kill Alexander Livinenko, a former Russian spy, in London in 2006. He died after drinking tea with two Russians; the tea contained Po-210.[565]

Fires, explosions, and other catastrophes caused by humans, whether intentionally or inadvertently, or by accident. The list is endless, so I will mention, as examples, only one of each type of event that was caused by humans. The fire in the Coconut Grove nightclub in Boston in 1942 was a devastating event for hundreds of families and also for those who took care of the victims. With 492 dead, it was the worst nightclub fire in U.S. history. The almost total destruction of Halifax, Nova Scotia, in 1917 was originally thought to be sabotage by Germans, but it was in fact a preventable catastrophe due to poor navigation by the two ships that were involved. About 2000 people were killed in what was the largest explosion in world history prior to the bombing of Hiroshima in 1945. The ignition of a truckload of ammonium nitrate fertilizer in a terrorist attack on the Alfred P. Murrah Federal Building in Oklahoma City in 1995, killing at least 168 people, was made possible because the fertilizer was easily obtained and could be converted with little difficulty into an explosive. It was the deadliest act of domestic terrorism in American history. The massive explosion in Beirut, Lebanon, in 2020, causing about 190 deaths, was caused by about 2,750 tons of ammonium nitrate fertilizer that had been stored improperly in an unguarded building on the waterfront. Whether this explosive chemical was ignited spontaneously, or accidentally, or by terrorists, may never be known. We could also mention events in wartime, especially in World War II. Hundreds of civilians died in bombings of cities in Europe, such as Coventry, England, by the Germans; and in Cologne and Dresden, Germany, by the R.A.F.; and hundreds more died as "collateral damage" when atom bombs were dropped by the U.S. on Hiroshima and Nagasaki, Japan.[566]

Deaths from uncertain causes: Here is a theoretical question: A man with cancer leaves home to hike on a familiar trail in the White Mountains and he doesn't return. He is found dead a few days later, at the bottom of a cliff near the trail. Did he commit suicide, or was it an accident?

Natural causes, such as volcanic eruptions, hurricanes and floods, and wild fires: The earth's temperature has undergone long periods of alternating warm and cold temperatures. The so-called Little Ice Age cannot be dated precisely, but colder temperatures than usual occurred in many years from the 14th to the end of the 19th centuries. The entire 17th century was cold, but the worst year is said to have been 1750, in the 18th century. Some summers were cold enough to interfere with crop growth and thus led to starvation. The eruption of Mount Tambora in Indonesia in 1815 produced a cloud of ash which blocked the light of the sun. The result was the "Year Without a Summer" in 1816. Global temperatures in 1816 decreased by 0.4-0.7 C. and major food shortages occurred throughout the Europe and North America. A volcanic eruption in 1883 of Krakatoa, an island in Indonesia, is said to have caused more than 30,000 deaths, and the cloud of ash also produced another world-wide loss of crops. The "perfect storm" of 2012 in the northeastern United States was a combination of high tide and severe tropical rainstorm in Superstorm Sandy, October 25, 2012. However, typhoons, cyclones, and tsunamis have caused many more deaths in the Pacific and Indian Oceans. Dams burst, sometimes drowning hundreds of people; the Johnstown flood in Pennsylvania in 1889 is a good example. Fires were common in the dry grasses of the Heartland of America in the nineteenth century, and farmers learned to prepare firebreaks and backfires to save their families, their livestock, and their homes. The backfire technique was not employed in time to save the 13 firefighters who were burned to death in the Mann Gulch in Montana in 1949. Their sad story is told in the book by Norman Maclean, *Young Men and Fire*.[567]

Poisons are discussed dispassionately in the *Encyclopaedia Britannica*. It is difficult to read the article entitled "poison" in the *Encyclopaedia* and not to imagine the purpose, the agony, and the deception involved in this murderous act. If a poison is taken by accident, it is a tragedy; if the poison is self-administered, it becomes a choice; if it is intentionally applied or administered surreptitiously, it is repugnant. Poisoning is said to be an ancient Oriental art, and that may be true, although it would now seem to be a racist statement: the hauteur of the West, in condescension of the East. We cannot possibly do justice to the subject of poisons in this brief essay, so but a few examples must suffice. Typically, most poisons are given by the oral route, disguised in food or beverages – bitter strychnine slipped into sugar for tea; arsenic, given in slowly increasing doses until the outcome is death; or by accident, as decorators licked their brush tips as they applied leaded paint in the porcelain industry in England, or when the "radium girls" did the same when they painted watch dials in New Jersey. Poison from some mushrooms – the toadstools – are famously lethal, and some tropical fish contain a poison known as ciguatoxin, which is a rapid killer. Barbiturates or narcotics would be possible, but a large dose is required, so they rarely are used as poisons; more often, they appear as causes of accidental death from overdose, or suicide. If wood alcohol is substituted for ethyl alcohol in a beverage, it usually passes the taste test, yet it blinds or kills the victim. Many biological weapons are available for poisonous uses, and can be lethal, dead or alive; for instance, cholera, botulinum, ricin, and even a high dose of enterotoxic *E. coli* (ETEC). A deadly poison can be given by inhalation, as carbon monoxide or methane gas, especially when the intended victim is asleep. Or it can be applied to the skin, as thallium. Many other chemicals are fatal to humans, such as mercury, lead, phosgene (poison gas), and dioxin, which was a contaminant in Agent Orange. None of these other chemicals are likely to be used by murderers, whose intent is to poison secretly and to be undetected.[568]

Ricin, obtained from castor beans, is a deadly poison, but it has rarely been used an intentional poison, and then only by professional assassins. The Bulgarian dissident, Georgi Markov, was stabbed with an umbrella containing a pellet of ricin in London, presumably by Bulgarian or Russian operatives. However, his assassin was never identified. The Russian opposition figure Alexi Navalny was poisoned with the nerve agent Novichok in October 2020. The *New York Times* apparently was prepared for this, for it immediately published a review of poisonings associated with Russian intelligence operations since 2002, and some of the poisons developed by the Soviet Union that are "tasteless and untraceable."[569]

Domestic violence: An all too typical scene: a man is dead, having shot his wife, their children, and himself. She had asked for a restraining order against him. He and the wife had many fights, which he usually won. The children are innocent victims. The Second Amendment to the U.S. Constitution states, in eighteenth century language: "A well regulated Militia, being necessary to the security of a free State, the right of the people to keep and bear Arms, shall not be infringed." The language, punctuation, and syntax of the Second Amendment have led to endless arguments about what it means, and how to interpret it. The Second Amendment is used as an argument to permit widespread ownership of a variety of weapons – of pistols and long guns and semiautomatic rifles – that are used for hunting, for personal protection, collections, and target shooting. Easy availability of guns also contributes to deaths from suicides, accidents, and escalating arguments. Federal and local laws have restricted ownership of some weapons, such as such as machine guns and howitzers. However, the National Rifle Association has a strong lobby which has succeeded in preventing many attempts to reduce the numbers and types of weapons in American homes. Many Americans are hunters and gun collectors.[570]

Assassination: There have been countless assassinations in history, and only a few can be mentioned here: King Philip II of Macedon, father of Alexander "the Great," who was killed in public by a jilted male lover. U.S. Presidents Abraham Lincoln, killed by John Wilkes Booth, and John F. Kennedy, killed by Lee Harvey Oswald. Other U.S. presidents have been assassinated, too: Garfield and McKinley; and attempts were made on the lives of Presidents Theodore Roosevelt (after he left office), Gerald Ford, and Ronald Reagan. The assassination of Archduke Franz Ferdinand of Austria and his wife Sophie, Duchess of Hohenberg, on June 28, 1914, by Gavrilo Princip, in Sarajevo, was the spark that began World War I. Three assassinations in the 1960s changed American history: President John F. Kennedy, his brother Robert Kennedy; and Martin Luther King.[571]

Cannibalism, briefly mentioned: Occasional reports in the news media of gruesome murders and cannibalism by serial criminals. The Fore people of Papua New Guinea formerly had a fatal degenerative disease known as *kuru* (meaning "trembling"), which progressed to dementia and death. The disease was caused by an infection with a prion – a protein – that accumulates in the brain, which was transmitted by cannibalistic rituals in which the brains of the dead were eaten. When the rituals were discontinued, the disease disappeared. The Donner Party, stranded in the Sierra Mountains in 1846, reportedly resorted to cannibalism, but only from parts of travelers who died from starvation or hypothermia. On the other hand, there are stories, supposedly true, of men lost at sea, drawing lots to see who would be sacrificed to feed the others. The navigator was spared because he would be the one who could find the way to a safe landing. However, dead men tell no tales, and survivors didn't like to talk about these things. A rare psychiatric condition known as autophagia is a form of self-cannibalism. The weird possibility of apparent death with dignity for elderly humans, followed by recycling them into food for younger people, was explored in the science fiction movie *Soylent Green* (1973).[572]

Murders, Duels, and Mass murders: By gunshots, especially in the United States, there are so many that the numbers are staggering. They are almost countless, but a few in recent years are especially memorable: the elementary school in Newtown, Connecticut, which ended in the shooter's suicide; the Stoneman School in Florida, in which the shooter walked away but was captured; and the massacre in Las Vegas in which the shooter used a "bump stock" to modify his semi-automatic rifle, enabling it to fire rapidly. Other mass murders have been committed recently with guns in Norway and New Zealand, by deranged men who claimed right wing political motives. In other instances, such as at the U.S. Navy base in Pensacola, Florida, at a military recruiting station in California, and a U.S. Army base in Texas, the shooters were inspired by terrorist organizations in the world of radical Islam. Various modifications of the AK-47 automatic rifle, which was designed in the Soviet Union by Kalashnikov in World War II, were used in most of these mass shootings. For example, the AR-15, which looks like the AK-47. It is not very accurate, but it fires rapidly and has a large magazine. The shooters were often armed with many additional weapons, such as pistols, shotguns, and grenades, and explosives that were intended to be used as suicide bombs. The public health risk of guns is obvious, but the Second Amendment to the U.S. Constitution guarantees the "right to bear arms." There is a never-ending battle between those who wish to study the problem and to place restraints on gun ownership, versus those who are bitterly opposed to anything that appears to limit any access to guns.[573]

The National Rifle Association (N.R.A.) is unyielding, and it derives support from sportsmen and those who hunt for food for their families. About 1,000 people have been shot to death by police in the U.S. every year for the five years preceding 2020; that number was revealed in connection with the death in Minneapolis on May 25, 2020, of George Floyd, who died with a policeman's knee on the back of his neck. Many law enforcement unions have vigorously defended current police tactics and officers who have been charged with crimes.[574]

Duels were once an exercise in formality, a deadly dance, in which one or both of the duelers may be killed. Most duels were fought by men, one or both of whom felt that his honor was challenged. The choice of a weapon – swords or pistols – was made by one combatant, and the other would have the chance to choose which of the two he would use. The most famous duel in American history was Aaron Burr's challenge to Alexander Hamilton for slander. In 1804, Burr, who was Vice President of the United States, fatally wounded Hamilton in Weehauken, New Jersey. Hamilton was taken across the Hudson River and died in New York City. Dueling was illegal in both states, and Burr was charged with murder in New Jersey and New York. Burr fled and was never tried, but his reputation was ruined.[575]

Thrill killings: There are many grisly instances of "thrill" killings, but one of the most famous is that of Nathan Leopold and Richard Loeb in Chicago in 1924. Both men were from wealthy families, and their victim was totally innocent, just a plaything. Countless others have gotten thrills from killing.[576]

Suicide and murder: A strange episode recently involved both suicide and murder, when a woman drove her minivan off of a cliff in California, killing her wife [sic] and several adopted and foster children, without a clear motive. An enormous event in which both murder and suicide were partners took place in Guyana in 1978. The Reverend Jim Jones gave Kool-Aid laced with cyanide to more than 900 followers of his religious sect, the Peoples Temple. He then shot himself. To "drink the Kool-aid" then become a meme for a false belief in a dangerous idea, although most people wouldn't recognize its origin. One more mass murder, and that will be enough: Charles Manson was the charismatic leader of a band of young women (and a few men) who lived near Los Angeles. The Manson gang, inspired by its leader, killed two groups of people, including the actress, Sharon Tate, pregnant wife of the director Roman Polanski, and the coffee heiress, Abigail Folger. Even though he had not been present at the killings, Manson was found guilty and spent the rest of his life in prison.[577]

Medical errors resulting in death is an important issue. We need to be confident that physicians and others who provide health care will make good decisions and ensure that they are properly carried out. Unfortunately, accidents, neglect, and coverup of bad results clouds this issue. How many are injured or die as the result of medical errors? Even one is one too many, but the exact number is difficult to ascertain. Reports range from a high of 250,000 to only 22,000, with only 7,150 of these being in previously healthy people. The first estimate would make medical errors the third leading cause of death in the United States.[578]

Mass murders committed by **medical professionals** must be mentioned at this point, along with the possibility of accidental deaths caused by medication errors. Some of the saddest and most mysterious deaths in recent history have been committed by physicians, nurses, and others in the health professions. Some have apparently been "mercy" killings, of those whose life was nearly at an end, while others were "thrill" killings. Doctors and nurses have access to medications that can be lethal and often undetectable. Intravenous potassium causes the heart to relax and stop, and intravenous calcium causes the heart to contract and stop. Solutions of these minerals are readily available in hospital pharmacies, and neither is likely to be detected at autopsy. Insulin is injected in syringes that are labelled with the dose, but if the wrong syringe is selected, the dose may be too late, and fatal. Undetectable. Neither the nurse who administered it, nor the pathologist who does the autopsy would recognize that an error had occurred. It would appear to be a sudden untimely death of a person with diabetes. Digitalis is another drug in common use, which can be lethal if even one extra dose is administered. That would be easy to accomplish, intentionally or accidentally, if the patient is already receiving digitalis. It would cause fatal contraction of the heart muscle. The opposite effect would be produced by an excessive dose of atropine – which is a purified form of the ancient poison, belladonna (from nightshade, *Atropa belladonna*). That would cause the heart to relax, to stop beating; and that, too, probably would not be detected at autopsy. Several paralytic drugs that are used in anesthesia would cause death that would be difficult to detect at autopsy, unless the drug was specifically looked for.[579]

Medical hoaxes: Laetrile, also known as amygdalin, was touted as a cancer chemotherapeutic agent in the late 1960s by a small but vocal group of physicians, and it is still available in Mexico. Laetrile releases cyanide in the presence of acid, such as hydrochloric acid which is present in the stomach. It was never shown to be effective. Before Laetrile, there was another expensive anti-cancer drug – Krebiozen – which was highly touted, but it only consisted of a simple amino acid, creatinine, dissolved in mineral oil. Krebiozen's supporters included a prominent physician, Dr. Andrew Ivy, and Senator Paul Douglas. Ivy's status was trashed because of his support of Krebiozen, although Senator Douglas' reputation remained intact.[580]

Medical professionals were not without fault in the so-called "Burke and Hare" body-snatcher problem in Edinburgh in 1828. Medical schools needed cadavers for their students to dissect, and surgeons wanted cadavers on which to practice new forms of surgery. William Burke and William Hare were recruited to bring bodies to surgeon Robert Knox for dissection, and they found what they needed by robbing graves of recent burials. They were called "resurrection men." When the demand exceeded the number that they could find who were deceased, they found unwitting persons to dispatch who could serve their needs. Burke and Hare committed 16 murders; Hare turned state's evidence, and Burke was hanged.[581]

Beheading: The most famous beheading is that of John the Baptist, but others come to mind – Anne Boleyn and Mary Queen of Scots, who were axed; and Louis XIV and his Queen, Marie Antoinette, who knelt under the blade of the guillotine. The guillotine was more efficient than the axe, which is why it was used in France during the period after the Revolution that was known as The Terror. The death of the martyred patron saint of England is celebrated on June 22 each year at the Cathedral of St. Albans by a parade in the city square leading to the steps of the cathedral, where a giant puppet of St. Alban is beheaded.[582]

Punishment: Execution by beheading was a gift of a presumably painless death for Royalty and Lords in England who were accused of the most heinous of crimes, which was treason. However, English gentry who were guilty of treason, and lesser folk who were guilty of whatever might be a crime that was punishable by death, would suffer public humiliation with such methods as "hanged, drawn and quartered." The unfortunate victim would first be pulled up with a rope around his neck; he would be lowered while he was still struggling; his abdomen would be sliced open; his intestines would be drawn out of his abdomen and burned "before his eyes"; and his arms and legs would be tied to four large horses and pulled from his body as they were driven in different directions. His head would then usually be placed on a stake and displayed for several weeks. The traditional method was observed by the Royalists, post mortem, when they returned to power: Oliver Cromwell had died a natural death in 1658, but he was exhumed in 1660 and his head was staked. That would be a quicker death, however, than to be placed in a cage, dying slowly without food or water, piteously crying, high on the outside of a cathedral, as in Toledo, Spain.[583]

Torture: Native Americans were said to use a slow death to give the subject a chance to show courage. After running the gauntlet, a captive would be tied to a stake and roasted above a low fire, with small sticks passed through his skin and set ablaze. Vlad the Impaler used a stake thrust into the nether part of the body. The unfortunate victim would then be hoisted to an erect position, where he would struggle hopelessly. Death would occur slowly over a period of several days.[584]

Electric chair: Thomas Edison, in competition with his rival George Westinghouse, devised a method to demonstrate the lethality of alternating current. He called it "Westinghouse-ing," but it soon became known as the "electric chair." It was considered to be more humane than hanging, but repeated charges of electricity were sometimes needed to finish the job, and the inmate struggled helplessly.[585]

Hanging was supposed to be lethal as the result of dislocation of the cervical vertebra – a broken neck – when the body dropped, but on many occasions, a person just swung and strangled at the end of the rope. That was the fate of many of the older women who were hanged at Salem in 1692, including my ancestor Rebecca Towne Nurse ("Goody Nurse"). There were 13 women and six men who were hanged that year in Salem, and also one man who was pressed to death under heavy stones. Perhaps they were the lucky ones. Many others languished in jail and died of neglect in Salem and elsewhere in Essex County, Massachusetts. The heroism of Nathan Hale, who was hanged as a spy by the British in New York during the American Revolutionary War, is commemorated in statues in Washington, D.C., and New Haven, Connecticut. Hale's hands are tied behind him, and he is standing proudly erect. His final words are unknown, but they are said to have been: "I regret that I have but one life to give for my country." A spy was traditionally hanged, because he had been captured wearing civilian clothing or a false uniform. A soldier in his own uniform who committed an offense punishable by death was traditionally shot by a firing squad. According to legend, one soldier would have a blank round in his rifle, so anyone in the firing squad might think he was the one who did not participate in the execution. The officer in charge ended the grisly episode with a *coup de grâce*, a pistol shot in the head.[586]

Burning at the stake: In England, France, and Spain, apostacy and witchcraft were crimes that were punished by burning in a public ceremony – in the town square, or in front of a church. A slow fire was often used to torment the victim. It was common in Europe, though not in the English colonies of North America. The most famous, of course, is Joan of Arc, burned in front of the Rheims cathedral.[587]

Lynching: One of the great shames of the American republic is the lynching of thousands of African Americans in the decades following the Civil War. The victims – men, women, and sometimes children – would be tortured, hanged, and then burned, all while still alive and dying slowly. The grisly event sometimes became a celebration or picnic by white people, who were pleased to be photographed while holding parts of the victim. The Ku Klux Klan (KKK) was a major sponsor of lynching and terror of African American communities. The number of lynchings began to rise after Reconstruction was repealed in 1877, and the awful practice continued throughout the first half of the twentieth century.

The lives of African Americans have been shortened in many other ways than by lynch mobs. All-cause death rates are higher for men and women who identify as Black than those who identify as white, and lives are much shorter in Blacks than in whites. There are many causes for the discrepancy in mortality rates, but they begin with segregation and enforced poverty, and they are manifested in poor school systems, difficulty in obtaining employment, increased exposure to environmental toxins, unhealthy diets, and a higher rate of incarceration for Blacks than whites.[588]

Appendix B

Parasitology and Microbiology

The malaria parasite is one of several species of the genus *Plasmodium*. The species that are infective to humans include the most dangerous, *P. falciparum*, and the most common, *P. vivax*; and also *P. malariae* and *P. ovale*. The malaria parasite is transmitted by the bite of a female *Anopheles* mosquito, in which the parasite undergoes part of its life cycle. Falciparum malaria causes most of the deaths from malaria – over 400,000 per year. The relapsing nature of vivax malaria is responsible for much of the chronic illness – the morbidity – from malaria in the world. Prevention and treatment of illnesses and deaths from malaria is a significant world-wide problem.[589]

Leishmania (leishmaniasis) is a protozoal parasitic disease. It is transmitted by the bite from one of more than 90 species of female sandflies, causing more than 1,000,000 new cases per year. Three forms of leishmaniasis are recognized: visceral, cutaneous, and mucocutaneous. The visceral form, known as kala-azar, is usually fatal if untreated; the cutaneous form is disfiguring and leads to societal rejection; and the muco-cutaneous form causes destruction of the mucous membranes of the nose and mouth.[590]

Entamoeba histolytica is one of several species of *Entamoeba*, which have only one cell with a single nucleus. *E. histolytica* causes amoebiasis, including amoebic dysentery and amoebic liver abscesses. Both forms are deadly. Amoebiasis affects hundreds of thousands of people, mostly in developing countries.

Balantidium coli is a single celled organism that infects the colon, and is transmitted through fecal contamination of food and water. It is a devastating diarrheal disease that is widespread in developing countries.

Giardia species infect the colon, causing diarrhea and malabsorption, sometimes with a fatal outcome. *G. lamblia* is a typical example. Giardia are tiny swimmers; they have flagella and two nuclei in a single cell. Giardiasis is transmitted by ingestion of contaminated food and water.

Trypanosoma cruzi is the parasite that causes Chagas disease. It is a deadly disease with a complicated life cycle. The parasite spends part of its life cycle in a blood-sucking bug known as a "kissing bug," because it usually bites at night, near the face. Chagas disease can also be transmitted through blood transfusions. It causes death from cardiac or intestinal complications.[591]

Diseases of humans that are caused by multicellular parasitic worms include schistosomiasis, filariasis, ascariasis, hookworm, tapeworm, river blindness, and trichinosis. The adult forms of many of these creatures are known scientifically as helminths, and they can be seen by the naked eye when they are expelled from the body. Some are enormous. Most humans find them to be repulsive, dead or alive.

Schistosoma (flukes), also known as trematodes, include *S. mansoni* and *S. japonicum*. With snails as the intermediate host, the disease is usually transmitted by contact with infected water, as in bathing, swimming, or fishing. Schistosomiasis is said to be the most widespread of parasitic diseases in humans, and it is a leading cause of death in Egypt. The parasite thrives in the beautiful clear water of the lower Nile, near Cairo.[592]

Wuchereria bancrofti causes a disease known as filariasis. The tiny parasites infect the lymphatic system, blocking the circulation of lymph, causing swelling of the legs and, in males, the scrotum. When the swelling is longstanding, the grotesque condition is called elephantiasis. Imagine a miserable man pushing a wheelbarrow, carrying his scrotum. The photos are so repulsive that they have been purged from Google Images as if they were pornography.[593]

Ascaris lumbricoides (giant roundworm) is one of several species of nematodes that are parasitic on humans. The worms, which may be several inches in length, lodge in the intestines and can cause obstruction of the intestines or the biliary tract. When treatment is successful, large numbers of dead, black-striped grayish worms, two or three inches in length, are expelled in feces.[594]

Strongyloides is a disease caused by a roundworm which usually enters the body through bare feet, lodging in the intestinal tract, causing death from diarrhea. It is also a superinfection producing multi-organ failure that develops in patients who have immune suppression disorders, such as HIV/AIDS, and COVID-19. Treatment includes anti-helminthic drugs such as ivermectin and corticosteroids such as prednisone and dexamethasone.[595]

Necator americanus (hookworm). Hookworm is a debilitating disease in which these tiny roundworms typically penetrate the bare feet of children who are playing in the dirt. The worms migrate to the lining of the intestines and feast on blood, producing a debilitating degree of iron-deficiency anemia.[596]

Enormous tapeworms of three species, *Taenia saginata* (beef tapeworm), *T. solium* (pork) and *T. asiatica* (Asiatin), live in the intestinal tract and migrate to the muscles of the body, producing a disease known as cysticercosis. Infected patients have abdominal pain, weight loss, and obstruction of bile and pancreatic ducts. Tapeworms may be up to ten meters in length – yes, that's 30 feet – and their segments are often passed in the stools.

Onchocerca volvulus is a tiny roundworm. It is the cause of "river blindness" in Africa. Onchocerciasis is transmitted to humans by the bite of a black fly that lives near rivers. Attempts to control the disease have met with some success, using ivermectin and doxycycline. The Nobel Prize for Physiology or Medicine was awarded to William C. Campbell in 2015 for the discovery of ivermectin.[597]

Algae

Algae rarely cause human disease, but immunocompromised persons, such as those with HIV (human immunodeficiency virus) or AIDS (acquired immunodeficiency syndrome), are at risk for a disease known as Protothecosis, caused by members of the genus *Prototheca*. These are colorless algae that ordinarily are not pathogenic for humans. Reports of algae infecting the brain have been seen in patients who use saline nasal wash with tap water. Several types of shellfish harbor blue-green algae that are toxic to humans. These toxins may also be found in tap water.[598]

Fungi[599]

Fungal Diseases

Aspergillosis. More than 100 species exist of *Aspergillus*, a mold that is common in the environment, both indoors and outdoors. A green aspergilloma caused by *A. fumigatus* may develop in the lung as a "fungal ball," or aspergillosis may appear as a black sticky discharge in the ear canal of a springer spaniel, caused by *A. niger*. The drug of choice is an "azole" such as Itraconazole, or for intractable cases, a soluble form of amphotericin. Surgery is usually required for pulmonary aspergillomas.[600]

Blastomycosis is a rare infection that is caused by a fungus, *Blastomyces*. The fungus is present in moist soil and in decomposing organic matter such as wood and leaves. In the United States, the fungus is prevalent in the river valleys of the mid-west and south. Infections usually occur in patients with depressed immunity, or after exposure to a very large amount of the fungus. The infections may be localized, and treated with topical anti-fungal agents. Systemic infections can be deadly, requiring treatment with amphotericin B and other systemic fungicides.[601]

Candidiasis is a fungal infection caused by the *Candida*, a yeast, which normally lives on the skin and inside the body, in places such as the mouth, throat, gut, and vagina, without causing any problems. *Candida* may cause infections of the internal organs such as the kidney, heart, or brain. Candidiasis that develops in the mouth or throat is called thrush or oropharyngeal candidiasis. Candidiasis in the vagina is commonly referred to as a yeast infection.[602]

Coccidioidomycosis. Commonly called Valley Fever, "coccie" is an infection caused by spores of the fungus *Coccidioides*. The fungus is mainly located in the soil of the southwestern United States and parts of Mexico and further south in Latin America. People who live or travel through these areas commonly inhale the spores without any problem, although some people will get a transient flu-like illness. In some cases, pulmonary or meningeal coccidioidomycosis develops, which can be fatal.[603]

Ergotism – also known as St. Anthony's Fire. The fungus *Clavicepts purpurea* infects rye, producing a black mass of fungal filaments as the grain ripens. The mass is the source of the drug ergonovine, which produces profound constriction of arterial blood vessels. This is useful in the treatment of migraine and for control of hemorrhage in obstetrics, but it also causes miscarriage, temporary insanity, and death from gangrene. Ergot is the source from which lysergic acid diethylamide (LSD) is synthesized. Some people have speculated that the girls who gave false testimony in Salem in 1692 were deranged from ergotism, acquired from eating moldy bread.[604]

Fungal eye infections. These are rare but they are given a special place in the list of fungal diseases of humans. They are difficult to treat and can have a devastating, though rarely fatal, outcome. These infections of the eye are usually caused by a species of *Aspergillus* or *Candida*.

Histoplasmosis. Histoplasmosis is an infection caused by the fungus *Histoplasma*, which lives principally in soil that contains large amounts of bird or bat droppings. *Histoplasma* is located in the valley of the Ohio River and of the eastern drainage of the Mississippi River. A skin test has been developed, which shows that histoplasmosis is widespread among residents in this area. It is usually only a mild illness which may leave a residual small nodule in the lung.[605]

Mucormycosis is a serious but rare fungal infection caused by a group of molds which live in soil and in decaying organic matter, such as leaves, compost piles, or rotten wood. Mucormycosis is usually seen only in patients with depressed immunity, such as those who have had organ transplants. A slimy reddish infection of the skin is the clue to diagnosis.

Pneumocystis pneumonia (PCP) is a serious infection caused by the fungus *Pneumocystis jirovecii*. Most people who get PCP have a depressed immune system, such as HIV/AIDS, or are being treated with immunosuppressive medications. Antiretroviral therapy (ART) has reduced the risk of PCP.

Sporotrichosis (also known as "rose gardener's disease") is an infection caused by a fungus called *Sporothrix* which lives in soil and on plant matter such as rose bushes. Skin infection is the most common form of the disease. Sporotrichosis rarely infects internal organs, but when it does, the outcome is similar to the fungal infections noted above.

Antibiotics[606]

Antibiotic is defined by *Britannica* as a "chemical substance produced by a living organism, generally a microorganism, that is detrimental to other microorganisms." These organisms show the beneficial effects of some fungi on human illnesses, instead of the troublesome and lethal diseases described above.

Two antibiotics, gramicidin and tyrocidin, produced by *Bacillus*, were discovered in 1939 by Rene Dubos. They are too toxic for internal use, but are valuable for treating surface infections. Penicillin, obtained from the mold *Penicillium notatum*, was the first antibiotic found to be useful for a wide variety of infections. First used in 1942, penicillin was spectacularly effective against both streptococcus and staphylococcus. However, drug resistance soon appeared in staphylococcus. By the 1950s, derivatives were synthesized that expanded the spectrum of action of penicillin. So-called second and third generation penicillin derivatives have barely kept pace with resistance that has subsequently developed to antibiotics.[607]

Other classes of fungal-derived antibiotics have since been discovered. Streptomycin, derived from *Streptomyces griseus*, was found in 1943 to be active against the tuberculosis bacillus, and also typhoid. *S. venezuelae* is the source of the important antibiotic, chloramphenicol, which is used to treat malaria. Tetracycline (Achromycin) is derived from *S. aureofaciens*. *S. nodosus* is the source of amphotericin B (Fungizone). Neosporin, a powerful combination in an ointment of three antibiotics, is used for surface infections; they are neomycin, from *S. fradie*, bacitracin, and polymyxin. Other combinations of non-absorbable antibiotics include gramicidin. Cephalosporins, such as Cefalexin (Keflex), which are related to penicillin, are produced by *Cephalosporium acremonium*, and are often used in combination with Ciprofloxacin and Azithromycin. Drug resistance has become a world-wide problem, which has been accelerated by the indiscriminate use of antibiotics and from veterinary use of antibiotics in the food of domesticated animals such as hogs and cattle.[608]

Bacteria

Some examples of bacteria that affect humans and the diseases that they cause are:
Gram positive cocci:
> *Enterococcus*, including *E. faecalis*, "fecal" bacteria, which spreads infections from the colon.
> *Staphylococcus aureus*, "staph," causes boils, carbuncles, and antibiotic-resistant sepsis.
> *Streptococcus pyogenes* or "strep" is a major cause of death in the world, from scarlet fever, cellulitis, "flesh-eating" bacteria, rheumatic fever – afflicting the heart, joints, and kidneys – with meningitis, and pneumonia.
> *Streptococcus pneumoniae*, pneumococcus, caused lobar pneumonia, once known as the "old man's friend" because it permitted death to occur before senility. It can be prevented by Pneumovax.

Gram positive rods:
> *Clostridium botulinum* (anaerobe) causes "botulism," fatal paralysis; also used to paralyze facial muscles to mask the appearance of aging. It is present in poorly prepared food and in unpasteurized honey, and it may be lethal for children and others with no gastric acid to destroy the bacillus.
> *Clostridium perfringens* (anaerobe) causes "gas gangrene," a dreaded complication of wounds in World War I. It is rarely seen now. Antitoxin is an effective treatment. Equine antitoxin is raised in horses by repeated injections of attenuated living (toxin) or killed bacteria (toxoid). It is serum obtained from these horses. Antitoxins were used for several other deadly bacterial diseases that now respond to antibiotics and can be prevented with vaccines. Antitoxin is still the treatment of choice for bites of venomous snakes. Antitoxins prepared in horses sometimes produces a serious allergic reaction in humans. Convalescent (immune) human plasma is therefore preferred, when it is available.[609]
> *Clostridium tetani* (anaerobe), causes tetanus, "lock jaw"; it is a spore-former, like *C. botulinum*. Treatment originally was with antitoxin, but DPT vaccine is effective for prevention of tetanus, so the disease is now rarely seen. DPT vaccine prevents diphtheria, pertussis (whooping cough), and tetanus. It should be given to children, and repeated as scheduled, even in adults.[610]
> Diphtheria, caused by *Corynebacterium diphtheriae*, was one of the most common causes of death in America in the nineteenth century. The bacterium is ordinary a silent occupant of the mouth, but it can suddenly attack with vengeance.

Gram negative cocci:
> *Neisseria gonorrhoeae*, causes gonorrhea, "the clap," a venereal infection with secondary ramifications, such as ectopic pregnancy; it is now a "superbug."
> *Neisseria meningitidis*, meningococcus; normally present in about ten percent of people, but suddenly can cause fatal meningitis; a vaccine is available.

Gram negative coccobacillus:
> *Haemophilus influenzae*, a major cause of fatal influenza in children, and of other infections, causing miscarriage in pregnancy, and ear infections.
> Tularemia, caused by *Francisella tularensis,* is found in wild animals such as squirrels and rabbits, and is easily transmitted to humans, where it can be fatal. It is a potential bioweapon.

Gram negative rods:
> *Borrelia* species cause various forms of relapsing fevers, and Lyme disease, acquired from the bite of a blacklegged deer tick, producing a "bull's eye" rash and a wide range of bizarre miseries.

Brucellosis, in several species, causes undulant (recurring) fever and deaths; one species is *Brucella abortis,* the name of which shows its mode of misery in cattle, which miscarry before calving, to the distress of farm families.

Cholera is caused by *Vibrio cholerae*, a small bacterium which infects only humans, causing profuse diarrhea. Spread by infected sewage, it has caused enormous epidemics which millions of deaths.

Escherichia coli, E. coli. The most common commensal bacteria, quietly residing in the colon. Entero-toxic strains, known as ETEC, are a frequent cause of traveler's diarrhea and death.

Klebsiella aerogenes, formerly known as *Enterobacter*, is relatively harmless, but devastating infections can occur in debilitated patients.

Legionellosis or Legionnaire's disease; pneumonia, caused by *Legionella pneumophila*, was first seen at an American Legion convention in Philadelphia in 1976.

Leptospira causes leptospirosis, a disease common to many animals, and transmitted to humans who work with them, such as veterinarians, or in water that is contaminated. Unless treated promptly, it can cause kidney failure, and it has a high mortality rate.

Pasteurella multocida and other related *Pasteurella* are animal diseases that can be transmitted by bite or scratch to humans, and can be deadly.

Pertussis, "whooping cough," caused by *Bortadella pertussis*, which only infects humans. Vaccination with DPT is given to as many children as possible to insure herd immunity for all.[611]

Proteus mirabilis, a facultative anaerobe, is a major cause of urinary tract infections, especially in patients with indwelling catheters. It is resistant to many antibiotics, including second generation derivatives of penicillin, such as ampicillin. *Proteus* is a rapid swarmer in the laboratory.[612]

Pseudomonas aeruginosa and other pseudomonads are increasing due to their antibiotic resistance and genetic adaptability, supplanting weaker germs.

Shigella cause shigellosis (dysentery), which are major causes of death in the world. *Shigella* live in the lining of the intestinal tract, producing diarrhea. *S. dysenteriae and S. flexneri* are the major types.

Salmonella disease, salmonellosis, is now usually due to infections acquired from poorly cooked eggs or backyard poultry. *Salmonella enterica typhi* is the cause of typhoid fever, a potentially fatal disease, famously transmitted by "Typhoid Mary" in the U.S. A variant, paratyphoid, is similar.[613]

Spirochaeta. Spirochetes are an unusual order of gram-negative bacteria, some of which are visible without a microscope. They are coiled like corkscrews and are motile, with flagella. Some live in the mouth as commensals, but several species are serious pathogens.

Treponema pallidum is the cause of syphilis, known as the "great pox" when it first appeared in Europe, in contrast to the viral disease known as smallpox. Syphilis is usually a venereal disease, but it can be contracted in other ways, such as infants in the birth canal, which causes congenital syphilis. The disease passes through three distinct phases: chancre (the "genital sore"); then a transient rash; and tertiary syphilis, which mimics many other diseases and leads to a long, slow death. For example: *tabes dorsalis*, with excruciating back and leg pain; general paresis, with psychosis and dementia; and tumors of the heart, known as gummas.

Treponema pertenue cause yaws, a chronic disease that first was observed in America. It may have been transported to Europe, where it became the great pox (syphilis), and there is cross-immunity in the two diseases. Like syphilis, yaws, too, passes through three stages.

Yersinia pestis, formerly *Pasteurella pestis*, is the cause of plague. Three types are known: pneumonic, septicemic, and bubonic. The plague bacillus resides in the rat, and it is transmitted to humans by the Oriental rat flea, *Xenopsylla cheopsis*.[614]

Acid-fast bacteria: Discovered with new types of staining, and new methods for growing bacteria.

Mycobacterium tuberculosis, known as TB, is one of the most important problems of infectious disease at this time. "Consumption," as tuberculosis was formerly called, was the leading cause of death in Europe and North America from the 18th to the 20th century. Tuberculosis decreased with improved hygiene and antibiotics in the 1940s, but drug-resistant TB has again become a problem, as it infects patients debilitated with diseases such as HIV.

Mycobacterium leprae is the cause of leprosy, also known as Hansen's disease. It is usually a very slowly progressive disease, characterized by painless, disfiguring skin ulcerations. The peripheral nerves are damaged by the disease. Patients are permanently quarantined, and "leper" is a meme for a shunned person. Chemotherapy has been helpful.[615]

Mycobacterium bovis, also known as TB, is similar to *M. tuberculosis*, but it is transmitted in milk, instead of through the respiratory tract, so it has a different mode of progression through the body. TB testing of cows has controlled it, because cows that show a positive test are euthanized.

Filterable Infectious Agents[616]

Filterable infectious agents include *Mycoplasma*, Rickettsia, viruses, and prions. These agents remain infectious after passing through a diatomite or porcelain filter. Viruses were discussed in Chapter 9.

Mycoplasma

Mycoplasma are filterable agents. Nevertheless, they are considered to be bacteria, and they are among the smallest of that group of microorganisms. Mycoplasma must be cultured on chicken eggs, rather than on simple chemical media. Mycoplasma infect the lungs, joints, and the mucous membranes, causing disability but rarely death. *M. pneumoniae* is a cause of primary atypical pneumonia (PAP), also known as one form of "walking pneumonia" and also pleuropneumonia, which does not respond to traditional antibiotics, and can be fatal.[617]

Rickettsia[618]

Three genera of the family of Rickettsia are recognized: *Rickettsia, Coxiella,* and *Rochalimaea*. The Rickettsia are similar to gram-negative bacteria, but they cannot be cultured on chemical media and are usually grown on chicken eggs. Some are rod-shaped; others are variably spherical. Smaller than bacteria, they range from 0.3 to 0.5 micrometers in size. Most forms can only reproduce within animal cells, and cell culture is therefore crucial to their study in vitro. The Rickettsia are treatable with antibiotics, including several tetracyclines, and chloramphenicol for resistant cases.

Rickettsia, the largest genus of Rickettsia, is divided into three groups: typhus, spotted fever, and scrub typhus. Various species of *Rickettsia* cause the diseases known as epidemic typhus, endemic typhus, Brill-Zinsser disease, Rocky mountain spotted fever, and scrub typhus.[619]

Coxiella is the cause of Q fever. First recognized in Queensland, Australia, in 1935, and since then in various parts of Australia. It was seen during World War II in troops in Italy.

Rochalimaea, transmitted by the body louse, was the cause of trench fever in World War I.

Prions

Prions are subviral particles that cause a terrifying group of brain diseases, dementias, of humans and other mammals which are known as "transmissible spongiform encephalopathies." In humans, one form of the disease is known as Creutzfeldt-Jakob disease. Kuru, which was discovered in indigenous peoples in Papua New Guinea, is probably now extinct. Prion diseases also include "mad cow disease" and "scrapie" in sheep, and chronic wasting disease of mule deer and elk. These prion diseases are always fatal, and the course is long, slow, and difficult.

"Prion" is an acronym for "**pr**ote**i**nace**ou**s **in**fectious particle." Prions are formed as normal proteins of the brain are folded into abnormal shapes, by a process that is not fully understood. The infection is transmitted by contact with infected brain tissue. The disease has a long latent period, during which it can be passed to others who are susceptible. Prions are unusual infectious agents because they contain neither DNA or RNA, and they are therefore resistant to killing by ultraviolet light, which normally would destroy nucleic acids.[620]

Appendix C

More Doctors Afield

Actors: Physicians are rarely seen as actors on stage or in film. One exception is Sir Jonathan Miller, M.B., B.Chir., CBE (1934-2019). Miller trained as a gastroenterologist, but he became famous as an actor and director on stage and in films. Another exception is Haing S. Ngor (1940-66), a surgeon and gynecologist, who won the Academy Award for Best Supporting Actor in 1985. His life story is tragic. He barely survived in prison camps in Cambodia, where his wife died during delivery of their child, who also died. After he escaped to Thailand and he came as a refugee to the United States. Without previous acting experience, he obtained a role in *The Killing Fields* (1984), and was in several more films. He was murdered in a botched robbery. It is interesting that so few physicians have chosen to be professional actors, either part-time, or as a new career, because acting is an important part of the practice of medicine. It may be "method acting" (to inhabit the part), or "classic acting" (to appear to show empathy or imperturbability). Acting is a necessary aspect of the professional role of a physician, although perfection is elusive. A wise physician learns to don "the mask," figuratively speaking, to show a good bedside manner, if need be, but the mask of imperturbability can also hide impending burnout.[621]

Advocate: Dr. Nawal el Saadawi (1931-2021) was a physician, author and teacher. Having been subjected to genital mutilation herself as a child, she became an advocate for women's rights in the Arab world. She received her medical degree from Cairo University in 1954, and she practiced as a village physician as well as serving in the Health Ministry of Egypt. She persisted in spite of death threats.[622]

Anthropology: One might think there would be many physician-anthropologists, because anthropology is the academic field of the study of human beings. But as it was with actors, it is rare to encounter the name of famous anthropologist who was, or who became, a physician. The reason for this is probably because the field of medical anthropology developed recently and it is still a discipline in its growth phase. A search for those who are well-known outside the field in two recently published books reveals no familiar names. No single source is ever complete, however, and the name of Paul Farmer (b. 1959), M.D., Ph.D., Chairman of Global Health and Social Medicine at Harvard Medical School, should be mentioned. He has a doctorate in anthropology. The late Charles L. Bosk (c.1942-2020), Ph.D., M.D., was Professor of Sociology and Anesthesiology at the University of Pennsylvania. In his book, *Forgive and Remember*, Bosk described himself as an anthropologist who became a physician in order to study the profession of medicine.[623]

Architect: Alistair Mackenzie (1870-1934), F.R.C.S., was a landscape architect. He designed more than 50 golf courses, several of which are in the top ten golf courses in the world. He was also an outstanding *camofleur*, who designed camouflage for military purposes in World War I.

Athletes: James Naismith (1861-1939) invented the game of basketball in 1891. Nine years later, he received his M.D. degree from the University of Colorado. Sir Roger Bannister (1929-2013) ran the first 4-minute mile. He was knighted for his service as a physician.

Authors: This is the area in which more physicians appear as "Doctors Afield" with contributions outside of the fields of medicine and science. Claude Bernard (1813-1878), wrote a play, *Arthur de Bretagne*, as his first contribution to literature. It was a valiant effort, but it had limited success. His genius appeared later, as was mentioned in Part Two, when his writings focused on medical research and surgery. Bernard's scientific discoveries were carried forward in America by Walter Bradford Cannon (1871-1945). Cannon was the most important figure in the field of human physiology in America in the early twentieth century. His contributions were mentioned in Part One. Cannon's deceptively simple writing style enabled his autobiography, *The Way of an Investigator* (1945), to be a successful model for students and others who were interested in science. A contemporary of Cannon's on the faculty of Harvard Medical School, Hans Zinsser (1878-1940), was also a gifted writer, in addition to his career as a physician-scientist. His discoveries in microbiology were mentioned in Part One, as was his contribution to scientific writing for the lay public in *Rats, Lice and History*. His fictionalized memoir is unique. It was written in the third person as *As I Remember Him: The Biography of R. S.* (Gloucester, Mass.: Peter Smith, 1970).[624]

Sir William Osler (1849-1919), Bt., a Canadian physician, was one on the four founding professors of the medical school at Johns Hopkins University. He was later Regius Professor of Medicine at Oxford, where he founded the Medical History Society. Osler was a prolific writer, noted for his *Principles and Practice of Medicine* (1892) and for the essay *Aequanimitas*. Osler was devastated by the death of his only surviving son from wounds in World War I, and he soon died thereafter from complications of influenza. Sir William Osler was beloved by all who knew him. His biography was written by his protégé, Dr. Harvey Cushing (1869-1939), who has everlasting fame as the founder of the field of neurosurgery. Cushing's *The Life of Sir William Osler* (1925) won the Pulitzer Prize. Cushing's Disease and Cushing's Syndrome, named for him, are conditions that result from adrenal cortical hyperactivity, and the syndrome is also produced by excessive amounts of cortisone. Cushing was a surgeon with the Harvard Medical School unit in France in World War I. In his book, *From a Surgeon's Journal* (1936), Cushing tells of the sad story in which, by an astounding coincidence, he was called to operate on Sir William's son, Lieutenant Revere Osler. Cushing was promoted to colonel and was awarded the Army's Distinguished Service Medal. In contrast to Osler, Harvey Cushing was said by his contemporaries to have been uncooperative and ruthless. No tears were shed when he retired as Professor of Surgery at Harvard. Cushing moved back to his alma mater, Yale, with his immense collection of rare books, leaving only one small shelf of books at the Harvard Medical School library.[625]

Sir Arthur Conan Doyle (1859-1930) began his successful career with Sherlock Holmes stories in 1887. He continued to practice medicine. He was affected by the deaths of his brother and other members of his family during and shortly after World War I, and he became an advocate for spiritualism. Anton Chekov (1860-1904), Russian playwright and short story writer; author of *Uncle Vanya* and *The Cherry Tree*; he continued to practice medicine as he wrote. Another physician-playwright is William Carlos Williams (1883-1963), who was a family doctor in Paterson, New Jersey. In his practice, between patient visits in his office and after delivering babies walk-up apartments, he scribbled and typed poetry and wrote plays. He was Poet Laureate of the United States in 1952 and he received the Pulitzer Prize in 1963. William Somerset Maugham (1874-1965), who omitted his first name as an author, was a popular author of many novels. A. J. (Archibald Joseph) Cronin (1896-1981), Scottish physician and novelist; best known for *The Citadel* (1937), based on the life of a fictional village doctor who became a successful London physician. Lewis Thomas (1913-1993) was a prominent physician administrator and research scientist; was dean of the Yale Medical School and president of Memorial Sloan Kettering Cancer Institute; won many literary prizes for his essays, including *The Lives of a Cell: Notes of a Biology Watcher* (1974). Sherwin Nuland (1930-2014) was a surgeon at Yale University and the author of many award-winning books, including *The Art of Healing* (1992) and *How We Die: Reflections on Life's Final Chapter* (1994). His lectures for the Teaching Company were entitled *Doctors: The History of Scientific Medicine Revealed Through Biography* (2013). Oliver Sacks (1933-2015), CBE, FRCP, was a neurologist and author. His long list of publications includes *Awakenings*, which was adapted for a film of the same name starring Robin Williams (1990).

Business: Paul Adriann Jan, Baron Janssen (1926-2003), a Belgian physician with additional training in pharmacology, founded Janssen Pharmaceutica. His company developed more than 80 new drugs, including haloperidol, for schizophrenia; fentanyl; and Lomotil, which comforts travelers with loose stools. Both fentanyl and Lomotil are narcotics. Janssen is now a subsidiary of Johnson & Johnson. Three brothers, Arthur, Mortimer, and Raymond Sackler, were sons of an immigrant from Ukraine who established a grocery business in Brooklyn. The three brothers became physicians and specialized in psychiatry. In 1952, they purchased Purdue-Frederick, a small pharmaceutical company. Arthur Sackler was responsible for marketing, and the younger brothers ran the business. Arthur died in 1987, and his share was purchased from his estate by the younger brothers. They turned it into the company known as Purdue Pharma. In 1996, Purdue Pharma introduced the drug OxyContin, a slow-release form of oxycodone, which is a powerful oral semi-synthetic derivative of the opium poppy. OxyContin was originally praised by physicians and patients for its ability to control pain. However,

OxyContin became the centerpiece of the opioid epidemic that has killed more than 450,000 people in the United States in the past two decades.[626]

Criminals: It is sad to say, but there are many, so a few must suffice to illustrate the various ways that physicians have gone astray. Several others are mentioned elsewhere in this essay. Dr. H. H. (Herman Mudgett) Holmes (1861-1896) was "America's first known serial killer." He built a house that became known as "Murder Castle." Holmes is estimated to have killed more than 200 people before he was arrested in 1893 and sentenced to death. Dr. Marcel Petiot (1897-1946) had a good reputation with his patients as a doctor before World War II in Paris, but he was also killing and burning others, especially women and Jews, after stealing their money. Thirty corpses were found in his basement when he was arrested. He was guillotined. Jack Kevorkian (1928-2011), "Dr. Death," was a proponent of assisted suicide, and was sent to prison for his many assists using his unique "Suicide machine." Kevorkian was eventually released and he died at home. Dr. Harold Shipman (1946-2004) was a general practitioner in Lancashire, England, in the 1970s who murdered more than 236 patients. He apparently began with the intent of shortening lives that were unbearable, but he began to enjoy the work. A thrill killer, he hanged himself in prison. Dr. John Bodkin Adams (1899-1983) got away with it. No less than 163 of his patients died in coma, and 132 listed him in their wills. He was tried for murder, but he was found guilty only of minor offenses such as prescription fraud and lying on cremation forms. His trial was "one of the greatest murder trials of all time," but he regained his license to practice.[627]

Criminal insanity is demonstrated vividly, and sadly, in the case of William Chester Minor (1834-1920), an American Army surgeon who served in the Civil War and then moved to England. While in London, he developed schizophrenia with paranoid delusions, and he shot a man who he believed was breaking into his room. He was confined to a mental hospital from 1872 to 1910, where he retained access to his large personal library. He used the library to become a major contributor to the first edition of the Oxford English Dictionary. His bizarre behavior continued, however, and he amputated his own penis. Winston Churchill ordered his release and repatriation to America and he died in Connecticut.[628]

One of the most infamous physicians in fiction is "Dr. Hannibal Lecter," portrayed in several movies as a brilliant and eerily likeable gentleman, who serves his guests elegant dinners that are composed of well-prepared pieces of previous guests. Lecter's character, played by Anthony Hopkins in *The Silence of the Lambs* (1991) is believed to have been based on the careers of several serial killers, none of whom were physicians. I have not found conclusive evidence that shows any physician was a cannibal. That is a bit of good news, following the preceding accounts of murders and dismemberments by physicians.[629]

The questionable business affairs of some physicians and the illegality of billing practices of some group practices is discussed in the Health Care Industry.

Educators: William Danforth (1926-2020), Chancellor of Washington University, St. Louis; and Calvin Plimpton (1918-2007), President of Amherst College and of SUNY-Downstate Medical Center.

Espionage: The most successful spies are those that are unknown. In the 1960s and for several decades thereafter, the U.S. Navy required all Medical Officers to file a "Report of Ports and Countries Visited" when they returned from an overseas trip. The requirement and format for the report was included in a Naval Medical Command Instruction (NAVMEDCOMIST). That Instruction has vanished without a trace. Medical officers – physicians – have an opportunity to observe everything, while doing their usual work. Medical intelligence can be useful, for it reveals problems in regard to the health of a community or nation. If this is being done now for the United States is unknown to me. For a believable look at physician-spies, see the novels by Patrick O'Brian, CBE (1914-2000). He wrote several books that told of the adventures of an officer in the Royal Navy and his companion in arms, a ship's surgeon, at the end of the 18th century. Unknown to Captain Jack Aubrey, his surgeon – the fictional Doctor Stephen Maturin, FRS – was also a spy. *Master and Commander* and *The Far Side of the World* were two of these books. The plots were conflated in the script of the movie, which was filmed in the Galapagos Islands.[630]

Explorers: Eliza Kent Kane (1820-1857) was an Assistant Surgeon in the Navy. He commanded the ship *Advance*, which sailed further north than any ship had previously gone. Frozen into ice, wintering over, he returned to a hero's welcome in Philadelphia. Kane Basin at the northwest coast of Greenland is named for him. Arctic and Antarctic explorer Dr. Frederick Cook (1865-1940) was President of the Explorers Club. He reported that he was the first to summit Mt. McKinley (Denali) and that he reached the North Pole before Robert Peary. He published as his own work a dictionary of the Native islanders of Tierra del Fuego that was compiled by a missionary, but his claims are still debated.

Historians: Many physicians have distinguished themselves in the field of the history of medicine, and in the history of science as it is involved in medicine. These physicians are all familiar with history in general. However, I am unable to find a record of any physician who has published or gained repute as a teacher in the field of academic history, outside of medicine. An illuminating article by Howard Kushner discusses the separation of "academic medical historians" from "academic history." It was published in *The Lancet* in 2008. To mention but a few of the physicians who have made contributions to the history of medicine: Drs. John Shaw Billings (1838-1913), who created the National Library of Medicine and the *Index Medicus*; Fielding H. Garrison (1870-1935), who followed Billings as the Director of the National Library of Medicine, authored *Introduction to the History of Medicine* and with Leslie Morton, *A Medical Bibliography*; Sir William Osler (1849-1919), mentioned below; Owsei Temkin (1902-2002), Professor of the History of Medicine at Johns Hopkins University; and Ralph Major (1884-1970), Professor of the History of Medicine at Kansas University School of Medicine, whose work on the *History of Medicine* has been quoted many times in *Health Matters*.[631]

Humanitarians: Sir Wilfred Thomason Grenfell (1865-1940), KCMG, was a medical missionary to Newfoundland. He was awarded the first-ever honorary Doctorate in Medicine from Oxford. Grenfell's many books tell delightful stories of life in the frontier province of Canada. They were illustrated with his own water color sketches. Dr. Albert Schweitzer (1875-1985) was a true polymath, and also a theologian and humanitarian. He became famous as an organist in Germany for his interpretations of Bach, and he then became a doctor to the indigenous people in Labaréné, French Equatorial Africa. He was the author of *Aus meinem Leben und Denken*, and he received the Nobel Peace Prize in 1952. He inspired others to follow the same path, most famously William "Larry" Mellon (1910-1989), M.D., who used his personal fortune to establish a similar hospital in Haiti. Bernard Lown (1921-2021) and Yevgeniy Chazov (b. 1929) shared the Nobel Peace Prize in 1997 for forming the International Physicians for the Prevention of Nuclear War (IPPNW).

Inventors: Dr. W. K. (William Keith) Kellogg (1852-1943), was a physician, nutritionist, and inventor. Kellogg was the director of the Battle Creek Sanitarium and a member of the Seventh-Day Adventist Church. He established the Kellogg Company to manufacture corn flakes as a healthy breakfast food. William E. Upjohn (1853-1952) graduated in 1875 from the University of Michigan medical school. While practicing medicine, he began to experiment with ways to formulate friable pills. The inventions were marketed by his company, the Upjohn Pharmaceutical Company, in Kalamazoo, Michigan. The Upjohn company later developed a method for large scale production of cortisone. Upjohn has been a major benefactor in Kalamazoo. The company merged in 1995 with Pharmacia AB, and it was owned by Pfizer from 2015 until 2020. In that year, it merged with Mylan to form Viatris. Dr. Homer Stryker (1894-1980) was a surgeon and a brilliant inventor. He founded the Stryker Corporation in Kalamazoo, Michigan, which manufactures many useful orthopedic products. The company has also been a major benefactor for the people of Kalamazoo and the surrounding area.

Law: It may come as a surprise, but there is no one to offer as a physician-lawyer who is well known in history in either one field or the other, or as both a lawyer and physician. There have been many men and women with both degrees, M.D. and J.D. (formerly L.L.B.), but none have been famous throughout the world in either field. It appears to be rare to practice both simultaneously as both a lawyer and a physician. A typical person with these two degrees will be practicing malpractice law, usually confined to litigation on one side or the other; either for patients who allege malpractice, or for physicians, who are defendants in a suit. These are typically civil suits, alleging torts; if the physician is accused of a crime, such as an illegal abortion or tax evasion, a lawyer specializing in criminal law will usually be requested. The American Society of Law, Medicine and Ethics (ASLME) is a non-profit organization based in Boston, Mass., which draws its membership from both the legal and medical professions. It publishes two journals in this field. Recent presidents of the ASLME are drawn from one field or the other. There is also an organization known as the American Society of Legal Medicine, whose presidents all have had the degrees of MD and JD.[632]

Martyrs: The Roman Catholic Church has compiled a long list of physicians who were martyrs and gruesome accounts of their deaths. Some of their stories require suspension of belief in reality. The twins Cosmos and Damien were tortured to death in about 300 A.D. Not usually mentioned in the Church's official account of their life and death is the reason that they are the patron saints of surgeons. These brothers are said to have performed the first leg transplant, from a Black Moor who had just died to a white man from the Middle East whose leg was amputated for cancer. The hybrid recipient has been the subject of interesting works of art. The story of Saint Martin de Porres (d. 1639) is an inspiring exception to the general rule. A "half-caste" poor boy in Panama, Martin was apprenticed to a barber-surgeon. He became a Dominican lay-brother who founded a hospital, and is revered throughout the Americas for his gentle good works. His icon usually shows him as a Black man in a long frock with a broom in his hand. Saint Martin de Porres apparently did not die for his faith but he is nevertheless listed with the Catholic martyrs. Closer to the present, there are accounts of hundreds of physicians who have been persecuted and died in recent centuries, in their homes, in prisons, in open fields, and in concentration camps. One example must suffice: A list of 2,465 Polish Jewish physicians who died in the Holocaust.[633]

Military: Doctor Mary Edwards Walker, a surgeon with the Union Army in the Civil War, is the only woman to have been awarded the Medal of Honor. Vice Admiral Joel T. Boone, won the Medal of Honor as a young Navy medical officer with the Marines in World War I. Lieutenant Corydon M. Wassell, U.S. Navy, was awarded the Navy Cross for heroism in the Battle of Java in World War II; a movie, "*Dr. Wassell*" starred Gary Cooper.

Music: Hector Berlioz (1803-1869) was the son of a French provincial doctor. He attended medical school in Paris, but did not complete the course. His work as a composer and conductor was spectacular but he was considered to be independent. He won the Prix de Rome, but continued to be non-traditional. He is remembered for such works as the *Symphonie fantastique* and *La Damnation de Faust*. Alexander Borodin (1833-1887) was the illegitimate son of a Russian nobleman. Although his nominal father was a serf, Borodin was given the opportunity by his biological father to have a good education. He attended medical school in Saint Petersburg, and after graduation, he underwent additional medical training for several years. In 1862, he began to study musical composition. For the rest of his life, he mixed a successful academic career in medicine and chemistry with both the practice of medicine and with music. His most important musical works were *In the Steppes of Central Asia*, a symphonic poem, and an opera, *Prince Igor*.

Nursing: Colonel Christine E. Haycock (1924-2008), R.N., M.D., F.A.C.S., graduated from Presbyterian Hospital's nursing school and served in the Cadet Nurse Corps in World War II. She continued her registration as a nurse while attending medical school at Downstate Medical Center, from which she graduated in 1952. She was a trauma surgeon at the New Jersey Medical School, and she founded and was president of the American Medical Women's Association. She retired from the U.S. Army Reserve Medical Corps Reserve.

Politics and Government: Pope John XXI was an ophthalmologist and medical school faculty member in Siena before he was elected Pope in 1276. Dr. John Pott(s), who died in 1651, was the Crown Governor of Jamestown in 1629-30. He received the M.A. from Oxford 1605 and was the physician to the Virginia Company of London. Georges Clemenceau (1841-1929), Prime Minister of France, demanded that the Versailles Treaty include severe reparations from Germany, and thus contributed to the return to war in 1939. He received his medical degree in Paris in 1865, and it was there as a student that he became a political activist. He continued to practice medicine during his early career. Mohammad Najibullah (1947-1996), commonly known as Najibullah, and sometimes as Dr. Najib, was the brutal ruler of Afghanistan during the period when the USSR was dominant in that country. He qualified as a physician (MBBS) in 1965, but never practiced medicine. He was captured and killed by the Taliban. Other physicians, now deceased, who became Head of State, were Sun Yat-sen (1866-1925), first president of the Republic of China, briefly in office in 1912; Hastings Banda (1898-1997), president of Malawi from 1966-94; and Francois Duvalier (1907-1971), infamous president of Haiti from 1957-71.

Several other physicians who became Head of State as president or prime minister are still alive. Newspaper publisher Ernest Gruening (1887-1994), graduated from Hotchkiss and from college and medical school at Harvard. He found a career in journalism instead of medicine. He was elected as the first U.S. Senator from Alaska in 1969 and served in the Senate for ten years.[634]

Revolutionaries: In the American Revolutionary War, Benjamin Rush (1746-1813), a signer of the Declaration of Independence and surgeon in a front-line hospital at the Battle of Trenton; Gen. Hugh Mercer (1726-1777), a physician, was a line officer when he was killed at the Battle of Princeton; Dr. John Warren (1741-1775), a prominent Massachusetts leader, who fought as a private and was killed at the Battle of Bunker Hill. Counties in New Jersey are named for Mercer and Warren. Che Guevara, M.D., (1928-1967) was a prominent leader of the Cuban Revolution.

Other Stories about Physicians

Parenthetically, it is often instructive to read about physicians when their lives are viewed from the perspective of those who are not members of the medical profession. The writing may be realistic fiction, as in the life of "Will Kennicott" a doctor in a small town in the Midwest, which was told by Sinclair Lewis in *Main Street* (1920). The story is told through the eyes of his wife, "Carol." The book is perhaps the most famous of Lewis' novels. In 1930, Lewis (1885-1951) became the first American to win the Nobel Prize for Literature. Sinclair Lewis inspired many college students in the 1950s to become pre-meds with his true-to-life novel *Dr. Arrowsmith*, about a heroic although fictional physician. Or it may be one of the best accounts ever written of the profession of surgery, which in this case was composed by a non-physician, Jürgen Thorwald (1915-2006), as *The Century of the Surgeon* (1956). Thorwald was the runner up to Truman Capote for the Edgar Allen Poe award in 1966. Thorwald was the *nom de plume* of Heinz Bongartz, who was a propaganda writer for the Nazis. He had a comfortable life after the war in spite of his Nazi background. It is an example of how to admire the art, not the artist, as we do with Picasso and Wagner. The Nobel Prize-winning author, Boris Pasternak (1890-1960), wrote the novel, *Dr. Zhivago* (1957) about "Yuri Zhivago," a county doctor and poet in the Soviet Union prior to World War II. The book became an immensely popular movie in 1965, starring Julie Christie and Omar Shariff, with the haunting music of "Lara's Theme," accompanied by a solitary zither.[635]

Two Remarkable Doctors

Major General Leonard Wood (1860-1927), a country boy, born in New Hampshire and raised in a small town in Massachusetts, and with financial assistance he graduated from Harvard Medical School in 1884. After an internship in Boston, he found it difficult to earn a living as a physician in that city, which was crowded with doctors. He succeeded in competition to win a position as a contract physician with the U.S. Army. He worked his way up in the Army in a way that none before him, nor any after, has ever done. Physically strong, combative, and driven by ambition to succeed, he won the Medal of Honor as a physician on the successful expedition to capture Geronimo. The award of the medal was not automatic; Wood lobbied for years to receive it. He used his fame to become the White House physician for Presidents Grover Cleveland and William McKinley. He soon became acquainted with a fellow Harvard alum, Assistant Secretary of the Navy Theodore Roosevelt. They enjoyed recreational boxing with each other. In the meantime, Wood had transferred to become an Army line officer, though still a Volunteer.

Wood was Roosevelt's superior when T.R. led the Reserve regiment in the Spanish-American War that he had recruited known as the "Rough Riders." For his successful leadership of the charge to reach the summit of San Juan Hill, T.R. would belatedly, posthumously, receive the Medal of Honor. Wood was commander of American forces in Cuba in 1898, and after the war he was appointed Governor General of Cuba. He oversaw the work of the chief medical officer and later Army Surgeon General, Dr. William Gorgas (1854-1920), who authorized the research that was conducted by Dr. Walter Reed (1851-1902) in search of the cause of yellow fever. Wood, Gorgas, and Reed were successful. The disease was convincingly shown to be transmitted by the bite of an *Aedes* mosquito. It was accomplished with the loss of life of a volunteer nurse, Clara Maass, who died from a yellow fever-infected mosquito. This caused an immediate cessation in Reed's experiments. The discovery showed the necessity to create a mosquito-free environment in the jungle of Central America, enabling the U.S. to construct the Panama Canal.

At the time Leonard Wood was Governor General of the Philippines, he oversaw the brutal suppression of the islanders, while also helping control the problem of leprosy. The Leonard Wood Memorial of the American Leprosy Missions is named for him. In 1901, T.R. became Vice President when McKinley was elected for a second term. When McKinley was assassinated six months later, T.R. became president, and Wood continued with his upward trajectory. He became a Brigadier General in the Regular Army in 1901. Two years later, he was promoted to Major General and he continued with that rank on the Retired list in 1921. Wood's connection with high-level members of the Republican party enabled him to become Chief of Staff of the Army in 1910. Wood was sidelined by the Wilson administration, and he failed to achieve a leadership role in World War I. As a friend and colleague of Theodore Roosevelt, and with the support of T.R.'s politically well-connected daughter, Alice (Roosevelt) Longworth, Leonard Wood almost became the Republican Party's nominee for President in 1920. After many votes, with no clear winner, a compromise was made, and Warren G. Harding became the Republican candidate. Wood's end came at the Peter Bent Brigham Hospital in Boston from blood loss during a failed attempt by his friend, Dr. Harvey Cushing, to remove a recurrent benign brain tumor. It was said at Harvard to be one of the few times when Cushing showed emotion. Leonard Wood was famous when he was alive, but *Sic transit gloria mundi*.[636]

Michael Crichton (1942-2008) was also a graduate of the Harvard Medical School, but his career was vastly different from that of General Leonard Wood. The general was famous, but Crichton was a celebrity. Most people who read Crichton's books and see his films would never imagine that he was trained as a physician and that he took postgraduate training in medical research at the Salk Institute. Crichton began writing at an early age, and he published his first letter to the *New York Times* at the age of 14. He continued to write short stories and novels as he progressed through school to earn an undergraduate degree in anthropology at Harvard, *summa cum laude*. His first six novels, all published before he completed medical school, were written using a pseudonym, "John Lange." He then began to write using his own name, and in 1969, the year he received his M.D. degree, Crichton published his blockbuster novel, *The Andromeda Strain*, about the rapid spread of an imaginary new form of bacteria. It was a plausible and therefore supremely scary movie when it opened in 1971. By that time, Crichton had decided to make a career as a writer and film maker, so he never obtained a license to practice medicine. The pattern set in his early novels continued throughout the rest of his life. They combined, to varying degrees, elements of science, science fiction, dystopia, technology, suspense, and crime. Some were also leavened by a bit of humor. His science fiction novel, *Jurassic Park* (1990), based on cloning dinosaurs, was also made into a movie, with huge success. Crichton published 26 novels, several of which were incomplete at the time of his death and were published posthumously. His other works include a non-fiction study, *Five Patients* (1970), based on his experiences as a medical student, and *The Great Train Robbery* (1978). This was a fictional thriller based on an actual train robbery in the 19th century in England. It was made into a movie starring Sean Connery, which Crichton directed. Crichton knew the Hollywood system. He could either function as an independent producer, making "Indie" movies and films for television, or he could work and bargain with major film companies. Crichton was married five times and had two children; he died at age 66 of lymphoma, which was diagnosed earlier in that year. Though he is deceased, Michael Crichton is still a Hollywood celebrity.[637]

Appendix D

COVID-19

Listed Chronologically Within Sections as Shown Below

The Environment

• Lawrence Wright, The plague year, *New Yorker* (4 & 11 January 2021), 20-59, quotes from Matthew Pottinger on COVID-19, summarizing the disease from the fall of 2019 to January 2021. One month later, the origin of the virus was still unclear.

• Alina Chan and Matt Ridley, The world needs a real investigation into the origins of Covid-19, *The Wall Street Journal* (16-17 January 2021), C4: "The present pandemic of COVID-19 (coronavirus disease 2019) shows how modern travel has facilitated the spread of one biotic, a virus known as SARS-CoV-2 (severe acute respiratory syndrome coronavirus 2)."

• Gerry Shih and Emily Rauhala, WHO team no closer to learning origins of novel coronavirus, *Washington Post*, 10 February 2021, A17.

Social Connections

• August 2020 Sturgis Bike Rally linked to 260,000 COVID-19 cases. See: https://khn.org/morning-breakout/sturgis-biker-rally-linked-to-260000-covid-cases/ (accessed February 19, 2021).

• Mark Walker and Jack Healy, A motorcycle rally in a pandemic? *New York Times* (6 November 2020), at: https://www.nytimes.com/2020/11/06/us/sturgis-coronavirus-cases.html (accessed February 19, 2021); and https://www.facebook.com/SturgisBikeRally2021/ (accessed February 19, 2021).

• On August 27, 2020, the U.S. Environmental Protection Agency (EPA) gave emergency approval for a patented disinfectant, SusrfaceWise2, made by Allied BioScience. The active ingredient is said to be "a quaternary ammonium polymer coating," in a ratio that is a "trade secret." Mitigation includes hand sanitizing, which may be by cleansing the hands with soap or alcohol, or some other disinfectant. A concentration of 62.5 to 70 percent ethyl alcohol is in most hand sanitizers.

• Steven Mufson and Meryl Kornfield, Chemical experts question EPA's approval of coronavirus disinfectant, *Washington Post*, 27 August 2020, A7.

• Luisa A. Ikner, et al, A continuously active antimicrobial coating effective against human coronavirus 229E, at https://www.medrxiv.org/content/10.1101/2020.05.10.20097329v1.full.pdf (accessed August 27, 2020).

COVID-19 Chronology

• Anon., History's deadliest pandemics, from ancient Rome to modern America, *Washington Post*, 12 and 25 April 2020.

• Orhan Pamuk, What plague novels tell us, *New York Times*, 26 April 2020, 6.

• Kate Murphy, Why Zoom is terrible, *New York Times*, 29 April 2020.

• Megan Craig, The courage to be alone, *New York Times*, 3 May 2020, 10.

• Ruchir Shrama, How the pandemic is turning us inward, *New York Times*, 4 May 2020, A23.

• Anon., *New York Times*, 7 May 2020, 1: As hunger grows, G.O.P. pushes back over food stamps. Millions struggling during pandemic; Democrats seek to raise benefits.

• Michele L. Norris, *Washington Post*, 7 May 2020, A25: "We're normalizing the threat of chaos and violence."

• An Pan, Li Liu, Chaolong Wang, et al, Association of public health interventions with the epidemiology of the COVID-19 outbreak in Wuhan, China, *JAMA* 323 (no. 19, May 10, 2020): 1915-23 [12 authors]:

"A series of multifaceted public health interventions was temporally associated with improved control of the COFVID-19 outbreak in Wuhan, China."
- "COVID-19 Special Edition" was published by Alpha Omega Alpha Honor Medical Society in September 2020: *The Pharos* (Summer 2020) 1-64. Notable articles include Richard L. Byyny [editor of *Pharos*], All things considered… The future of the U.S. health care "system," (pages 3-10) [ellipses in original; Byyny is the editor of *Pharos*]; Richard Bronson, Penumbra (p. 11, a poem); Richard B. Gunderman, Courage in the time of coronavirus (pp. 12-15); Edward C. Halperin, A summer reading list for new medical students during a pandemic (pp. 16-20); Charles S. Bryan, COVID-19: What would Osler say? (pp. 21-24); and Steven A. Wartman, Intimations of mortality (pp. 26-30), with two charts that show the timeline of history and mortality of pandemics from the Antonine Plague of 165-180 CE to COVID-19 (pp 2, 38).
- David Quammen, Consider the virus's point of view, *New York Times*, 20 September 2020, SR5: "Measured by the cold logic of evolution: The career of SARS-CoV-2 so far is, in Darwinian terms, a great success story … Bad luck for us. But evolution is not rigged to please Homo sapiens. … Will we ever be rid of it entirely, now that it's a human virus? Probably not? Will we ever get past the travails of this Covid-19 emergency? Yes."
- In November, 2020, the journal *JAMA* published two articles which showed the impact of COVID-19 at that time. The personal view from a physician working during the crisis was seen in Stephane Parks Taylor, Shear forces, *JAMA* 324 (no. 19, November 17, 2020): 1943-4: "I too felt intense, oppositional forces simultaneously applied to the competing priorities of work and family, and it seemed to be tearing me apart." A comment from the Chief of the NIAID [Fauci] was given by Andrea M. Lerner, Gregory K. Folkers, and Anthony S. Fauci, Preventing the spread of SARS-CoV-2 with masks and other "low-tech" interventions, *JAMA* 324 (no. 19, November 17, 2020):1935-6: "Return to normalcy will require the widespread acceptance and adoption of mask wearing and other inexpensive and effective interventions as part of the COVID-19 prevention toolbox."
- In December 2020, COVID problem in prisoners was mentioned by Christopher Blackwell, Covid-19 is rampant in prisons like mine. We need the vaccine early, *Washington Post*, 13 December 2020, B1-4.
- Steven H. Woolf, Derek A. Chapman, and John Hyung Lee, COVID-19 as [sic] the leading cause of death in the United States, *JAMA* 325 (no. 2, January 12, 2021):123-4: "With COVID-19 mortality rates now exceeding these thresholds, this infections disease has become deadlier than heart disease and cancer." On January 20, 2021, the total of deaths from COVID-19 in the United States reached approximately 400,000. This was the date on which Joseph R. Biden was inaugurated as President. The authors amplified the information in April 2021: Steven H. Woolf, Derek A. Chapman, Roy T. Sabo, et al., Excess deaths from COVID-19 and other causes in the US, March 1, 2020, to January 2, 2021, *JAMA*. Published online April 2, 2021. Doi:10.1001/jama.2021.5199: "A study analyzing US mortality in March-July 2020 reported a 20% increase in excess deaths, only partly explained by COVID-19. …Between March 1, 2020, and January 2, 2021, the US experienced 2,801,439 deaths, 22.9% more than expected, representing 522,368 excess deaths."
- Lyz Lenz, Welcome to Iowa, a state that just doesn't care if you live or die, *Washington Post*, 15 February 2021, B4: "Our governor is pretending that we defeated the pandemic … Last weekend, Iowa Gov. Kim Reynolds (R) lifted all pandemic restrictions. There was no explanation, no warning. … Iowa ranks as the 47th worst state for per capita vaccine distribution from the federal government and 46th-worst in the rate of administering doses to residents. ... But the reality is that 'Iowa nice' has become nothing more than Iowa do-nothingness: a passive acceptance of the carnage."
- A day-by-day log of first year of COVID-19 was the subject of Reis Thebault, Tim Meko and Junne Alcantara, Sorrow, stamina, defiance, despair: A pandemic year, *Washington Post* (14 March 2021), A1, 16-17. Three graphs show the numbers for the past year in the U.S. of total cases (29,354,140; yesterday 52,691); deaths (total 532,229; yesterday 1,085); and vaccine doses administered (total 105,703,501; yesterday 4,575,496).
- Another look at the first year of COVID-19 was published as a collection of personal stories and pictures in *New York Times*, Sunday Review (14 March 2021), 1-14. The lead story was Leslie Jamison,

We longed for the "Before Times." It was accompanied by a silhouette of a mother and child, looking sadly out of a mostly shuttered window.

Irrational Behavior
▪ Opposing views were seen in the *Washington Post* on 14 November 2020. Robert Barnes, In stern speech, Alito laments restrictions on freedoms during pandemic, *Washington Post*, 14 November 2020, A5. Samuel Alito is an Associate Justice of the Supreme Court. His lecture was considered to be an unusual political statement when it was made by a high court justice. In contrast: Editorial, It isn't hard to mandate masks: Republican Governors are wrong to rely on 'personal responsibility' alone, *Washington Post*, 14 November 2020, A18.

Choices
▪ Sarah Watson, et al, A new front in America's pandemic: College towns, *New York Times*, 6 September 2020: "'If people get sick, they get sick — it happens,' Mady Hanson, a 21-year-old exercise science major [at the University of Iowa], said last week on campus. She added that she and her household had survived Covid-19 and that she resented town's 'ridiculous' restrictions. *'We're all farmers and don't really care about germs*, so if we get it, we get it and we have the immunity to it'." From https://www.nytimes.com/2020/09/06/us/colleges-coronavirus-students.html (accessed September 9, 2020).

Endemic – Epidemic – Pandemic
▪ In the first two months after patients with COVID-19 were diagnosed in Wuhan, China, the disease spread quickly around the world. The impact of the disease varied greatly. On February 26, 2020, the CDC reported only 61 cases in the U.S.: https://emergency.cdc.gov/han/2020/han00428.asp (accessed January 9, 2021). This soon changed, "During a 3-week period in late February to early March, the number of U.S. COVID-19 cases increased more than 1,000-fold": https://www.cdc.gov/mmwr/volumes/69/wr/mm6918e2.htm (accessed January 9, 2021). On March 11, the World Health Organization (WHO) "declared that the COVID-19 outbreak is a pandemic": https://www.alnap.org/help-library/gender-alert-for-covid-19-outbreak-march-2020 (accessed January 9, 2021).
▪ Jeffrey F. Addicott, COVID-19 pandemic: policy and legal Issues, *Officer Review, The Military Order of the World Wars* (March-April 2020), 7-9.
▪ Rochelle P. Walensky and Carlos de Rio, From mitigation to containment of the COVID-19 pandemic: Putting the SARS-CoV-2 genie back in the bottle, *JAMA* 323 (no. 19, May 19, 2020): 1889-90. Walensky was appointed to be the Chief of the Centers of Disease Control (CDC) by President Biden.
▪ By May 2020, a cost of $500 billion and $30 billion in Medicare and Medicaid expenses due to COVID appeared to be possible, and because of the decrease expected in Gross Domestic Product (GDP), "health care would comprise 20% of GDP next year." See Sherry Glied and Helen Levy, The potential effects of coronavirus on national health expenditures, *JAMA* 323 (no. 20, May 26, 2020): 2001-2. The current status of COVID-19 in that month was summarized by Saad B. Omer, Preeti Malani, and Carlos del Rio, The COVID-19 pandemic in the U.S.: A clinical update, *JAMA* 323 (no. 18, May 12, 2020): 1767-8. "The estimated timeline for availability of an initial vaccine is between early and mid-2021."
▪ Poignant comments about COVID patients' deaths and the impact on survivors soon became commonplace in newspapers and magazines. Four examples: Elliot Rosenberg, A case of polio-covid double jeopardy, *Washington Post*, 23 May 2020, A17. Somini Sengupta, Disasters with twice the misery: When global warming collides with a pandemic, *Washington Post* (May 24, 2020), A19. David von Drehle, How to honor our new memories, *Washington Post*, 24 May 2020, A25. [von Drehle survived COVID-19] Whitney Ellenby, The coronavirus forced me to explain death to my autistic son, *Washington Post*, 26 May 2020, A19. The pandemic caused others to reflect on eschatology and the meaning of life. Roger Cohen, No return to the "Old Dispensation," *Washington Post*, 13 May 2020, A26.
▪ Six months into the pandemic, *JAMA* summarized the problem for patients: Anon., What is COVID-19? *JAMA* 324 (no. 8, August 25, 2020): 816.

- Many unintended consequences of COVID-19 have been reported. Two examples are: Jay A. Pandit, Memento mori, *JAMA* 324 (no. 17, November 3, 2020): 1731-2; and Frances Stead Sellers, "Science in real time": From funding to publishing, crisis rewrites the rules, *Washington Post*, 25 October 2020, A23.
- Jesse L. Goodman, John D. Grabenstein, and M. Miles Braun, Answering key questions about COVID-19 vaccines, *JAMA* 324 (no. 20, November 24, 2020), 2027-8.
- Saad B. Omer, Inci Yildirim, and Howard P. Forman, Herd immunity and implications for SARS-CoV-2 control, *JAMA* 324 (no. 20, November 24, 2020): 2095-6.
- Alyssa Bilinski and Ezekiel J. Emanuel, COVID-19 and excess all-cause mortality in the US and 18 comparison countries, *JAMA* 324 (no. 20, November 24): 2.
- Jeffrey H. Toney and Stephanie Ishack, A pandemic of confusion, *American Scientist* 108 (November-December 2020): 344-5.
- COVID-19: The first patients with the disease now known as COVID-19 were treated in Wuhan, China, in December 2019, and were reported on December 30 by an ophthalmologist, Dr. Li Wenliang (1986-2020). Dr. Li died in his own hospital on February 7. The Chinese government secretly controlled all information about his death (see *New York Times*, 20 December 2020). On March 11, 2020, the Director General of the World Health Organization (WHO) declared that COVID-19 was a pandemic. Anthony Fauci, quoted by J. R. McNeill, Covid-19 can protect us from the next pandemic, *Washington Post*, 30 July 2020, A21. McNeill said that COVID-19 has caused "more than 650,000 deaths worldwide and counting."
- Howard Bauchner, 2020-a year that will be remembered, *JAMA* 324 (no. 3, July 21, 2020): 245. Bauchner was the editor of *JAMA*.
- George Will, A year [1942] as disruptive as 2020, *Washington Post*, 26 July 2020, A23.
- By September 2020, the world-wide incidence of COVID-19 cases had reached 33.2 million, with nearly 1 million deaths, and 7.1 million cases and 204,000 deaths in the United States. *JAMA* 324 (no. 12, September 22/24, 2020): 1153-6.
- *New York Times Book Review*, 15 November 2020, 1, 20: David Quammen, Our pandemic future, reviewing Nicholas A. Christakis, *Apollo's Arrow: The Profound and Enduring Impact of Coronavirus on the Way We Live* (Boston: Little, Brown Spark, 2020), predicts an ominous future.
- "Fever greater than 99.9F" at: https://yalehealth.yale.edu/covid-19-monitor-your-health (accessed February 2, 2021). Cape Cod Health: "The U.S. Centers for Disease Control and Prevention (CDC) lists fever as one criterion for screening for COVID-19 and considers a person to have a fever if their temperature registers 100.4 or higher." From: https://www.capecodhealth.org/medical-services/infectious-disease/coronavirus/is-temperature-a-good-marker-for-covid-19/ (accessed January 2, 2021).
- On a single day, in February 2021, inequities and uncertainties were reported from Maryland to Massachusetts. Hallie Miller, Alex Mann and Jean Marbella, Vaccine numbers add to confusion, *Baltimore Sun*, 13 February 2021, 1.
- Lola Fadulu and Antonio Olivo, Va. pauses shot sign-ups to launch new system," *Washington Post*, 13 February 2021, B1.
- Colbert I. King, D.C.'s vaccine disparity didn't have to happen, *Washington Post*, 13 February 2021, A19.
- Ellen Barry, Taking 75-year old for vaccine is new way to qualify for one, *New York Times*, 13 February 2021, 1.
- David von Drehle, What 500,000 covid-19 deaths means, *Washington Post*, 21 February 2021, A29. He pointed out that a death toll of 480,000 or more in one year had been predicted by James Lawler at the University of Nebraska Medical Center in February 2020.
- Controversy over the management of the COVID-19 crisis by the Trump administration is reflected in the paper by Philip A. Pizzo, David Spiegel, and Michelle M. Mello, When physicians engage in practices that threaten the nation's health, *JAMA* 325 (no. 8, 23 February 2021): 723-4. The only physician named was Dr. Scott Atlas, who was appointed to the White House Coronavirus Task Force in 2020. "Nearly all public health experts were concerned that his recommendations could led to tens of thousands (or more) of unnecessary deaths in the US alone." There were also a "number of leaders in federal, state, and local

government … who ignored or dismissed science, refused to promote sensible, effective practice such as mask wearing and social distancing [and] contributed to the US having more infections and deaths than other developed nations in proportion to population size."

▪ Viral variants began to appear as early as March and April 2020, with a new variant called D614G. The situation was reviewed a year later by John P. Moore and Paul A. Offit, SARS-CoV-2 vaccines and the growing threat of viral variants, *JAMA* 325 (no. 9, 2 March 2021): 821-2. The mutation of greatest concern in March 2021 was the N501Y change in the B.1.1.7 variant, which was "sufficient to almost ablate the activity of several nMABs" (virus neutralizing antibodies).

▪ April 2021, a fourth wave of infection appeared to be rising in the U.S., fueled by the B.1.1.7 variant.

▪ Carlos del Rio and Preeti Malani, COVID-19 in 2021: Continuing uncertainty, *JAMA* 325 (no. 14, 13 April 2021): 1389-90. "More than a year has passed since the first confirmed case of SARS-CoV-2 infection in the US was reported on January 20, 2020." The authors discuss eight topics to "perform calculations to balance competing risks." A week later: Athalia Christie, Sarah A. Mbaeyi, and Rochelle P. Walensky, CDC Interim recommendations for fully vaccinated people: An important first step, *JAMA* 325 (no. 15, 20 April 2021): 1501-2: "CDC still recommends … for all people …a well-fitting mask when in public [and] postponing travel."

▪ May 13, 2021: Rochelle Walensky, now head of CDC, announced that "Fully vaccinated people need not wear masks or physically distancing in most cases" and they "can resume activities that they did prior to the pandemic." The sudden change in CDC policy caught the White House by surprise. See Editorial, A pandemic turning point, *Washington Post* (16 May 2021), A32. The exceptions were for such locations as hospitals and clinics, and for those who were expected to be immunocompromised. No requirement to prove vaccination status was included in the CDC announcement.

▪ July 2021. Eva Dou, Lyric Li, Chico Harlan and Rick Noack, The global search for covid-19's patient zero, *Washington Post* (8 July 2021). "On December 8, 2019, the accountant began to feel ill. He did not frequent Wuhan's Huanan seafood market." Patient SO1, China's first confirmed case, surnamed Chen, was said by Li Wenliang to have fallen ill on December 16, and another account says that he fell ill on Dec. 20. But on Dec 5, 2019, a 5-year-old boy in Milan, Italy, tested positive for coronavirus RNA – a finding discovered many months later. Researchers in France have found hints of the virus in November 2019, and antibodies were later detected in patients in Italy in September 2019. As of 8 July 2021, 33,754, 027 cases had been reported in the U.S., and 605,694 deaths. Daniel E. Slotnik, World's official Covid-19 death toll passes 4 million amid vaccine inequities, *Washington Post* (9 July 2021), A4: but this is "widely believed to undercount pandemic-related deaths."

Heath Care Industry

▪ Vaccines against COVID-19 were developed much earlier than was expected, but the availability failed to meet expectations. Annette Rid and Mark Lipsitch, The ethics of continuing placebo in SARS-CoV-2 vaccine trials, *JAMA* 325 (no. 3, 19 January 2021):219-20.

▪ Steven Joffe, Evaluating SARS-CoV-2 vaccines after emergency use authorization or licensing of initial candidate vaccines, *JAMA* 325 (no. 3, 19 January 2021): 221-2.

Appendix E

Hippocratic Oath Variations

From the National Library of Medicine[638]

I swear by Apollo the physician, and Asclepius, and Hygieia and Panacea and all the gods and goddesses as my witnesses, that, according to my ability and judgement, I will keep this Oath and this contract:

To hold him who taught me this art equally dear to me as my parents, to be a partner in life with him, and to fulfill his needs when required; to look upon his offspring as equal to my own siblings, and to teach them this art, if they shall wish to learn it, without fee or contract; and that by the set rules, lectures, and every other mode of instruction, I will impart a knowledge of the art to my own sons, and those of my teachers, and to students bound by this contract and having sworn this Oath to the law of medicine, but to no others.

I will use those dietary regimens which will benefit my patients according to my greatest ability and judgement, and I will do no harm or injustice to them.

I will not give a lethal drug to anyone if I am asked, nor will I advise such a plan; and similarly, I will not give a woman a pessary to cause an abortion.

In purity and according to divine law will I carry out my life and my art.

I will not use the knife, even upon those suffering from stones, but I will leave this to those who are trained in this craft.

Into whatever home I go, I will enter them for the benefit of the sick, avoiding any voluntary act of impropriety or corruption, including the seduction of women or men, whether they are free men or slaves. Whatever I see or hear in the lives of my patients, whether in connection with my professional practice or not, which ought not to be spoken of outside, I will keep secret, as considering all such things to be private.

So long as I maintain this Oath faithfully and without corruption, may it be granted to me to partake of life fully and the practice of my art, gaining the respect of all men for all time. However, should I transgress this oath and violate it, may the opposite be my fate.

Another Classic Version of the Hippocratic Oath[639]

I swear by Apollo Physician and Asclepius and Hygieia and Panaceia and all the gods and goddesses, making them my witnesses, that I will fulfil according to my ability and judgment this oath and this covenant:

To hold him who has taught me this art as equal to my parents and to live my life in partnership with him, and if he is in need of money to give him a share of mine, and to regard his offspring as equal to my brothers in male lineage and to teach them this art - if they desire to learn it - without fee and covenant; to give a share of precepts and oral instruction and all the other learning to my sons and to the sons of him who has instructed me and to pupils who have signed the covenant and have taken an oath according to the medical law, but no one else.

I will apply dietetic measures for the benefit of the sick according to my ability and judgment; I will keep them from harm and injustice.

I will neither give a deadly drug to anybody who asked for it, nor will I make a suggestion to this effect. Similarly, I will not give to a woman an abortive remedy. In purity and holiness, I will guard my life and my art.

I will not use the knife, not even on sufferers from stone, but will withdraw in favor of such men as are engaged in this work.

Whatever houses I may visit, I will come for the benefit of the sick, remaining free of all intentional injustice, of all mischief and in particular of sexual relations with both female and male persons, be they free or slaves.

What I may see or hear in the course of the treatment or even outside of the treatment in regard to the life of men, which on no account one must spread abroad, I will keep to myself, holding such things shameful to be spoken about.

If I fulfil this oath and do not violate it, may it be granted to me to enjoy life and art, being honored with fame among all men for all time to come; if I transgress it and swear falsely, may the opposite of all this be my lot.

A Modern Version of the Hippocratic Oath[640]

I swear to fulfill, to the best of my ability and judgment, this covenant:

I will respect the hard-won scientific gains of those physicians in whose steps I walk, and gladly share such knowledge as is mine with those who are to follow.

I will apply, for the benefit of the sick, all measures which are required, avoiding those twin traps of overtreatment and therapeutic nihilism.

I will remember that there is art to medicine as well as science, and that warmth, sympathy, and understanding may outweigh the surgeon's knife or the chemist's drug.

I will not be ashamed to say "I know not," nor will I fail to call in my colleagues when the skills of another are needed for a patient's recovery.

I will respect the privacy of my patients, for their problems are not disclosed to me that the world may know. Most especially must I tread with care in matters of life and death. If it is given me to save a life, all thanks. But it may also be within my power to take a life; this awesome responsibility must be faced with great humbleness and awareness of my own frailty. Above all, I must not play at God.

I will remember that I do not treat a fever chart, a cancerous growth, but a sick human being, whose illness may affect the person's family and economic stability. My responsibility includes these related problems, if I am to care adequately for the sick.

I will prevent disease whenever I can, for prevention is preferable to cure.

I will remember that I remain a member of society, with special obligations to all my fellow human beings, those sound of mind and body as well as the infirm.

If I do not violate this oath, may I enjoy life and art, respected while I live and remembered with affection thereafter. May I always act so as to preserve the finest traditions of my calling and may I long experience the joy of healing those who seek my help.

Note: This version of the Hippocratic Oath omits the promise in the Classic versions not to use a "deadly drug," or not to cause an "abortion," or to use "the knife." It also states that a physician may have the "awesome responsibility" to "take a life."

Bibliography

Books

Adams, Charles Francis. *Familiar Letters of John Adams and His Wife Abigail Adams, During the Revolution with a Memoir of Mrs. Adams.* Boston: Houghton Mifflin Company, 1875.

Altman, Lawrence K. *Who Goes First: The Story of Self-Experimentation in Medicine.* New York: Random House, 1987.

Arendt, Hannah, *Eichmann in Jerusalem: A Report on the Banality of Evil.* Munchen: Piper, 1945.

Ambrose, Stephen. *Band of Brothers: E Company, 506th Regiment, 101st Airborne: From Normandy to Hitler's Eagle's Nest.* New York: Simon & Schuster, 1992.

_____. *Undaunted Courage: Meriwether Lewis, Thomas Jefferson, and the Opening of the American West.* New York: Simon & Schuster, 1996.

Anderson, Hans Christian. *Anderson's Fairy Tales Told in Words of One Syllable.* 1835. Akron, Ohio: Saalfield Publishing Co., n.d. [c. 1931].

Aronson, Marc, and Marina Budhos, *Sugar Changed the World: A Story of Magic, Spice, Slavery, Freedom, and Science.* New York: Clarion Books, 2010.

Atkinson, Rick. *The Guns at Last Light: The War in Western Europe, 1944-1945.* New York: Henry Holt and Company, 2013.

Bacon, John U. *The Great Halifax Explosion: A World War I Story of Treachery, Tragedy, and Extraordinary Heroism.* New York: HarperCollins, 2017.

Baker, David W. *The Joint Commission's Pain Standards: Origins and Evolution.* Oakbrook Terrace, Ill: The Joint Commission, 2017.

Baldwin, Neal. *Edison: Inventing the Century.* New York: Hyperion, 1995.

Baron, Samuel, ed. *Medical Microbiology.* 4th ed. Galveston, Tex.: University of Texas Medical Branch, 1996.

Barry, John M. *The Great Influenza: The Story of the Deadliest Pandemic in History.* New York: Penguin, 2005. New York: Penguin Random House LLC, 2018.

Baum, L. Frank. *Wizard of Oz.* New York: Grosset & Dunlap, 1944.

Bernard, Claude. *Introduction à la médecine expérimentale (An Introduction to the Study of Experimental Medicine).* 1865.

_____ and Charles Huette, *Illustrated manual of operative surgery and surgical anatomy* [title translated]. 1855.

Besse, Joseph. *A Collection of the Sufferings of the People called Quakers for the Testimony of a Good Conscience.* London: Luke Hinde, 1753.

Blaser, Martin J. *Missing Microbes: How the Overuse of Antibiotics is Fueling Our Modern Plagues.* London: Picador, 2015.

Bosk, Charles S. *Forgive and Remember: Managing Medical Failure.* Chicago: University of Chicago Press, 1979.

Bradford, William. *Of Plymouth Plantation, 1620-1647.* Edited and introduced by Samuel Eliot Morison. Franklin Center, Pa.: Franklin Library, 1983.

Brands, H. W. *The Zealot and the Emancipator: John Brown, Abraham Lincoln, and the Struggle for American Freedom.* New York: Doubleday, 2020.

Breverton, Terry. *Immortal Words: History's Most Memorable Quotations and the Stories Behind Them.* London: Quercus Publishing Plc., 2009.

Brokaw, Tom. *The Greatest Generation.* New York: Penguin Random House, 1998.

Bronte, Emily. *Wuthering Heights.* London: Thomas Cautley Newby, 1847.

Brown, Dee. *Bury My Heart at Wounded Knee: An Indian History of the American West.* New York: Henry Holt, 1970.

Browne, Sir Thomas. *Religio Medici.* 1643.

Bryson, Bill. *A Short History of Almost Everything.* New York: Broadway Books, 2003.
Buckner, Fillmore. *Versatile Physicians.* Heritage Books, 2002.
_____. *Versatile Physicians II: Physicians the Medical Historians Forgot.* Heritage Books, 2009.
Bugliosi, Vincent, and Curt Gentry. *Helter Skelter: The True Story of the Manson Murders.* New York: W. W. Norton & Company, 1974.
Burdick, Eugene, and William Lederer. *The Ugly American.* New York: Norton, 1958.
Butler, Thomas. *Plague and Other Yersinia Infections.* New York: Plenum Publishing Corp., 1983.
Butterfield, Herbert. *The Whig Interpretation of History.* 1931. New York: W. W. Norton & Company, 1965.
Bynum, William. *A Little History of Science.* New Haven: Yale University Press, 2012.
_____. *The History of Medicine: A Very Short Introduction.* Oxford: Oxford University Press, 2008.
Byrd, Richard Evelyn. *Alone.* New York: G. P. Putnam's Sons, 1938.
Caesar, Julius. *Commentarii.* Trans. H. J. Edwards. *The Gallic War.* Cambridge, Mass.: Harvard University Press, 2015.
Camus, Albert. *La Peste* [*The Plague*]. Paris: Gallimard, 1947.
Cannon, LeGrand, Jr. *Look to the Mountain.* 1942. New York: Golden Apple Publishers, 1983.
Cannon, Walter B. *The Wisdom of the Body.* New York: W. W. Norton, 1932.
_____. *The Way of an Investigator.* New York: W. W. Norton, 1945.
Capote, Truman. *In Cold Blood.* New York: Random House, 1966.
Carson, Rachel. *Silent Spring.* New York: Houghton Mifflin Co., 1962.
Carroll, Lewis [Charles Dodgson]. *Alice's Adventures in Wonderland.* London: Macmillan, 1865.
Cather, Willa. *Oh, Pioneers.* Boston: Houghton, Mifflin Co., 1913.
_____. *My Ántonia.* Boston: Houghton Mifflin Harcourt, 1918.
Chaucer, Geoffrey. *The Canterbury Tales,* trans. Nevill Coghill. New York: Penguin Group, 1951.
Cherry-Garrard, Apsley. *The Worst Journey in the World.* London: Constable & Co., 1922.
Christie, Agatha. *The Pale Horse.* London: Collins Crime Club, 1961.
Churchill, Winston. *The World Crisis.* vol. 1, *1911-1914.* New York: Scribner's, 1924.
_____. *The Second World War.* 6 vols. Boston: Houghton Mifflin Co., 1948-1953. vol. 1. *The Gathering Storm,* 1948. vol. 5. *Triumph and Tragedy,* 1953.
Clancy, Tom. *Executive Orders.* New York: G. P. Putnam's Sons, 1996.
Coffin, J. M., S. H. Hughes, and H. E. Varmus, eds. *Retroviruses.* Cold Spring Harbor, N.Y.: Cold Spring Harbor Laboratory Press, 1997.
Collins, Wilkie. *The Moonstone.* London, Tinsley Brothers, 1868.
Conrad, Joseph. *Heart of Darkness.* London: Blackwood's Magazine, [serial 1899] 1902.
Cooper, Kenneth. *Aerobics.* New York: Bantam Books, 1968.
Crosby, Alfred W., Jr. *The Columbian Exchange: Biological and Cultural Consequences of 1492.* 1973. Westport, Conn.: Praeger Publishers, 2003.
Curran, Mary G. McCrea, Howard Spiro, and Deborah St. James, eds. *Doctors Afield.* New Haven, Conn.: Yale University Press, 1999.
Cushing, Harvey. *The Life of Sir William Osler,* 3vols. Oxford: Oxford University Press, 1926.
_____. *From a Surgeon's Journal, 1915-1918.* Boston: Little Brown and Co., 1936.
Cutler, Elliot, and Robert M. Zollinger. *Atlas of Surgical Operations.* New York: Macmillan, 1944.
Darnton, Robert Choate. *The Forbidden Best-Sellers of Pre-Revolutionary France.* New York: Norton, 1996.
Darwin, Charles. *On the Origin of Species by Means of Natural Selection, or the Preservation of Favoured Races in the Struggle for Life.* London: John Murray, 1859.
_____. *The Descent of Man.* London: John Murray, 1871.
Daschle, Tom, S. S. Greenberger and J. M. Lambrew. *Critical: What We Can Do About the Health Care Crisis.* New York: Thomas Dunne Books, 2008.
Dawson, Kate Winkler. *Death in the Air: The True Story of a Serial Killer, the Great London Smog, and the Strangling of a City.* New York: Hachette Books, 2017.

de Kruif, Paul. *Microbe Hunters:* New York: Harcourt, Brace, 1926.

Demos, John Putnam. *A Little Commonwealth: Family Life in Plymouth Colony*. New York: Oxford University Press, 1970.

_____. *Entertaining Satan: Witchcraft and the Culture of Early New England*. New York: Oxford University Press, 1982.

_____. *The Unredeemed Captive: A Family Story from Early America*. New York: Vintage, 1994.

Descartes, Rene. *Discourse on the Method*, 1637.

DeVoto, Bernard. *The Year of Decision, 1846*. Boston: Houghton Mifflin, 1942.

Diamond, Jared. *Guns, Germs, and Steel: The Fates of Human Societies*. New York: W. W. Norton, 1997.

Dickens, Charles. *Oliver Twist*. London: Richard Bentley, 1839.

_____. *A Christmas Carol*. London: Chapman and Hall, 1843.

_____. *Bleak House*. London: Bradbury & Evans, 1853.

_____. *A Tale of Two Cities*. London: Chapman and Hall, 1859.

Donnachie, Ian, and George Hewitt. *Historic New Lanark: The Dale and Owen Industrial Community since 1785*. Edinburgh: Edinburgh University Press, 1993.

Dostoyevsky, Fyodor. *Crime and Punishment*. 1867.

_____. *The Brothers Karamazov.* 1880.

Douglas, Ed. *Himalaya: A Human History.* New York, W. W. Norton, 2020.

Douglas, Mary. *Purity and Danger: An Analysis of Concepts of Pollution and Taboo.* New York: Praeger Publishers, 1996.

Douglas, Mary, and Aaron Wildavsky. *Risk and Culture: An Essay on the Selection of Technical and Environmental Dangers.* Berkeley: University of California Press, 1982.

Doyle, Arthur Conan. *A Study in Scarlet.* London: Ward Lock & Co., 1887.

_____. *The Adventures of Sherlock Holmes.* London: George Newnes, 1892.

Draper, William. *History of the Conflict between Religion and Science.* New York: D. Appleton and Co., 1874

Du Mez, Kristen Kobes. *Jesus and John Wayne: How White Evangelicals Corrupted a Faith and Fractured a Nation.* New York: W. W. Norton, 2020.

Dulles, Foster Rhea. *The American Red Cross.* New York: Harper and Brothers, 1950.

Durant, Will, and Ariel Durant. *The Story of Civilization.* 11 vols. New York: Simon & Schuster, 1935-1975.

Ebers papyrus. c.1500 BCE. *The Papyrus Ebers: The Greatest Egyptian Medical Document.* Translated by Bendix Ebbell. Copenhagen: Levin & Munksgaard, 1937.

Eight Translation New Testament. The New Testament of Our Lord and Saviour Jesus Christ. Wheaton, Ill.: Tyndale House Publishers, Inc., 1974.

Enders, Gordon. *Foreign Devil: The Adventures of an American 'Kim' in Modern Asia.* New York: Simon & Schuster, 1942.

Engels, Friedrich. *Die Lage der arbeitenden Klasse in England.* 1845.

Fall, Bernard. *Street without Joy. Indochina at war, 1946-54.* Harrisburg: Stockpole Co., 1961.

Farmer, Paul. *Infections and Inequalities: The Modern Plagues.* Berkeley, University of California Press, 1999.

_____. *Pathologies of Power: Health, Human Rights, and the New War on the Poor.* Berkeley, University of California Press, 2003.

Faulkner, William. *Requiem for a Nun.* New York: Random House, 1951.

Faust, Drew. *This Republic of Suffering.* New York: Vintage Books, 2009.

Fay, Sidney Bradshaw. *The Origins of the World War.* 2 vols. New York: The Macmillan Company, 1928.

Fenn, Elizabeth. *Pox Americana: The Great Smallpox Epidemic of 1775-82.* New York: Hill and Wang, 2001.

Feynman, Richard. *Feynman's Lost Lecture: The Motion of Planets Around the Sun.* New York: W. W. Norton, 1996.

Fisher, David Hackett. *Albion's Seed: Four British Folkways in America.* New York: Oxford University Press, 1989.

_____. *Washington's Crossing.* New York: Oxford University Press, 2004.

Fitzgerald, F. Scott. *The Great Gatsby.* New York: Charles Scribner's Sons, 1925.

Follett, Ken. *The Pillars of the Earth.* New York: Macmillan, 1989.

_____. *A Column of Fire.* New York: Penguin Random House, LLC, 2017.

Foote, Shelby. *Shiloh.* New York: Dial Press, 1952.

Foster, Feather Schwartz. *The First Ladies: From Martha Washington to Mamie Eisenhower, an Intimate Portrait of the Women Who Shaped America.* Naperville, Ill.: Sourcebooks, 2011.

Foucault, Michel. *The History of Sexuality.* New York: Pantheon Books, 1978.

Fox, Robin Lane. *The Invention of Medicine: From Homer to Hippocrates.* New York: Basic Books, 2020.

Frank, Anne. *The Diary of Anne Frank.* 1947. trans. New York: Doubleday & Co., 1952.

Franklin, Benjamin. *The Autobiography of Benjamin Franklin.* 1791. Boston: Houghton Mifflin & Co., 1928.

Frazer, J. G. [James George]. *The Golden Bough: A Study in Magic and Religion.* 1890. New York: Oxford University Press, 1994.

_____. *The Golden Bough: A Study in Magic and Religion*, edited with an Introduction and Notes by Robert Fraser. 1890. Oxford: Oxford University Press, 2009.

Fulton, John Farquhar. *Harvey Cushing A Biography.* Springfield, Illinois: Charles C Thomas, 1946.

Fussell, Paul. *The Great War and Modern Memory.* 1974. New York: Sterling, 2009.

Galton, Francis. *Hereditary Genius: An Inquiry into Its Laws and Consequences.* London: Macmillan, 1869.

Geison, Gerald. *The Private Science of Louis Pasteur.* Princeton, N.J.: Princeton University Press, 1995.

Gibbon, Edward. *The History of the Decline and Fall of the Roman Empire.* 6 vols. London: Strahan & Cadell, 1776-1789.

Gilbo, Patrick F. *The American Red Cross: The First Century.* New York: Harper and Row, 1981.

Glemser, Bernard. *Mr. Burkitt and Africa.* New York: World Publishing Co., 1970

Godfrey-Smith, Peter. *Metazoa: Animal Life and the Birth of the Mind.* New York: Farrar, Straus & Giroux, 2020.

Goldfarb, Ben. *Eager: The Surprising Secret Life of Beavers and Why They Matter.* White River Junction, Vt.: Chelsea Green Publishing, 2018.

Goldsmith, Donald, and Tobias Owen. *The Search for Life in the Universe.* 3rd ed. Sausalito, Calif.: University Science Books, 2001.

Gordon-Reed, Annette. *Thomas Jefferson and Sally Hemings: An American Controversy.* Charlottesville, Virginia: University of Virginia Press, 1997.

_____. *The Hemingses of Monticello: An American Family.* New York: W. W. Norton & Co., 2008.

Gottlieb, Robert. *Forcing the Spring: The Transformation of the American Environmental Movement.* Washington, D.C.: Island Press, 1993.

Gutierrez, Ramon A. *When Jesus Came, the Corn Mothers Went Away: Marriage, Sexuality, and Power in New Mexico, 1500-1846.* Stanford, California: Stanford University Press, 1991.

Gwande, Atul. *The Checklist Manifesto: How to Get Things Right.* New York: Henry Holt and Company, 2009.

Hagedorn, Hermann, *Leonard Wood: A Biography.* New York: Harper & Brothers, 1931.

Hammett, Dashiell. *The Maltese Falcon.* New York: Alfred A. Knopf, 1930.

Hardin, Jeff, Ronald L. Numbers, and Ronald A. Binzley. *The Warfare between Science & Religion: The Idea That Wouldn't Die.* Baltimore: Johns Hopkins University Press, 2018.

Hardy, Thomas. *Far from the Madding Crowd.* London: Cornhill Magazine, 1874.

_____. *Tess of the d'Urbervilles: A Pure Woman Faithfully Presented.* London: James R. Osgood, McIlvaine & Co., 1891.
Harris, S. H. *Factories of Death: Japanese Biological Warfare, 1932—1945, and the American Cover-up.* New York: Routledge, 2002.
Harris, Thomas. *The Silence of the Lambs.* New York: St. Martin's Press, 1988.
Harvey, William. *De Motu Cordis.* 1628.
Hawthorne, Nathaniel. *The Scarlet Letter.* Boston, Mass.: Ticknor, Reed & Fields, 1850.
_____. *House of the Seven Gables.* Boston, Mass.: Ticknor and Fields, 1851.
Heffer, Simon. *The Age of Decadence: A History of Britain, 1860-1914.* New York: Pegasus Books, 2021.
Heinlein, Robert A. *The Moon Is a Harsh Mistress.* New York: G. P. Putnam's Sons, 1966.
Hemingway, Ernest. *The Sun Also Rises.* New York: Scribner's, 1926.
_____. *A Farewell to Arms.* New York: Scribner's, 1929.
Henrich, Joseph. *The Weirdest People in the World: How the West Became Psychologically Peculiar and Particularly Prosperous.* New York: Farrar, Straus & Giroux, 2020.
Hersey, John. *Hiroshima.* New York: Alfred A. Knopf, 1946.
Hill, George J. *Leprosy in Five Young Men.* Boulder: Associated Press of the University of Colorado, 1970.
_____. *Outpatient Surgery.* Philadelphia: W. B. Saunders Co., 1973.
_____, with John Horton. *Clinical Oncology.* Philadelphia: W. B. Saunders Co., 1977.
_____. *Edison's Environment: The Great Inventor Was Also a Great Polluter*, 3d ed. 2007. Berwyn Heights, Md.: Heritage Books, 2107.
_____. *Proceed to Peshawar.* Annapolis: Naval Institute Press, 2013.
_____. *Rolling with Patton: The Letters and Photographs of Field Director Gerald L. Hill, 303rd Infantry Regiment, 97th "Trident" Division, 1943-1945.* Berwyn Heights, Md.: Heritage Books, 2020.
_____. *The Home Front in World War II: From the Letters of Essie Mae Hill to Field Director Gerald L. Hill.* Berwyn Heights, Md.: Heritage Books, 2020.
_____. *War Letters, 1917-1918: From Dr. William T. Shoemaker, A.E.F., in France, and His Family in Philadelphia.* Berwyn Heights, Md.: Heritage Books, 2021.
Hill, Helene Z. *Hidden Data: The Blind Eye of Science.* 3d ed. 2016. Baltimore, Maryland: Bookwhip, 2019.
Hitler, Adolph. *Mein Kampf* [*My Struggle*]. Munich: Franz Eher Nachfolger, 1925-1926.
Homer, *The Iliad.* c.8th c. BCE.
_____, *The Odyssey.* c.7–8th c. BCE.
Horton, John, and George J. Hill. *Clinical Oncology.* Philadelphia: W. B. Saunders Co., 1977.
Hughes, Thomas Proctor. *Medicine in Virginia, 1607-1689* (Hamburg: Trendition Classics, 2012).
Huxley, Aldous. *Brave New World.* London: Chatto and Windus, 1932.
Isaacson, Walter. *Benjamin Franklin: An American Life.* New York: Simon & Schuster, 2003.
Irving, Washington. "The Legend of Sleepy Hollow" and 'Rip Van Winkle," in *The Sketch Book of Geoffrey Crayon, Gent. No. 1.* New York: C. S. Van Winkle, 1819.
James, William. *Principles of Psychology.* New York: Henry Holt and Company, 1890.
Jacobsen, Ann M. *Operation Paperclip: The Secret Intelligence Program that Brought Nazi Scientists to America.* Boston: Little, Brown, 2014.
Jacobson, Michael. *Salt Wars: The Battle Over the Biggest Killer in the American Diet.* Boston: MIT Press, 2020.
James, P. D. [Phyllis Dorothy, Baroness, OBE]. *The Children of Men.* New York: Alfred A. Knopf, 1992.
Josephson, Matthew. *The Robber Barons: The Great American Capitalists, 1861-1901.* New York: Harcourt, Brace and Company, 1934.
_____. *Edison: A Biography.* New York: McGraw Hill, 1959.
Joyce, James. *Ulysses.* Paris: Shakespeare and Company, 1922.

Julian, John, ed. *A Dictionary of Hymnology: Setting for the Origin and History of Christian Hymns of all Ages and Nations.* Second revised edition. N.p. 1907. New York: Dover Publications, 1957.

Junger, Sebastian. *The Perfect Storm: A True Story of Men Against the Sea.* New York: W. W. Norton, 1997.

Kafka, Franz. *Der Prozess* [*The Trial*]. Leipzig: Kurt Wolff Verlag, 1925.

_____. *Das Schloss* [*The Castle*]. Leipzig: Kurt Wolff Verlag, 1926.

Karlsen, Carol F. *The Devil in the Shape of a Woman: Witchcraft in Colonial New England.* 1987. New York: Random House, 1989.

Keefe, Patrick Radden. *Empire of Pain: The Secret History of the Sackler Dynasty.* New York: Doubleday, 2010.

Keller, Werner. trans. William Neil. *The Bible as History: A Confirmation of the Book of Books.* 13th ed. 1956. New York: William Morrow and Company, 1964.

_____. *The Bible as History in Pictures.* 1963. New York: William Morrow and Company, 1964.

Kinsey, Alfred C., Wardell B. Pomeroy, and Clyde E. Martin. *Sexual Behavior in the Human Male.* Philadelphia: W. B. Saunders Co., 1948.

_____, with Paul Gebhard. *Sexual Behavior in the Human Female.* Philadelphia: W. B. Saunders Co., 1953.

Kipling, Rudyard. *Kim.* 1901. Mineola, N.Y.: Dover Publications, 2005.

Klass, Perri. *A Good Time to be Born: How Science and Public Health Gave Children a Future.* New York: W. W. Norton & Company, 2020.

Kline, Adam. *The Current War: A Battle Story Between Two Electrical Titans, Thomas Edison and George Westinghouse.* Np.: CreateSpace, 2017.

Kuhn, Thomas S. *The Structure of Scientific Revolutions.* Introductory Essay by Ian Hacking. 1962. 4th ed. Chicago: The University of Chicago Press, 2012.

Laennec, René T. H. *Traité de l'auscultation mediate.* 1819.

Lansing, Alfred. *Endurance: Shackleton's Incredible Voyage.* London: Hodder & Stoughton. 1959.

Leakey, Meave, with Samira Leakey. *The Sediments of Time: My Lifelong Search for the Past* (Boston: Houghton Mifflin Harcourt, 2020.

Lebo, Kate. *The Book of Difficult Fruit: Arguments for the Tart, Tender, and Unruly (with Recipes).* New York: Farrar, Straus & Giroux, 2021.

Lee, Harper. *To Kill a Mockingbird.* Philadelphia, Pa.: J. B. Lippincott Co., 1960.

_____. *Go Set a Watchman.* New York: HarperCollins, 2015.

Lewis, Sinclair. *Main Street.* New York: Harcourt, Brace & Co., 1920.

_____. *Arrowsmith.* New York: Harcourt Brace & Co., 1925.

Lieberman, Daniel E. *Exercised: Why something We Never Evolved to Do is Healthy and Rewarding.* New York: Parthenon, 2020.

Lincoln, Abraham. *Gettysburg Address.* 1863. In Edward Everett, *An Oration Delivered on the Battlefield of Gettysburg (November 19, 1863).* New York: Baker & Godwin, 1863.

Lindberg, David C. *The Beginnings of Western Science: The European Scientific Tradition in Philosophical, Religious, and Institutional Context, Prehistory to A.D. 1450.* 1992. 2nd ed. Chicago: The University of Chicago Press, 2007.

Lindsay, David. *Mayflower Bastard: A Stranger Among the Pilgrims.* New York: St. Martin's Press, 2002.

Loewen, James W. *Lies My Teacher Told Me: Everything Your American History Textbook Got Wrong.* 1995. New York: Simon & Schuster, 2007.

Logevall, Fredrik. *JFK: Coming of Age in the American Century, 1917-1956.* New York: Random House, 2020.

London, Jack. *White Fang.* New York: Macmillan, 1906.

Longfellow, Henry Wadsworth. *Evangeline, A Tale of Acadie.* Boston: William D. Ticknor and Company, 1847.

Maclean, Norman. *Young Men and Fire*. Chicago: University of Chicago Press, 1992.
Mahan, Alfred Thayer. *The Influence of Sea Power upon History, 1660-1783*. Boston: Little, Brown and Co., 1890.
Mailer, Norman. *The Naked and the Dead*. New York: Rinehart & Company, 1948.
Margulis, Lynn. *Symbiotic Planet: A New Look at Evolution*. New York: Basic Books. 1998.
Major, Ralph H. *A History of Medicine*. 2 vols. Springfield, Ill.: Charles C. Thomas, 1954.
Malthus, Thomas Robert [originally anon.]. *Essay on the Principle of Population as It Affects the Future Improvement of Society, with Remarks on the Speculations of Mr. Godwin, M. Condorcet, and Other Writers*, 1798.
Mather, Cotton. *The Angel of Bethesda: An Essay upon the Common Maladies of Mankind*, c.1632. Gordon W. Jones, ed. Barre, Mass.: American Antiquarian Society, 1972.
Melville, Herman. *Moby Dick*. London: Richard Bentley, 1851.
Michener, James A. *Chesapeake*. New York: Random House, 1978.
Miller, Arthur. *The Crucible*. 1952. Introduction by Christopher Bigsby. New York: Penguin Books, 1995.
Miller, Perry. *Errand into the Wilderness*. Cambridge, Mass.: Harvard University Press, 1956.
Mann, Thomas. *Der Tod in Venedig* [*Death in Venice*]. Berlin: S. Fischer Verlag, 1912.
_____. *Der Zauberberg* [*The Magic Mountain*]. 1924. trans. Helen Tracy Lowe-Porter. London: Secker and Warburg, 1927.
Martin, Betty. *Miracle at Carville*. Garden City: Doubleday, 1950.
Marx, Karl Heinrich. *Manifest der Kommunistischen Partei*, 1848.
_____, completed by Friedrich Engels. *Das Kapital*, 1867.
McMurtry, Larry. *Dead Man's Walk*. New York: Simon & Schuster, 1995.
McNeill, John Robert. *Mosquito Empires: Ecology and War in the Greater Caribbean, 1640–1914*. New York: Cambridge University Press, 2010.
McNeill, William H. *Plagues and Peoples*. 1975. Garden City, N.Y.: Random House, Inc., 1998.
McPhee, John. *Coming in to the Country*. New York: Farrar, Straus, and Giroux, 1976.
Miles, Jack. *God: A Biography*. New York: Knopf, 1995.
Miller, BJ [sic], and Soshana Berger. *A Beginner's Guide to the End: Practical Advice for Living Life and Facing Death*. New York: Simon & Schuster, 2021.
Milton, John. *Paradise Lost*, 1667.
Mintz, Sidney W. *Sweetness and Power: The Place of Sugar in Modern History*. New York: Wiley, 1985.
Mitford, Jessica. *The American Way of Death*. New York: Simon & Schuster, 1963.
Montgomery, Lucy Maud. *Ann of Green Gables*. Boston: L. C. Page & Co., 1908.
Moore, Kate. *The Radium Girls: The Dark Story of America's Shining Women*. Naperville, Ill.: Sourcebooks, Inc. 2017.
Moran, Lord. See: Wilson, Sir Charles.
[Morton, George] *Mourt's Relation*, 1622. Probably edited and published by George Morton.
Mukherjee, Siddhartha. *The Emperor of All Maladies: A Biography of Cancer*. New York: Scribner's, 2010.
Mumford, Lewis. *Technics and Civilization*. Chicago: University of Chicago Press, 1934.
Murphy, Bryan. *81 Days Below Zero: The Incredible Survival Story of a World War II Pilot in Alaska's Frozen Wilderness*. New York: Hachette Books, 2015.
Nabokov, Vladimir. *Lolita*. Paris: Olympia Press, 1955.
Nasar, Sylvia. *A Beautiful Mind*. New York: Simon & Schuster, 1998.
Nestor, James. *Breath: The New Science of a Lost Art*. New York: Penguin Random House Riverhead Books, 2020.
Noble, David F. *America by Design: Science, Technology, and the Rise of Corporate Capitalism*. New York: Alfred A. Knopf, 1977.
Nordhoff, Charles, and James Hall, *Mutiny on the Bounty*. Boston: Little, Brown and Company, 1932.
Norton, Mary Beth. *In the Devil's Snare*. New York: Random House, 2002.

O'Brian, Patrick. *Master and Commander*. Philadelphia: Lippincott, 1969.

_____. *The Far. Side of the World*. London: Collins, 1984.

Offit, Paul. *The Cutter Incident: How America's First Polio Vaccine Led to the Growing Vaccine Crisis*. New Haven: Yale University Press, 2007.

One Thousand and One Nights. 8th – 14th Century. trans. Malcolm C. Lyons and Ursula Lyons. 3 vols. New York: Penguin Classics, 2003.

Orwell, George. *Animal Farm: A Fairy Story*. London: Secker and Warburg, 1945.

_____. *Nineteen Eighty-four*. London: Secker and Warburg, 1949.

Osler, Sir William. *The Principles and Practice of Medicine*. New York: D. Appleton & Co., 1892.

_____. *Aequanimitas*. 1889. Philadelphia: P. Blakiston's & Co., 1910.

Pasternak, Boris. *Dr. Zhivago*. trans. New York: Pantheon Books, 1957.

Pattison, Kermit. *Fossil Men: The Quest for the Oldest Skeleton and the Origins of Humankind*. New York: William Morrow, 2020.

Payer, Lynn. *Medicine and Culture: Notions of Health and Sickness in Britain, the U.S., France and West Germany*. New York: Macmillan, 1989.

Philbrick, Nathaniel. *Mayflower: A Story of Courage, Community, and War*. New York: Viking Pilgrim, 2006.

Poe, Edgar Allen. *The Complete Tales and Poems of Edgar Allan Poe*. New York: Vintage Books, 1975. Includes: "The Pit and the Pendulum," 1842. "The Masque of the Red Death," 1842. "The Premature Burial," 1844. "The Murders in the Rue Morgue,"1841.

Porter, Roy. *The Greatest Benefit to Mankind: A Medical History of Humanity*. 1997. New York: W. W. Norton, 1999.

Rabelais, Francois. *The Histories of Gargantua and Pantagruel*, trans. John Michael Cohen. New York: Penguin, 1955.

Raushway, Eric. *Why the New Deal Matters*. New Haven: Yale University Press, 2021.

Reisman, David, Nathan Glazer and Reuel Denney. *The Lonely Crowd: A Study of the Changing American Character*. New Haven, Conn.: Yale University Press, 1950.

Reiterman, Tom, and John Jacobs. *Raven: The Untold Story of Rev. Jim Jones and His People*. New York: E. P. Dutton, 1982.

Rothwell, Jonathan. *A Republic of Equals: A Manifesto for a Just Society*. Princeton: Princeton University Press, 2019.

Rose, Jonathan F. P. *The Well-Tempered City: What Modern Science, Ancient Civilizations and Human Nature Teach Us About the Future of Urban Life*. New York: HarperCollins, 2016.

Ross, Elizabeth Kubler, and David Kessler, *On Grief and Grieving: Finding the Meaning of Grief Through the Five Stages of Loss*. 1969. New York: Scribner's, 2005.

Rouché, Berton. *Eleven Blue Men and Other Narratives of Medical Detection*. Boston: Little, Brown, and Co., 1953.

_____. *The Incurable Wound*. New York: Berkley Publishing Corp., 1958.

Rowlandson, Mary. *A True History of the Captivity and Restoration of Mrs. Mary Rowlandson, a Minister's Wife in New England*. 1682. N.p.: Createspace, 2017.

Rowling, J. K. *Philosopher's Stone*. London: Bloomsbury Publishing. 1997. The first Harry Potter book.

Rubenfeld, Sheldon, and Daniel P. Sulmasy (eds.). *Physician-Assisted Suicide and Euthanasia: Before, During and After the Holocaust*. Lanham, Md: Lexington Books, 2020.

Rubenstein, Howard. *Romance of the Western Chamber*. La Jolla, Calif.: Granite Hills Press, 2020.

Rush, Benjamin. *Medical Inquiries and Observations upon the Diseases of the Mind*, 1812.

Russo, Jean B., and J. Elliott Russo. *Planting an Empire: The Early Chesapeake in British North America*. Washington, D.C: Smithsonian Libraries, 2012.

Saadawi, Nawal el. *The Hidden Face of Eve: Women in the Arab World*, 1977. trans. Sherif Hetata. New York: Zed Books, 1980.

Sachs, Oliver. *Awakenings*. New York: Duckworth and Co., 1973

_____. *The Man Who Mistook His Wife for a Hat*. London: Gerald Duckworth, 1985.
Safina, Carl. *Becoming Wild: How Animal Cultures Raise Families, Create Beauty, and Achieve Peace*. New York: Henry Holt & Co., 2020.
Sagan, Carl. *Cosmos*. New York: Random House, 1980.
Saillant, Francine, and Serge Genest. *Anthropologie médicale. Ancrages locaux, défis globaux (Medical anthropology. Local roots, global challenges)*. In French. Quebec: Les presses de l'Université Laval, 2005.
_____. *Medical Anthropology: Regional Perspectives and Shared Concerns*. Malden, Mass.: Blackwell, 2007.
Sala, Enric. *The Nature of Nature: Why We Need the Wild*. Washington, D.C.: National Geographic Partners, LLC, 2020.
Sanger, Jonathan. *Making the Elephant Man: A Producer's Memoir*. Jefferson, N.C.: McFarland & Co., 2016.
Schiff, Stacy. *A Great Improvisation: Franklin, France, and the Birth of America*. New York: Henry Holt, 2005.
_____. *Cleopatra: A Life*. Boston: Little Brown & Co., 2010.
Sebba, Anne. *American Jennie: The Remarkable Life of Lady Randolph Churchill*. New York: W. W. Norton & Co., 2007.
Segal, Nancy L. *Born Together – Reared Apart*. Cambridge: Harvard University Press, 2012.
Seton, Anya. *The Winthrop Woman*. London: Hodder & Stoughton, 1958.
Seuss, Dr. *Cat in the Hat*. New York: Random House, 1957.
Severin, Tim. *The Ulysses Voyage: The Search for the Odyssey*. 1987. London: Hutchinson, 1988.
Shakespeare, William. *The Yale Shakespeare*. Many vols. New Haven, Conn.: Yale University Press, 1918-1966.
Sherwin, Martin J. *Gambling with Armageddon: Nuclear Roulette from Hiroshima to the Cuban Missile Crisis, 1945-1962*. New York: Alfred A. Knopf, 2020.
Shillace, Brandy. *Mr. Humble and Dr. Butcher: A Monkeys Head, the Pope's Neuroscientist, and the Quest to Transplant the Soul*. New York: Simon & Schuster, 2021.
Shorto, Russell. *The Island at the Center of the World*. New York: Vintage Books, 2005.
_____. *Descartes' Bones: A Skeletal History of the Conflict Between Faith and Reason*. New York: Random House, 2008.
Singer, Charles. *A Short History of Science to the Nineteenth Century*. 1941. Mineola, N.Y.: Dover Publications, Inc., 1997.
Skloot, Rebecca. *The Immortal Life of Henrietta Lacks*. New York: Crown Publishers, 2010.
Smith, Adam. *An Inquiry into the Nature and Causes of the Wealth of Nations*. 1776.
Smith, Geddes. *Plague on Us*. New York: The Commonwealth Fund, 1940.
Smith, Mychal Denzel. *Stakes is [sic] High: Life After the American Dream*. Hachette Group: Bold Type Books, 2020.
Smith Papyrus. *The Edwin Smith Papyrus: Updated Translation of the Trauma Treatise and Modern Medical Commentaries*. trans. Gonzalo M. Sanchez and Edmund S. Meltzer. Atlanta, Ga.: Lockwood Press, 2012.
Snow, C. P. *The Two Cultures and the Scientific Revolution: The Bede Lecture, 1959*. New York: Cambridge University Press, 1959. Reprint. Mansfield Centre, CT: Martino Publishing, 2013.
_____. *The Two Cultures and A Second Look*. 1964. New York: Cambridge University Press, 1979.
Snowden, Frank M. *Epidemics and Society: From the Black Death to the Present*. 2019. New Haven: Yale University Press, 2020.
Snyder, Timothy. *Our Malady: Lessons in Liberty from a Hospital Diary*. New York: Crown, 2020.
Solzhenitsyn, Aleksandr. *A Day in the Life of Ivan Denisovich*. trans. H. T. Willetts. New York: New American Library, 1962.
_____. *The Gulag Archipelago: An Experiment in Literary Investigation*. Paris: Éditions du Seuil, 1973.

Starr, Paul. *The Social Transformation of American Medicine: The Rise of a Sovereign Profession and the Making of a Vast Industry.* New York: Basic Books, 1984.
Stegner, Wallace. *Crossing to Safety.* New York: Random House, 1987.
Stevenson, Byran. *Just Mercy: A Story of Justice and Redemption.* New York: Spiegel & Grau, 2014.
Stone, Irving. *Lust for Life.* New York: Grosset and Dunlap, 1934.
Stowe, Harriet Beecher, *Uncle Tom's Cabin.* Boston: John P. Jewett & Company, 1852.
Suyin, Han. *A Many-Spendoured Thing.* London: Jonathan Cape, 1952.
Swan, Shanna H., and Stacey Colino. *Count Down: How Our Modern World Is Threatening Sperm Counts, Altering Male and Female Reproductive Development, and Imperiling the Future of the Human Race.* New York: Simon and Schuster, 2021.
Swanson, Doug J. *Cult of Glory: The Bold and Brutal History of the Texas Rangers.* New York: Viking, 2020.
Taylor, Roger, and Edward Wakeling. *Lewis Carroll, Photographer.* Princeton, N.J.: Princeton University Press, 2002.
The Book of Common Prayer and Administration of the Sacraments and Other Rites and Ceremonies of the Church. New York: Harper and Brothers, 1952.
The Book of Common Prayer and Administration of the Sacraments and Other Rites and Ceremonies of the Church. revised ed. New York: New York: Seabury Press, 1979.
The Koran. trans. N. J. Dawood. 1956. New York: Penguin Books, 1974.
The Layman's Parallel Bible: Comparing Four Popular Translations in Parallel Columns. Grand Rapids, Mich.: The Zondervan Corp., 1973.
The Methodist Hymnal. New York: The Methodist Publishing House, 1939.
The New York Times Complete World War II, 1939-1945. New York: Black Dog & Leventhal, 2013.
The Presidential Commission for the Study of Bioethical Issues. *"Ethically Impossible" STD Research in Guatemala from 1946 to 1948.* Washington, D.C.: Government Printing Office, 2011.
The Satyricon of Petronius Arbiter. trans. W. C. Fierbaugh. New York: Liveright Publishing Co., 1922.
The Torah: The Five Books of Moses. A New Translation of The Holy Scriptures According to the Masoretic Text. Philadelphia: The Jewish Publication Society, 1962.
Thesinger, Wilfred. *Arabian Sands.* London: Longmans, 1959.
Thomson, Elizabeth H. *Harvey Cushing: Surgeon, Author, Artist.* New York: Henry Schuman, 1950.
Thorndike, Lynn. *A History of Magic and Experimental Science During the First Thirteen Centuries of Our Era.* 1923. New York: Columbia University Press, 1958.
Thorwald, Jürgen. trans. *The Century of the Surgeon.* New York: Pantheon Books, 1957.
Thucydides, *History of the Peloponnesian War.* c.4th Century BCE.
Tolstoy, Leo. *War and Peace.* Moscow: Russian Messenger, 1869.
Trump, Mary L. *Too Much and Never Enough: How My Family Created the World's Most Dangerous Man.* New York, Simon & Schuster, 2020.
Tuchman, Barbara. *The Guns of August: The Outbreak of World War I.* New York: Macmillan, 1962.
Twain, Mark [Samuel Clemens]. *The Celebrated Jumping Frog of Calaveras County and Other Sketches.* 1867.
_____. *Huckleberry Finn.* London: Chatto & Windus, 1884.
Ulrich, Laurel Thatcher. *A Midwife's Tale: The Life of Martha Ballard, 1785-1812.* New York: Random House, 1990.
Vallery-Radot, René. *The Life of Pasteur.* Trans. Mrs. R. L. Devonshire. London: Constable, 1919.
Van Engen, Abram C. *City on a Hill: A History of American Exceptionalism.* New Haven: Yale University Press, 2020.
Vesalius, Andreas. *De humani corporis fabrica libri septem* ("On the fabric of the human body in seven books"). 1543.
Virgil, *The Aeneid.* trans. Robert Fitzgerald. 1981. New York: Vintage Classics, 1983.
Vonnegut, Kurt. *Slaughterhouse Five* or *The Children's Crusade: A Duty-Dance with Death.* New York: Dell Publishing, 1969.

Walker, Matthew. *Why We Sleep: Unlocking the Power of Sleep and Dreams*. New York: Scribner's, 2017.
Wallace, Anthony F. C., *Rockdale: The Growth of an American Village in the Early Industrial Revolution.* New York: Alfred A. Knopf, 1978.
Warrick, Joby. *Red Line: The Unraveling of Syria and America's Race to Destroy the Most Dangerous Arsenal in the World.* New York: Doubleday, 2020.
Weinberg, Steven. *Third Thoughts: The Universe We Still Don't Know.* Cambridge, Mass.: Harvard University Press/Belknap Press, 2019.
White, Andrew Dickson. *A History of the Warfare of Science with Theology in Christendom.* 2 vols. London: Macmillan and Company, 1896.
White, Richard. *The Organic Machine.* New York: Hill and Wang, 1995.
Wilde, Oscar. *The Ballad of Reading Gaol and Other Poems.* New York: Dover Publication, 1992.
Wilder, Laura Ingalls. *The Little House.* 1932ff. 9 vols. New York: Harper Collins, 2016.
Willkie, Wendell. *One World.* New York: Simon & Schuster, 1943.
Wilson, Sir Charles [Lord Moran]. *The Anatomy of Courage.* London: Constable, 1945.
_____. *Churchill: Taken from the Diaries of Lord Moran. The Struggle for Survival, 1940-1945.* Boston: Houghton Mifflin Company, 1966.
Winchell, Mike. *The Electric War: Edison, Tesla, Westinghouse, and the Race to Light the World.* New York: Henry Holt and Co., 2019.
Winchester, Simon. *The Professor and the Madman: A Tale of Murder, Insanity and the Making of the Oxford English Dictionary.* New York: HarperCollins, 1998.
_____. *The Alice Behind Wonderland.* London: Oxford University Press, 2011.
Winegard, Timothy C. *The Mosquito: A Human History of Our Deadliest Predator.* New York: Dutton/Penguin Random House LLC, 2019.
Wister, Owen. *The Virginian.* New York: Macmillan, 1902.
Withering, William. *A Botanical Arrangement of all the Vegetables Naturally Growing in Great Britain.* 1766.
Wright, Lawrence. *The Plague Year: America in the Time of Covid.* New York: Penguin/ Random House, 2021.
Zimmer, Carl. *Life's Edge: The Search for What It Means to Be Alive.* New York: Dutton, 2021.
Zimmermann, Warren. *First Great Triumph: How Five Americans Made Their Country a World Power.* New York: Farrar, Straus and Giroux, 2002.
Zinsser, Hans. *A Textbook of Microbiology.* New York: Appleton, 1910.
_____. *Rats, Lice and History: A Study in Biography.* 1935. New York: Pocket Books, 1945.
_____. *As I Remember Him: The Biography of R. S.* 1940. Gloucester, Mass.: Peter Smith, 1970.
Zola, Émile. *Germinal*, 1885.
_____. *J'Accuse*, 1896.
Zollinger, Robert M., and Robert M. Zollinger, Jr. *Atlas of Surgical Operations.* New York: Macmillan. N.d.
Zollinger, Robert M., Jr., and E. C. Ellison, *Atlas of Surgical Operations.* New York: Macmillan. 10th edition. 2016.

Reference Works

A Manual for Writers of Term Papers, Theses, and Dissertations. 1st ed., Kate L. Turabian. 6th ed. rev. John Grossman and Alice Bennett. Chicago: The University of Chicago Press, 1996.
Britannica.com
Encyclopædia Britannica Deluxe Edition. Chicago: Encyclopædia Britannica, 2013.
Forward Day by Day
Handbook. Boy Scouts of America
Holy Bible, King James Version.

My personal source is *The Holy Bible* London: Collins' Cleartype Press, 1941.

Home and Holiday Verse: 800 Poems of the Home, Mother, Father, Children, Gardens, Pets, Friends, Memories, Birthdays, Weddings, and Holidays. edit Louella D. Everett. New York: Halcyon House, 1939.

Guinness Book of World Records.

Merriam-Webster. Dictionary and Thesaurus. https://www.merriam-webster.com. (accessed January 15, 2020).

Oxford English Dictionary. OxfordLanguages. https://languages.oup.com/dictionaries (accessed August 8, 2020).

Stanford Encyclopedia.

The Oxford Dictionary of Quotations. 2d ed. Oxford: Oxford University Press, 1955.

The Oxford Universal Dictionary on Historical Principles, ed. C. T. Onions, et al. Oxford: Clarendon Press, 1955.

Webster's Collegiate Dictionary. 5th ed. Springfield, Mass.: G. & C. Merriam Co., 1948.

Webster's New Twentieth Century Dictionary Unabridged. William Collins Publishers, 1972.

Webster's New Twentieth Century Dictionary of the English Language Unabridged, 2d ed. 1979.

Word Virus: The William S. Burroughs Reader. New York: Grove/Atlantic, Inc., 2007.

Journals

Abele, Donald C., John E. Tobie, George J. Hill, Peter Contacos, and Charles B. Evans. 1965. Alterations in serum proteins and 19S antibody production during the course of induced malarial infections in man. *Amer J Trop Med Hyg.* 14: 191-7.

Alexander, Eben, Jr. Donald Darrow Matson. 1969. *Journal of Neurosurgery* 31 (no. 3, September): 249-50.

Andrews, Justin M., Griffith E. Quinby, and Alexander D. Langmuir. 1950. Malaria Eradication in the United States. *American Journal of Public Health* 40 (November): 1405-10.

Androutsos, G., A. Diamantis, and L. Vladimiros. 2008. The first leg transplant for the treatment of a cancer by Saints Cosmas and Damian. *J. Buon* 13 (no. 2, April-June): 297-304.

Anon. 1963. Medical Intelligence. *N Engl J Med* 268 (20 June): 1417.

_____. 2019. First do no harm: The impossible oath. *BMJ* 366: 14734.

_____. 2020. Understanding brain death. *JAMA* 323 (no. 21, 2 June): 2139-40.

_____. 2020. History of pandemics. *The Pharos* (Summer): 2.

_____. 2020. News from the Food and Drug Administration. *JAMA* 324 (no. 11, 15 September): 1026.

_____. 2020. What is COVID-19? *JAMA* 324 (no. 8, 25 August): 816.

_____. 2020. COVID-19. *JAMA* 324 (no. 12, 22/24 September): 1153-6.

Avery, Harold. 1966. Plague churches, monuments and memorials. *Proceedings of the Royal Society of Medicine* 59 (no. 2, February): 110-16.

Ballantyne, E. E. 1944. Gas gangrene antitoxin production. *Canadian Journal of Comparative Medicine* 3 (no. 4, April): 109-10.

Baker, David W. 2017. History of The Joint Commission's pain standards: Lessons for today's prescription opioid epidemic. *JAMA* 317 (no. 11): 1117-8.

Bauchner, Howard. 2020. 2020-A year that will be remembered. *JAMA* 324 (no. 3, 21 July): 245.

Benmoussa, Nadia, John-David Rebibo, Patrick Conan, and Philippe Chartier. 2019. Chimney-sweeps' cancer – early proof of environmentally driven tumourigenicity. *The Lancet* 20 (no. 3, 1 March): 338.

Bernhoft, Robin A. 2012. Mercury toxicity and treatment: A review of the literature. *J. Environ. Public Health*: 460508. Published online 2011 Dec 22. doi: 10.1155/2012/460508.

Bilinski, Alyssa, and Ezekiel J. Emanuel. 2020. COVID-19 and excess all-cause mortality in the US and 18 comparison countries. *JAMA* 324 (no. 20, 24 November): 2.

Blanchard, D. Pope John XXI, ophthalmologist. 1995. *Doc Ophthalmol.* 89 (no. 1-2): 75-84.

Bowman, D. M. J. S., et al. 2009. Fire in the earth system. *Science* 324 (no. 5926): 481-4.

Brainard, Jeffrey, and Jia You. 2018. What a massive database of retracted papers reveals about science publishing's "death penalty" *Science* (25 October).

Braunwald, Eugene. 1985. Effects of digitalis on the normal and the failing heart. *J. Am. Coll. Cardiol.* 5 (May, Suppl A,): 51A-9A.

Burch, Druin. 2010. Astley Paston Cooper (1768-1841): Anatomist, radical and surgeon. *Journal of the Royal Society of Medicine* 103 (no. 12, 1 December): 505-508.

Byerley, Julie Story. 2020. Mentoring in the era of #MeToo. *JAMA* 323 (no. 17, 5 May): 17-8.

Byyny, Richard L., et al. 2020. COVID-19 special edition. *Pharos* 83 (no. 3, Summer): 1-64.

Byyny, Richard L. 2021. Now is the time to enact a U.S. health care system. *Pharos* 84 (no. 2, Spring):3.

Christie, Athalia, Sarah A. Mbaeyi, and Rochelle P. Walensky. 2021. CDC Interim recommendations for fully vaccinated people: An important first step, *JAMA* 325 (no. 15, 20 April): 1501-2.

Coulehan, Jack. 2021. *Pharos* 84 (no. 2, Spring): 45. Review of Sheldon Rubenfeld and Daniel P. Sulmasy (eds.), *Physician-Assisted Suicide and Euthanasia: Before, During and After the Holocaust* (Lanham, Md.: Lexington Books, 2020).

Cui, Liwang, Sungano Mharakurwa, Daouda Ndiaye, Pradipsinh K. Rathod, and Philip J. Rosenthal. 2015. Antimalarial drug resistance: Literature review and activities and findings of the ICEMR network. *Am. J. Trop. Med. Hyg.* 93 (3 Suppl., 2 September): 57–68.

Cummings, Mike. 2021. Study offers earliest evidence of humans changing ecosystems with fire. *Yale News* (5 May).

del Rio, Carlos, and Preeti Malani. 2021. COVID-19 in 2021: Continuing uncertainty. *JAMA* 325 (no. 14, 13 April): 1389-90.

Davydov, Liya. 2011. Maggot therapy in wound management in modern era and a review of published literature. *J Pharm Prac.* 24 (no. 1, February): 89-93.

Durmus, Saliha, and Kutlu O. Ulgen. 2017. Comparative interactomics for virus-human protein-protein interactions: DNA viruses versus RNA viruses. *FEBS Open Bio* 7 (no. 1, January): 96-107.

Ehrenkranz, N. Joel, and Deborah A. Sampson. 2008. Origin of the Old Testament plagues: Explications and implications. *Yale Journal of Biology and Medicine* 81 (no. 1, March): 31-42.

Fallingborg, J. 1999. Intraluminal pH of the human gastrointestinal tract. *Dan. Med. Bull.* 46 (no. 3): 183-96.

Farber, Steven A. 2008. U.S. scientists' role in the eugenics movement (1907-1939): A contemporary biologist's perspective. *Zebrafish* 5 (no.4): 243-5.

Fee, Elizabeth. 2015. The first American medical school: The formative years. *Lancet* 385 (no. 9981, 16 May): 1917-2014.

Feinstein, R. N., R. J. Fry, and E. F. Staffeldt. 1978. Carcinogenic and antitumor effects of aminotriazole on acatalasemic and normal catalase mice. *J. Natl Cancer Inst.* 60 (no. 5, May): 1113-6.

Freemon, Frank R. 2005. Bubonic plague in the Book of Samuel. *J. Royal Soc. Med.* 98 (no. 9, September): 436.

Gallagher, Richard E. 2014. In memoriam, George J. Hill, M.D., Ph.D." *Journal of Cancer Education* 29: 213.

_____. 2015. Erratum to: In memoriam, George J. Hill, M.D., Ph.D. *Journal of Cancer Education* 30: 815.

Ghiselin, Michael T. 1968. The economy of the body. *The American Economic Review* 68 (no. 2, May): 233-7.

Glied, Sherry, and Helen Levy. 2020. The potential effects of coronavirus on national health expenditures. *JAMA* 323 (no. 20, 26 May): 2001-2.

Goodman, Jesse L., John D. Grabenstein, and M. Miles Braun. 2020. Answering key questions about COVID-19 vaccines. *JAMA* 324 (no. 20, 24 November): 2027-8.

Gowlett, J. A. J., and R. W. Wrangham. 2013. Earliest fire in Africa: towards the convergence of archaeological evidence and the cooking hypothesis. *Azania: Archaeological Research in Africa* 48 (no. 1): 5-30.

Greer, David M., Sam D. Shermie, Ariane Lewis, et al. 2020. Determination of brain death/death by neurologic criteria: The world brain death project. *JAMA* 324 (no. 11, 15 September): 1078-97.

Haley, Danielle F., and Richard Saitz. 2020. The opioid epidemic during the COVID-19 pandemic. *JAMA* 324 (no. 16, 27 October), 1615-7.

Hill, George J., William T. Butler, Paul T. Wertlake, and John P. Utz. 1962. The renal histopathology of amphotericin B toxicity in man and the dog: A study of biopsy and post-mortem specimens. *Clinical Research* 10: 249. Abstract.

_____, William T. Butler, Charles F. Szwed, and John P. Utz. 1963. Comparison of renal toxicity of two preparations of amphotericin B. *Amer Rev Resp Dis*. 88: 342-6.

_____, William T. Butler, Charles F. Szwed, and Sarah U. Moore. 1963. Lethal toxicity and dose-related azotemia due to amphotericin B in dogs. *Proc Soc Exper Biol and Med*. 114: 76-9.

_____, Vernon Knight, G. Robert Coatney, and Donald K. Lawless. 1963. Vivax malaria complicated by aphasia and hemiparesis." *A.M.A. Arch Intern Med*. 112: 863-8.

_____, Vernon Knight, and G. M. Jeffrey. 1964. Thrombocytopenia in vivax malaria. *Lancet* 1: 240-1.

_____, Manuel G. Herrera-Aceña; Guillermo Arboleda, and Rafael Montoya. 1973. Surgical education in a developing country: Participation of a rural community hospital in Colombia. *Arch. Surg.* 106: 356-8.

_____, Thomas Shine, Helene Z. Hill, and Catherine Miller. 1976. Failure of amygdalin to arrest B16 melanoma and BW5147 AKR leukemia. *Cancer Research* 36: 2102-9.

_____, 1977. Testimony on Laetrile, in "Laetrile: The Commissioner's Decision," HEW publication No. 77-3056. Superintendent of Documents, U.S. Government Printing Office, Washington, DC 20402. Supreme Court of the United States, *United States et al v. Rutherford et al*, No. 78-605, p. 11, June 18, 1979, quoted in 442 U.S. 544 (1979), No. 78-605, p. 557; 42 Fed. Reg. 39768, 39787, 1977.

_____. 1979. "Lerne and gladly teche": A view of the Vietnam Medical Education Project. *Military Medicine* 144: 124-8.

_____. 2007. Intimate relationships: Secret affairs of church and state in the United States and Liberia, 1925-1945. *Diplomatic History* 31 (no. 3, June): 465-503.

_____. 2021. Diamond anniversary for the AACE. Presented to Annual Meeting, American Association for Cancer Education, October 12-16, College Park, Md. Abstract 4-B, presented by prerecorded Zoom and live Zoom discussion on October 16, 2020. To be published in *Journal of Cancer Education*.

Hill, Helene Z., R. Backer, and George J. Hill. 1980. Blood cyanide levels in mice after administration of amygdalin. *Biopharmaceutics and Drug Disposition*. 1: 211-20.

Hoffman, Brian F., and Donald H. Singer. 1964. Effects of digitalis on electrical activity of cardiac fibers. *Progress in Cardiovascular Diseases* 7 (no. 3, November): 226-60.

Hublin, Jean-Jacques et al. 2017. New fossils from Jebel Irhoud Morocco and the pan-African origin of *Homo sapiens*. *Nature* 546 (no. 7657, 7 June): 289-92.

Hutton, E. K., and Hassan E. S. 2007. Late vs early clamping of the umbilical cord in full-term neonates: systematic review and meta-analysis of controlled trials. *JAMA* 297 (no. 11, March): 1241–52.

Joffe, Steven. 2021. Evaluating SARS-CoV-2 vaccines after emergency use authorization or licensing of initial candidate vaccines. *JAMA* 325 (no. 3, 19 January): 221-2.

Keiichi, Tsuneishi. trans. John Junkerman. 2005. Unit 731 and the Japanese Imperial Army's biological warfare program. *Asia Pacific Journal* 3 (no. 11, 24 November).

Klemmer, Philip, Clarence E. Grim, and Friedrich C. Luft. 2014. Who and what drove Walter Kempner? The rice diet revisited. *Hypertension* 64 (no. 4, 7 July): 684-8.

Koonin, E. V., and Y. I. Wolf. 2016. Just how Lamarckian is CRISPR-Cas immunity? The continuum of evolutionary mechanisms. *Biology Direct* 11 (no. 1, February): 9.

Larson, Eric B., and Xin Yao 2005. Clinical empathy as emotional labor in the patient-physician relationship. *JAMA* 293 (no. 9, 2 March): 1100-1106.

Lerner, Andrea M., Gregory K. Folkers, and Anthony S. Fauci. 2020. Preventing the spread of SARS-CoV-2 with masks and other 'low-tech' interventions. *JAMA* 324 (no. 19, 17 November): 1935-6.

Levitt, Larry. 2020. Trump vs. Biden on health Care. *JAMA* 324 (no. 14, 13 October):1384-5.

Li, Kuanrong, Ling Li, Xianfeng Wang, et al. 2020. Comparative analysis of clinical features of SARS-CoV-2 and adenovirus infection among children. *Virology Journal* 17 (10 December): 193.

Lippman, Alan J. 2017. Facilitated natural death: An approach to death with dignity, *MDAdvisor* 10 (no. 3): 16-19.

Liscum, Emmanuel, et al. 2014. Phototropism: Growing towards an understanding of plant movement. *Plant Cell* 26 (no. 1, January): 38–55. Published online 2014 Jan 30. doi:10.1105/tpc.113.119727.

London, Jack. 1902. To build a fire. In *The Youth's Companion* 76 (29 January).

Machugh, David E., Greger Larsen, and Ludovic Orlando. 2016. Taming the past: Ancient DNA and the study of animal domestication. *Annual Review of Animal Biosciences* 5: 329-351.

MacLatchy, Laura M., William J. Sanders, and Craig L. Wuthrich. 2015. Hominoid origins. *Nature Education Knowledge* 6 (no. 7): 4.

Manning, Joseph G., Francis Ludlow, Alexander R. Stine, et al. 2017. Volcanic suppression of Nile summer flooding triggers revolt and constrains interstate conflict in ancient Egypt. *Nature Communications* 8.

Mayr, Astrid. 2007. Human protothecosis. *Clin. Microbiol. Rev.* 20 (no. 2, April): 230-42.

McCrobie, Susan Evans. 2021. Chirurgian, phisique and the sicke: The art and history of Jamestown medicine. *Jamestowne Society Magazine* 45 (no. 1, Spring): 23-4.

McHugo, Gillian P., Michael J. Dover, and David E. Machugh. 2019. Unlocking the origins and biology of domestic animals using ancient DNA and paleogenomics. *BMC Biology* 17 (no. 1): 98.

Miles, Steven H. Hippocrates and informed consent. 2009. *The Lancet* 374 (no. 9698, 17 Oct):1322-3.

Mordechai, Lee, Merle Eisenberg, Timothy P. Newfield, et al. 2019. The Justinianic plague: An inconsequential pandemic? *Proceedings of the National Academy of Sciences* 1116 (no. 51, 17 December): 25546-54.

Mufson, Maurice A., Michael A. Manko, James R. Kingston, et al. 1961. Eaton agent pneumonia: Clinical features. *JAMA* 178 (no. 4): 369-74.

Murray, Barbara E., Karl E. Anderson, Keith Arnold, et al. 2005. Destroying the life and career of a valued physician-scientist who tried to protect us from plague: Was it really necessary? *Clinical Infectious Diseases* 40 (no. 11, 1 June): 1644-48.

Nahas, Gabriel G. 1982. Hashish in Islam, 9th to 18th Century. *Bull. N.Y. Acad. Med.* 58 (no. 9, December): 814-31.

Nathawani, Amit C., James F. Down, John Goldstone, et al. 2016. Polonium-210 poisoning: A first hand account. *Lancet* 388 (no. 100049, 10 September): 1075-1080.

Newman, Laura. 2001. Lynn Payer. *BMJ* 323 (no. 7317, 13 October): 871.

Omer, Saad B., Preeti Malani, and Carlos del Rio. 2020. The COVID-19 pandemic in the U.S.: A clinical update. *JAMA* 323 (no. 18, 12 May): 1767-8.

_____, Inci Yildirim, and Howard P. Forman. 2020. Herd immunity and implications for SARS-CoV-2 control. *JAMA* 324 (no. 20, 24 November): 2095-6.

_____. 2020. The discredited doctor hailed by the anti-vaccine movement. *Nature* 586 (27 October): 668-9.

O'Shea, J. G. 1990. Two minutes with venus, two years with mercury: Mercury as an antisyphilitic chemotherapeutic agent. *Journal of the Royal Society of Medicine* 83 (June): 392-5.

Pan, An, Li Liu, Chaolong Wang, et al. 2020. Association of public health interventions with the epidemiology of the COVID-19 outbreak in Wuhan, China. *JAMA* 323 (no. 19, 10 May): 1915-23.

Pandit, Jay A. 2020. Memento Mori. *JAMA* 324 (no. 17, 3 November): 1731-2.

Parsons, Mikeal C., and D. Thomas Hanks, Jr. 2001. When the salt lost its savour: A brief history of Matthew 5.13/Mark 9.50/Luke 14.34 in English translation. *The Bible Translator* 52 (no. 3): 320.

Peacock, Andrew J. 1998. Oxygen at high altitude. *BMJ* 317 (no. 7165, 17 October): 1063-66.

Pearce, J. M. S. 2016. Sydenham on hysteria. *Eur Neurol* 76:175-181.

Pray, Leslie A. 2008. Discovery of DNA structure and function: Watson and Crick. *Nature Education* 1 (no. 1): 100.

Putnam, Emily E., and Andrew L. Goodman. 2020. B vitamin acquisition by gut commensal bacteria. *PLoS Pathog* 16 (no. 1, January): e1008208.

Quammen, David. 2021. How viruses shape our world, *National Geographic* 239 (no. 2, February):41-67.

Rasio, E. A., George J. Hill, J.S. Soeldner, and Manuel G. Herrera. 1967. The effect of pancreatectomy on glucose tolerance and extracellular fluid insulin in the dog, *Diabetes*, 16: 551-6.

Rehder, Roberta, Subash Lohani, and Alan R. Cohen. 2015. Unsung hero: Donald Darrow Matson's legacy in pediatric neurosurgery. *J. Neurosurg. Pediatr.* 16 (no. 5, November): 483-94.

Reisch, Mark S. 2015. EPA limitations on hydrofluorocarbons give Honeywell an opportunity for an environmentally acceptable substitute. *Chemical and Engineering News* 93 (no. 42, 26 October).

Rennie, Drummond. 1997. Thyroid storm. *JAMA* 277 (no. 15, 16 April): 1238-43.

Rid, Annette, and Mark Lipsitch. 2021. The ethics of continuing placebo in SARS-CoV-2 Vaccine trials. *JAMA* 325 (no. 3, 19 January): 219-20.

Riedel, Stefan. 2005. Edward Jenner and the history of smallpox and vaccination. *Proc (Bayl Univ Med Cent)* 18 (no. 1, January): 21-5.

Sala, Enric. 2020. The cost of harming nature. *National Geographic* 238 (no. 3, September): 15-18.

Sabbatani, S., and S. Fiorino. 2009. The Antonine Plague and the decline of the Roman Empire. *Infexz Med.* 17 (no 4, 17 December): 261-75. Article in Italian.

Segall, H. N. 1985. William Osler and Thomas Browne, a friendship of fifty-two years; Sir Thomas pervades Sir William's library. *Korot* 8 (nos. 11-12, Summer): 150-65.

Simmons, James S. 1944. American mobilization for the conquest of malaria in the United States. *J. Nat. Malaria Soc.* 3 (1944): 7-11.

Stark, Stephen D. The four days that made Tv news. 1997. *American Heritage* 48 (no. 3, May/June).

Stauffer, William M., Jonathan D. Alpern, and Patricia F. Walker. 2020. COVID-19 and dexamethasone: A potential strategy to avoid steroid-related *Strongyloides* hyperinfection. *JAMA* (30 July). doi:10.1001/ jama.2020.

Stephen, Alison M., and J. H. Cummings. 1980. The microbial contribution to human faecal mass. *Journal of Medical Microbiology* 13 (no. 1, 1 February): 45-56.

Stephenson, Kathryn E., Mathieu Le Gars, Jerald Sadoff, et al. 2021. Immunogenicity of the Ad26.COV2.S Vaccine for COVID-19. *JAMA* 325 (no. 15, 20 April): 1535-1544.

Stone, Marvin J. 1998. Henry Bence Jones and his protein. *Journal of Medical Biography* 6 (1 February): 53-7.

Stratton, Jennifer. 2020. CRISPR vs COVID-19: How can gene editing help beat a virus? *Biotechniques* 69 (no. 5, 2 November): 327-9.

Taylor, Stephane Parks. 2020. Shear forces. *JAMA* 324 (no. 19, 17 November): 1943-4.

Tello-Martin, R., K. Dzul-Rosado, J. Zavala-Castro, and C. Lugo-Caballero. 2018. Approaches for the successful isolation and cell culture of American *Rickettsia* species. *Journal of Vector Borne Diseases* 55 (no. 4): 258-64.

Thomas, Elaine. 2021. Book Review of Martin J. Blaser, *Missing Microbes* (London: Picador, 2015). *Pharos* 84 (no. 2, Spring 2021): 43.

Tipton, Charles M. 2014. The history of "Exercise Is Medicine" in ancient civilizations. *Adv. Physiol. Educ.* 38 (no. 2, June): 109-17.

Tobie, John E., Donald C. Abele, George J. Hill, Peter Contacos, and Charles B. Evans. 1966. Fluorescent antibody studies on the immune response in sporozoite-induced vivax malaria and the relationship of antibody production to parasitemia. *Amer J Trop Med Hyg.* 15: 676-83.

Toney, Jeffrey H., and Stephanie Ishack. 2020. A pandemic of confusion. *American Scientist* 108 (November-December): 344-5.

Truog, Robert D., Kandamaran Krishnamurthy, and Rebert C. Tasker. 2020. Brain death: Moving beyond consistency in the diagnostic criteria. *JAMA* 324 (no. 11, 15 September): 1045-7.

Walensky, Rochelle P., and Carlos de Rio. 2020. From mitigation to containment of the COVID-19 pandemic: Putting the SARS-CoV-2 genie back in the bottle. *JAMA* 323 (no. 19, 19 May): 1889-90.

Weisse, Allen B. 2012. Self-experimentation and its role in medical research. *Tex Heart Inst J.* 39 (no. 1): 51-4.

Wendland, Claire L. Physician anthropologists. 2020. *Annual Review of Anthropology* 48: 187-205.

Wilson, Adrian, and T. G. Ashplant. 1988. Whig history and present-centered history. *The Historical Journal*, 31 (no. 1, March): 1–16.

Wolinetz, Carrie D., and Francis S. Collins. 2020. Recognition of research participants' need for autonomy: Remembering the legacy of Henrietta Lacks." *JAMA* 324 (no. 11, 15 September): 1027-8.

Wood, Bernard, and Alexis Williams. 2020. Meet your exotic, extinct close relative. *American Scientist* 108 (November-December): 348-55.

Woolf, Steven H., Derek A. Chapman, and John Hyung Lee. 2021. COVID-19 as [sic] the leading cause of death in the United States." *JAMA* 325 (no. 2, 12 January): 123-4.

_____. Derek A. Chapman, Roy T. Sabo, et al. 2021. Excess Deaths from COVID-19 and other causes in the US, March 1, 2020, to January 2, 2021. *JAMA*. Published online April 25, 2021. doi:10.1001/jama.2021.5199.

Wright, Lawrence. The plague year. *New Yorker* (4 & 11 January 2021), 20-59.

Yancy, Clyde W., and Howard Bauchner. 2021. Diversity in Medical Schools: Need for a new bold approach, *JAMA* 325 (no. 1, 5 January): 31-2.

Magazines

Forward Day by Day (Cincinnati, Ohio: Forward Movement, 2020). *Good Housekeeping. Harvard Magazine. National Geographic. Nature. Naval History. New York Review of Books* [*NYR*] *Officer Review, The Military Order of the World Wars. Popular Science. Population Connection. Playboy. Smithsonian. The Atlantic. The Bulletin of the Atomic Scientists. The Old Farmer's Almanac*

Newspapers

Indianapolis Star. International Business Times. New York Times. USA Today. Washington Post

Theatrical Productions

Gounod, Charles. *Romeo and Juliet.* Miller, Arthur. *The Crucible. Death of a Salesman.* Mozart, Wolfgang Amadeus. *Don Giovanni.* Puccini, Giacomo. *La Bohème. Turandot.* Sherriff, R[obert]. C[edric]. *Journey's End* (1929). Shakespeare, William. *Hamlet. King Lear. The Tempest. The Merchant of Venice.* Verdi, Giuseppe. *Nabucco. Aida. La Traviata. Madama Butterfly.*

Poetry, Short Stories, and Music

Bach, Johann Sebastian. "Alle Menschen müssen sterben." 1714,
Benet, Stephen Vincent. "John Brown's Body." 1928.
Brian's Escape. "The Journey: An Account of S. A. Andrée's Arctic Expedition of 1897." 2010.

Browning, Elizabeth Barrett. "How do I remember thee." 1850.
Chopin, Frederick. "Funeral March." 1840.
Debussy, Claude. *Prélude à l'après-midi d'un faune* (*Prelude to the Afternoon of a Faun*). 1894.
Dvořák, Antonin. Symphony No. 9, "From the New World." 1893.
Elgar, Arthur. "Pomp and Circumstance March." 1901.
Eliot, T[homas]. S[tearns]. "The Hollow Men." 1925.
Foster, Stephen. "Jeanie with the Light Brown Hair," 1854. "My Old Kentucky Home." 1853.
Frost, Robert. "Stopping by Woods on a Snowy Evening." 1923.
Gilbert, W. S., and Sir Arthur Sullivan. "Pirates of Penzance." 1879.
Graves, Robert "The Soldier." 1915.
Higley, Brewster M. "Home on the Range." 1874.
Howe, Julia Ward. "Battle Hymn of the Republic." 1861.
Jones, Isham, and Gus Kahn. "I'll See You in My Dreams." 1924.
Kellette, John and "Jaan Kenbrovin," a pseudonym for James Kendis, James Brockman, and Nat Vincent. "I'm forever blowing bubbles." 1918.
Kipling, Rudyard. "Gunga Din." 1890.
Livingston, Jay, and Ray Evans. "Que Sera, Sera." 1956. For the Alfred Hitchcock movie, *The Man Who Knew Too Much*.
Longfellow, Henry Wadsworth. "A Psalm of Life." 1838.
Lynn, Vera. We'll Meet Again." 1939. "A Nightingale Sang in Berkeley Square." 1939. "(There'll Be Bluebirds Over) The White Cliffs of Dover." 1942.
Mahler, Gustav. "Das Lied von der Erde." 1912.
Massenet, Jules. "Méditation" from the opera *Thaïs*. 1894.
McRae, John. "In Flanders Fields." 1915.
Mussorgsky, Modest. "Pictures at an Exhibition." 1874.
Owen, Wilfred. "Anthem for Doomed Youth." 1917.
Powell, Felix, and George Henry Powell. "Pack up your troubles in your old kit bag and smile, smile, smile," 1915.
Saint-Saëns, Camille. "Danse Macabre." 1874.
Sassoon, Siegfried. "The Kiss." 1917.
Seeger, Alan. "I have a Rendezvous with Death." 1916.
Stevenson, Robert Louis, "Requiem." 1890.
Strauss, Richard. "Death and Resurrection." (Tod und Verklärung). 1899.
Tennyson, Alfred, Lord. "In Memoriam A.H.H." 1850.
Tchaikovsky, Pyotr Ilyich. "The Year 1812 Solemn Overture." 1880.
Whitman, Walt. "Leaves of Grass." 1855.
_____. "Oh Captain, My Captain." 1865.
Wordsworth, William. "My Heart Leaps Up." 1802.

Songs

As Time Goes By. Carry me back to ol' Virginny. Clementine. Crossing over into Jordan. Deep River. Dem Bones, dem dry bones. John Brown's Body. Last Post. Lili Marlene. Luck, Be a Lady Tonight. Song of Roland. Taps.

Movies

2001: A Space Odyssey. A Beautiful Mind. All is Lost (2013). *Andrea Gail* (2000). *Awakenings. Bataan. Birdman of Alcatraz* (1962). *Blair Witch Project. Braveheart* (1995). *Casablanca* (1942). *Diana* (2013), about Lady Diana, Princess of Wales. *Doc Martin* (BBC TV), 2010ff. *Double Indemnity.*

Dunkirk. Gaslight. Glory (1989). *God Knows Where I Am* (2016). *Grease. Hair* (1979), based on the 1969 musical of the same name. *Harry Potter. Her Majesty, Mrs. Brown* (1997), in which "Mrs. Brown" is Queen Victoria. *High Noon. I'll See You in My Dreams* (1951). *Jaws. La Cage aux Folles. La Strada. Love Is a Many-Splendored Thing* (1955). *Love Story. Lust for Life* (1956). *Magnificent Obsession. Master and Commander* (2003). *Mrs. Miniver. Mutiny on the Bounty. Oh, Pioneers. Pasteur. Paths of Glory. Penn and Teller: Fool Us* (TV, 2010ff). *Rebecca. Rosemary's Baby. Saving Private Ryan. Schindler's List. Silence of the Lambs. Silence of the Lambs. South Pacific. Soylent Green* (1973). *Star Wars. Sunset Boulevard* (1950). *Tess of the d'Urbervilles. Texas Chain Saw Massacre. The Best Years of Our Lives. The Crown* (series, 2016-2020). *The Lone Ranger. The Longest Day. The Lost Weekend. The Maltese Falcon* (1941). *The Man with the Golden Arm. The Pianist. The Raiders of the Lost Ark* (1981). *The Sands of Iwo Jima. The Sun Also Rises* (1956), based on the novel of the same name, published in 1926. *The Virginian. The Witches of Eastwick. They were Expendable. Three Sovereigns for Sarah* (1985). *Titanic* (1997). *To Build a Fire* (1969). *Tora Tora Tora. Unbroken. Whatever Love Means* (2005), about Prince Charles and Camilla, Duchess of Cornwall. *White Fang* (1925), and many times thereafter.

Internet Sources

7 duels between women. Mentalfloss.com. https://www.mentalfloss.com/article/75944/7-duels-between-women (accessed January 31, 2021).

9-11 Attacks. Topics. History.com. https://www.history.com/topics/21st-century/9-11-attacks (accessed June 15, 2020).

Adenovirus. Respiratory viruses. Merckmanuals.com. https://www.merckmanuals.com/professional/infectious-diseases/respiratory-viruses/adenovirus-infections (accessed January 12, 2021).

African American History. Smithsonian. Smisonianmag.com. https://www.smithsonianmag.com/smithsonian-institution/national-museum-african-american-history-and-culture-interactive-museum-tour/ (accessed June 14, 2020).

Agassiz. Darwin. Ucmp.berkeley.edu. https://ucmp.berkeley.edu/history/agassiz.html (accessed December 22, 2020).

Al Islam. Polygamy. https //www.alislam.org/question/polygamy-in-islam/ (accessed January 25, 2021).

All That's Interesting. Rockefeller, Nelson. https://allthatsinteresting.com/nelson-rockefeller-death (accessed January 23, 2021).

American Cancer Society. Cancer.org. https://www.cancer.org/about-us/ (accessed July 20, 2020).

American College of Legal Medicine. https://www.aclm.org/Past-Presidents (accessed July 11, 2021).

American Red Cross. ICRC. Icrc.org. https://www.icrc.org/en/who-we-are/movement (accessed November 27, 2020).

Annas, George. Lawyer. Quora.com. https://www.quora.com/Are-there-people-who-are-both-lawyers-and-doctors (accessed March 16, 2021).

Antibiotics. Prokaryotes. Bio.libretexts.org. https://bio.libretexts.org/Bookshelves/Microbiology/Book%3A_Microbiology_(Boundless)/13%3A_Antimicrobial_Drugs/13.3%3A_Commonly_Used_Antimicrobial_Drugs/13.3D%3A_Antibiotics_from_Prokaryotes (accessed February 1, 2021).

Antibiotics. Human health. Ncbi.nlm.nih.gov. https://www.ncbi.nlm.nih.gov/books/NBK216502/ (accessed August 22, 2020).

Antifreeze Poisoning. Healthline.com. https://www.healthline.com/health/antifreeze-poisoning (accessed January 31, 2021).

Antonine Plague. Pubmed.ncbi.nlm.nih.gov. https://pubmed.ncbi.nlm.nih.gov/20046111/ (accessed January 5, 2021).

Arboviruses. Cdc.gov. www.cdc.gov>nndss>conditions>case-definition (Arboviral Diseases, Neuroinvasive and Non-neuroinvasive) (accessed July 10, 2020).

Ark of the Covenant. New Testament. Fountainoflifetm.com. http://www.fountainoflifetm.com/2017/08/31/why-isnt-the-the-ark-of-the-covenant-in-the-new-testament/ (accessed August 5, 2020).

Articles. Ncbi.nlm.nih.gov. https://www.ncbi.nlm.nih.gov/pmc/articles/PMC2117903/ (accessed June 14, 2020).

Attila the Hun. Ancient.eu. https://www.ancient.eu/Attila_the_Hun/ (accessed November 3, 2020).

Avery, Harold. Plague. Ncbi.nlm.nih.gov. https://www.ncbi.nlm.nih.gov/pmc/articles/PMC1900794/pdf/procrsmed00186-0033.pdf (accessed November 29, 2020).

Ayahuasca. Drug. Healthline.com. https://www.healthline.com/nutrition/ayahuasca (accessed February 6, 2021).

Bacterial infections. Gram negative bacteria. Merckmanuals.com. https://www.merckmanuals.com/home/infections/bacterial-infections-gram-negative-bacteria/overview-of-gram-negative-bacteria (accessed June 30, 2020).

Baker, Peter. Harding. Nytimes.com. https://www.nytimes.com/2015/08/13/us/dna-is-said-to-solve-a-mystery-of-warren-hardings-love-life.html (accessed December 12, 2020).

Baron. Medical Microbiology. Ncbi.nlm.nih.gov. https://www.ncbi.nlm.nih.gov/books/NBK7864/ (accessed July 5, 2020).

Bat, honey nectar. Animalia.bio. http://animalia.bio/long-tongued-nectar-bat (accessed February 17, 2021).

Battle Hymn of the Republic. Theatlantic.com. https://www.theatlantic.com/entertainment/archive/2010/11/the-battle-hymn-of-the-republic-americas-song-of-itself/66070/ (accessed June 13, 2020).

Bayer. Bayer.com. https://www.bayer.com/en/history/1881-1914 (accessed October 26, 2020).

Beirut. Explosion. Nytimes.com. https://www.nytimes.com/2020/08/05/world/middleeast/beirut-lebanon-explosion.html (accessed September 2, 2020).

Benmoussa, Nadia. Chimney sweep's cancer. Thelancet.com. https://www.thelancet.com/journals/lanonc/article/PIIS1470-2045(19)30106-8/fulltext#%20 (accessed December 13, 2020).

Berman, Bob. Crescent Moon. Almanac.com. https://www.almanac.com/content/captivating-crescent-moon (accessed November 4, 2020).

Bernhoft, Robin. Mercury. Ncbi.nlm.nih.gov. https://www.ncbi.nlm.nih.gov/pmc/articles/PMC3253456/ (accessed October 31, 2020).

Bible. Babylonian Exile. Biblestudytoolscom. https://www.biblestudytools.com/bible-study/topical-studies/who-was-king-nebuchadnezzar-in-the-bible.html (accessed November 7, 2020).

_____. Crimes. Biblegateway.com. https://www.biblegateway.com/resources/encyclopedia-of-the-bible/Crimes-Punishments (accessed November 9, 2020).

Blum, Arlene. Green Science Policy Institute. Greenactioncentre.ca. https://greenactioncentre.ca/clean-energy-environment/myth-is-24-d-a-risk. (accessed August 20, 2020).

Blumberg, Baruch. Hepatitis B. Hepb.org. https://www.hepb.org/about-us/baruch-blumberg-md-dphil/ (accessed July 5, 2020).

Body Composition. Oxford University Press. Encyclopedia.com: https://www.encyclopedia.com/medicine/encyclopedias-almanacs-transcripts-and-maps/composition-body (accessed June 28, 2020).

_____. Cleveland Clinic. My.clevelandclinic.org. https://my.clevelandclinic.org/health/articles/4182-fat-and-calories (accessed February 22, 2021).

Bohmbach, Karla. Jephthah. Jwa.org. https://jwa.org/encyclopedia/article/daughter-of-jephthah-bible (accessed August 26, 2020).

Bologna. Oldest. Mastersavenue.com. https://www.mastersavenue.com/articles-guides/good-to-know/the-10-oldest-universities-in-the-world (accessed November 13, 2020).

Boy Scouts of America. Scout Oath and Law. Scouting.org. https://www.scouting.org/about/faq/. (accessed January 12, 2021).

_____. Scout Slogan. Boyscouttrail.com. https://www.boyscouttrail.com/boy-scouts/boy-scout-slogan. (accessed January 12, 2021).

_____. Scout Motto. Scoutingmagazine.org. https://blog.scoutingmagazine.org/be-prepared/ (accessed January 12, 2021).

Brain, Marshall. "What if an Asteroid Hit Earth?" Science How Stuff Works.com. https://science.howstuffworks.com/nature/natural-disasters/asteroid-hits-earth.htm (accessed August 18, 2020).

Brown fat. Metabolism. Nih.gov. https://www.nih.gov/news-events/nih-research-matters/how-brown-fat-improves-metabolism (accessed February 20, 2021).

Burch, Druin. Cooper, Astley. Ncbi.nlm.nih.gov. https://www.ncbi.nlm.nih.gov/pmc/articles/PMC2996521/ (accessed November 26, 2020).

Bushido Code. History. Invaluable.com. https://www.invaluable.com/blog/history-of-the-bushido-code/ (accessed August 27, 2020).

Business Insider. Electoral Maps. Businessinsider.com. https://www.businessinsider.com/2016-2020-electoral-maps-exit-polls-compared-2020-11#the-electoral-vote-count-from-2016-to-2020-basically-flipped-1 (accessed January 25, 2021).

Butler. Plague. Academic.oup.com. https://academic.oup.com/cid/article/40/11/1644/446159 (accessed February 21, 2021).

Butterfield. Whig history. Univ.ox.ac.uk. https://www.univ.ox.ac.uk/book/the-whig-interpretation-of-history/ (accessed February 23, 2020).

_____. Present Whig history. Nybooks.com. https://www.nybooks.com/articles/2015/12/17/eye-present-whig-history-science/(accessed February 23, 2020).

Campbell, Joseph. Religion. Jcf.org. https://www.jcf.org/ (accessed March 19, 2021).

Campbell, William C. Nobelprize.org. https://www.nobelprize.org/prizes/medicine/2015/press-release/ (accessed June 29, 2020).

Cancer. Seven Warning Signs. Medicinenet.com. https://www.medicinenet.com/the_seven_warning_signs_of_cancer/article.htm (accessed April 1, 2021).

Cathedrals. Gothic. touropia.com. https://www.touropia.com/gothic-cathedrals/ (accessed November 12, 2020).

Chagas disease. Centers for Disease Control. Cdc.gov. https://www.cdc.gov/parasites/chagas/gen_info/detailed.html (accessed June 29, 2020).

Cherry laurel. Homeguides.sfgate.com. https://homeguides.sfgate.com/poisonous-cherry-laurel-tree-67400.html (accessed October 24, 2020).

Centers for Disease Control. Leading Causes of Death. https://www.cdc.gov/nchs/fastats/leading-causes-of-death.htm (accessed July 20, 2020).

Cherry, Kendra. "Stages of Prenatal Development." Verywellmind. https://www.verywellmind.com/stages-of-prenatal-development (accessed January 17, 2021).

Chi-squared. Statistics. Socscistatics.com https://www.socscistatistics.com/tests/chisquare/default2.aspx (accessed September 5, 2020).

Churchill Project. Hillsdale College. "In Search of Lord Randolph Churchill's Purported Syphilis." https://winstonchurchill.hillsdale.edu/in-search-of-lord-randolph-churchills-purported-syphilis/ (accessed May 20, 2020).

Clinton. Vote. Abcnews.go.com. https://abcnews.go.com/Politics/hillary-clinton-officially-wins-popular-vote-29-million/story?id=44354341 (accessed December 21, 2010).

Cirillo, Vincent. Turpentine. Mhsnj.org. https://www.mhsnj.org/event-4093300 (accessed January 1, 2021).

Civil War Casualties. Battlefields.org. https://www.battlefields.org/learn/articles/civil-war-casualties (accessed June 13, 2020).

Civil War Facts. Battlefields.org. https://www.battlefields.org/learn/articles/civil-war-facts#How%20many%20soldiers%20fought%20in%20the%20Civil%20War? (accessed April 1, 2021).

Cleveland, Grover. Surgery. Ahsl.arizona.edu. http://ahsl.arizona.edu/about/exhibits/presidents/cleveland (accessed December 11, 2020).

Climate Agreement. Paris. Unfccc.int. at: https://unfccc.int/process-and-meetings/the-paris-agreement/the-paris-agreement (accessed March 29, 2021).

Clostridium. Equine antitoxin. Emedicine.medscape.com. https://emedicine.medscape.com/article/217943-overview (accessed September 2, 2020).

CN gas. Pepper spray. Cen.acs.org. https://cen.acs.org/policy/chemical-weapons/Tear-gas-and-pepper-spray- (accessed February 18, 2021).

Cocoanut Grove Fire. Nightclubs. Nfpa.org. https://www.nfpa.org/Public-Education/Staying-safe/Safety-in-living-and-entertainment-spaces/Nightclubs-assembly-occupancies/The-Cocoanut-Grove-fire (accessed September 2, 2020).

Cocoanut. Health. Medicalnewstoday.com. https://www.medicalnewstoday.com/articles/323743 (accessed February 18, 2021).

Concordance. Bible. Learnthebible.org. http://www.learnthebible.org/bible/concordance/ (accessed August 12, 2020).

Contac. Antitussive. Webmd.com. https://www.webmd.com/drugs/2/drug-54534-1096/contac-oral/non-opioid-antitussive-w-decongestant-oral/details (accessed January 2, 2021).

COVID-19. CRISPR. Future-science.com. https://www.future-science.com/doi/10.2144/btn-2020-0145 (accessed December 23, 2020).

_____. Deaths. Excess Causes. Jamanetwork.com. https://jamanetwork.com/journals/jama/fullarticle/2778361?utm_source=silverchair&utm_campaign=jama_network&utm_content=covid_weekly_highlights&utm_medium=email (accessed April 3, 2021).

_____. Emergency. Cdc.gov. https://emergency.cdc.gov/han/2020/han00428.asp (accessed January 9, 2021).

_____. False Death Reports. Nbcnews.com. https://www.nbcnews.com/think/opinion/truth-about-cdc-s-covid-19-death-rate-conspiracies-undermining-ncna1241343 (accessed February 21, 2021).

_____. Fever. Monitor. Yalehealth.yale.edu. https://yalehealth.yale.edu/covid-19-monitor-your-health (accessed February 2, 2021).

_____. MMWR. Cdc.gov. https://www.cdc.gov/mmwr/volumes/69/wr/mm6918e2.htm (accessed January 9, 2021).

_____. Outbreak. March 2020. Alnap.org. https://www.alnap.org/help-library/gender-alert-for-covid-19-outbreak-march-2020 (accessed January 9, 2021).

_____. Temperature. Marker. Capecodhealth.org. https://www.capecodhealth.org/medical-services/infectious-disease/coronavirus/is-temperature-a-good-marker-for-covid-19/ (accessed January 2, 2021).

Cro-Magnon. Geology. Bgs.ac.uk. https://www.bgs.ac.uk/discoveringGeology/time/timeline/croMagnon.html (accessed September 13, 2020).

CS gas. Effects. Ncbi.nlm.nih.gov. https://www.ncbi.nlm.nih.gov/pmc/articles/PMC539444/

da Gama, Vasco. Biography. Biography.com. https://www.biography.com/explorer/vasco-da-gama (accessed January 15, 2020).

Death. National Cemeteries. Nps.gov. https://www.nps.gov/nr/travel/national_cemeteries/Death.html# (accessed June 13, 2020).

Deaths. Cdc.gov. https://www.cdc.gov/nchs/fastats/deaths.htm (accessed January 21, 2021).

Department of Defense. Defense.gov. (accessed July 21, 2020).

DNA. Watson and Crick. Nature.com. https://www.nature.com/scitable/topicpage/discovery-of-dna-structure-and-function-watson (accessed December 21, 2020).

Doudna, Jennifer. Wolf Prize. Dailycal.org. https://www.dailycal.org/2020/01/23/uc-berkeley-professor-jennifer-doudna-wins-2020-wolf-prize-in-medicine (accessed September 15, 2020).

Douglass, Jane Dempsey. Predestination. Presbyterianmission.org. https://www.presbyterianmission.org/what-we-believe/predestination/ (accessed August 31, 2020).

DreamWorks Water Park. Americandream.com. https://www.americandream.com/venue/dreamworks-water-park (accessed January 19, 2021).

Drug Resistance. Antibiotics. Cdc.gov. https://www.cdc.gov/drugresistance/food.html (accessed August 22, 2020).

Edison effect. Dictionary.com. https://www.dictionary.com/browse/edison-effect (accessed September 15, 2020).

Egypt, ancient. History.com. https://www.history.com/topics/ancient-history/ancient-egypt (accessed November 6, 2020).

Electoral. Maps. Businessinsider.com. https://www.businessinsider.com/2016-2020-electoral-maps-exit-polls-compared-2020 (accessed December 21, 2010).

Elephantiasis. Azquotes.com. https://www.azquotes.com/quote/1336316 (accessed July 17, 2020).

Environmental Protection Agency. Pesticide Products. epa.gov/ingredients-used-pesticide-products/24 (accessed August 20, 2020).

Essential amino acids, from Webster's Dictionary, https://www.merriam-webster.com/dictionary/essential amino acid (accessed June 28, 2020).

FDR. Popularity. Mises.org. https://mises.org/library/real-reason-fdrs-popularity (accessed April 28, 2021).

Fecal Mass. Microbial. Microbiologyresearch.org. https://www.microbiologyresearch.org/content/journal/jmm/10.1099/00222615-13-1-45 (accessed February 22, 2021).

Fee, American Medical School. Thelancet.com. https://www.thelancet.com/journals/lancet/issue/vol385no9981 (accessed February 13, 2021).

Fickle finger. Laugh In. timescall.com. https://www.timescall.com/2017/10/09/ralph-josephsohn-the-fickle-finger-of-fate (accessed February 15, 2021).

Fildes. The Doctor. Tate.org.uk. https://www.tate.org.uk/art/artworks/fildes-the-doctor-n01522 (accessed February 7, 2021).

Filsinger, Amy Lynn. Smallpox. George Washington. Loc.gov. https://www.loc.gov/rr/scitech/GW&smallpoxinoculation.html (accessed November 25, 2020).

Filterable virus. Dictionary. Merriam-Webster.com. https://www.merriam-webster.com/dictionary/filterable%20virus (accessed July 2, 2020).

Fire. Pleistocene. News.yale.edu. https://news.yale.edu/2021/05/05/study-offers-earliest-evidence-humans-changing-ecosystems-fire (accessed May 12, 2021).

Fleas. University of Kentucky. Uky.edu. https://entomology.ca.uky.edu/ef602 (accessed June 29, 2020).

Flint. Water crisis. Nrdc.org. https://www.nrdc.org/flint (accessed December 5, 2020).

Fossett, Steve. Plane crash. Usatoday.com. http://usatoday30.usatoday.com/news/ nation/2008-11-03-3668149862_x.htm (accessed September 7, 2020).

Fungal Diseases. Cdc.gov. https://www.cdc.gov/fungal/diseases/ (accessed July 18, 2020).

Garrity, Amada. Robotic pets. Goodhousekeeping.com https://www.goodhousekeeping.com/life/pets/a28353484/hasbro-joy-for-all-robotic-pets-for-seniors/ (accessed September 30, 2020).

Gaslighting. Pri.org. Stories. https://www.pri.org/stories/2016-10-14/heres-where-gaslighting-got-its-name (accessed July 12, 2020).

Gastrointestinal. pH. Pubmed.ncbi.nlm.nih.gov. https://pubmed.ncbi.nlm.nih.gov/10421978/ (accessed February 20, 2021).

Gettysburg Museum. Visitor Center. Gettsburgfoundation.org. https://www.gettysburgfoundation.org/museum-visitor-center (accessed June 14, 2020).

Ghee. India. Feastingathome.com. https://www.feastingathome.com/how-to-make-ghee/ (accessed January 11, 2021).

Girgis, Linda. Evil Doctors. Physiciansweekly.com. https://www.physiciansweekly.com/top-14-most-evil-doctors-of-the-last-two-centuries/ (accessed March 16, 2021): "Top 14 most evil doctors of the last two centuries," *Physicians Weekly* (25 October 2019).

Gray, Theodore. Radiation. Popsci.com. https://www.popsci.com/scitech/article/2004-08/healthy-glow-drink-radiation/ (accessed October 31, 2020).

Great Influenza. Pandemic. Cdc.gov. https://www.cdc.gov/flu/pandemic-resources/1918-pandemic-h1n1.html (accessed April 4, 2021).

Green. Heraldic. Thetreemaker.com. https://www.thetreemaker.com/design-coat-of-arms-symbol/meaning-of-colors.html (accessed March 6, 2021).

Greshko, Michael. Rats. Black Death. Nationalgeographic.com. https://www.nationalgeographic.com/news/2018/01/rats-plague-black-death-humans-lice-health-science/ (accessed November 14, 2020).

H1N1 Pandemic. Cdc.gov/flu https://www.cdc.gov/flu/pandemic-resources/2009-h1n1-pandemic.html (accessed July 15, 2020).

Hadid, Diaa. Hajj. Nytimes.com. https://www.nytimes.com/2016/09/16/world/middleeast/hajj-mecca-saudi-arabia.html (accessed August 23, 2020).

Halal. Muslim. Waht.nhs.uk/en. http://www.waht.nhs.uk/en-GB/NHS-Mobile/Our-Services/?depth=4&srcid=2004 (accessed August 5, 2020).

Halifax Harbor. News. Washingtonpost.com. https://www.washingtonpost.com/news/retropolis/wp/2017/12/06/two-ships-collided-in-halifax-harbor-one-of-them-was-a-3000-ton-floating-bomb/ (accessed September 2, 2020).

Hals, Tom. Sackler. Reuters.com. https://www.reuters.com/article/us-purdue-pharma-bankruptcy-factbox/where-the-purdue-pharma-sackler-legal-saga-stands-idUSKBN1ZS1H3 (accessed October 30, 2020).

Hansen's Disease. Health Resources and Services Administration. Hrsa.gov. https://www.hrsa.gov/hansens-disease/history.html (accessed February 1, 2021).

Health Line. Milk. https://www.healthline.com/health/is-milk-bad-for-you (accessed 10/31/2020).

Henry VIII. Greensleeves. Classicfm.com. https://www.classicfm.com/discover-music/greensleeves-did-henry-viii-write-song/ (accessed February 19, 2021).

Herbal supplements. Bay laurel. Herbal-supplement-resource.com. https://www.herbal-supplement-resource.com/bay-laurel-benefits (accessed October 26, 2020).

Herd immunity. Gypsyamber D'Souza and David Dowdy. Jhsph.edu. https://www.jhsph.edu/covid-19/articles/achieving-herd-immunity-with-covid19.html (accessed July 18, 2020).

Heroin. Narcotics. Medlineplus.gov. https://medlineplus.gov/ency/article/000949.htm (accessed October 30, 2020).

Hill, George J. Health and History. Mhsnj.org. www.mhsnj.org/online-publications (accessed January 17, 2021).

_____. Marshall University. Mds.marshall.edu. https://mds.marshall.edu/sc_finding_aids/344/ + 0789: George J. Hill Collection, 1889-2011 (accessed November 23, 2020).

Hippocrates. Oath. North. Nlm.nih.gov. https://www.nlm.nih.gov/hmd/greek/greek_oath.html (accessed March 14, 2021).

_____. Oath. Edelstein. Medicinenet.com. https://www.medicinenet.com/hippocratic_oath/definition.htm (accessed April 24, 2021).

_____. Oath. Lasagna. Medicinenet.com. https://www.medicinenet.com/hippocratic_oath/definition.htm (accessed April 24, 2021).

History. 15th. Fsmitha.com. from http://www.fsmitha.com/time/ce15.htm (accessed January 15, /2020).
_____. 17th. Fsmitha.com. from http://www.fsmitha.com/time/ce17.htm (accessed November 20, 2020).
Agent Orange. History.com. https://www.history.com/topics/vietnam-war/agent-orange-1 (accessed August 20, 2020).
_____. Centuries 11-16. 13th. Fsmitha.com. http://www.fsmitha.com/time/ce13.htm (accessed November 13, 2020).
Hoffman, Jan. Ant-Vaccine sentiment. Nytimes.com. https://www.nytimes.com/2019/09/23/health/anti-vaccination-movement-us.html (accessed September 8, 2020).
Holocaust Museum. Information. Ushmm.org. https://www.ushmm.org/information/about-the-museum (accessed June 14, 2020).
Hominid. Origins. Nature.com https://www.nature.com/scitable/knowledge/library/hominoid-origins (accessed September 13, 2020).
Honey bat. Animalia. Animalia.bio. http://animalia.bio/long-tongued-nectar-bat (accessed February 17, 2021).
Hookworm. CDC. Cdc.gov. https://www.cdc.gov/dpdx/hookworm/index.html (accessed June 29, 2020).
Humans, archaic. Biology. Excellup.com. https://www.excellup.com/InterBiology/eleven_history/archaic-humans.aspx (accessed September 13, 2020).
Ice and the Density of Water. ThoughtCo.com. https://www.thoughtco.com/why-does-ice-float-604304 (accessed January 20, 2021).
ICRC. Red Cross. Icrc.org. https://www.icrc.org/en/who-we-are/movement (accessed November 27, 2020).
Ikner, Luisa A. "A Continuously Active Antimicrobial Coating effective against Human Coronavirus 229E." Medrxiv. https://www.medrxiv.org/content/10.1101/2020.05.10.20097329v1.full.pdf (accessed 8/27/2020).
INRI. The Catholic Miscellany. https://themiscellany.org/2017/07/22/what-does-inri-stand-for/ (accessed July 10, 2010).
International Monetary Fund. Investopedia.com. https://www.investopedia.com/terms/g/groupoften.asp (accessed July 20, 2020).
_____. List of Countries. Wikipedia.org. https://en.wikipedia.org/wiki/List_of_countries_by_GDP_(nominal)_per_capita (accessed July 20, 2020). There is no primary source given by Wikipedia for this consolidated list.
Internet Encyclopedia of Philosophy. Golden Rule. https://iep.utm.edu/goldrule/ (accessed August 25, 2020).
Jacobs, Fred. Lawyer. Doctor. Tapinto.net. https://www.tapinto.net/towns/livingston/sections/health-and-wellness/articles/jacobs-retiring-after-long-career-with-saint-barn (accessed March 16, 2021).
Jewish clothing. Article. Myjewishlearning.com. https://www.myjewishlearning.com/article/jewish-clothing/ (accessed August 23, 2020).
Jewish. Martyred Physicians. Jewishgen.org. https://www.jewishgen.org/databases/Holocaust/0065_Polish_Martyred_Physicians.html (accessed March 12, 2021).
Leishmaniasis. World Health Organization. Who.int. https://www.who.int/news-room/fact- sheets/detail/leishmaniasis (accessed June 28, 2020).
Lilford, Richard. Physicians. Heads of State. Wordpress.com. https://richardlilfordsfridayblog.wordpress.com/2013/07/19/doctors-and-natural-scientists-who-became-head-of-state/ (accessed March 15, 2021).
Kennedy. Berlin. Wsj.com. https://www.wsj.com/articles/ich-bin-ein-berliner-jfk-got-it-righthe-was-no-jelly-doughnut-11573152244 (accessed February 18, 2021).
King. Thyroid. Wsj.com. https://www.wsj.com/articles/SB861137272686553500 (accessed December 22, 2020).
Koran. Quod.lib. Umich.edu. https://quod.lib.umich.edu/k/koran/simple.html (accessed August 12, 2020).

Krebiozen. Quack. Chicagotribune.com. https://www.chicagotribune.com/ opinion/commentary/ct-perspec-flashback-cancer-cure-krebiozen-quack-fraud-0930-20180925-story.html (accessed July 9, 2020).

Laetrile. About Cancer. Cancer.gov. https://www.cancer.gov/about-cancer/treatment/cam/hp/laetrile-pdq. (accessed 6/20/2020).

Leading Causes of Death. Cdc.gov. https://www.cdc.gov/nchs/fastats/leading-causes-of-death.htm (accessed July 20, 2020).

Lee, Harper. Biography. m Biograpy.com: https://www.biography.com/writer/harper-lee (accessed February 19, 2021).

Let's Talk Science. Iceberg. https://letstalkscience.ca/educational-resources/hands-on-activities/how-much-iceberg-on-top-water (accessed January 21, 2021).

Levine, Amy-Jill. Tanakh. Bibleodyssey.org. https://www.bibleodyssey.org/en/tools/bible-basics/what-is-the-difference-between-the-old-testament-the-tanakh-and-the-hebrew-bible (accessed November 8, 2020).

Lewis, John L. Congressman. Biography.com. https://www.biography.com/political-figure/john-lewis (accessed December 15, 2020).

Lincoln, Abraham. Smallpox. Reuters.com. https://www.reuters.com/article/us-smallpox-lincoln/lincoln-came-near-death-from-smallpox-researchers (accessed December 8, 2020).

Lind, James. Scurvy. Bbvopenmind.com. https://www.bbvaopenmind.com/en/science/leading-figures/james-lind-and-scurvy-the-first-clinical-trial-in-history/ (accessed November 24, 2020).

Luke. Jesus. Todayintheword.org. https://www.todayintheword.org/issues/2020/march/question-and-answer/question-2/ (accessed March 14, 2021).

_____. Saints. Fiamc.org. https://www.fiamc.org/faith-prayer/saints/physician-saints-of-the-catholic-church/ (accessed March 13, 2021).

Luther, Martin. Theses. Uncommon-travel-germany.com. https://www.uncommon-travel-germany.com/martin-luther-95-theses.html (accessed August 31, 2020).

Maass, Clara. History. Aahn.org. https://www.aahn.org/maass (accessed August 27, 2020).

Maggot. WebMD.com. https://www.webmd.com/skin-problems-and-treatments/qa/how-is-maggot-therapy-used-to-treat-gangrene (accessed June 29, 2020).

Manifest Destiny. Polk. Teachinghistory.org. https://teachinghistory.org/history-content/ask-a-historian/22205 (accessed January 1, 2021).

Masonic. Great Seal. Greatseal.com. https://www.greatseal.com/symbols/reverse.html; https://greatseal.com/mythamerica/notmasonic.html (accessed December 3, 2020).

MedlinePlus. Intersex. https://medlineplus.gov/ency/article/001669.htm (accessed May 20, 2020).

Memorial Sloan Kettering Cancer Center. Mskcc.org. https://www.mskcc.org/ (accessed July 20, 2020).

Memorials. National Mall. Washington.org. https://washington.org/visit-dc/must-see-memorials-monuments-national-mall (accessed June 17, 2020).

Merovingian. Dynasty. Merovingiandynasty.org. http://www.merovingiandynasty.org/ (accessed November 12, 2020).

MERS. Coronavirus. Cdc.gov. https://www.cdc.gov/coronavirus/mers/index.html (accessed July 4, 2020).

Microbiome. Stat. Statnews.com. https://reports.statnews.com/ (accessed April 28, 2021).

Milk. India. Financialexpress.com. https://www.financialexpress.com/economy/on-world-milk-day (accessed August 24, 2020).

Mormon. Faith. Pbs.org. https://www.pbs.org/mormons/faqs/ (accessed December 19, 2020).

Mosher, Dave, and Morgan McFall-Johnsen. Business Insider. https://www.businessinsider.com/car-size-asteroid-2020qg-missed-earth-by-2000-miles-2020-8 (accessed August 19, 2020).

Mullai Mani Mozhi, J. "Urbanization and its impact on environment in Pudukkottai, Tamilnadu, India," Thesis, May 2010. Shodh Bibtex. http://hdl.handle.net/10603/5081 (accessed January 18, 2021).

Muniz, Hannah. What is the Rainbow Color Order? PrepScholar, https://blog.prepscholar.com/rainbow-color-order (accessed January 19, 2021).

Mutualism. Symbiosis. Thoughtco.com. https://www.thoughtco.com/mutualism-symbiotic-relationships-4109634 (accessed February 20, 2021).

Nathawani, Amit C. Lancet. Thelancet.com. https://www.thelancet.com/journals/lancet/article/PIIS0140-6736(16)00144-6/fulltext (accessed July 12, 2020).

National Cancer Institute. Cancer.gov. (accessed July 21, 2020).

National Cancer Institute. National Cancer Act. Cancer.gov. https://www.cancer.gov/about-nci/overview/history/national-cancer-act-1971 (accessed February 1, 2021).

National Health Service. Lactose Intolerance. https://www.nhs.uk/conditions/lactose-intolerance/ (accessed 10/31/2020).

National Human Genome Research Institute. Genomics. https://www.genome.gov/about-genomics/fact-sheets/Deoxyribonucleic-Acid-Fact-Sheet (accessed June 28, 2020).

National Institutes of Health. Nih.gov. (accessed July 21, 2020).

National WW2 Museum. New Orleans. Nationalww2museum.org. https://www.nationalww2museum.org/ (accessed June 14, 2020).

Navy.Mil. Navydata. https://www.navy.mil/navydata/nav_legacy.asp?id=172 (accessed June 10, 2020).

Nelson, Lord. Blind eye. Thetimes.co.uk. https://www.thetimes.co.uk/article/how-turning-a-blind-eye-won-the-battle-for-nelson (accessed August 25, 2020).

Neolithic. Pre-history. History.com. https://www.history.com/topics/pre-history/neolithic-revolution (accessed September 13, 2020).

Netflix. Octopus Teacher. Netflix.com. https://www.netflix.com/title/81045007 (accessed March 19, 2021).

New York Times. Harris, Jean. Nytimes.com. https://www.nytimes.com/2012/12/29/nyregion/jean-s-harris-killer-of-scarsdale-diet-doctor-dies-at-89.html (accessed January 23, 2021).

Newman, Laura. National Library of Medicine. Lynn Payer. https://www.ncbi.nlm.nih.gov/pmc/articles/PMC1121410/ (accessed January 24, 2021).

Newton. Calculus. Grc.nasa.gov. https://www.grc.nasa.gov/www/k-12/airplane/newton2c.html (accessed December 30, 2020)

_____. Second Law. Howthingsfly.si.edu. https://howthingsfly.si.edu/ask-an-explainer/what-difference-between-fma (accessed December 30, 2020).

North, Michael. Greek. Nlm.nih.gov. https://www.nlm.nih.gov/hmd/greek/greek_oath.html (accessed August 12, 2020).

Oklahoma City bombing. Topics. History.com. https://www.history.com/topics/1990s/oklahoma-city-bombing (accessed September 2, 2020).

Opioid. Oxycodone. Dea.gov. https://www.dea.gov/factsheets/oxycodone (accessed March 16, 2021).

_____. Oxycodone. Medlineplus.gov. https://medlineplus.gov/druginfo/meds/a682132.html (accessed March 16, 2021).

Organ. 78. Byjus.com. https://byjus.com/biology/what-are-the-78-organs-in-the-human-body/ (accessed February 20, 2021).

Organ system. Eleven. Biologydictionary.net. https://biologydictionary.net/organ/ (accessed February 20, 2021).

Osler, Margaret J. Scientific Revolution. Britannica.com. https://www.britannica.com/science/Scientific-Revolution (accessed November 26, 2020).

Pain. Joint Commission. Jointcommission.org. https://www.jointcommission.org/-/media/tjc/documents/resources/pain-management/pain_std_history_web_version_05122017pdf.pdf?db (accessed March 16, 2021).

Parasite. Saprophyte. Differencebetween.net. http://www.differencebetween.net/ science/difference-between-parasite-and-saprophyte (accessed June 27, 2020).

Parasitology. National Center for Biotechnology Information. Ncbi.nlm.nih.gov. https://www.ncbi.nlm.nih.gov/books/NBK8262/ (accessed June 28, 2020).

Paris Agreement. Climate. Unfccc.int. https://unfccc.int/process-and-meetings/the-paris-agreement (accessed February 16, 2021).

Pandemics. Visualcapitalist.com. https://www.visualcapitalist.com/history-of-pandemics-deadliest/ (accessed January 5, 2020).

Pasteur. Spontaneous generation. Immunology.org. https://www.immunology.org/pasteurs-col-de-cygnet-1859 (accessed March 26, 2021).

Pestsäule, Vienna. Plague. Atlasobscura.com. https://www.atlasobscura.com/places/vienna-pestsaule-plague-column (accessed November 29, 2020).

Pietrangelo, Ann. "Left Brain vs. Right Brain: What Does This Mean for Me." Healthline.com. https://www.healthline.com/health/left-brain-vs-right-brain (accessed January 17, 2021).

Plasmodium. Malaria. Who.int. https://www.who.int/news-room/fact-sheets/detail/malaria (accessed June 28, 2020).

Poison. Five deadliest poisons. Theconversation.com. https://theconversation.com/handle-with-care-the-worlds-five-deadliest-poisons-56089 (accessed July 19, 2020).

Police shootings database. Washingtonpost.com. https://www.washingtonpost.com/graphics/investigations/police-shootings-database/ (accessed January 31, 2021).

Population. Connection. Populationconnection.org. https://www.populationconnection.org/ (accessed February 6, 2021).

Prokaryotes. Biology. Openstax.com. https://opentextbc.ca/biology2eopenstax (accessed December 23, 2020).

Protothecosis. Ncbi.nlm.nih.gov. https://www.ncbi.nlm.nih.gov/pmc/articles/PMC1865593/ (accessed February 1, 2021).

Rabies. Biologic. Who.int. https://www.who.int/rabies/resources/other_rabies_biolog_product/en/ (accessed January 12, 2021).

Reagan, Nancy. Astrology. Atlasobscura.com. https://www.atlasobscura.com/articles/a-brief-history-of-nancy-reagan-and-astrology (accessed August 24, 2020).

Rennie, Drummond. Thyroid. Jamanetwork.com. https://jamanetwork.com/journals/jama/article-abstract/415402 (accessed December 22, 2020).

Respiratory viruses. Infectious diseases. Merkmanuals.com. https://www.merckmanuals.com/professional/infectious-diseases/respiratory-viruses (accessed January 12, 2021).

Retraction Watch. Database. Sciencemag.org. https://www.sciencemag.org/news/2018/10/what-massive-database-retracted-papers-reveals-about-science-publishing-s-death-penalty (accessed March 26, 2021).

Reye's syndrome. Mayoclinic.org. https://www.mayoclinic.org/diseases-conditions/reyes-syndrome/ (accessed October 26, 2020).

Ricin. Markov as Spy. Rferl.org. https://www.rferl.org/a/no-agent-bulgarian-spies-letter-refutes-talk-of-umbrella-murder-victim-markov-as-spy/29772449.html. (accessed July 9, 2020).

Rivard, Laura. Genetics Forum. Nature.com. https://www.nature.com/scitable/forums/genetics-generation/america-s-hidden-history-the-eugenics-movement-123919444/ (accessed May 17, 2020).

Rockwell, Norman, Museum. Golden Rule. Nrm.org. http://www.nrm.org/thinglink/text/GoldenRule.html (accessed August 25,2020).

Roser, Max, et al. "World Population Growth." Our World in Data. https://ourworldindata.org/world-population-growth (accessed August 20, 2020).

Roswell Park. Roswellpark.org. https://www.roswellpark.org/about-us/ (accessed July 20, 2020).

Rush, Bobby. Emmett Till. Chicago Tribune. https://www.chicagotribune.com/politics/ct-nw-emmett-till-lynching-act-bobby-rush-20200226-r5qpkwjikvednbrkxvkncpudiy-story.html (accessed May 20, 2020).

Sackler. Opioid. Abcnews.go.com. https://abcnews.go.com/US/sackler-family-pay-42-billion-opioid-lawsuit-settlement/story?id=76485141 (accessed March 16, 2021).

Sahih Muslim, Book: 9. The Book of Divorce. Iium.edu. https://www.iium.edu.my/deed/hadith/muslim/009_smt.html (accessed January 25, 2021).

Saleh, Naveed. Notorious doctors. Mdlinx.com. https://www.mdlinx.com/article/10-notorious-doctors-in-history/lfc-3448 (accessed March 16, 2021). "10 notorious doctors in history," *MDlinx* (24 February 2019).

Saltin, Bengt. ExercisePhysiology.net. http://www.exercisephysiology.net/Bengt_Saltin.asp (accessed September 6, 2020).

Santayana. History repeating. Liberalarts.vt.edu. https://liberalarts.vt.edu/magazine/2017/history-repeating (accessed February 15, 2021).

Schwarzkopf, Fabian. Sauer Organ. YouTube. https://www.youtube.com/watch?v=77CP5YitoGk (accessed July 18, 2020).

Science of the 10 plagues. Livescience.com. https://www.livescience.com/58638-science-of-the-10-plagues.html (accessed June 8, 2020).

Scopolamine. Drugs. Drugs.com. https://www.drugs.com/illicit/devils-breath.html (accessed October 26, 2020).

Scrofula. Tuberculosis. History.rcplondon.ac.uk/. https://history.rcplondon.ac.uk/blog/touching-kings-evil-short-history (accessed August 25, 2020).

Segall, H. N. Thomas Browne. Pubmed.ncbi.nlm.nih.gov. https://pubmed.ncbi.nlm.nih.gov/11614038/ (accessed November 20, 2020).

Serratore, Angela. "President Cleveland's Problem Child." Smithsonianmag.com. https://www.smithsonianmag.com/history/president-clevelands-problem-child-100800/ (accessed December 12, 2020).

Silence of the Lambs. Film. Documentarylovers.com. https://documentarylovers.com/film/silence-of-lambs-true-story/ (accessed July 10, 2020).

Sleep. Healthy. Mayoclinic.org https://www.mayoclinic.org/healthy-lifestyle/adult-health/in-depth/sleep-aids/art-20047860 (accessed January 2, 2021).

Smallpox. History. Ncbi.nlm.nih.gov. https://www.ncbi.nlm.nih.gov/pmc/articles/PMC1200696/ (accessed February 19, 2021).

_____. Washington, George. History.com. https://www.history.com/news/smallpox-george-washington-revolutionary-war (accessed February 24, 2021).

Stone, Marvin J. Henry Bence Jones. Journals.sagepub.com. https://journals.sagepub.com/doi/abs/10.1177/096777209800600112?journalCode=jmba (accessed December 13, 2020).

Sturgis, S.D., Bike Rally. Khn.org. https://khn.org/morning-breakout/sturgis-biker-rally-linked-to-260000-covid-cases/ (accessed February 19, 2021).

_____. Facebook.com. https://www.facebook.com/SturgisBikeRally2021/ (accessed February 19, 2021).

_____. Nytimes.com. https://www.nytimes.com/2020/11/06/us/sturgis-coronavirus-cases.html (accessed February 19, 2021).

Sydenham. Hysteria. Karger.com. https://www.karger.com/Article/FullText/450605 (accessed April 8, 2021).

Tampa, Mercia. Brief History of Syphilis. Ncbi.nlm.nih.gov. https://www.ncbi.nlm.nih.gov/pmc/articles/PMC3956094 (accessed January 23, 2021).

TED. Technology. Ideas worth spreading. Ted.com. https://www.ted.com/ (accessed February 14, 2021).

The Kings Bible. King James Bible. Thekingsbible.com. http://thekingsbible.com/Concordance (accessed January 18, 2021).

The Presidential Commission for the Study of Bioethical Issues. "Ethically Impossible" STD Research in Guatemala from 1946 to 1948. Government Printing Office. www.bioethics.gov (accessed July 10, 2020).

Thomas, Dana. Washington Post. https://www.washingtonpost.com/archive/politics/1995/01/19/cave-paintings (accessed January 9, 2021).

Time and tide. Dictionary.com. https://www.dictionary.com/browse/time-and-tide-wait-for-no-man (accessed September 2, 2020).

_____. Phrase Finder. Phrases.org. https://www.phrases.org.uk/meanings/time-and-tide-wait-for-no-one.html (accessed September 2, 2020).

Time. Content Time.com. http://content.time.com/time/specials/packages/article/0,28804,1859513_1859526_1859518,00.html (accessed May 17, 2020).

TMC. Texas Medical Center. Tmc.edu. https://www.tmc.edu/ (accessed March 1, 2021).

Tory. Loyalist. Uelac.org. http://www.uelac.org/Loyalist-Trails/Loyalist-Trails-index.php (accessed November 27, 2020).

Turner, Bambi. Elephant graveyards. Howstuffworks.com. https://animals.howstuffworks.com/animal-facts/are-there-really-elephant-graveyards.htm (accessed March 19, 2021).

Twain. Death. Mentalfloss.com. https://www.mentalfloss.com/article/562400/reports-mark-twains-quote-about-mark-twains-death-are-greatly-exaggerated (accessed February 21, 2021).

Twins. Epigenetics. Theatlantic.com. https://www.theatlantic.com/science/archive/2018/05/twin-epigenetics/560189/ (accessed August 30, 2020).

United States Public Health Service. Usphs.gov. (accessed July 21, 2020).

Urey. Oparin. Life Origin. Khanacademy.org. https://www.khanacademy.org/science/ap-biology/natural-selection/origins-of-life-on-earth/a/hypotheses-about-the-origins-of-life#:~:text (accessed April 6, 2021).

Veterans Administration. Agent Orange. https://www.publichealth.va.gov/exposures/agentorange (accessed August 20, 20200).

Vietnam War Timeline. History.com. https://www.history.com/topics/vietnam-war/vietnam-war-timeline (accessed June 13, 2020).

Voyager. Spacecraft. Earthsky.org. https://earthsky.org/space/nasa-reestablishes-contact-with-voyager2-spacecraft-oct2020# (accessed December 4, 2020).

Walter Reed Medical Center. Tricare.mil (accessed July 21, 2020).

Warren, John Collins. Anesthesia. Collections.countway.harvard.edu. http://collections.countway.harvard.edu/onview/exhibits/show/family-practice/john-collins-warren--1778-1856 (accessed December 13, 2020).

Watson, Sarah. Pandemic. Nytimes.com. https://www.nytimes.com/2020/09/06/us/colleges-coronavirus-students.html (accessed September 9, 2020).

Weinberg. Silverstein. Nybook.com. https://www.nybooks.com/articles/2016/02/25/the-whig-history-of-science-an-exchange/ (accessed February 23, 2020).

_____. Thony. Thonyc.wordpress.com. https://thonyc.wordpress.com/2015/08/19/to-explain-the-weinberg-the-discovery-of-a-nobel-laureates-view-of-the-history-of-science/ (accessed February 23, 2020).

Weisse. Self-experimentation. https://www.ncbi.nlm.nih.gov/pmc/articles/PMC3298919/ (accessed February 8, 2012).

Welcome Fleet. Welcomesociety.org. https://www.welcomesociety.org/ancestors.html (accessed November 23, 2020).

WHO. World Health Organization. Coronavirus. Who.int. https://www.who.int/health-topics/coronavirus (accessed March 1, 2021).

Winthrop. City upon a hill. neh.gov. https://www.neh.gov/article/how-america-became-city-upon-hill (accessed February 6, 2021).

Zakat. Islam. Islamic-relief.org. https://www.islamic-relief.org/zakat (accessed August 31, 2020).

_____. Calculator. Muslimaid.org. https://www.muslimaid.org/ zakat-calculator/ (accessed August 31, 2020).

Zika. Cdc.gov. https://www.cdc.gov/zika/index.html (accessed July 6, 2020).

Zimmermann, Corinne. Washington Post. Legacy.com. https://www.legacy.com/obituaries/washingtonpost/obituary.aspx?n=corinne-zimmermann-teeny&pid=190177314. (accessed July 11, 2020).

Zinsser. Typhus. https://www.encyclopedia.com/people/medicine/medicine-biographies/hans-zinsser (accessed February 8, 2021).

Zoroastrians. Water. Fire. Lumenlearning.com. https://courses.lumenlearning.com/suny-hccc-worldcivilization/chapter/zoroastrianism (accessed March 31, 2021).

Miscellaneous

Addams, Charles Samuel. *Addams Family* cartoons.
Anon. *Mother Goose*. "Sleeping Beauty."
Anon. "Ring around the Roses."
"Call the Midwife." BBC TV.
Capp, Al. "Li'l Abner" (comic strip)
Munch, Edvard *The Scream* (painting)
Non Sequitur (comic strip)
Rodin, Auguste. *The Burghers of Calais* (sculpture)
Roe v Wade
Regents of the University of California v Bakke, 438 U.S. 265 (1978)

Notes

Introduction

[1] The cover portrait: "In 1890 Sir Henry Tate (1819-98) commissioned a painting from Luke Fildes, the subject of which was left to his own discretion. The artist chose to recall a personal tragedy of his own, when in 1877 his first son, Philip, had died at the age of one in his Kensington home. Fildes' son and biographer wrote: 'The character and bearing of their doctor throughout the time of their anxiety, made a deep impression on my parents. Dr. Murray became a symbol of professional devotion which would day inspire the painting of *The Doctor*' ... The composition of this study is similar to a smaller oil study of the painting in the Robert Packer Hospital in Sayre, Pennsylvania." From: From https://www.tate.org.uk/art/artworks/fildes-the-doctor-n01522 (accessed February 7, 2021).

The principal source used in this essay is "Britannica 2013 Deluxe DVD," Encyclopædia Britannica Deluxe Edition (Chicago: Encyclopædia Britannica, 2013), shortened to *Britannica*. The text and notes of *Health Matters* utilize the guidelines of the *Chicago Manual of Style*, as in Kate L. Turabian, *A Manual for Writers of Term Papers, Theses, and Dissertations* (Chicago: The University of Chicago Press, 1996). Unless otherwise stated, Biblical references are quoted from the King James Bible (KJB). The Merriam-Webster dictionary is cited as *Merriam-Webster* and *Webster's New Twentieth Century Dictionary of the English Language Unabridged*, 2d ed. (1979), shortened to *Merriam-Webster* and *Webster's*. An earlier version was published as: George J. Hill, "Health and History," in Member's Papers, Articles, and Talks, at www.mhsnj.org/online-publications, www.mhsnj.org/online-publications (accessed January 17, 2021).

[2] Lewis Mumford, *Technics and Civilization.* (Chicago: University of Chicago Press, 1934).

[3] J. G. Frazer, *The Golden Bough: A Study in Magic and Religion* [1890] (New York: Oxford University Press, 1994). The term "early healer" is often used instead of "witch doctor," which was formerly used to denote a healer in early human society, because the term is usually used now as a derogatory epithet.

Joseph J. Campbell (1904-87) was a professor of literature at Sarah Lawrence College. He studied comparative religion and mythology. Campbell's most famous quotation is, "Follow your bliss." From https://www.jcf.org/ (accessed March 19, 2021).

[4] This paragraph summarizing the development of human civilization is based on many books, especially Mumford, *Technics and Civilization*; and Jonathan F. P. Rose, *The Well-Tempered City: What Modern Science, Ancient Civilizations and Human Nature Teach Us About the Future of Urban Life* (New York: HarperCollins, 2016).

[5] Thomas S. Kuhn, *The Structure of Scientific Revolutions*, with an Introductory Essay by Ian Hacking. 4th ed. (1962. Chicago: The University of Chicago Press, 2012); Alfred Thayer Mahan, *The Influence of Sea Power upon History, 1660-1783* (Cambridge, University Press, 1890). Robert Darnton lectured in about the year 2000 at Drew University, after publishing *The Forbidden Best-Sellers of Pre-Revolutionary France* (New York: Norton, 1996).

[6] The word "life" comes to us from the Nordic word *lif,* which became *lif* or *lyf* in Middle English. The word "health" has its origin in Nordic and Old English as *hælth,* meaning "whole." Words that convey the meanings of life and health are probably present in every language. For instance, in French, *vie* (life) and *santé* (health), and *vita* (life) and *salutem* (health) in Latin. And ZΩH (*zoi*) (life), and υγεία (ygeía) (health) in Greek.

Part One – Human Health – The Components of Health

[7] Life and death are recurring themes throughout this essay. Life is a characteristic of higher organisms – plants and animals – but the use of the term "life" becomes problematic in reference to some very small particles, such as viruses. The nature of life is the subject of Carl Zimmer's recent book, *Life's Edge: The Search for What It Means to Be Alive* (New York: Dutton, 2021), reviewed by Siddhartha Mukherjee, Look alive, *New York Times Book Review*, 4 April 2021, 1, 20. Zimmer ponders, "Is 'life' the resistance of death?" He points out that metabolism "is crucial to all living things." Yet he answers the question of What is life? with a tautology: "Life *is* what life *does*." In *Health Matters*, I chose to focus on the avoidance of Death instead of prolongation of Life. Life and Death represent the ancient problem depicted in the two faces of the Roman god, Janus.

[8] The appearance of mourning behavior in elephants has been shown on *Nature* and *National Geographic* films for television in recent years. Our inability to understand their communications limits what we can say about this behavior. The ability of primates to grasp with their hands – with thumb and fingers – has changed what humans can do about the future, in contrast to animals, such as elephants, that lack that capability. It is a persistent legend that elephants go to a special place to die persists, but it has never been confirmed by science. See, for example: Bambi Turner, Are there really elephant graveyards? How Stuff Works, https://animals.howstuffworks.com/animal-facts/are-there-really-elephant-graveyards.htm (accessed March 19, 2021). The Netflix film, "My Octopus

Teacher," shows the death of a wild octopus, who in anthropomorphic terms, has become the friend of a man. The octopus appears to anticipate her death, as she crawls into a crevice and dies. It is a curiously haunting film. See: https://www.netflix.com/title/81045007 (accessed March 19, 2021)

[9] Healthquest was the name that was originally planned for the essay. However, the words Healthquest and Health Quest have been used in recent years for commercial enterprises, and may be protected by trademarks.

The double meaning of "health" (as adjective and noun) and "matters" (as noun and verb) appears in *Webster's*. Health (noun): "1. Physical and mental well-being; soundness; freedom from defect, pain, or disease; normality of mental and physical functions." An example of "health" as an adjective is shown in its use as "health officer." Matter (noun) has 12 meanings, including "7. (a) an important affair; thing of some moment or significance; (b) importance; moment; significance; as It's of no *matter*." As an intransitive verb, "matter" appears in both *Webster's Unabridged* and in Merriam-Webster's *Dictionary and Thesaurus* from *Britannica* (2020) as "to be of importance." This essay uses the plural form of the word "matter."

[10] Although history is always moving forward as the "fickle finger of fate," it is important to remember that history also seems in some ways to repeat itself. George Santayana is quoted as saying, "Those who cannot remember the past are condemned to repeat it." Another sober view of history was expressed by William Faulkner, "The past is never dead. It's not even past." A more felicitous expression was given by Azeem Ibrahim, "History rhymes, but it never repeats itself exactly." The "Flying Fickle Finger of Fate" award was a goofy trophy made famous by the 1960s TV show "Laugh-In," at: https://www.timescall.com/2017/10/09/ralph-josephsohn-the-fickle-finger-of-fate (accessed February 15, 2021); https://liberalarts.vt.edu/magazine/2017/history-repeating (accessed February 15, 2021); Faulkner, *Requiem for a Nun* (New York: Random House, 1951). Ibrahim, Why democracy in Myanmar was so easily crushed, *Washington Post*, 16 January 2021, A19.

What Humans Have – the Needs, Urges, Wants, and Exceptions

[11] Professor Christopher Sellers taught two courses about the Human Body and the Environment at Rutgers-Newark in 1996-7, and Professor Richard Sher taught a course on the Environment at New Jersey Institute of Technology (NJIT). These courses shaped some of my thoughts on this part of *Health Matters*. The term *milieu intérieur* was coined by Claude Bernard (1813-1878). This was the basis for the concept of homeostasis, which was proposed by Walter Bradford Cannon (1871-1945).

[12] Mind and Body are discussed separately, but the two are connected in many ways; for instance, in exercise. Humans have a unique quality of endurance. See: Daniel E. Lieberman, *Exercised: Why Something We Never Evolved to Do is Healthy and Rewarding* (New York: Parthenon, 2020), reviewed by Jen A. Miller, Muscle memory, *New York Times Book Review*, 10 January 10, 2021, 15: "Happily, there are ways to get your mind and body past the fact that exercise can be unpleasant." In *Born to Run* (New York: Vintage Books, 2009) Christopher McDougall traced this quality to humans' superior ability in food-gathering. See: Gretchen Reynolds, Bodies like ours, maybe we were born to run, *New York Times*, 16 February 2021, D6.

The uncertain future of the human body is foretold in Debora L. Spar, The poly-parents are coming, *New York Times*, 16 August 2020, SR9. Spar is past president of Barnard College and she is now a professor at Harvard Business School. She comments on reproductive biology, with in vitro fertilization (I.V.F.) and in vitro gametogenesis (I.V.G.): "In vitro gametogenesis is likely to reshape basic ideas about family."

Chapter 1   The Haves   A. The Body

[13] Lear also said, "I fear I am not in my perfect mind" (Shakespeare, *King Lear*, Act 4, Scene 7).

[14] The continuing debate over abortion is partly dependent on defining the moment when human life begins. This is therefore not only a biological question, but also one of religion and philosophy.

[15] To "cut the cord" is an ancient synonym for independence, although humans can never "cut the cord" completely from each other. See E. K. Hutton and Hassan E. S., Late vs early clamping of the umbilical cord in full-term neonates: Systematic review and meta-analysis of controlled trials, *JAMA*, 297 (no. 11, March 2007): 1241–52.

[16] The division of pregnancy into these three parts is shown in Kendra Cherry, Stages of prenatal development, Verywellmind, https://www.verywellmind.com/stages-of-prenatal-development (accessed January 17, 2021).

[17] *Britannica*, Prenatal development; Genetics, human.

[18] "Call the Midwife" on BBC TV (2012ff), is a semi-fictional adaptation of the memoir of an English midwife. It shows the perils and wonders of pregnancy, childbirth, and early parenthood, in a difficult environment. The programs are set beginning in 1957 and continue into the early 1960s.

[19] "The child is father of the man" is said to be a phrase translated from Hindi, and it has since been used by poets and songwriters in English. For example, William Wordsworth in "My Heart Leaps Up" (1802). Also: English to Hindi Dictionary. "The Child is the Father to the Man Meaning in Hindi." AmBoli.com. https://www.aamboli.com/dictionary/the-child-is-the-father-to-the-man-meaning-in-hindi (accessed January 16, 2021).

[20] For mutualism, commensalism, and symbiosis, see: https://www.thoughtco.com/mutualism-symbiotic-relationships-4109634 (accessed February 20, 2021). For the eleven organ systems, see: https://biologydictionary.net/organ/ (accessed February 20, 2021). They are Integumentary, Skeletal, Muscular, Circulatory, Respiratory, Digestive, Urinary, Immune, Nervous, Endocrine, and Reproductive. For the 78 organs, see https://byjus.com/biology/what-are-the-78-organs-in-the-human-body/ (accessed February 20, 2021). (accessed February 20, 2021).

For one example of the bacterial contents of feces, see: Alison M. Stephen and J. H. Cummings, The microbial contribution to human faecal mass, *Journal of Medical Microbiology* 13 (no. 1, 1 February 1980): "the bacterial component of faecal material may be larger than previously thought. Previous estimates of the bacterial component of the wet faecal mass are 30-40%."

I do not know the origin of the term, but it appears in Michael T. Ghiselin, The economy of the body, *The American Economic Review* 68 (no. 2, May 1968): 233-7. It is consistent with homeostasis (see below).

[21] J. Fallingborg, Intraluminal pH of the human gastrointestinal tract, *Dan. Med. Bull.* 46 (no. 3, 1999): 183-96. At: https://pubmed.ncbi.nlm.nih.gov/10421978/ (accessed February 20, 2021).
"How brown fat improves metabolism" (September 10, 2019), from https://www.nih.gov/news-events/nih-research-matters/how-brown-fat-improves-metabolism (accessed February 20, 2021). White fat is an efficient way for the body to store calories. The caloric content of fat is about twice as great, per gram, as the caloric content of protein or carbohydrate: https://my.clevelandclinic.org/health/articles/4182-fat-and-calories (accessed February 22, 2021).

[22] See: Andreas Vesalius, *De humani corporis fabrica libri septem* ("On the fabric of the human body in seven books"), 1543. Vesalius was an outstanding anatomist, and he was one of the first to perform dissections of the human body.

B. The Mind

[23] *Britannica*, Descartes, René.

[24] The sentence, "We only see…" is unattributed. The sign was posted in the conference room adjacent to the office of Professor Francis D. Moore at what was then the Peter Bent Brigham Hospital (now Brigham and Women's). Dr. Moore never referred to the sign, but many of his students believe that he posted the phrase as a warning to all who read it. The expression "We only see…" is also relevant in respect to the emergency use of convalescent plasma to treat COVID-19 patients by Adriane Fugh-Berman, M.D., in a letter to the *Washington Post*, 28 August 2020, A26: "When patients and physicians know what therapy a patient is getting, expectations can affect result and evaluations can be skewed … Randomization reduces the influence of hope, expectation and bias in evaluating differences between groups." Fugh-Berman directs PharmedOut at Georgetown University.

[25] *Britannica*, Nervous system, human."

[26] The most important aspect of the human brain is probably to think, which means to work as a mind and to consider the future. This is a higher function than simply being the center of automatic responses. A contrary view was expressed by Lisa Feldman Barrett, a psychologist, who traced the development of the brain to a "tiny sea creature" about five hundred million years ago, when a "command center" first appeared. See Barrett, Your brain isn't made for thinking, *New York Times*, 24 November 2020, A23.

[27] Oliver Sachs, *The Man Who Mistook His Wife for a Hat* (London: Gerald Duckworth, 1985), described a rare neurological condition known as "visual agnosia," in which the patient cannot recognize or name faces or common objects. Sylvia Nasar, *A Beautiful Mind* (New York: Simon & Schuster, 1998), is based on the life of John Nash (1928-2015), a brilliant mathematician who had delusional paranoid psychosis. The so-called left brain-right brain theory has been challenged, so I have omitted including it in this discussion. See: Ann Pietrangelo, Left brain vs. right brain: What does this mean for me, Healthline, https://www.healthline.com/health/left-brain-vs-right-brain (accessed January 17, 2021).

[28] Joseph Henrich, *The Weirdest People in the World: How the West Became Psychologically Peculiar and Particularly Prosperous* (New York: Farrar, Straus & Giroux, 2020), reviewed by Daniel C. Dennett, Mapping the mind, *New York Times Book Review*, 11 October 2020, 10. The indulgences, which enriched the Church, are documented in colonial America by Ramon A. Gutierrez, *When Jesus Came, the Corn Mothers Went Away: Marriage, Sexuality, and Power in New Mexico, 1500-1846* (Stanford, California: Stanford University Press, 1991).

For the future of *Homo sapiens*, see the speculation by Tali Sharot, The shortlist: The brain, *New York Times Book Review*, 23 May 2021, 22, discussing Jeff Hawkins, *A Thousand Brains: A New Theory of Intelligence* (New York: Basic Books, 2021). Sharot: "Part of Hawkins motivation for developing 'true' A.I. is to prepare for human extinction."

[29] *Britannica*, Habits, in psychology. Also, Felix Powell and George Henry Powell, "Pack Up Your Troubles in Your Old Kit Bag and Smile, Smile, Smile" (1915).

[30] Adapted from "DNA Policy Guidelines," General Society of Mayflower Descendants, Plymouth, Mass. (20 August 2020).

C. The Environment

[31] See George J. Hill, *Edison's Environment: The Great Inventor Was Also a Great Polluter*, 2007. 3d Ed. (Berwyn Heights, Md.: Heritage Books, 2107), 324-365. The most important works cited in *Edison's Environment* are: David F. Noble, *America by Design: Science, Technology, and the Rise of Corporate Capitalism* (New York: Alfred A. Knopf, 1977); Richard White, *The Organic Machine* (New York: Hill and Wang, 1995); Mary Douglas, *Purity and Danger: An Analysis of Concepts of Pollution and Taboo* (New York: Praeger Publishers, 1996); Mary Douglas and Aaron Wildavsky, *Risk and Culture: An Essay on the Selection of Technical and Environmental Dangers* (Berkeley: University of California Press, 1982); Rachel Carson, *Silent Spring* (New York: Houghton Mifflin Co., 1962); and Robert Gottlieb, *Forcing the Spring: The Transformation of the American Environmental Movement* (Washington, D.C.: Island Press, 1993).

[32] Lewis Mumford, *Technics and Civilization* (New York: Harcourt, Brace & World, 1934), 169-70.

[33] Lynn Margulis (1938-2011) was unpredictable, and she enjoyed controversy. She received the National Medal of Science in 1999. She was twice married and divorced; her first husband was the astronomer, Carl Sagan. James Lovelock (b.1919) is long lived.

[34] *Britannica*, Environment. Also see: J. Mullai Mani Mozhi, "Urbanization and its impact on environment in Pudukkottai, Tamilnadu, India," Thesis (May 2010), at Shodh, Bibtex, http://hdl.handle.net/10603/5081 (accessed January 18, 2021).

[35] Marshall Brain, What if an asteroid hit earth? Science How Stuff Works, https://science.howstuffworks.com/nature/natural-disasters/asteroid-hits-earth.htm (accessed 8/19/2020): "There are obvious craters on Earth (and the moon) that show us a long history of large objects hitting the planet." Dave Mosher and Morgan McFall-Johnsen, Business Insider, https://www.businessinsider.com/car-size-asteroid-2020qg-missed-earth-by-2000-miles-2020-8 (accessed August 19, 2020). "A car-size asteroid flew within 1,830 miles of Earth over the weekend [on 17 August 2020]; — the closest pass ever — and we didn't see it coming."

[36] Max Roser, et al, "World Population Growth": The population of the world is estimated to have been 1 billion in 1800; it is now approximately 7.7 billion. See: https://ourworldindata.org/world-population-growth (accessed August 20, 2020). "The Paris Agreement is a legally binding international treaty on climate change. It was adopted by 196 Parties at COP 21 in Paris, on 12 December 2015 and entered into force on 4 November 2016. Its goal is to limit global warming to well below 2, preferably to 1.5 degrees Celsius, compared to pre-industrial levels." From https://unfccc.int/process-and-meetings/the-paris-agreement (accessed February 16, 2021). The discharge of chemical pollutants is the likely cause of many of the other threats to species of plants and animals.

The honey nectar bat is described on Animalia at http://animalia.bio/long-tongued-nectar-bat (accessed February 17, 2021).

[37] For recent actions to address the rise in the world's temperature, see: "The Paris Agreement," at: https://unfccc.int/process-and-meetings/the-paris-agreement/the-paris-agreement (accessed March 29, 2021).

Britannica: Great Smog of London (1952). Also, Kate Winkler Dawson, *Death in the Air: The True Story of a Serial Killer, the Great London Smog, and the Strangling of a City* (New York: Hachette Books, 2017). See R. N. Feinstein, R. J. Fry, and E. F. Staffeldt, Carcinogenic and antitumor effects of aminotriazole on acatalasemic and normal catalase mice, *J. Natl Cancer Inst.* 60 (no. 5, May 1978):1113-6: "Dietary 3-amino-1H-1,2,4-triazole (AT), [was] carcinogenic when administered alone," at https://pubmed.ncbi.nlm.nih.gov/642030/ (accessed January 13, 2021).

Mark S. Reisch, EPA limitations on hydrofluorocarbons give Honeywell an opportunity for an environmentally acceptable substitute, *Chemical and Engineering News* 93 (no. 42, October 26, 2015). https://cen.acs.org/articles/93/i42/Global-Warming-Concerns-Put-Pressure.html (accessed August 20, 2020).

[38] 2-4D is 2,4-Dichlorophenoxyacetic acid, sold under various brand names. For a discussion of the risks of 2-4D, and why its use is banned in Canada, see Arlene Blum, Green Science Policy Institute, "Green Action Centre" https://greenactioncentre.ca/clean-energy-environment/myth-is-24-d-a-risk/ (accessed August 20, 2020).

Agent Orange was used in Operation Ranch Hand in Vietnam. See: epa.gov/ingredients-used-pesticide-products/24 (accessed August 20, 2020). Also, see https://www.history.com/topics/vietnam-war/agent-orange-1 (accessed August 20, 2020), and https://www.publichealth.va.gov/exposures/agentorange/ (accessed August 20, 20200).

The world's best-selling herbicide is Monsanto's Roundup®. It is marketed in various forms and with different concentrations of the active ingredient, glyphosate, which is not named on the containers in which it is sold. From https://www.consumernotice.org/environmental/pesticides/roundup/ (accessed February 17, 2021).

[39] Tests showed that the ingredients in baby foods showed high levels of arsenic, lead, and other heavy metals. See: Laura Reiley, Heavy metals unsafe for child development found in baby foods, study says, *Washington Post*, 5 February 2021, A15.

"Tear gas" comes in several forms. One of the first was MACE. It was originally phenacyl chloride (CN), but it is now marketed in combination with "OC Pepper formula." See: https://www.mace.com/collections/pepper-spray-with-tear-gas. The most commonly used at this time is CS gas (2-chlorobenzylidene malonitrile). Y. G. Karagama, J. R. Newton, and C. J. R. Newbegin, Short-term and long-term physical effects of exposure to CS spray, *J. R. Soc. Med.* 96 (no. 4, April 2003): 172-174. Note the different chemical formulas for CN in the two sources. From: https://cen.acs.org/policy/chemical-weapons/Tear-gas-and-pepper-spray- (accessed February 18, 2021).

[40] The movement of plants, animals, and microbes from one continent to another will be discussed later in this essay. My principal references are Hans Zinsser, *Rats, Lice and History: A Study in Biography* (1935. New York: Pocket Books, 1945); William H. McNeill (*Plagues and Peoples* (1975. Garden City, N.Y.: Random House, Inc., 1998); Alfred W. Crosby, Jr., *The Columbian Exchange: Biological and Cultural Consequences of 1492* (1973. Westport, Conn.: Praeger Publishers, 2003); and Jared Diamond, *Guns, Germs, and Steel: The Fates of Human Societies* (New York: W. W. Norton, 1997).

Also see Enric Sala, *The Nature of Nature: Why We Need the Wild* (Washington, D.C.: National Geographic Partners, 2020); and Sala, The cost of harming nature, *National Geographic* 238 (no. 3, September 2020), 15-18. See Appendix D for references regarding COVID-12.

[41] For beavers, see William Cronon, *Changes in the Land: Colonists and the Ecology of New England* (New York: Hill and Wang, 1983); and Ben Goldfarb, *Eager: The Surprising Secret Life of Beavers and Why They Matter* (White River Junction, Vt.: Chelsea Green Publishing, 2018). Goldfarb also appreciates other animals, writing in "Animal Planet" about birds, eels, and horses, *The New York Times Book Review*, 23 August 2020, 22.

[42] The arguments surrounding the issues of affirmative action, meritocracy, and equal opportunity were discussed in the news media before and after the decision was issued by the Supreme Court in the case of *Regents of the University of California v. Bakke*, 438 U.S. 265 (1978). The court upheld the principle of affirmative action, and it said that race could be considered in college admissions. However, the court ruled that specific racial quotas were not permissible.

Clyde W. Yancy and Howard Bauchner, Diversity in Medical Schools: Need for a new bold approach, *JAMA* 325 (no. 1, 5 January 2021): 31-2.

[43] Thomas Robert Malthus, FRS, *An Essay on the Principle of Population* (1798). The essay was originally anonymous. For *Bulletin of the Atomic Scientists*, see: https://thebulletin.org/ (accessed 8/21/2020).

Chapter 2 The Needs

[44] My four-sided card has a brilliant crimson cover with a large image of Lung-ta. The card from the Tibet Collection™ was made in Nepal using handmade paper, created from Himalayan lokta or daphne bark. The legend of the prayer flags is said to date from the 11th century CE.

By happy coincidence, green is also the academic color for the profession of medicine. The origins are obscure, but it apparently was chosen first by Harvard, and the rest of the academic world followed dutifully along. "Heraldic color for Medicine: Green – Vert: Signifies abundance, joy, hope and loyalty in love." From https://www.thetreemaker.com/design-coat-of-arms-symbol/meaning-of-colors.html (accessed March 6, 2021).

Charles Singer, *A Short History of Science*, 24-5: Empedocles of Agrigentum in Sicily (c.500-c.430 BCE) also proposed that "Love and Strife alternately held sway over all things."

[45] *Britannica*, Buddhism. For an early 20th century Englishman's view of a Yellow Hat Tibetan monk on his spiritual journey, known as "The Way," see Rudyard Kipling's novel, *Kim* (1901. Mineola, N.Y.: Dover Publications, 2005), which is set in the mid-19th century. Gordon Enders published his memoir in 1942: *Foreign Devil: The Adventures of an American 'Kim' in Modern Asia* (New York: Simon & Schuster).

A. Air and Breath

[46] Rev. 7:1 is the book of Revelation, Chapter 7, Verse 1. Neither "wind" nor "air" in the KJV relate to air for breathing, or for air as being necessary for life. From: The Kings Bible, http://thekingsbible.com/Concordance (accessed January 18, 2021).

[47] *Britannica*, air. There are 10 atmospheric gases that are present in steady concentrations. Of these, two comprise 99.03 percent of the atmosphere: nitrogen (N) = 78%; oxygen (O_2) = 20.9%. Air, in *Merriam Webster Dictionary*, has 10 meanings as a noun and 5 meanings as a verb. Inspire, in *Oxford Languages*, https://languages.oup.com/dictionaries (accessed August 8, 2020), includes: "Middle English *enspire*, from Old French *inspirer*, from Latin *inspirare* 'breathe or blow into' from *in-* 'into' + *spirare* 'breathe'. The word was originally used of a divine or supernatural being, in the sense 'impart a truth or idea to someone'."

[48] *Britannica*, photosynthesis; respiration; mitochondrion; Euglena. In the mitochondria, carbon dioxide is absorbed and oxygen is released. The amount of O_2 and CO_2 exchanged in respiration in plants is small, in comparison to the amount of CO_2 and O_2 exchanged in photosynthesis. Many scientists have been fascinated with Euglena. One of them, Dr. Helene Hill, wrote a Ph.D. thesis and published four papers about Euglena. The last of these consolidated her previous papers: Helene Z. Hill and David W. Alling, A model for ultraviolet and photo reactivating light effect in Euglena, *Biophys. J.* 9 (1969): 347-69.

[49] *Britannica*, respiration, human. Also, "Atmospheric pressure and inspired oxygen pressure fall roughly linearly with altitude to be 50% of the sea level value at 5500 m and only 30% of the sea level value at 8900 m (the height of the summit of Everest)."

Andrew J. Peacock, Oxygen at high altitude, *BMJ* 317 (no. 7165, 17 Oct 1998): 1063-1066. "The normal range of oxygen saturation for adults is 94 to 99 percent. Anyone with an oxygen saturation level below 90 percent will likely require supplemental oxygen … There are two common ways of measuring oxygen saturation: an arterial blood gas (ABG) test and a pulse oximeter. Of the two, the pulse oximeter is more commonly used." From https://lunginstitute.com/blog/oxygen-saturation-means/ (accessed August 7, 2020). Also, James Nestor, *Breath: The New Science of a Lost Art* (New York: Penguin Random House Riverhead Books, 2020).

The Centers for Disease Control (CDC)'s leading causes of death in the USA in 2017 were: Heart disease: 647,457; Cancer: 599,108; Accidents (unintentional injuries): 169,936; Chronic lower respiratory diseases: 160,201; Stroke (cerebrovascular diseases): 146,383; Alzheimer's disease: 121,404; Diabetes: 83,564; Influenza and pneumonia: 55,672. From https://www.cdc.gov/nchs/fastats/leading-causes-of-death.htm (accessed July 20, 2020). If we combine the two types of pulmonary disease (chronic lower respiratory diseases, and influenza + pneumonia), pulmonary diseases become the third most common cause of death in the U.S.

The difficulty in distinguishing between seasonal allergies, (due to pollen), other allergies (such as to animals and dust), and the common cold, which is usually caused by an adenovirus (DNA) or a coronavirus (RNA), can be a problem for both physicians and their patients. Patients often demand treatment when they feel miserable with a sore throat, nasal congestion, and cough; and physicians are quick to respond.

[50] *Britannica*, phlogiston; Occam's Razor. However, the idiomatic language of humans is inconsistent with current scientific theory. We still say that the sun and moon rise in the east and set in the west, and that the stars revolve around the sky. This is inconsistent with the theory of a heliocentric solar system. And by thinking that the sun and moon "revolve," we forget that it is the earth that is turning. Furthermore, the stars are moving away from the earth; they do not revolve around it, regardless of their appearance in the sky at night.

[51] Jon Krakauer, *Into Thin Air: A Personal Account of the Mt. Everest Disaster* (New York: Villard, 1997); *Sunset Boulevard* (1950); *Titanic* (1997).

B. Sun and Light

[52] *Britannica*, Solar system, written by Tobias C. Owen, Professor of Astronomy, University of Hawaii, and co-author with Donald Goldsmith of *The Planetary System: The Search for Life in the Universe* (2001).

[53] *Britannica*, physics. Also, Richard Feynman (1918-1988), *Feynman's Lost Lecture: The Motion of Planets Around the Sun* (New York: W. W. Norton, 1996), and other books for non-scientists by Feynman. Also, biographies of some of the great men in the distant past, such as Galileo and Newton.

[54] *Britannica*, sun: "As the Sun rotates, one half is moving toward us, and the other away."
Britannica, moon: "The Moon and Earth presently orbit the barycentre in 27.322 days, the sidereal month, or sidereal revolution period of the Moon. … the time from one full moon to the next is 29.531 days, the synodic month, or synodic revolution period of the Moon. … As the stars appear to move westward because of Earth's daily rotation and its annual motion about the Sun, so the Moon slowly moves eastward, rising later each day and passing through its phase."

[55] *Britannica*, light. The arc of a rainbow is based on the wavelengths of the colors. The long red arc is at the top of the rainbow; the short violet arc is at the bottom. From Hannah Muniz, What is the rainbow color order? PrepScholar, https://blog.prepscholar.com/rainbow-color-order (accessed January 19, 2021).

[56] For Rickets and Vitamin D: "Vitamin-D deficiency rickets, a disorder that becomes apparent during infancy or childhood, is the result of insufficient amounts of vitamin D in the body." See: https://rarediseases.org/rare-diseases/rickets-vitamin-d-deficiency/ (accessed August 10, 2020). "Vitamin D is a fat-soluble vitamin that is naturally present in very few foods, added to others, and available as a dietary supplement," from https://ods.od.nih.gov/factsheets/VitaminD (accessed August 10, 2020). The usual source of Vitamin D for vegans is artificially "fortified" food, such as soy milk and orange juice, or pills containing Vitamin D. See: https://www.healthline.com/health/vegan-vitamin-d#vegan-sources (accessed August 12, 2020). Melanoma in Australia: "Australia has one of the highest rates of melanoma in the world, and melanoma is often referred to as 'Australia's national cancer'." See: https://www.melanoma.org.au/understanding-melanoma/melanoma-facts-and-

statistics/ (accessed August 10, 2020). Hyperbilirubinemia: "Neurotoxicity is the major consequence of neonatal hyperbilirubinemia." See: https://www.merckmanuals.com/professional/pediatrics/metabolic-electrolyte-and-toxic-disorders-in-neonates/neonatal-hyperbilirubinemia (accessed August 10, 2020).

[57] Jimmie Davis wrote "You Are My Sunshine" in 1938. See: https://genius.com/Jimmie-davis-you-are-my-sunshine-lyrics (accessed January 19, 2021). Ernest Hemingway, *The Sun Also Rises* (New York: Scribner's, 1926), is a *roman à clef*.

C. Sleep and Dreams

[58] Matthew Walker, *Why We Sleep: Unlocking the Power of Sleep and Dreams* (New York: Scribner's, 2017), which the cover blub states is "The first sleep book by a leading scientific expert."

[59] *Britannica*, sleep. The *Britannica* article on Sleep is 24-pages, authored by Thien + Thand Dang-Vu, et al, with additional comments by two of the co-authors, David Foulkes and Rosalind D. Cartwright.

[60] *Britannica*, King, Martin Luther, Jr. Stephen Foster (1826-1864) wrote "I dream of Jeanie with the light brown hair" in 1854. Isham Jones and Gus Kahn wrote "I'll see you in my dreams" in 1924; it has been recorded since then by many vocalists. The 1951 movie based on Kahn's life had the same title. Prospero: "We are such stuff / As dreams are made on" in Shakespeare's *The Tempest*, Act 4, Scene 1, 148-158. DreamWorks Water Park, American Dream, https://www.americandream.com/venue/dreamworks-water-park (accessed January 19, 2021). *The Maltese Falcon* (1941) starred Humphrey Bogart; it was based on Dashiell Hammett's book *The Maltese Falcon* (1930). Shakespeare, "What's past," from Antonio's speech in *The Tempest*, Act 2, Scene 1.

Chapter 3. The Urges

[61] *Britannica*, Pasteur, Louis (1822-1895). Pasteur's quote is from his Inaugural Address as the recently appointed Professor and Dean at the opening of the new Faculté des Sciences at the University of Lille, France, on December 7, 1854. Citation from René Vallery-Radot, *The Life of Pasteur*, translated by Mrs. R. L. Devonshire (1919), 76, at https://todayinsci.com/P/Pasteur_Louis/PasteurLouis-Quotations.htm (accessed January 20, 2021). The quotation and a translation are from Goodreads, Louis Pasteur, https://www.goodreads.com/quotes/354678-dans-les-champs-de-l-observation-le-hasard-ne-favorise-que (accessed January 20, 2021); Pinterest, https://www.pinterest.com/pin/532198880957687838/ (accessed January 20, 2021).

[62] Bryan Wendell, Scouting Magazine, Be Prepared, at https://blog.scoutingmagazine.org/2017/05/08/be-prepared-scout-motto-origin (accessed January 20, 2021).

[63] Bryan Murphy, *81 Days Below Zero: The Incredible Survival Story of a World War II Pilot in Alaska's Frozen Wilderness* (New York: Hachette Books, 2015). See other examples in Wilfred Thesinger, *Arabian Sands*; Alfred Lansing, *Endurance*; Apsley Cherry-Garrard, *The Worst Journey in the World*; John McPhee, *Coming in to the Country*; and Charles Nordhoff and James Hall's novel about William Bligh, *Mutiny on the Bounty*.

A. Water

[64] One of the most puzzling verses in the Bible quotes Jesus as saying, "Ye are the salt of the earth: but if the salt have lost his savour, wherewith shall it be salted?" (Matthew 5:13). The word "savour" becomes "taste" in the Revised Standard Version and other translations. The subject is discussed in Mikeal C. Parsons and D. Thomas Hanks, Jr., When the salt lost its savour: a brief history of Matthew 5.13/Mark 9.50/Luke 14.34 in English translation, *The Bible Translator* 52 (no. 3, 2001): 320.

[65] Karen Sandstrom, Salt: The dietary danger that's easy to ignore, *Washington Post*, 13 December 2020, B6; Review of Michael Jacobson, *Salt Wars: The Battle Over the Biggest Killer in the American Diet* (Boston: MIT Press, 2020).

Hypertension was difficult to treat until anti-hypertensive agents were developed in the late 1950s. A salt-free diet was the best choice. It appeared to work but it was difficult to get patients to stick with it. A "rice diet" was started at Duke University as one way to achieve it. For the "rice diet," see: Philip Klemmer, Clarence E. Grim, and Friedrich C. Luft, Who and what drove Walter Kempner? The rice diet revisited, *Hypertension* 64 (no. 4, 7 Jul 2014):684-688.

[66] *Britannica*, iceberg. The part of an iceberg that is above the water surface is known as "freeboard," and the part below the surface is known as the "draft," as in the draft of a ship. See *Britannica*, Titanic. One reader commented that, "It is verging on miraculous that ice floats - expands from 4C to 0C. If it didn't, the planet would be an ice ball." "Ice floats because it is about 9% less dense than liquid water." From ThoughtCo., Ice and the Density of Water, https://www.thoughtco.com/why-does-ice-float-604304 (accessed January 20, 2021). From Let's Talk Science, https://letstalkscience.ca/educational-resources/hands-on-activities/how-much-iceberg-on-top-water (accessed January 21, 2021): "[B]ecause the difference in relative density between ice and sea water is small, only some of the iceberg floats above the water. In fact, on average only 1/10th of an iceberg is above the surface of the water." For "Health benefits from cocoanut milk," see: https://www.medicalnewstoday.com/articles/323743

(accessed February 18, 2021). The word "geyser" comes from the Icelandic word, "geysir," which is the name of the Great Geysir of that island country.

[67] The term Minimal Infective Dose (MID) is usually employed in discussing viral disease, but the concept also applies to bacterial diseases. See: Joel Rybicki, Eva Kisdi, and Jani V. Anttila, Model of bacterial toxin-dependent pathogenesis explains infective dose, *PNAS* 115 (no. 42, 16 October 2018): 10690-95.

[68] Zorastrians, at https://courses.lumenlearning.com/suny-hccc-worldcivilization/chapter/zoroastrianism (accessed March 31, 2021). The river known as Ganges in English is Ganga in Sanskrit, named for Ganga, a Hindu Goddess.

Noah (Genesis 7). Other religious ceremonies are referenced later in this essay.

[69] Boundary waters are important in protection of population groups, because amphibious invasions are less likely to succeed than invasions by land. Mahan's *Sea Power* is based in part on the role that fleets of warships have in overcoming the protection that seas afford to the land. "Singin' in the Rain" (1952), was an unforgettable movie that starred Gene Kelly, Donald O'Connor, and Debbie Reynolds. Talia is a Hebrew girl's name meaning "gentle dew from heaven."

[70] Rachel Carson, *Silent Spring* (New York: Houghton Mifflin Co., 1962).

B. Food

[71] And, "Give us this day our daily bread" (Matthew 6:11).

[72] Walter B. Cannon, *The Wisdom of the Body* (New York: W. W. Norton, 1932) and *The Way of an Investigator* (New York: W. W. Norton, 1945). A milk diet is sufficient for children until the usual age of weaning. See: Health Line, Milk, https://www.healthline.com/health/is-milk-bad-for-you (accessed 10/31/2020).

[73] Lactose intolerance is caused by an insufficient production of lactase, the enzyme in the stomach that breaks down the complex sugar in milk (lactose) into two sugars (glucose and galactose), which are absorbed into the blood. See: https://www.nhs.uk/conditions/lactose-intolerance/ (accessed 10/31/2020).

[74] Sidney W. Mintz, *Sweetness and Power: The Place of Sugar in Modern History* (New York: Wiley, 1985).

[75] *Britannica*, Borlaug, Norman Ernest (1914-2009). An agricultural scientist, born in Iowa. His work laid the foundation for the Green Revolution, and he received the Nobel Peace Prize in 1970. Yield = production per acre.

[76] *Britannica*, metabolism.

C. Shelter

[77] *Britannica*, Martin Luther (1483-1546). He wrote *Ein Feste Burge* between 1527 and 1529. See: John Julian, ed., *A Dictionary of Hymnology: Setting for the Origin and history of Christian Hymns of all Ages and Nations*. 2nd revised ed., 1907; reprint (New York: Dover Publications, Inc., 1957.)

[78] *Online Etymology Dictionary*: *kae-id. It forms all or part of: abscise; avicide; biocide… chisel, -cide; circumcise …concise … decision … excision … genocide … homicide … incision … insecticide … pesticide … precision … suicide" At: https://www.etymonline.com/search?q=homicide (accessed 1/14/2021).

[79] Medical students learn the names and functions of the twelve cranial nerves from two mnemonic devices.

Britannica, taste: "the sensation of different tastes (i.e., salty, sweet, sour, bitter, or umami) is diverse not only within a single taste bud but also throughout the surface of the tongue." The sensation known as umami adds savor to foods; it corresponds to the flavor of glutamates, especially monosodium glutamate.

[80] Put the suffix "-er" on the name of a city, and you get food that is typical for that city: Hamburg becomes hamburger; Vienna (Wein) becomes wiener (with letters i and e reversed). President John F. Kennedy was advised show his support for those who lived in Berlin when he visited the city in 1963. JFK said, "Ich ben ein Berliner." The crowd laughed, and the Americans all laughed, too. The crowd in Berlin knew he meant well, but Kennedy's choice of the word "Berliner" was grammatically a double entendre. It also meant a Berlin jelly doughnut. Who knows what the Germans thought? See: https://www.wsj.com/articles/ich-bin-ein-berliner-jfk-got-it-righthe-was-no-jelly-doughnut-11573152244 (accessed February 18, 2021).

[81] Franz Kafka, *Das Schloss* (Leipzig: Kurt Wolff Verlag, 1926).

[82] Dana Thomas, Cave paintings from Ice Age found in France, *Washington Post*, 19 January 1995, at https://www.washingtonpost.com/archive/politics/1995/01/19/cave-paintings (accessed January 9, 2021). Thomas estimates that they were painted between 10,000 and 27,000 years ago. These paintings are similar to those in the caves in Lascaux, which were probably painted at about the same time. Avignon is about 200 km SE of Lascaux, in the Dordogne region of France, near Bordeaux. See also Barbara Morris, Otherworldly beauty, *Washington Post*, 23 May 2020, A22. A photograph published with her Letter to the Editor "of a herd of goats in France returning to their barn was stunning in its resemblance to the famous prehistoric cave drawings in the Dordogne region … of a cave 10,000 years ago."

D. Lust

[83] Oscar Wilde, *The Ballad of Reading Gaol and Other Poems* (New York: Dover Publication, 1992), 26. Wilde (1854-1900) was convicted for "gross indecency" with men in 1895 (i.e., sodomy), and he was in Reading prison from 1895-1897.

[84] Alfred Charles Kinsey (1894-1956) authored the Kinsey Reports, which were major instigators of the sexual revolution in the 1960s. The reports, which were co-authored by others, are: Alfred C. Kinsey, Wardell B. Pomeroy, and Clyde E. Martin, *Sexual Behavior in the Human Male* (Philadelphia: W. B. Saunders Co., 1948); and *Sexual Behavior in the Human Female* (Saunders, 1953), with Paul Gebhard as an additional co-author.

The meaning of "lust" has changed slightly over the past century. "Lust" is defined and synonyms given by *Merriam-Webster's* (1979) as (1) Usually intense or unbridled sexual desire: LASCIVIOUSNESS. (2a) an intense longing: CRAVING. (2b) ENTHUSIASM, EAGERNESS. (3) [obsolete] (a) PLEASURE, DELIGHT (b) personal inclination: WISH (viewed on-line, 5/9/20). In 1948, "Lust" was defined as 1. *Obs.* a. Pleasure; liking b. Inclination, desire 2. Sensuous desire; bodily appetite; commonly, sexual desire as a degrading passion. 3. Longing or eagerness to enjoy. From *Webster's Collegiate Dictionary,* 5th ed. (Springfield, Mass.: G. & C. Merriam Co., 1948). "Lasciviousness" is more powerful way to express "lust" than "sensuous desire ... sexual desire as a degrading passion."

The novel by Irving Stone, *Lust for Life* (New York: Grosset and Dunlap, 1934) about the life of Vincent Van Gogh was made into a movie in 1956, starring Kirk Douglas as the painter. In 1934 and 1956, the word "lust" was intended to have the older meaning of "craving" or "longing or eagerness to enjoy."

The lust for power is usually different from the lust for sex, although a person seeking power may also seek sex, or use power to achieve the lust for sex. History tells us of medieval Popes who achieved goals of both power and sex. On the other hand, Oliver Cromwell achieved his goal of power but was apparently indifferent to sex. Risk-taking in the search for power will be discussed at a later point in this essay; it is one of the risks that are undertaken, consciously or unconsciously, in defiance of the normal human search for health.

[85] A reader commented, "It is interesting that two 'sins', drink and lust can create such an enormous number of euphemisms."

[86] The erogenous zones are well-known, but they are not usually referred to by this bland anatomical term. They are principally what are euphemistically called "private parts"; the breasts, organs for producing and dispensing milk (especially in the female); and areas of the skin, such as the sole of the foot, which when stroked, arouse interest in sex. Other parts of the body that cause arousal when stimulated are referred to as the object of fetishes. The erogenous zones were biologically intended to assist copulation for propagation of the species. However, these zones are sometimes utilized by one person, acting alone, or by a group of men, or women, or both sexes; this is known as masturbation. Views of these activities were once thought to be of interest only to voyeurs, and they were called pornography; but the film industry has gradually relaxed its censorship, and there are now hundreds of titles available for the titillating delectation of the public. In Oxford Dictionary: The "id" refers to "the part of the mind in which innate instinctive impulses and primary processes are manifest," or "the conflict between the drives of the id and the demands of the cultural superego." Anatomically, the id resides in the amygdala. The superego is the conscience, residing anatomically in the forebrain.

[87] The ancient requirement for "heterosexual conjugation" is no longer an absolute necessity. In the late 20th century, various methods were developed to enable birth to occur without the ancient sexual act, including in vitro fertilization (IVF) with sperm or DNA, and surrogate motherhood.

[88] Homer, *Iliad* and *Odyssey.* Also, Tim Severin, *The Ulysses Voyage: The Search for the Odyssey* ([1987] London: Hutchinson, 1988).

[89] Charles Darwin, *On the Origin of Species by Means of Natural Selection, or the Preservation of Favoured Races in the Struggle for Life* (London: John Murray, 1859).

Lewis Carroll [Charles Dodson] was the author of *Alice's Adventures in Wonderland* (London: Macmillan, by Oxford University Press, 1865). The book of nude or nearly nude juvenile girls is not shown in the list of "important publications" by Dodgson on the website of the Lewis Carroll Society (http://lewiscarrollsociety.org.uk/, accessed 5/12/2020), and there is nothing on that website about Dodgson's unusual sexuality. The book has probably been withdrawn from libraries and references to it have been scrubbed. See speculation about Dodgson's sexuality in Simon Winchester, *The Alice Behind Wonderland* (London: Oxford University Press, 2011); and Roger Taylor and Edward Wakeling, *Lewis Carroll, Photographer* (Princeton, N.J.: Princeton University Press, 2002).

[90] The influence of syphilis on history is given by Mircea Tampa, et al., Brief history of syphilis, *Journal of Medicine and Life* 7 (no. 1, March 15): 4-10, from https://www.ncbi.nlm.nih.gov/pmc/articles/PMC3956094 (accessed January 23, 2021). I have been informed by one reader that "venereal means hunting, from the Norman love of hunting," and that "a chowder of cats or a murder of crows are venereal terms."

[91] Lot's daughters' incest in Genesis 19:30-38; clever Rachel in Genesis 31:35. The four brothers of Jesus (James, Joseph/Joses, Judas/Jude, and Simon), and his sisters (unnamed) are mentioned in Mark 6:3 and Matthew 13:55-56.

[92] Stacy Schiff, *Cleopatra: A Life* (Boston: Little Brown & Co., 2010). Some say that Caesar's philandering may well have added to his list of enemies.

[93] *The Satyricon of Petronius Arbiter*, trans. by W. C. Fierbaugh (New York: Liveright Publishing Co., 1922), 242-5. Priapus was the lusty Greek god of fertility. He was the son of Dionysus, the god of wine, and of Aphrodite or another nymph. Priapus had an enormous phallus; he was the god of sailors, and the ass (a double meaning, too) was sacrificed in his honor. Priapism, the medical term for an unpleasant sustained erection, is named for him.

[94] Geoffrey Chaucer, *The Canterbury Tales*, trans. Nevill Coghill (New York: Penguin Group, 1951); Francois Rabelais, *The Histories of Gargantua and Pantagruel*, trans. John Michael Cohen (New York: Penguin, 1955); Nathaniel Hawthorne, *The Scarlet Letter* (Boston, Mass.: Ticknor, Reed & Fields, 1850); and David Lindsay, *Mayflower Bastard: A Stranger Among the Pilgrims* (New York: St. Martin's Press, 2002). Some of the cultural differences in the English settlers in the American Colonies are explored in David Hackett Fisher, *Albion's Seed: Four British Folkways in America* (New York: Oxford University Press, 1989). The situation of a woman in New Netherlands is one of the topics explored by Russell Shorto, in *The Island at the Center of the World* (New York: Vintage Books, 2005). Mrs. Edeson, the Dutch ancestor of Thomas Edison, was a widow from the Netherlands. She chose to come to New Jersey because under the civil code of that colony, which was formerly part of New Netherlands, she was allowed to keep her assets. Her son, John Edeson, who came with his mother, was Thomas Edison's great-grandfather. See: Neal Baldwin, *Edison: Inventing the Century* (New York: Hyperion, 1995).

The story of the Royal Bastard, Richard More, is a curious one. He was the product of an unhappy marriage between two cousins who were distant descendants of the Royal family of England.

[95] The reference is to the Vedas and Bhagavad Gita, and to the principal Hindu gods: Brahma (the creator), Vishnu (the preserver), and Shiva (the destroyer); and to Ganesh, the elephant-headed god of beginnings, who is able to overcome any problem. Uma (aka Parvati), goddess of fertility, is the consort or wife of Shiva.

Howard Rubenstein, *Romance of the Western Chamber* (La Jolla, Calif.: Granite Hills Press, 2020), tells the story of an arranged marriage that was superseded by the meeting of two lovers in a thirteenth century Chinese story. It was told in English as an opera, and then published as a children's book.

[96] *The Yale Shakespeare* (New Haven, Conn.: Yale University Press, 1918-1966).

[97] Victoria's son succeeded her as King Edward VII, who ruled from 1901-1910. The Edwardian Period was the beginning of what Simon Heffer called *The Age of Decadence: A History of Britain, 1860-1914* (New York: Pegasus Books, 2021). He was succeeded by his second son, George V. The eldest son of George V became Edward VIII. He ruled for an even shorter period. Edward was determined to marry a divorced woman, Mrs. Wallis Simpson, and he was forced to abdicate to do this. This Edward, as Prince of Wales, visited India, where his guide, pimp, and future equerry was Edward Dudley "Fruity" Metcalfe (1887-1957), MC, MVO. Setting aside the "tribute" movies, some of the others are: *Diana* (2013); *Her Majesty, Mrs. Brown* (1997); *Whatever Love Means* (2005), about Charles and Camilla; *The Crown* (series, 2016-2020).

[98] What is accepted at one place at one time can be dangerous in a different time and place. For example, pederasty and pedophilia, including men with boys, was common in the Classical Greek period, though it is now forbidden. Eyebrows are now raised when reading about the obsession of "Humbert Humbert" with his 12-year old step-daughter in Vladimir Nabokov's *Lolitia* (Paris: Olympia Press, 1955). Multiple sex partners, such as those described in *1000 and One Nights*, and harems in Asia, are considered to be immoral in the Christian world; yet we have records of Kings of England who had serial Queens, and who also acknowledged having many illegitimate children (who were allowed to show the "bar sinister" on their escutcheon), and other casual contacts with unnamed young women, who were simply regarded as *droit du seigneur*. Bestiality was a hanging offense in Puritan New England, but it is now considered to be a subject for jokes, such as "Why does that young woman have a Great Dane?" (Don't ask her), and "Why does a sheepherder have an extra pair of boots?" (For his favorite sheep's hind legs, of course).

Emily Bronte, *Wuthering Heights* (London: Thomas Cautley Newby, 1847) was made into at least 14 films from 1920 to 2011. Thomas Hardy, *Tess of the d'Urbervilles: A Pure Woman Faithfully Presented* (London: James R. Osgood, McIlvaine & Co., 1891), has been adapted for the theatre, television, and at least eight movies.

[99] *Britannica*, Sickles, Daniel Edgar. *Britannica*, Rockefeller, Nelson, does not mention his death, nor is there an entry in *Britannica* for Jean Harris and Herman Tarnower. For Rockefeller, see: https://allthatsinteresting.com/nelson-rockefeller-death (accessed January 23, 2021). For Harris and Tarnower, see: https://www.nytimes.com/2012/12/29/nyregion/jean-s-harris-killer-of-scarsdale-diet-doctor-dies-at-89.html (accessed January 23, 2021).

[100] Annette Gordon-Reed, *Thomas Jefferson and Sally Hemings: An American Controversy* (Charlottesville, Va.: University of Virginia Press, 1997). Angela Serratore, President Cleveland's problem child, *Smithsonian Magazine* (September 26, 2013). https://www.smithsonianmag.com/history/president-clevelands-problem-child-100800/ (accessed January 25, 2021).

[101] In 1976, Jimmy Carter said in an interview with *Playboy* magazine, "I've looked on a lot of women with lust. I've committed adultery in my heart many times," contravening Matthew 5: 28: "I tell you that anyone who looks on a woman with lust in his heart has already committed adultery." This confession seemed strange to many people. http://content.time.com/time/specials/packages/article/0,28804,1859513_1859526_1859518,00.html (May 17, 2020). President Trump's braggadocio about women can be believed, although as president he made thousands of false claims. See Glenn Kessler, As President, Trump made 30, 573 false claims, *Washington Post*, 24 January 2021, A1, 4. Donald Trump's political base stayed with him throughout his presidency, and it may even have increased. His popular vote in 2016 was 62,984,828 (46%) and it was 73,466,544 (47%) in 2020.

[102] For a change in China's "one child" policy, see: China formally abolishes decades-old one-child policy. *International Business Times*, 27 December 2015.

"The Pill" is an oral contraceptive containing derivatives of hormones that are made in the ovaries – estrogen and progesterone. The latter is usually given in the form of a derivative, progestin; or sometimes progestin is given alone. Research that led to the development of oral contraceptives began in 1951 by Gregory Pincus, a reproductive physiologist in Worcester, Mass. In 1952, he enlisted the aid of John Rock, a gynecologist at the Free Hospital for Women in Brookline, Mass., which later became part of the Brigham and Women's Hospital. They developed a combination of two synthetic hormones, noretynodrel and mestranol, called Enovid, which suppressed ovulation. In 1957, the FDA approved Enovid for use in "menstrual disorders." Early trials with Enovid as a contraceptive were conducted in a so-called "Fertility Clinic" at the Brigham. Use of "the Pill" has been enormously controversial, but there is no doubt that it has changed the lives of women and men and their families. "The Pill" has changed society throughout the world.

[103] Karen Tumulty, In Colorado politics, power has a new look, *Washington Post*, 14 April 2019, A21: "In the current legislative session, more than half of the state representative – 34 out of 65 – are women . . . Only once before and only briefly has any legislature in the country experienced a female majority in even one of its chambers."

[104] A recent essay is subtitled, "The father of evolutionary theory took a dim view of women's potential, with one notable exception." The essay's author, Michael Sims, points out that as a young man, Charles Darwin was enchanted with a cigar-smoking journalist named Harriet Martineau. She presided over her salons "despite deafness that required visitors to all but shout into her ear trumpet, while rebutting the notion that femininity was a handicap." From Sims, Darwin and the second sex, *New York Times Book Review*, 7 February 2021, 12. "Survival of the fittest" is often attributed to Darwin, but it was actually Herbert Spencer who coined the term.

Francis Galton, *Hereditary Genius: An Inquiry into Its Laws and Consequences* (London: Macmillan, 1869). Laura Rivard (moderator), "Genetics Generation" posted 18 September 2018 by Genetics Forum: https://www.nature.com/scitable/forums/genetics-generation/america-s-hidden-history-the-eugenics-movement-123919444/ (accessed May 17, 2020).

Steven A. Farber, U.S. scientists' role in the eugenics movement (1907-1939): A contemporary biologist's perspective, *Zebrafish* 5 (no.4, 2008): 243-5: https://www.ncbi.nlm.nih.gov/pmc/articles/PMC2757926/ (accessed 5/17/2020).

[105] Edward Hyde, 3rd Earl of Clarendon (1661-1723), Viscount Cornbury from 1674-1709, a close relative of English monarchs, was Royal Governor of New York and New Jersey from 1701-1708. His troubled tenure in politics is now less remembered than accusations that he was a cross-dresser and possibly transsexual. His alleged portrait in elaborate women's clothing was probably painted posthumously, but the salacious rumors still persist.

[106] In medicine, one form of bisexuality is known as Klinefelter's syndrome. The biology of a variety of conditions now known as "intersex" is summarized by the National Library of Medicine as follows: Intersex is a group of conditions where there is a discrepancy between the external genitals and the internal genitals (the testes and ovaries). See: MedlinePlus, Intersex, https://medlineplus.gov/ency/article/001669.htm (accessed May 20, 2020).

[107] The Me Too movement has had positive effects for women. See Julie Story Byerley, Mentoring in the era of #MeToo, *JAMA* 323 (no. 17, 5 May 2020), 17-18. Her article concluded with, "[B]uilding relationships across lines that sometimes divide us must be encouraged."

[108] The story of Emmett Till is the most dramatic recent instances of lynching. It led to the passage of an act that made lynching a federal crime, though it took 65 years. Matthew Daly, Emmett Till Antilynching Act makes lynching a federal crime, 65 years after Chicago teen was murdered in Jim Crow South, *Chicago Tribune* (February

26, 2020). https://www.chicagotribune.com/politics/ct-nw-emmett-till-lynching-act-bobby-rush-20200226-r5qpkwjikvednbrkxvkncpudiy-story.html (accessed May 20, 2020).

Harper Lee, *To Kill a Mockingbird* (Philadelphia, Pa.: J. B. Lippincott Co., 1960). The story in this famous novel was fictious. We now know that it was altered by Harper Lee from her original plan, because the editor suggested changes to make it more marketable. Her earlier work, *Go Set a Watchman* (New York: HarperCollins), was not published until 2015. "*Go Set a Watchman* features *Mockingbird's* Scout as a 26-year-old woman on her way back home to Maycomb, Alabama, from New York City. Scout's father Atticus, the upstanding moral conscience of *To Kill a Mockingbird*, is portrayed as a racist with bigoted views and ties to the Ku Klux Klan." From Biograpy.com: https://www.biography.com/writer/harper-lee (accessed February 19, 2021).

[109] The enormous volume of literature on the "great pox" (syphilis) includes many curious stories, and some with strange twists. One is the recent discovery that questions the long-held belief that Winston Churchill's father, Randolph Churchill, had tertiary syphilis, although it was not transmitted to Winston's mother, Jenny (Jerome) Churchill, or to Winston. On April 12, 2019, John H. Mather, wrote that "there is enough medical information to consider syphilis a most unlikely cause of Lord Randolph's death," and that Lord Randolph probably died of a slow-growing brain tumor. See: In search of Lord Randolph Churchill's purported syphilis, The Churchill Project of Hillsdale College, https://winstonchurchill.hillsdale.edu/in-search-of-lord-randolph-churchills-purported-syphilis/ (accessed May 20, 2020). For the commonly held cause of Lord Randolph's derangement and death due to tertiary syphilis, see: Anne Sebba, *American Jennie: The Remarkable Life of Lady Randolph Churchill* (New York: W. W. Norton & Co., 2007).

Tuskegee syphilis study, in *Britannica*. The men in the Tuskegee study were not told that this was a research project, and as a result, none gave permission for the study. The study was started before penicillin was recognized as a useful treatment for syphilis, but the men were never treated after penicillin became available.

[110] Infection of the mother with gonorrhea was the major cause of neonatal blindness until 1881, when Dr. Carl Credé introduced a successful method of prophylaxis with a 2% solution of silver nitrate eye drops. These eye drops were administered to all children born in American hospitals for many decades.

E. Social Connections

[111] The Golden Rule in Christianity suggests an ethic of reciprocity as "Do unto others as you would have them do unto you" (Matt. 7:12). A stronger expression, not usually stated as the Golden Rule, is the second great commandment of Jesus, "And the second is like unto it, Thou shalt love thy neighbour as thyself" (Matt. 22: 39). Golden Rule, in *Britannica*, discusses earlier expressions and negative forms of the principle in Deuteronomy, and in the writings of Plato, Aristotle, Isocrates, and Seneca. For others comments on the Golden Rule see: https://iep.utm.edu/goldrule/ (accessed August 25,2020); and http://www.nrm.org/thinglink/text/GoldenRule.html (accessed August 25, 2020).

[112] "Allah says: 'But if you feel you may not be able to deal justly between them, then marry only one.' *(Holy Qur'an, 4:4)*'." From Al Islam, Polygamy, https://www.alislam.org/question/polygamy-in-islam/ (accessed January 25, 2021); and Sahih Muslim, Book: 9, The Book of Divorce, https://www.iium.edu.my/deed/hadith/muslim/009_smt.html (accessed January 25, 2021).

In spite of his cruelty, the image of Henry VIII has long been ameliorated by the legend that he wrote the haunting words and/or the melody for "Greensleeves" when he was wooing Ann Boleyn to be his third wife. The story persists, though it is unlikely. See: Discover Music Home (23 April 2020): Who was Greensleeves – and did Henry VIII really write the song, at: https://www.classicfm.com/discover-music/greensleeves-did-henry-viii-write-song/ (accessed February 19, 2021).

[113] Annalee Newitz, Hunters weren't only men, *Washington Post*, 2 January 2021, P.A. 23: "As some recent archaeological studies suggest, women have been leaders, warriors and hunters for thousands of years."

[114] For Esther: *Forward Day by Day* (Cincinnati, Ohio: Forward Movement, 2020), 49: "Esther is a curious book to have a place in the Bible. The name of God does not occur in it; neither is there any mention of prayer ... Esther is the heroine of the tale, but it was her uncle Mordechai who spurred her on to greatness. Esther decided she had work to do, even if it cost her life to do it: 'If I perish, I perish'."

[115] C. P. Snow, *The Two Cultures and the Scientific Revolution: The Bede Lecture, 1959* (New York: Cambridge University Press, 1959; reprint Mansfield Centre, CT: Martino Publishing, 2013); and Snow, *The Two Cultures and A Second Look* (1964; New York: Cambridge University Press, 1979). C.P. Snow was Charles Percy Snow (1905-1980), Baron Snow.

[116] It is interesting to consider the various ways that children have been considered in different cultures and in different periods in history. The place of children in society thus may range from something like a domesticated animal to a small version of an adult. For a discussion, see: Perri Klass, *A Good Time to be Born: How Science and Public Health Gave Children a Future* (New York: W. W. Norton & Company, 2020), reviewed by Christie

Watson, "The luckiest parents in history": A doctor explores the modern world's impressive decline in child mortality, *New York Times Book Review*, 10 January 2021, 10: Watson says that Klass "reminds us that 'racism continues to blight the health and growth of children in many different ways'."

[117] The anatomical development of the organs involved in human speech, and the implications of this ability of humans to communicate verbally, is the subject of a wide-ranging discussion by John Colapinto, *This Is the Voice* (New York: Simon & Schuster, 2021); reviewed by Mary Roach, Out loud: An exploration of our vocal cords, why we have them and what humans have gained from our dexterity at making different sounds, *New York Times Book Review* (7 March 2021), 11: "Colapinto makes the case that our larynx may be the most important boost evolution bestowed." He "takes up Darwin's emphasis on prosody – the notion that the melody and rhythms of speech are what move us toward language. … The larynx of the Neanderthal man … sat higher than our own [which] kept them from producing the more gymnastic vowels and sound combinations that set language apart from utterance."

[118] *Britannica*, Adam Smith (1723-1790), *An Inquiry into the Nature and Causes of the Wealth of Nations* (1776); Karl Heinrich Marx (1818-1883), *Manifest der Kommunistischen Partei* (1848), commonly known as *The Communist Manifesto* (1848); and *Das Kapital* (1st ed.,1867), completed by Friedrich Engels (2d ed., 1885 and (3d ed., 1894).

[119] Richard Evelyn Byrd, *Alone* (New York: G. P. Putnam's Sons, 1938); and David Reisman, Nathan Glazer and Reuel Denney, *The Lonely Crowd: A Study of the Changing American Character* (New Haven, Conn.: Yale University Press, 1950). The *Guinness Book of World Records* says Rod Stewart's concert had an audience estimated at 3.5 million but the crowd swelled to 4.2 million to watch the fireworks at midnight.

[120] "The law of the pack" is part of the motto of the Cub Scout program in the Boy Scouts of America.

[121] In the movie "Braveheart" (1995), Scottish warrior William Wallace leads a rebellion against King Edward I of England. Willa Cather's book, *Oh, Pioneers* (Boston: Houghton, Mifflin Co., 1913), and movie with the same name in 1992, starring Jessica Lange. Wallace Stegner, *Crossing to Safety* (New York: Random House, 1987).

[122] *Britannica*, Stroud, Robert Franklin. *Birdman of Alcatraz* (1962) was a fictional film based on Stroud's life.

[123] Freud, Sigmund, in *Britannica*, for a brief discussion of Freud's concepts of the id, ego, and superego. These terms are highlighted for additional amplification in *Britannica*. The use of the word "conscience" in respect to the superego is what I learned in medical school; it is not in *Britannica*.

[124] TED: Ideas worth spreading, at: https://www.ted.com/ (accessed February 14, 2021).

[125] "altruism" in *Online Etymology Dictionary*, was "coined or popularized 1830 by the French philosopher Auguste Comte, with -ism + *autrui* (Old French *altrui*) "of or to others," from Latin *alteri*, dative of *alter* "other." It is opposed to "egoism": "Meaning 'doing or seeking of that which affords pleasure or advances interest' [1800] "opposed to *altruism*, but not necessarily 'selfish.' Meaning 'self-centeredness' is from 1840." Egoism is derived from "ego" (Latin = *ego*). https://www.etymonline.com/word/altruism; /egoism; /ego (accessed August 28, 2020). Altruism is considered to be the opposite of selfishness. "alt" = other, versus "self."

Michael Gerson recently called attention to what Darwin wrote about the evolution of altruism in tribal groups. Gerson said that Darwin wrote that "It benefits a tribe when its members are cooperative, brave and concerned for each other [and that] Darwin pointed to a number of means [which included] a particularly powerful 'stimulus to the development of social virtues [is] the praise and blame of our fellow men,' and that Darwin added that religion gives to these duties the aura of sacredness." Gerson, Healthy and reusing a covid vaccine? Be ashamed, *Washington Post*, 16 April 2021, A27. I have not been able to locate the precise source of the quotation in Darwin's works, nor the "aura of sacredness" that Darwin supposedly granted to religion. However, this would be consistent with what Darwin wrote elsewhere. After Mendel's description of heredity, altruism would be considered to be epigenetic behavior, not transmitted through individual genes.

[126] The movie *God Knows Where I Am* (2016) is a biopic documentary movie that tells the story of Linda Bishop, a schizophrenic woman, whose delusions were controlled by medication. After her lawyer argued successfully for her release from protective detention in a psychiatric hospital, she stopped taking her pills and hid in an abandoned house. The movie is based on the diary that she kept from October to January, while slowly dying of hunger and hypothermia. She ate nothing but apples for six weeks, and then consumed only water for another six weeks. It is a paradox that the lawyer won the case, but by doing so, he lost the patient.

[127] It may come as a surprise, but the origin of smallpox is still uncertain. Some believe that the Antonine Plague in Rome in about 165-180 A.D. may have been the first appearance of smallpox, whereas others trace it the disease to much earlier times. It is said by some to have left traces in Egyptian mummies, and that it may have originated 12,000 years ago. See: Stefan Riedel, Edward Jenner and the history of smallpox and vaccination, *Proc (Bayl Univ Med Cent)* 18 (no. 1, January 2005): 21-25: "The origin of smallpox as a natural disease is lost in prehistory. It is believed to have appeared around 10,000 BC, at the time of the first agricultural settlements in northeastern Africa." From https://www.ncbi.nlm.nih.gov/pmc/articles/PMC1200696/ (accessed February 19, 2021).

[128] Mitigation is intended to reduce the rate of transmission of COVID-19. The three components of mitigation are wearing a cloth face mask that covers the nose and mouth; social distancing, at least six feet apart in public; and hand sanitizing. Hand sanitizing, to prevent transmission by droplets, was initially believed to be most important, but in the early months of 2021, the importance of aerosol transmission was recognized, and wearing face masks was emphasized. Considerable resistance to mitigation was seen in some segments of the population.

[129] Thomas Robert Malthus, FRS, *An Essay on the Principle of Population* (1798). The essay was originally anonymous. An exception to Malthus' rules may be occurring at this time, for birth rates have gradually been decreasing for several decades in western Europe and in descendants of western Europeans in America. And in addition to this, there has also been a dramatic drop in fertility in some countries during the COVID-19 pandemic. Whether there will be a post-pandemic "baby boom" is unpredictable. However, the pre-existing decline in fertility suggests that birth rates will continue to decline in developed countries.

G. Fire

[130] *Britannica*, Fire. The earliest use of fire by hominids may have been about 1,420,000 years ago, and Peking man, about 500,000 BCE certainly used fire. The earliest fires were probably acquired from lightning strikes.

The earliest controlled use of fire is said by Jessica Thompson, et al., to have been some 92,000 years ago in east Africa. See Mike Cummings, Study offers earliest evidence of humans changing ecosystems with fire, *Yale News* (5 May 2021): "Mastery of fire has given humans dominance over the natural world. A Yale-led study provides the earliest evidence to date of ancient humans significantly altering entire ecosystems with flames. The study … combines archaeological evidence — dense clusters of stone artifacts dating as far back as 92,000 years ago — with paleoenvironmental data on the northern shores of Lake Malawi in eastern Africa. … They used fire in a way that prevented regrowth of the region's forests, creating a sprawling bushland that exists today." Thompson said, "It suggests that by the Late Pleistocene, humans were learning to use fire in truly novel ways. In this case, their burning caused replacement of the region's forests with the open woodlands you see today. This is the earliest evidence I have seen of humans fundamentally transforming their ecosystem with fire'." From: https://news.yale.edu/2021/05/05/study-offers-earliest-evidence-humans-changing-ecosystems-fire (accessed May 12, 2021).

Neolithic humans made fires in about 7000 BCE. The art on the walls of caves, such as Avignon, in France, are mute testimony to the use of fire. Another hominin that walked erect is *Paranthropus boisei*, which "is likely to have shared a common ancestor with the genus *Homo* relatively recently (between about 3 million and 2.5 million years ago)." However, *P. boisei* is not an ancestor of *Homo sapiens*. *P. boisei* "first appears in the fossil record approximately 2.3 million years ago … and it disappears around 1.3 million years ago, shortly before the first signs of the controlled use of fire." *P. boisei* lived in East Africa. From Bernard Wood and Alexis Williams, Meet your exotic, extinct close relative, *American Scientist* 108 (November-December 2020): 348-355.

P. boisei was a durophagus herbivore (i.e., with a strong bite). Its success was probably due to its ability to make use of food sources that other hominids couldn't use – until fire was mastered. Cooking negated the advantage of big jaws (From Professor Donald Esker, personal communication).

[131] J. A. J. Gowlett and R. W. Wrangham, Earliest fire in Africa: towards the convergence of archaeological evidence and the cooking hypothesis, *Azania: Archaeological Research in Africa* 48 (no. 1, 2013): 5-30; and D. M. J. S. Bowman, et al, Fire in the Earth system, *Science* 324 (no. 5926, 2009): 481-84.

[132] *Britannica*. Prometheus.

[133] Spontaneous combustion is not listed as a natural cause of fire by *Britannica*, but it certainly happens when piles of wet grass begin to smolder. Haymows filled with green hay often burst into flame throughout the Midwest and Far West.

[134] Boy Scouts learn to build fires without matches, with flint and steel or with a bow and a wood base, and how to keep a fire burning. Zoroastrian worship of fire persists in central Asia to the present day, with fresh fire pits seen in Khiva, Uzbekistan.

[135] PFAS (perfluoroalkyl and polyfluoroalkyl substances) summarized from News from the Food and Drug Administration, *JAMA* 324 (no. 11, September 15, 2020):1026; and Erik Vance, A parent's guide to scary chemicals, *New York Times*, 22 September 2020, A2PFAS has been used as a flame retardant in clothing and blankets, and to prevent grease from penetrating food packaging. PFAS is associated with many health risks, including weakened responses to vaccines and alterations to the endocrine system which adversely affect pregnancy and child development. These substances persist in humans after ingestion or exposure and cannot be removed by cooking or washing. Related chemicals acronyms include POB, PCB (polychlorinated biphenyls), PBDE, BPA, and phthalates. Three manufacturers have notified the U.S. Food and Drug Administration (FDA) that they have agreed to a 3-year phase out of PFAS from packaging of fast-food wrappers, and a fourth manufacturer has already halted production of PFAS packaging. PFAS continues to be used as a flame retardant, in spite of the reports of harm.

[136] Jack London, *To Build a Fire*, in *The Youth's Companion*, vol. 76, 28 May 1902.

H. Dogs and Other Animals

[137] "the master's table" (Matthew 15:27).

[138] Jack London, *White Fang* (New York: Macmillan, 1906). It has been adapted into many movies with the title, *White Fang*, beginning in 1925.

[139] Jonathan Shaw, Did milk build the Mongol empire? *Harvard Magazine*, October 2020, 13-14, with photographs from Christina Warinner. Shaw says that Warinner proposes that the horse was the key to the successful expansion of the Mongols on three occasions from c. 200 BC to the thirteenth century.

[140] Gillian P. McHugo, Michael J. Dover, and David E. Machugh, Unlocking the origins and biology of domestic animals using ancient DNA and paleogenomics, *BMC Biology* 17 (no. 1, 2019): 98; and David E. Machugh, Greger Larsen, and Ludovic Orlando, Taming the past: Ancient DNA and the study of animal domestication, *Annual Review of Animal Biosciences* 5 (2016): 329-351.

[141] Hans Zinsser, *Rats, Lice and History: A Study in Biography* (1935. New York: Pocket Books, 1945), 152-6: "More than any other species of animal, the rat and mouse have become dependent on man. …In following man about all over the earth, the rat has – more than any other living creature except man – been able to adapt itself to any conditions of seasonal changes or climate. … By the time of the Crusaders, it had begun to domesticate and consequently to follow human travel." Zinsser pointed out that "the established hegemony of the black rat [*Mus rattus*] was eventually wiped out with the incursion of the hordes of the brown rat, or *Mus decumanus* – the ferocious, short-nose, and short-tailed Asiatic that swept across the Continent in the early eighteenth century." Albino strains of the brown rat, which is also known as *Mus norvegicus*, and strains of the house mouse, *Mus musculis*, have been intentionally domesticated and inbred for use in laboratories and as pets.

[142] For insight into the culture of animals and the relationship that humans have had with some animal species, see: Carl Safina, *Becoming Wild: How Animal Cultures Raise Families, Create Beauty, and Achieve Peace* (New York: Henry Holt & Co., 2020); review by Alexandra Horowitz, Talk to the animals: The culture of macaws, sperm whales and chimpanzees, *New York Times Book Review*, 17 May 2020, 20.

Chapter 4. The Wants   A. Love

[143] The epigraph "Love Is a Many Splendored Thing" is an adaptation of the autobiographical novel, *A Many-Spendoured Thing*, by Han Suyin (1952), which was adapted for the romance film, *Love Is a Many-Splendored Thing* (1955), and a television soap opera series from 1967-73, without the hyphen. It was also the title of a popular song, based on Puccini's opera *Madama Butterfly*. It was first recorded by the Four Aces, and then by many other stars, including Bing Crosby, Ringo Starr, Frank Sinatra, and Nat King Cole; and in many films, including *Grease*.

[144] Love, in Merriam-Webster's *Dictionary*. "The quality of mercy" is from Portia's plea to Shylock in William Shakespeare, *The Merchant of Venice*, Act 4, Scene 1.

[145] Elizabeth Barrett Browning (1806-1861), Sonnet 43, from *Sonnets from the Portuguese* (1850). A sonnet is a poem of fourteen lines, typically having ten syllables per line. Her poem was addressed to her husband, the poet Robert Browning (1812-1889). Alfred, Lord Tennyson (1809-1892), "In Memoriam A.H.H." (1850), canto 27.

[146] A reader commented that, "the most accepted reason is that love in tennis is from to play for love rather than money." Platonic love, in Merriam-Webster's *Dictionary*. There is nothing about sex in the entry for Plato, in *Britannica*. However, the entry for Michel Foucault, in *Stanford Encyclopedia*, says, "The ancient Greeks' view was that sexual acts were natural and necessary, but subject to abuse. They emphasized the proper use (*chresis*) of pleasures, where this involved engaging in a range of sexual activities (heterosexual, homosexual, in marriage, out of marriage)."

[147] [KJV] *The Holy Bible* (London: Collins' Cleartype Press, 1941), in which the OT is 813pp, and the NT is 248pp. The quotations cited from the Concordance are: Genesis 27:4 "And make me savoury meat, such as I love, and bring it to me, that I may eat; that my soul may bless thee before I die." Genesis 29:20 "And Jacob served seven years for Rachel; and they seemed unto him but a few days, for the love he had to her." Revelation 2:4 "Nevertheless I have somewhat against thee, because thou hast left thy first love." Revelation 3:19: "As many as I love, I rebuke and chasten: be zealous therefore, and repent." See: http://www.learnthebible.org/bible/concordance/ (accessed 8/12/2020).

In the Torah, the First Commandment is translated from Exodus 20:1-3, "I the Lord am your God who brought you out of the land of Egypt, the house of bondage: You shall have no other gods beside Me." *The Torah: The Five Books of Moses* (Philadelphia: The Jewish Publication Society, 1962).

The quotation is from the Qur'an, "The Dinner Table" (5:54), translated as Koran in English. Another use of the word "love" appears as a warning in the "The Family of Imran" (3:14): "The love of desires, of women and sons and hoarded treasures of gold and silver and well bred horses and cattle and tilth, is made to seem fair to men." https://quod.lib.umich.edu/k/koran/simple.html (accessed 8/12/2020).

[148] *Britannica*, agape. The class of "those who are unable to care for themselves" in this essay includes persons who are born with defects such as Down syndrome, or who have the spectrum of autism behaviors, the elderly, persons with disabilities, and those who are in need of food and housing. These individuals would not be survivors in pre-human hominid groups.

B. Money

[149] Matthew 13:12, "For whosoever hath, to him shall be given, and he shall have more abundance: but whosoever hath not, from him shall be taken away even that he hath"; and Matthew 25:29, "For unto every one that hath shall be given, and he shall have abundance: but from him that hath not shall be taken away even that which he hath."

[150] "And there came a certain poor widow, and she threw in two mites, which make a farthing" (Mark 12:42). And he saw also a certain poor widow casting in thither two mites. And He said, Of a truth I say unto you, that this poor widow hath cast in more than they all: For all these have of their abundance cast in unto the offerings of God: but she of her penury hath cast in all the living that she had" (Luke 21:2-4).

[151] *The Oxford Universal Dictionary on Historical Principles*, ed. C. T. Onions, et al (Oxford: Clarendon Press, 1955): "token" is "a sign, a symbol" and "something given as an expression of affection, or to be kept as a memorial; a keepsake." *Webster's New Twentieth Century Dictionary Unabridged* (William Collins Publishers, 1972): "token 1. A sign, indication or symbol; as this gift is a *token* of my affection."

Roy Porter, in "The Roots of Medicine": "Hunter-gatherer bands were more likely to abandon their sick than to succor them. … With an emergent division of labour, medical expertise became the *métier* of particular individuals. Although the family remained the first line of defence against illness, it was bolstered by medicine men, diviners, witch-smellers and shamans, and in due course by herbalists, birth-attendants, bone setters, barber-surgeons, and healer-priests. When that first happened, we cannot be sure… in France, some 17,000 years ago… may be the oldest surviving images of medicine-men." This section concludes with a brief agreeable conversation between Dr. David Livingstone (1813-1873) and a Rain Doctor in Africa. From Roy Porter, *The Greatest Benefit to Mankind: A Medical History of Humanity* (New York: W. W. Norton Co., 1997), 31.

[152] The Hippocratic Oath, trans. Michael North, excerpt: "To hold him who taught me this art equally dear to me as my parents … to look upon his offspring as equals to my own siblings, and to teach them this art, if they shall wish to learn it, without fee or contract." https://www.nlm.nih.gov/hmd/greek/greek_oath.html (accessed 8/12/2020).

[153] William Harvey (1578-1657) was the author of *De Motu Cordis*, which described for the first time the circulation of the blood; it is one of the great landmarks of medical history. Examples of titled physicians include Sir Frederick Treves, 1st Baronet, FRCS (1853-1923), who treated the "Elephant Man" and Lord [Joseph] Lister, 1st Baron (1827-1912), who pioneered antiseptic surgery. William Upjohn's company is now part of Pfizer; Stryker is one of the largest medical implant companies in the world; and Kellogg is famous for many breakfast cereals.

[154] The subject of "the spiralling costs" of health care is discussed by Porter, *Greatest Benefit*, 658. The chart on p. 659 of *Greatest Benefit* compares health care expenditures as a share of Gross National Product for the 37 Organization for Economic Co-operation and Development (OECD) countries from 1970 to 1992, with the U.S. rising from 7.4 to 14.0 in that 12-year period. Porter: "Health became one of the major growth industries in America, encompassing the pharmaceutical industry, manufacturers of sophisticated and costly diagnostic apparatus, laboratory instruments and therapeutic devices, quite aside from medical personnel, hospitals and their penumbra of corporate finance, insurers, lawyers, accountants and so forth." The costs continue to rise. In 2008, health care comprised one-sixth (16.6%) of the U.S. economy, and by 2021, it was 17.7% of the U.S. GNP (from Richard L. Byyny, Now is the time to enact a U.S. health care system, *Pharos* 84 (no. 2, Spring 2021):3, quoting Tom Daschle, S. S. Greenberger and J. M. Lambrew, *Critical: What We Can Do About the Health Care Crisis* (New York: Thomas Dunne Books, 2008).

Also, David Brooks, Want to get really rich? Here's how? *New York Times*, 26 February 27, 2021, A21. Quoting Jonathan Rothwell, *A Republic of Equals: A Manifesto for a Just Society* (Princeton: Princeton University Press, 2019), Brooks says that it isn't STEM. "What profession is most likely to get you rich? Medicine! You get to save lives and make bank all at once! One third of doctors overall, including about 58.6 percent of surgeons, are in the top one percent of earners. There are more doctors and surgeons in the top one percent than any other job category." In Sweden, Spain and Iceland, physicians and surgeons earn twice as much as the average worker, but in the U.S. it is nearly five times as much.

[155] Health has become the elephant in the corner in American society, with many hands reaching into what appears to be a bottomless pot of money. Also see Porter, ibid. Canada's expenditure on health care is more efficient than that of the U.S.A. Canada does better than the U.S. in life expectancy and in the probability of dying under age five and between 15 and 60 years of age, yet Canada has a 79% lower per capita income, and its expenditure on health care is only 61% of that of the U.S.

[156] The reader may recognize that the word "enough" at this time, in the year 2020, had an additional meaning in America. See Mary L. Trump, *Too Much and Never Enough: How My Family Created the World's Most Dangerous Man* (New York, Simon & Schuster, 2020).

[157] Hyponatremia, from "low-sodium-blood" was formerly a rare condition, but it has recently been reported in young people who carry plastic bottles of water, from which they sip frequently; and in joggers, who believe that maintaining hydration is so important that they do it in excess. Rupture of the gastro-esophageal junction was described by Hermann Boerhaave (1668-2738); it is known as Boerhaave's syndrome. The deaths of solitary individuals in homes, often from a fall, are a sad commentary on living alone. "Medi-Alert" buttons worn by persons living alone has been helpful, but they are not necessarily used correctly by older people.

[158] This analogy to feedback refers to the "warfare conflict" between science and religion. And to what is called the Scientific Method: of Laws and Theories, and of hypotheses, experiments, and observations. And how "chance favors the mind that is prepared." It was an unintended "signpost" to that discussion, which is in a later section of *Health Matters*.

Chapter 5   Other Considerations   Pain, Exercise, Avocations

[159] For a discussion of pain from a medical perspective, with references, see: George J. Hill, "Excruciating Pain," Chapter 28, in Hill, *Outpatient Surgery*, 1st ed. (Philadelphia: W. B. Saunders, 1973), 977-93.

[160] David W. Baker, *The Joint Commission's Pain Standards: Origins and Evolution* (Oakbrook Terrace, Ill: The Joint Commission, 2017), and Ibid., History of The Joint Commission's pain standards: Lessons for today's prescription opioid epidemic, *JAMA* 317 (no. 11, 2017):1117-8. At: https://www.jointcommission.org/-/media/tjc/documents/resources/pain-management/pain_std_history_web_version_05122017pdf.pdf?db (accessed March 16, 2021).

[161] Daniel E. Lieberman, Active grandparenting, costly repair, *Harvard Magazine* (September-October 2020), 28-34; and Liberman, *Exercised: Why Something We Never Evolved to Do Is Healthy and Rewarding* (New York: Penguin Random House/Pantheon Books, 2020). A fine review of the subject of exercise in the history of medicine was published by the American Physiological Society: Charles M. Tipton, The history of "Exercise Is Medicine" in ancient civilizations, *Adv. Physiol. Educ.* 38 (no. 2, June 2014): 109-117. The quotation from Hippocrates is in Lipton, although he does not specify the location in the works of Hippocrates.

[162] Medawar and Sir Macfarlane Burnet shared the Nobel Prize for Physiology or Medicine in 1960 for the discovery of acquired immunological tolerance.

[163] The graph that accompanies this article includes lovely cartoons, but it is pseudo-scientific.

[164] Bengt Saltin (1935-2014) "coined and proved the term 'humans were meant to move' from the level of gene expression to heart and muscle function. His famous 'bed rest' study transformed medical practice on how people recover from heart attacks, general surgery, or injury. Saltin proved the importance and limits of the heart in athletes and cardiac patients, described and explained the genetic basis for why world-class marathoners and sprinters run so fast." http://www.exercisephysiology.net/Bengt_Saltin.asp (accessed September 6, 2020).

[165] The reader is encouraged at this point to think of other personal avocations or hobbies.

Chapter 6   The Exceptions   A. Unavoidable Exceptions

[166] Down syndrome was formerly known as Down's syndrome. It is also known as trisomy 21, from the genetic defect which is responsible for it. It was formerly known by the pejorative term, "Mongolism," because of the facial appearance of patients with Down syndrome. The syndrome was described by John Landown Down, and it is named for him. He used the unfortunate term "mongoloid."

B. Religion

[167] The principal references are *Britannica* (religion) and the King James Version of the Holy Bible (KJV). Also, *The Golden Bough*, *A History of the Warfare of Science with Theology*, and *God: A Biography*, although I do not specifically cite the latter two books, and I rarely quote the first. The recent collection of essays about *Warfare of Science*, edited by Hardin, et al, looks at the "conflict narrative" though the eyes of many scholars, from different perspectives. Also, Virgil, *The Aeneid*, trans. Robert Fitzgerald (New York: Vintage Classics, [1981] 1983), Book VI, lines 268-96. Fraser mentions the connection to Aeneas but he traces the legend of the golden bough back to earlier sources in which it is considered to be mistletoe. (Fraser, *Golden Bough*, 13, 796).

Bibliography: Andrew Dickson White, *A History of the Warfare of Science with Theology in Christendom* 2 vols. (London: Macmillan and Company, 1896); Jack Miles, *God: A Biography* (New York: Knopf, 1995); N. J. Dawood, *The Koran* (New York: Penguin Books, [1956] 1974); *The Torah: The Five Books of Moses. A New Translation of The Holy Scriptures According to the Masoretic Text* (Philadelphia: The Jewish Publication Society of America, 1962); *Eight Translation New Testament. The New Testament of Our Lord and Saviour Jesus Christ* (Wheaton, Ill.: Tyndale House Publishers, Inc., 1974); *The Layman's Parallel Bible: Comparing Four Popular Translations in Parallel Columns* (Grand

Rapids, Mich.: The Zondervan Corp., 1973); Jeff Hardin, Ronald L. Numbers, and Ronald A. Binzley, eds., *The Warfare Between Science & Religion: The Idea That Wouldn't Die* (Baltimore, Md.: The Johns Hopkins University Press, 2018); and James George Frazer, *The Golden Bough: A Study in Magic and Religion* [1890ff], edited with an introduction and notes by Robert Frazer (New York: Oxford University Press, [1994], 2009.

[168] For Religion(s), 42 "religious traditions" are cited alphabetically under the general rubric of religion in *Britannica*. For a discussion of the relationship between magic and science from the perspective of a historian, see Lynn Thorndike, *A History of Magic and Experimental Science During the First Thirteen Centuries of Our Era* (New York: Columbia University Press, [1923] 1958). *Britannica*, Frazer, Sir James George.

[169] Hemophobia is shown in the fictional TV series *Doc Martin* (BBC, 2010) about a doctor who must overcome panicking at the sight of blood. Hemophilia has nothing to do with hemophilia, though the two words suggest that the conditions are opposites. Hemophilia is a condition characterized by failure of blood to clot. It is not, as the meaning would imply, a love of blood. Hemophilia was transmitted in the female line to males who descended from Queen Victoria, including Alexi, Tsarevich of Russia, the unfortunate son of Nicholas II and Alexandra.

[170] *Merriam-Webster*, magic; mysticism. *Britannica*, magic; mysticism. *Britannica* does not mention "illusion," which I believe is a key aspect in magic. The art of illusion is beautifully demonstrated in the television series, *Penn and Teller: Fool Us*. Nancy (Davis) Reagan, wife of President Ronald Regan, believed in astrology. She was the step-daughter of Dr. Loyal Davis, one of most respected surgeons in America. See: https://www.atlasobscura.com/articles/a-brief-history-of-nancy-reagan-and-astrology (accessed August 24, 2020).

[171] *Britannica*, religion.

[172] The four roles of community leaders were seen in the Plymouth Colony which was formed from passengers on the *Mayflower* in 1620. The physician was Samuel Fuller; the religious leader was William Brewster; the governor was William Bradford; and the defense of the colony was led by the captain, Myles Standish.

[173] The sun does not actually "rise" in the east. Copernicus showed that the earth revolves around the sun, and the sun appears in earth's eastern sky as the earth turns toward the sun. The traverse of the sun from east to west takes place in the southern sky in the northern hemisphere, and at noon it is located at its height in the south, at 180 degrees on the compass ("true north," after correcting for magnetic declination). The traverse of the sun is in the northern sky in the southern hemisphere, and at noon, the sun is at 0 degrees, "true north."

[174] Until simplified by the Second Vatican Council, the Roman Catholic Church had eight prayers. Four were prayers that related to the coming or leaving of night: Vespers, at evening; Compline, at night; Matins, during the night; and Lauds, at dawn.

[175] Ritual use of water appears in several places in the Old Testament; five locations have been identified. Total immersion is used in several Christian denominations, including Baptists, Anabaptists; Seventh Day Adventists, and by the Church of Jesus Christ of Latter-Day Saints (LDS, often called Mormons).

[176] Muslims will eat only permitted food (halal) and will not eat or drink anything that is considered forbidden (haram). http://www.waht.nhs.uk/en-GB/NHS-Mobile/Our-Services/?depth=4&srcid=2004 (accessed August 5, 2020). During the month of Ramadan, Muslims will not eat or drink between sunrise and sunset. The pre-dawn meal (*suhur*) and the after-sunset meal (*iftar*) are special daily occasions, and the end of Ramadan is celebrated with the feast of *Eid-al-Fitr*.

[177] "Israel was holy to the Lord, the firstfruits of his harvest" (Jer. 2:3). "By his choice, he gave us birth by the word of truth so that we would be a kind of firstfruits of his creatures." (James 1:18).

[178] The Ark of the Covenant first appears in Exodus, and the story of its construction, use, loss, and recapture appears in many additional locations in the Old Testament. The Ark is not mentioned in the New Testament, supposedly because Jesus is the replacement for the Ark. See: http://www.fountainoflifetm.com/2017/08/31/why-isnt-the-the-ark-of-the-covenant-in-the-new-testament/ (accessed August 5, 2020). It reappeared in fiction in the popular film, *The Raiders of the Lost Ark* (1981).

[179] The Roman Catholic Church's required tributes to be paid for marriage, with various degrees of relationships, are described by Ramón A. Gutiérrez, *When Jesus Came, the Corn Mothers Went Away* (Stanford, Ca.: Stanford University Press, 1991).

[180] Men and women are often segregated during worship services in many religions. In Islam, men and women worship separately, but mixing is allowed in the hajj. See: Diaa Hadid, https://www.nytimes.com/2016/09/16/world/middleeast/hajj-mecca-saudi-arabia.html (accessed August 23, 2020). In 2020, "Under present law, any woman under the age of 45 seeking a hajj visa must travel with a *mahram*—a male 'guardian,' generally related by blood." (Ibid.)

Edward the Confessor (1042-1066) is said to have been the first to touch for the King's Evil, which was usually tuberculosis of the lymph glands of the neck (scrofula). See: https://history.rcplondon.ac.uk/blog/touching-kings-evil-short-history (accessed August 25, 2020).

[181] "Clothing has long played a significant role in Judaism, reflecting religious identification, social status, emotional state and even the Jews' relation with the outside world." From https://www.myjewishlearning.com/article/jewish-clothing/ (accessed August 23, 2020).

[182] Leviticus 16:10, "But the goat, on which the lot fell to be the scapegoat, shall be presented alive before the LORD, to make an atonement with him, *and* to let him go for a scapegoat into the wilderness." Luke 15:23, "And bring hither the *fatted calf,* and kill it; and let us eat, and be merry."

Zebuine beef cattle have spread from India to other continents. See: https://www.financialexpress.com/economy/on-world-milk-day (accessed August 24, 2020).

[183] Islamic Relief Worldwide: "And establish prayer and give Zakat, and whatever good you put forward for yourselves – you will find it with Allah." (2:110, Qur'an). From https://www.islamic-relief.org/zakat/ & https://www.muslimaid.org/ zakat-calculator/ (accessed August 31, 2020). Martin Luther's 95 theses are at https://www.uncommon-travel-germany.com/martin-luther-95-theses.html (accessed August 31, 2020).

[184] For Presbyterians and predestination: https://www.presbyterianmission.org/what-we-believe/predestination/ (accessed August 31, 2020).

[185] "I will take less" is commonly taught in the Midwest. As mentioned above, altruism" is from Latin *alteri*, dative of *alter* "other." It is opposed to "egoism." In ordinary language, altruism is the spirit of unselfishness; it is the opposite of selfishness. "alt" = other, versus "self."
Britannica, humanism; empathy. Molly Worther, The trouble with empathy, *New York Times*, 6 September 2020, SR4. Empathy is required for an actor who uses the technique known as "method acting."

[186] *Britannica*, Darwinism. Darwin introduced "survival of the fittest" in the fifth edition (1869) of *The Origin of Species*; it was a term first coined by Herbert Spencer after reading the first edition of *Origin* in 1859. The words, "Nature, red in tooth and claw" appeared prior to *Origin* in the poem by Alfred, Lord Tennyson, "In Memoriam A.H.H." (1850), but this phrase is emblematic of Darwin's theory of natural selection. For identical twins, see Nancy L. Segal, *Born Together – Reared Apart* (Cambridge: Harvard University Press, 2012), summarized by Erika Hayasaki, Identical twins hint at how environments change gene expression, *The Atlantic* (15 May 2018), at https://www.theatlantic.com/science/archive/2018/05/twin-epigenetics/560189/ (accessed August 30, 2020).

[187] The last five commandments are paraphrased from the ten in Exodus 20:17 and Deuteronomy 5:6-21. The two commandments of Jesus are: "Thou shalt love the Lord thy God with all thy heart, and with all thy soul, and with all thy mind," and "Thou shalt love thy neighbor as thyself." (Matthew 22:37-40). The Koran (Quran, Qur'an) commands: "Feed the poor" (22:36). The Buddhist nirvana = "a transcendent state in which there is neither suffering, desire, nor sense of self, and the subject is released from the effects of karma and the cycle of death and rebirth. It represents the final goal of Buddhism" (Oxford Languages). A discussion of nirvana should include the contrast and similarity to the apocalypse, which in the Christian tradition is the final destruction of the world, as described in the Book of Revelation.

[188] The Scout Oath, Law, Slogan, and Motto, of the Boy Scouts of America. The Scout Oath is: "On my honor I will do my best to do my duty to God and my country and to obey the Scout Law; to help other people at all times; to keep myself physically strong, mentally awake, and morally straight." The 12th point of the Scout Law is "Reverent = Be reverent toward God. Be faithful in your religious duties. Respect the beliefs of others." From https://www.scouting.org/about/faq/. The Boy Scout Slogan = "Do a good turn daily" from https://www.boyscouttrail.com/boy-scouts/boy-scout-slogan. The Scout Motto = "Be prepared," from: https://blog.scoutingmagazine.org/be-prepared/ (all accessed January 12, 2021).

[189] Many of the harrowing stories mentioned in this paragraph are well known as biopics or fictional movies. See also George J. Hill, *Rolling with Patton* (Berwyn Heights, Md.: Heritage Books, 2020).

[190] The "blind eye" is not mentioned in *Britannica*, Nelson. Nevertheless, "the most famous act of insubordination in British naval history [was when] On April 2, 1801 Nelson put a telescope to his blind eye and said, "I really do not see the signal" — the order from his commanding admiral, Sir Hyde Parker, to withdraw from the Battle of Copenhagen." See: https://www.thetimes.co.uk/article/how-turning-a-blind-eye-won-the-battle-for-nelson (August 25, 2020).

[191] The origin of the word "sacrifice" is from *sacrificium* from *sacer* (Latin = holy) + *facere* (Latin = to make, or to do)." *Merriam-Webster* defines sacrifice as "an act of offering to a deity something precious, especially the killing of a victim on an altar."

[192] *Britannica*, Sacrifice, Human Sacrifice, and other Sacrifices (Hindu, pre-historic, pre-Colombian, Roman, etc.) in *Britannica.* The word "sacrifice" appears in 205 verses in the King James Version of the Bible. The Old Testament has 182 verses that mention the word "sacrifice" and there are 23 in the New Testament. Much detail is provided about the purpose and details of the sacrificial act in the Torah, in which meat is burned on the altar. In later chapters of the OT, other forms of oblation are mentioned in comparison to the sacrifice. The few verses in the NT

show even less about sacrifice, and. the act becomes more of a symbol than a reality. Nevertheless, the NT repeats the statement in Genesis 4:1-18, in which the offer by Abel, a farmer, who gave "the fruit of the soil" as "a more excellent sacrifice" to God than that of Cain, a herdsman, who offered "firstlings of his flock."

I do not include the Jains and Zoroastrians in the religions in which sacrifice is or has been performed, actually or symbolically. I do not know enough about the details of their ceremonies to comment on this. Jains eschew all forms of killing of animal life.

[193] Karla Bohmbach, "Daughter of Jephthah" in *Encyclopedia of Jewish Women*, https://jwa.org/encyclopedia/article/daughter-of-jephthah-bible (accessed August 26, 2020). Bohmbach says that Jephthah's daughter should have known that her father would have made that vow, and this may have been a self-sacrifice by the girl.

[194] Cannibalism is the ceremonial climax in the Last Supper: "Lord Jesus the *same* night in which he was betrayed took bread: And when he had given thanks, he brake *it*, and said, Take, eat: this is my body, which is broken for you: this do in remembrance of me. After the same manner also *he* took the cup, when he had supped, saying, This cup is the new testament in my blood: this do ye, as oft as ye drink *it*, in remembrance of me. (1 Cor 11:24-5). All four synoptic gospels tell of the final meal, when Jesus speaks of consuming "his" bread and wine, although it was not called the "Last Supper" nor do all mention the Passover (Matt. 26:17-30, Mark 14:12-26, Luke 22:7-39; John 13:1-17). Many people believe that it was on Thursday evening at Seder in the week of Passover.

[195] Joseph Besse, *A Collection of the Sufferings of the People called Quakers for the Testimony of a Good Conscience* (London: Luke Hinde, 1753).

The story of John Proctor and his wife Elizabeth is told incorrectly in Arthur Miller's play, *The Crucible*. Miller, supposedly in order to add spice to the story in order to make it a success on Broadway, changed Proctor's character to be a flawed person. He portrayed Proctor as a pedophile and an adulterer, in order to have him redeem himself on the scaffold. See: Elizabeth and John Proctor in Carol F. Karlsen, *The Devil in the Shape of a Woman: Witchcraft in Colonial New England* (New York: Random House, [1987] 1989; Mary Beth Norton, *In the Devil's Snare* (New York: Random House, 2002); and Arthur Miller, *The Crucible* (New York: Penguin Books, [1952] 1995). Introduction by Christopher Bigsby, "The play is not history in the sense in which the word is used by the academic historian" (p.2).

[196] Most of the discussions about *bushido* fail to mention the warrior's self-sacrifice known as *seppuku* or hari-kari. For example, see: "History of the Bushido Code" https://www.invaluable.com/blog/history-of-the-bushido-code/ (accessed August 27, 2020). "Greater love" is John 15:13, and "Love thy neighbor" is Matthew 22:39.

[197] A sympathetic though incomplete history of Clara Mass is given by the American Association for the History of Nursing. The name of the German Hospital in Newark is now Clara Maass Hospital. She was originally buried in Cuba, but she was later re-buried in Fairmount Cemetery in Newark. See: https://www.aahn.org/maass (accessed (accessed August 27, 2020).

[198] Lawrence K. Altman, *Who Goes First: The Story of Self-Experimentation in Medicine* (New York: Random House, 1987); and Allen B. Weisse, Self-Experimentation and its role in medical research, *Tex Heart Inst J.* 39 (no. 1, 2012): 51-54. From https://www.ncbi.nlm.nih.gov/pmc/articles/PMC3298919/ (accessed February 8, 2012).

C. Irrational Behavior

[199] USA Today, "DNA links bones near plane crash site to Fossett" from http://usatoday30.usatoday.com/news/nation/2008-11-03-3668149862_x.htm (accessed September 7, 2020). The crash was attributed to a probable downdraft that occurred just as he was about to clear the ridge.

[200] The actions of "Ordinary civilians" are described in Stephen E. Ambrose, *Band of Brothers: E Company, 506th Regiment, 101st Airborne: From Normandy to Hitler's Eagle's Nest* (New York: Simon & Schuster, 1992), and Tom Brokaw, *The Greatest Generation* (New York: Penguin Random House, 1998).

[201] I plead guilty to the trap of choosing adventure and rationalizing it. My experiences in Vietnam are shown at my website, http://georgejhill.com/ (accessed February 21, 2021). Two pertinent references are George J. Hill, "Lerne and gladly teche": A view of the Vietnam Medical Education Project, *Military Medicine* 144 (1979): 124-8; and Bernard Fall, *Street without Joy. Indochina at war, 1946-54* (Harrisburg: Stockpole Co., 1961). To appreciate the risk, see Vietnam War timeline, at https://www.history.com/topics/vietnam-war/vietnam-war-timeline (accessed June 13, 2020).

[202] "Luck, Be a Lady Tonight" (1965) was made famous by Frank Sinatra. Stephen E. Ambrose, *Undaunted Courage: Meriwether Lewis, Thomas Jefferson, and the Opening of the American West* (New York, Simon & Schuster, 1962) tells of the Lewis and Clark expedition in 1803-1806, and of how the Ambrose family retraced the path of the explorers.

[203] The "white feather" has long been a symbol of cowardice, but it is best known from the creation of the Order of the White Feather by Admiral Charles Fitzgerald in Britain in World War I, to shame men into serving in uniform. Many abuses were recorded. One dictionary definition of "yellow" is coward, for reasons that are obscure.

Rudyard Kipling's poem (1890) "Gunga Din" is about a fictional native servant who is working with the British Indian Army on the North-West Frontier. His unit is besieged, and he dies carrying water from the Swat River back to the garrison. Gunga Din is posthumously buried in uniform, as a corporal, with one of the officers reciting the poem's memorable final line. 1 Samuel 17:20 is the climax of the story of David and the giant Goliath: "So David prevailed over the Philistine with a sling and with a stone, and smote the Philistine, and slew him; but there was no sword in the hand of David."

[204] The Bible does not say explicitly that the earth is the center of the universe, but it is implied in Genesis. For instance, Genesis 1: 16-17, "And God made two great lights; the greater light to rule the day, and the lesser light to rule the night: he made the stars also. And God set them in the firmament of the heaven to give light upon the earth."

The history of the anti-vax movement is sometimes traced to problems caused by the polio vaccines. Neither the inactivated polio vaccine (Salk, IPV) or oral polio vaccine (Sabin, OPV) is completely free of risk. The anti-vax movement was given another boost by the false report that vaccines containing mercury compounds as a preservative were associated with autism. The initial report by Dr. Andrew Wakefield was published in *Lancet* and then withdrawn much later when the British Medical Association determined that the author had been untruthful. But the damage was done. The result is that herd immunity to some common childhood diseases, such as measles, has been lost in many parts of the world that had been free of these diseases for many years. The anti-vax movement is financed and led by many misguided wealthy and powerful people such as Robert F. Kennedy, Jr. See Paul Offit, *The Cutter Incident: How America's First Polio Vaccine Led to the Growing Vaccine Crisis* (New Haven: Yale University Press, 2007); and Jan Hoffman, How anti-vaccine sentiment took hold in the United States, *New York Times*, 23 September 2019, at https://www.nytimes.com/2019/09/23/health/anti-vaccination-movement-us.html (accessed September 8, 2020).

[205] Opposing views were seen in the *Washington Post* on 14 November 2020. See Appendix D.

[206] The reader should proceed slowly and think of the terrors that are involved in these disturbances.

[207] On religious fanaticism: No one knows what was in the mind of Bishop James Pike (1913-1969), when he wandered in the Judean Wilderness. He is said to have intended to recreate the life of Jesus. He and his second wife drove into the desert unprepared; she escaped, but he died. He was a brilliant and multitalented man, but his behavior in the years shortly before the final episode are consistent with a diagnosis of bipolar disorder.

D. Benefits from Disregarding the Exceptions

[208] Jesus said, "Go, and do thou likewise" (Luke 10:37).

E. The Dark Side of Medicine

[209] See "Doctors Afield" (Part Two) for criminal behavior of psychotic physicians.

[210] Dr. Larry Nassar (b. 1963) and several others were involved with his egregious assaults on young women in the gymnastic program at Michigan State University and USA Gymnastics. See David Woods, Four years later, how the Larry Nassar and USA Gymnastics scandals continue, *Indianapolis Star* (24 June 2020).

For more on euthanasia, physician-assisted-suicide (PAS), and physician aid in dying (PAD), see the section below on Death with Dignity. Also, Sheldon Rubenfeld and Daniel P. Sulmasy (eds.), *Physician-Assisted Suicide and Euthanasia: Before, During and After the Holocaust* (Lanham, Md.: Lexington Books, 2020). Review by Jack Coulehan, *Pharos* 84 (no. 2, Spring 2021): 45, says PAD has gained "remarkable traction." Voluntary euthanasia is now legal in the Netherlands, Belgium, Luxembourg, Spain, Canada, Western Australia, and Columbia. PAS, "but not voluntary euthanasia" is now legal in Switzerland, German, Victoria (Australia), eight American states and the District of Columbia.

Chapter 7 Choices and Ambitions   A. Choices – Decisions

[211] The proverbial or idiomatic expression, "Time and tide wait for no man," is of uncertain origin. Some say it was first expressed by Geoffrey Chaucer in the *Prologue to the Clerk's Tale* (c. 1395): "For thogh we slepe, or wake, or rome, or ryde, Ay fleeth the tyme; it nyl no man abyde." However, Chaucer does not mention "tide." See: Dictionary.com https://www.dictionary.com/browse/time-and-tide-wait-for-no-man (accessed September 2, 2020). I favor an earlier expression attributed to St. Marher (1225), "And te tide and te time þat tu iboren were, schal beon iblescet." From the Phrase Finder, https://www.phrases.org.uk/meanings/time-and-tide-wait-for-no-one.html (accessed September 2, 2020). A suggestion has been made that "tide" at that time meant "noon-tide" although the expression now is interpreted to mean the diurnal ocean tides.

[212] "Social Science Statistics" provides a simple means to calculate the odds by entering data on line. It is much easier than previous methods, which required data entry in writing, followed by laborious calculations and the use of

books with tables. For Chi-squared, a four-way table and significance chosen allows a result to be obtained in a few minutes at https://www.socscistatistics.com/tests/chisquare/default2.aspx (accessed September 5, 2020).

[213] The drama of the decision made by Eisenhower appears in detail, with quotations from Eisenhower and his staff, in Rick Atkinson, *The Guns at Last Light: The War in Western Europe, 1944-1945* (New York: Henry Holt and Company, 2013), 34-6. Eisenhower, on the evening of June 4, 1944: "'I'm quite positive we must give the order,' he said, 'I don't like it, but there it is.' … They would reconvene before dawn on Monday, June 5, to hear Stagg's latest forecast, but the order would stand. 'Okay,' Eisenhower declared. 'We'll go'." The decision was crucial, because much of the success of the invasion depended on launching it on June 4-6, and a delay of two weeks would have been necessary in order to have the tides return to the correct point. The Germans were rapidly moving troops into Northern France to confront an expected invasion. One might say that the decision to drop atomic bombs on Japan was a more momentous decision, but that was made by Truman without full understanding of what he was authorizing. Vincent P. O'Hara, The greatest naval war ever fought, *Naval History* (October 2020), 12-19, said the "invasion of Normandy was 'the single most decisive naval event of World War II'." O'Hara opined that the failure of the German Navy to prevent the invasion of Normandy "secured Germany's defeat in the West."

The events of June 4-6 in Eisenhower's meetings with his British, French, and American staff are not described in Winston Churchill, *The Second World War: Triumph and Tragedy* (Boston: Houghton Mifflin Company, 1953), "D-Day", p.3, which begins with "Our long months of preparation and planning for the greatest amphibious operation in history ended on D-Day, June 6, 1944. During the preceding night…" Churchill says nothing about June 4-5, 1944.

[214] See more in Appendix D.

B. Ambition

[215] Napoleon (1769-1821) is chosen to represent the other end of the spectrum of human affairs from Saint Mother Teresa (1910-1997), who received the Nobel Peace Prize in 1979 and was canonized in 1996. Napoleon is revered in France, but among his many cruel deeds was the re-instatement of slavery in Haiti in 1802. It had been abolished by a slave rebellion in 1794. After the rebellion was put down in a reign of terror, slavery was re-instituted and it continued until it was finally abolished in 1848. See: Mariene L. Daut, Napoleon isn't a hero to celebrate, *New York Times* (22 March 2021), A21.

Chapter 8 Death   A. Death with Dignity

[216] C. P. Snow, *The Two Cultures and the Scientific Revolution*, 1959, p.7; and *The Two Cultures and A Second Look*, 1963, p. 6, 58-59. Lord Snow wrote in 1963 that in the four years since *Two Cultures* was published, it was attacked "with virulence" on many occasions, and that one of the "crudest" was one his choice of the phrase "We die alone."

[217] John Donne (1572-1631) probably had the Bible in mind when he wrote in *Divine Meditations*, "'Death be not proud' ~ death should not be feared; you can not be killed because death is like sleeping. We are really at rest when we die'." These words paraphrase "O death, where is thy sting? O grave, where is thy victory?" (I Corinthians) 15:15.

[218] BJ Miller, What is death, *New York Times*, 20 December 2020, SR4: "Rather than spend so much energy keeping pain at bay, you might want to suspend your judgment and let your body do what a body does. If the past, present and future come together, as we sense they must, then death is a process of becoming." From BJ Miller [sic] and Soshana Berger, *A Beginner's Guide to the End: Practical Advice for Living Life and Facing Death* (New York: Simon & Schuster, 2021).

[219] A woman dies of a stroke (cerebral ischemia) following a heart attack (myocardial infarction), due to coronary artery disease (thrombosis); also "natural cause" of death.

[220] The defibrillator was developed in the 1960s to assist with open chest cardiac massage. External defibrillation with "pads" eventually replaced the open chest procedure in most cases. This was followed by internal defibrillators and implantation of cardiac rhythm converters. One of the pioneers, who developed the first external pacemaker at the Beth Israel Hospital in Boston, was Dr. Bernard Lown (1921-2021). Emily Langer, "Bernard Lown, 99: Eminent cardiologist rallied doctors against nuclear war," *Washington Post*, 21 February 2021, C9.

[221] For a recent discussion of this topic in more depth, see Alan J. Lippman, Facilitated natural death: An approach to death with dignity, MDAdvisor 10 (no. 3, 2017): 16-19. Also, Katherine Ellison, Diane Rehm tackles "death with dignity" debate, this time in a film, *Washington Post*, 6 April 6, 2021, E1, E5. See Appendix E for versions of the Hippocratic Oath. The prohibition of performing abortion has also been removed.

An example of physician-assisted suicide is seen in the oblique language of the obituary of Corinne Chubb "Teeny" Zimmermann, who died "peacefully on July 15, 2018, courageously asserting her right to pre-empt the lung cancer that she had battled for more than a year … after a weekend with close family to say heartfelt good-byes, and drink one last champagne toast to a life well-lived." A fatal dose of barbiturates was legally prescribed for her. See:

https://www.legacy.com/obituaries/washingtonpost/obituary.aspx?n=corinne-zimmermann-teeny&pid=190177314 (accessed July 11, 2020).

B. Immortality

[222] *Britannica*, immortality. Also, James George Frazer, *The Golden Bough: A Study in Magic and Religion*, edited with an Introduction and Notes by Robert Fraser (1890. Oxford: Oxford University Press, 2009).

[223] The word "immortal" has taken on an additional meaning, meaning a meme. Nathan Hale's supposed last words, "I regret that I have but one life to give for my country," would now be considered to be his "immortal" words. For other examples, see: Terry Breverton, *Immortal Words: History's Most Memorable Quotations and the Stories Behind Them* (n.p.: Arcturus, 2010).

[224] Jesus's questions about resurrection are in Matthew 22:23-33, Mark 12: 18-27, and Luke 20:27-40. The Nicene Creed in the Episcopal Church's *Book of Common Prayer* begins with "We believe" and ends with "We look for the resurrection of the dead, and the life of the world to come. Amen" (p.359); and in The Committal for burial of the dead, "In sure and certain hope of the resurrection to eternal life … ashes to ashes, dust to dust" (p.501).

[225] For apoptosis, TNR and p53, see: https://www.ncbi.nlm.nih.gov/pmc/articles/PMC2117903/ (accessed June 14, 2020). *Britannica*, Lacks, Henrietta (1920-1951); HeLa. Also, Carrie D. Wolinetz and Francis S. Collins, "Recognition of research participants' need for autonomy: Remembering the legacy of Henrietta Lacks," *JAMA* 324 (no. 11, September 15, 2020):1027-8. The original records at the Johns Hopkins Hospital for Henrietta Lacks, who died in 1951, have disappeared, according to Rebecca Skloot, *The Immortal Life of Henrietta Lacks* (New York: Crown Publishers, 2010). Also, Jacques Kelly, Henrietta Lacks' Turner Station home slated for rehab, *Baltimore Sun* (13 February 2021), 3.

[226] Anon., Understanding brain death, *JAMA* 323 (no. 21, June 2, 2020): 2139-40. Robert D. Truog, Kandamaran Krishnamurthy, and Rebert C. Tasker, Brain death – Moving beyond consistency in the diagnostic criteria, *JAMA* 324 (no. 11, September 15, 2020):1045-7, which "addressed inconsistencies in clinical guidelines across different countries." In the same issue of *JAMA*, a special communication by 45 authors reviewed the criteria for brain death: David M. Greer, Sam D. Shermie, Ariane Lewis, et al, Determination of brain death/death by neurologic criteria: The World Brain Death Project, *JAMA* 324 (no. 11, September 15, 2020):1078-97.

Organ transplantation was but a dream for centuries, but it became reality in 1954, when a team led by Joseph E. Murray transplanted a kidney from one person to his identical twin. The subsequent development of this field will be discussed later in this essay. The possibility of transplanting a brain from a totally paralyzed individual into a cadaver was the goal of Robert White, who witnessed Murray's operation. White eventually succeeded in transplanting an entire head from one monkey into the decapitated body of another monkey. The hybrid creature lived for nine days. This was before anti-rejection drugs were developed, so there was no hope for long survival at that time. See: Brandy Shillace, *Mr. Humble and Dr. Butcher: A Monkeys Head, the Pope's Neuroscientist, and the Quest to Transplant the Soul* (New York: Simon & Schuster, 2021).

[227] *Encyclopædia Britannica Deluxe Edition*: cloning; DNA (chemical compound); RNA (biochemistry); genomics; epigenetics; eugenics; anthropology. The genome is the "entire set of genetic material of an organism." David Reich and Orlando Patterson, "DNA rewrites the telling of the Caribbean's past," *New York Times*, 26 Dec 2020, A24.

Chapter 9   Public Health

[228] Public Health was not a subject that was taught at Harvard Medical School in 1953-1957.

[229] The G-10 member countries are Belgium, Canada, France, Germany, Italy, Japan, the Netherlands, Sweden, Switzerland, the United Kingdom, and the United States, with Switzerland playing a minor role. See: https://www.investopedia.com/terms/g/groupoften.asp (accessed July 20, 2020). The International Monetary Fund (IMF) includes data for 121 countries 2019, placed in rank order and shown on a map of the world on https://en.wikipedia.org/wiki/List_of_countries_by_GDP_(nominal)_per_capita (accessed July 20, 2020).

The World Health Organization (WHO) has 194 member states. The WHO's reports are similarly opaque, presumably by choice, although perhaps because the reports are not intended to be read by non-scientists. For example, see the most recent report on health in the U.S.A., at: https://apps.who.int/gho/data/node.country.country-USA. The U.S. has not submitted data since 2015. At https://www.who.int/countries/usa/en/ (accessed 7/20/2020), the U.S. is shown to have a life expectancy at birth in 2016 of 76 years for men and 81 years for women (overall, 79). Data from the United Nations Development Program (UNDP) is at https://en.wikipedia.org/wiki/List_of_countries_by_life_expectancy (accessed July 20, 2020).

[230] The three leading causes (heart disease, cancer, pulmonary diseases) account for half of the deaths in the U.S.

[231] The American Cancer Society (ACS) was founded in 1913 as the American Society for the Control of Cancer (ASCC), which was reorganized and became the ACS in 1945. The ACS promulgated the Seven Warning Signs of Cancer, which still are useful. See: https://www.cancer.org/about-us/ (accessed July 20, 2020); and https://www.medicinenet.com/the_seven_warning_signs_of_cancer/article.htm (accessed April 1, 2021). Roswell

Park Comprehensive Cancer Center was the nation's first cancer center. It was founded as a research center in 1898 in Buffalo, N.Y., by Dr. Roswell Park, a surgeon at the University of Buffalo. See: https://www.roswellpark.org/about-us/ (accessed July 20, 2020). Memorial Sloan Kettering Cancer Center, in New York City, was founded in 1884 as New York Cancer Hospital, which later became Memorial Hospital. See: https://www.mskcc.org/ (accessed July 20, 2020). The history of the concept of cancer as one disease, is told by Siddhartha Mukherjee, *The Emperor of All Maladies: A Biography of Cancer* (New York: Scribner's, 2010). It won the Pulitzer Prize for non-fiction in 2011. Mukherjee told the story of cancer using a method created by Hans Zinsser, in *Rats, Lice and History: A Study in Biography* (1935), which told the "life history of Typhus Fever."

I am pleased to have conceived of a book about cancer that would be intended to be read by medical students, residents, and practicing physicians. It was published as *Clinical Oncology* (Philadelphia: W. B. Saunders Co., 1977), co-authored with John Horton, who independently developed the same idea. The early signs of cancer were discussed in this book by Horton and Denis Haut, "Detection and Recognition of Cancer," Chapter 4 (pp. 86-102). My most recent abstract was for a presentation and panel discussion at the International Cancer Education Conference in 2020: George J. Hill, "Diamond anniversary for the AACE." Presented to Annual Meeting, American Association for Cancer Education, October 12-16, College Park, Md. Abstract 4-B, presented by prerecorded Zoom and live Zoom discussion on October 16, 2020. *Journal of Cancer Education* (2021), in press.

A. Infectious Disease

[232] This brief summary of the history of the USPHS draws on the following sources (accessed 7/21/2020): usphs.gov/; usphs.gov/history; nih.gov/about-nih/; hhs.gov/ niaid.nih.gov/; cancer/gov; tricare.mil/mtf/walterreed; https://www.hrsa.gov/hansens-disease/history.html; defense.gov/Explore. For the National Cancer Institute, see: https://www.cancer.gov/about-nci/overview/history/national-cancer-act-1971 (accessed February 1, 2021).

The Department of Health, Education, and Welfare was created in 1953. It became the Department of Health and Human Services in 1979, when the Department of Education was established. The Clinical Center is Building 10 on the NIH campus in Bethesda, Maryland. It is across Wisconsin Avenue from the flagship hospital of the Department of Defense, which was formerly the National Naval Medical Center and is now the Walter Reed National Military Medical Center. The joint services Uniformed Services University of the Health Sciences (USUHS) is also on that campus. The Surgeon General of the USPHS, with the rank of Vice Admiral, reports to an Admiral in the USPHS who is the Assistant Secretary for Health in DHEW.

References for USPHS and NIH: Betty Martin, *Miracle at Carville* (Garden City: Doubleday, 1950); George J. Hill, *Leprosy in Five Young Men* (Boulder: Associated Press of the University of Colorado, 1970); Donald C. Abele, John E. Tobie, George J. Hill, Peter G. Contacos, and Charles B. Evans, Alterations in serum proteins and 19S antibody production during the course of induced malarial infections in man, *Amer J Trop Med Hyg.* 14 (1965): 191-7; Tobie, Abele, Hill, Contacos, and Evans, Fluorescent antibody studies on the immune response in sporozoite-induced vivax malaria and the relationship of antibody production to parasitemia, *Amer J Trop Med Hyg.* 15 (1966): 676-83; Hill, Vernon Knight, G. R. Coatney and Donald K. Lawless, Vivax malaria complicated by aphasia and hemiparesis, *A.M.A. Arch Intern Med.* 112 (1963): 863-8; Hill, Knight, and G. M. Jeffrey, Thrombocytopenia in vivax malaria, *Lancet* 1 (1964): 240-1; Hill, William T. Butler, Paul T. Wertlake and John P. Utz, The renal histopathology of amphotericin B toxicity in man and the dog: A study of biopsy and post-mortem specimens, *Clin Res.* 10 (1962: 249. (Abstract). Also: Hill, Butler, Charles F. Szwed, and Utz, Comparison of renal toxicity of two preparations of amphotericin B, *Amer Rev Resp Dis.* 88 (1963: 342-346; and Hill, Butler, Szwed, and Sarah U. Moore, Lethal toxicity and dose-related azotemia due to amphotericin B in dogs, *Proc Soc Exper Biol and Med.* 114 (1963): 76-9.

[233] One of many articles on the subject of the 10 plagues mentioned in Exodus is: N. Joel Ehrenkranz and Deborah A. Sampson, Origin of the Old Testament plagues: Explications and implications, *Yale Journal of Biology and Medicine* 81 (no. 1, March 2008): 31-42. The authors reviewed previous articles on this subject and they conclude that several of the plagues may have been caused by parasitic, bacterial, or viral diseases.

The story in I Samuel 5-6 is analyzed by Frank R. Freemon, Bubonic plague in the Book of Samuel" *J. Royal Soc. Med.* 98 (no. 9, September 2005): 436. Freemon concludes that the illness which affected the Israelites and Philistines may not have been plague, but that the disease which was described by a later writer in I Samuel, is convincingly that of plague.

[234] Virgil, *The Aeneid.* trans. Robert Fitzgerald (New York: Random House, 1983), Book III, lines 123-8. Virgil wrote in Latin, *plaga* which transliterates into English as "plague."

B. Endemic – Epidemic - Pandemic

[235] The bland definitions of endemic, epidemic, and pandemic are shown in https://www.merriam-webster.com/dictionary/ (accessed July 14, 2020).

[236] In 2009, the annual H1N1 influenza was called a pandemic by the U.S. Centers of Disease Control (CDC); this pandemic was considered to have ended in August 2010, but yearly episodes of influenza continue to persist: CDC, The 2009 H1N1 pandemic: A new flu virus emerges: "The (H1N1)pdm09 virus was very different from H1N1 viruses that were circulating at the time of the pandemic. On August 10, 2010, WHO declared an end to the global 2009 H1N1 influenza pandemic. However, (H1N1)pdm09 virus continues to circulate as a seasonal flu virus, and cause illness, hospitalization, and deaths worldwide every year." See: https://www.cdc.gov/flu/pandemic-resources/2009-h1n1-pandemic.html (accessed July 15, 2020).

[237] *Britannica*: pandemic; plague; influenza pandemic of 1918-19. CDC (previous reference); the virus of the H1N1 2009-10 pandemic was technically known as (H1N1)pdm09. *Yersinia pestis* is the plague bacillus. It resides in the rat, and it is transmitted to humans by the Oriental rat flea.

Estimates of the numbers of cases and deaths from the Great Influenza of 1918-1919 vary widely. The CDC currently estimates that there were 500,000,000 cases world-wide, one third of the world's population. CDC estimates that there were 50,000,000 deaths, 675,000 in the United States. See: https://www.cdc.gov/flu/pandemic-resources/1918-pandemic-h1n1.html (accessed April 4, 2021). *Britannica* estimates that the pandemic of 1918-19, the "Spanish flu," caused 25,000,000 deaths world-wide, and that it was caused by influenza A subtype H1N1.

William Bynum discusses plague (*History of Medicine*, 69-72), saying that "the Black Death was *a* plague," because that word had then and still does have a general use. He argues that the Black Death and subsequent European plagues were probably diseases caused by the same organism. It is now known as the plague bacillus, *Yersinia pestis*.

"Plague" is a metaphor for sickness on a massive scale in history, not specifically the diseases caused by *Yersinia pestis*. Much has been written about this phenomenon during the COVID-19 pandemic that began in December 2019, and continues into the year 2021. The wave of illness in Algiers which was described in fiction by Albert Camus in *La Peste* (1947), translated into English as *The Plague*, was actually cholera. The "plagues" of Athens in 430 BC and in Venice in 1630 are mentioned by James P. Lenfestey, "Pandemics Past," *New York Times Book Reviews*, 14 June 2020, Letters, 6.

Twenty pandemics, with years and mortalities are shown in a chart, "History of Pandemics," *The Pharos* (Summer 2020), 2. *Pharos* says it was taken from https://www.visualcapitalist.com/history-of-pandemics-deadliest/ (accessed January 5, 2020). The Antonine Plague is not mentioned in *Britannica* as a specific topic, or in the entry on Galen. From S. Sabbatani and S. Fiorino, The Antonine Plague and the decline of the Roman Empire, *Infez Med*. 17 (no 4. December 17, 2009): 261-75, at https://pubmed.ncbi.nlm.nih.gov/20046111/ (accessed January 5, 2021).

The variation in the public's response to COVID-19 is similar to ancient plagues, according to Marc Fisher, Plagues and extremism part of ancient pattern, *Washington Post*, 16 February 2021, A1, A6.

C. Biology and Biochemistry – The Chemistry of Life

[238] *Britannica*: life; parasitism (biology); parasitology (biology); eukaryote; prokaryote; organic compound; photosynthesis; respiration; biology. A parasite is usually a eukaryote; a saprophyte can be either a eukaryote or a prokaryote. http://www.differencebetween.net/ science/difference-between-parasite-and-saprophyte (accessed June 27, 2020). "Metazoa" paraphrased from Peter Godfrey-Smith, *Metazoa: Animal Life and the Birth of the Mind* (New York: Farrar, Straus & Giroux, 2020), reviewed by Aimee Nezhukumatathil, Deep dive, *New York Times Book Review*, 27 December 2020, 8.

Emmanuel Liscum, et al., Phototropism: Growing towards an understanding of plant movement, *Plant Cell* 26 (no. 1, January 2014): 38–55. Published online 2014 Jan 30. doi: 10.1105/tpc.113.119727. This discussion of phototropism in birds and humans is based on my own concept of the term. I have not seen it previously described as phototropism.

[239] Hans Zinsser wrote that "infectious disease is one of the great tragedies of living things – the struggle for existence between different forms of life ... Incessantly, the pitiless war goes on ... of species against species [and] in the imperfect development of cohabitation on a crowded planet, the habit of eating one another – dead and alive – has become a general custom." (Zinsser, *Rats, Lice and History*, 4-5).

Britannica, symbiosis; prion.

[240] Body Composition, from Oxford University Press: https://www.encyclopedia.com/medicine/encyclopedias-almanacs-transcripts-and-maps/composition-body (accessed June 28, 2020). National Human Genome Research Institute, online: https://www.genome.gov/about-genomics/fact-sheets/Deoxyribonucleic-Acid-Fact-Sheet (accessed June 28, 2020). DNA is usually a right-handed double helix. Essential amino acids, from Webster's Dictionary, https://www.merriam-webster.com/dictionary/ essential amino acid (accessed June 28, 2020). Four small molecules have been proposed as the basis for life itself: water, methane, ammonia, and hydrogen. They are composed of atoms of hydrogen, carbon, oxygen and nitrogen, and they are assembled into amino acids. The Book of Genesis describes the origin of life as Religion would have it. But in a chemistry laboratory, without a Guiding Hand, these

molecules were combined to produce amino acids with an electrical spark. See Britannica, Oparin, Aleksandr; and Urey, Harold C. The possible origin of life which was proposed by J.B.S. Haldane and Aleksandr Oparin was confirmed by Harold Urey and Stanley Miller in 1953. Not mentioned by *Britannica*, the Urey-Miller experiment is described in detail in "Hypotheses about the origins of life: The Oparin-Haldane hypothesis, Miller-Urey experiment, and RNA world," Khan Academy, AP.BIO:SYI-3 (EU), SYI-3.E (LO), SYI-3.E.1 (EK), SYI-3.E.2 (EK), at: https://www.khanacademy.org/science/ap-biology/natural-selection/origins-of-life-on-earth/a/hypotheses-about-the-origins-of-life#:~:text (accessed April 6, 2021).

[241] One of the problems faced by vegans is the lack of Vitamin B-12, which causes folic acid deficiency, producing anemia and a slow, insidious neurological disease.

D. Parasitology and Microbiology

[242] Parasitology from NCBI (National Center for Biotechnology Information): https://www.ncbi.nlm.nih.gov/books/NBK8262/ (accessed June 28, 2020).
Britannica, Microbiology, includes Protozoa and Amoebas in the field of Microbiology. This classification also includes parasites such as *Entamoeba*, *Balantidium*, and *Giardia*.

[243] An American rock group created a seven-track record: Brian's Escape, *The Journey: An Account of S. A. Andrée's Arctic Expedition of 1897* (2010).

[244] *Britannica*, parasitism.

[245] One of the Flexner brothers, who co-authored the Flexner Report that changed American medical education, fell onto his face at his home in New York City in 1958. He bled into his face, and then treated himself with leeches.

[246] Hans Zinsser, *Rats, Lice, and History* (1935. New York: Pocket Books, 1945).

[247] Fleas, from University of Kentucky: https://entomology.ca.uky.edu/ef602 (accessed June 29, 2020).

[248] *Britannica*, tick; tropism.

[249] Timothy C. Winegard, *The Mosquito: A Human History of Our Deadliest Predator* (New York: Dutton/Penguin Random House LLC, 2019); Rachel Carson, *Silent Spring* (New York: Houghton Mifflin, 1962).

[250] "Maggot" from WebMD: https://www.webmd.com/skin-problems-and-treatments/qa/how-is-maggot-therapy-used-to-treat-gangrene (accessed June 29, 2020). Liya Davydov, Maggot therapy in wound management in modern era and a review of published literature. *J Pharm Prac.* 24 (no. 1, February 2011): 89-93.

E. Microbiology

[251] *Britannica*, microbiology = includes Protozoa and Amoebas in the field of Microbiology. This classification includes *Entamoeba*, *Balantidium*, and *Giardia*, which are discussed above as parasites.

[252] *Britannica*, microbiology: Types of microorganisms. OpenStax, *Biology 2e*: Prokaryotes from: https://opentextbc.ca/biology2eopenstax (accessed December 23, 2020).

[253] Bacteria, from *Encyclopædia Britannica Deluxe Edition* (Chicago: Encyclopædia Britannica, 2013)

[254] Merck Manual – Overview of Gram-Negative Bacteria, at https://www.merckmanuals.com/home/infections/bacterial-infections-gram-negative-bacteria/overview-of-gram-negative-bacteria (accessed June 30, 2020). Emily E. Putnam and Andrew L. Goodman, B vitamin acquisition by gut commensal bacteria, *PLoS Pathog* 16 (no. 1, January 2020): e1008208. Regrettably, the proven importance of gut commensal bacteria was not mentioned by Markham Heid, Can we learn to love germs again? *New York Times*, 25 April 2021, Sunday Review 1, 4-5. In this long article, Heid failed to provide any example of benefit from germs. He said, without any documentation, that "The pandemic has left us with a collective germophobia. We're going to have to get over it – for our health." Nevertheless, I can cite one organism: the present view of many food scientists and gastroenterologists is that *Lactobacillus* species are useful in preserving and restoring the normal ecology of the human intestinal tract. Eat yogurt, which contains living *Lactobacillus*. Also see: Stat Reports, *Good bacteria: The microbiome, its vast therapeutic potential, and the challenges ahead*: "In the late 1950s a radical idea was born: What if a patients' gastrointestinal inflammation could be cured by implanting a healthier gut? The result, now known as a fecal microbiota transplant, is the foundation, 60 years later, of the microbiome industry. This report examines the science behind this nascent industry, fleshing out what we know about the ecology of the human microbiome and the various interventions scientists are studying to help keep or make it healthy." From https://reports.statnews.com/ (accessed April 28, 2021). The normal ecology of the gut varies from one part of the world. People who live in Mexico presumably have accommodated to their usual gut flora. However, Americans who go to Mexico are warned to avoid leafy vegetables to protect against "Montezuma's Revenge." The leaves are presumably contaminated by farm workers' feces. Travelers from the U.S. to Asia are encouraged to take a prescribed bottle of antibiotics in case they develop traveler's diarrhea. It may not be the result of fecal contamination in these different countries; the normal gut flora may be different in different parts of the world.

Another book on this subject is Martin J. Blaser, *Missing Microbes: How the Overuse of Antibiotics is Fueling Our Modern Plagues* (London: Picador, 2015). He asks "Why does administration cause livestock (and possible people) to grow larger and fatter." Elaine Thomas, Book Review, wrote that "Blaser's conclusions sometimes run ahead of the data" *Pharos* 84 (no. 2, Spring 2021): 43.

[255] See also David Quammen, How viruses shape our world, *National Geographic* 239 (no. 2, February 2021): 41-67, with illustrations by Craig Cutler. "They kill us by the millions. But without them, life is impossible." The cover shows *Mimivirus*, one of the largest known viruses. The Contents page is confusing, because it erroneously says it is "February 2020."

[256] *Britannica*, virus: The infectious part of any virus is its nucleic acid, either DNA or RNA but never both. In many viruses, but not all, the nucleic acid alone, stripped of its capsid, can infect (transfect) cells, although considerably less efficiently than can the intact virions.

The classification of viruses continues to evolve, especially in respect to DNA viruses and reverse transcribing viruses. See, for example: Saliha Durmus and Kutlu O. Ulgen, Comparative interactomics for virus-human protein-protein interactions: DNA viruses versus RNA viruses, *FEBS Open Bio* 7 (no. 1, Jan 2017): 96-107. Published online Jan 4. doi: 10.1002/2211-5463.12167 (accessed July 6, 2020).

Arboviruses: www.cdc.gov>nndss>conditions>case-definition (Arboviral Diseases, Neuroinvasive and Non-neuroinvasive) (accessed July 10, 2020). Arboviruses discussed in this essay are Yellow fever, Dengue, and West Nile virus. See the cdd.gov website for Rift Valley Fever, Japanese encephalitis, Tick-borne encephalitis, and Eastern Equine Encephalitis.

[257] Ronald B. Johnson, "Viral Diseases," in *Weedon's Skin Pathology Essentials*, 2d ed. (2017) at https://www.sciencedirect.com/topics/neuroscience/dna-viruses, classifies RNA viruses as: paramyxovirus (measles, mumps), picornavirus (Coxsackie), rhabdovirus (rabies), retrovirus (HIV), and togavirus (rubella).

[258] *Britannica*, rabies; vaccine; Pasteur. Also, Berton Rouché, *The Incurable Wound* (Boston, Little Brown, 1958).

The World Health Organization (WHO) states: "The combination of local treatment of the wound, passive immunization with rabies immunoglobulins and vaccination is recommended for all severe (category III) exposures to rabies. https://www.who.int/rabies/resources/other_rabies_biolog_product/en/ (accessed January 12, 2021). The terms "anaphylaxis and serum sickness" are allergic reactions to products that are "heterologous," meaning from a different species. For a discussion of Pasteur's work, see: Gerald Geison, *The Private Science of Louis Pasteur* (Princeton, N.J.: Princeton University Press, 1995).

[259] *Britannica*, measles; smallpox. See: Alfred W. Crosby, Jr., *The Columbian Exchange: Biological and Cultural Consequences of 1492* (1973. Westport, Conn.: Praeger Publishers, 2003). The Persian physician ar-Razi, known in Europe as Rhazes, in 900 AD "clearly described the symptoms of smallpox and distinguished it from measles"

[260] *Britannica*, dengue.

[261] *Britannica*, yellow fever. For the disease in Liberia, see George J. Hill, Intimate relationships: Secret affairs of church and state in the United States and Liberia, 1925-1945, *Diplomatic History* 31 (no. 3, June 2007): 465-503.

[262] *Britannica*, West Nile virus. It is especially dangerous for people over age 50. *Britannica* does not mention Zika, another Flavivirus, which is similar to dengue and West Nile virus infections. It is transmitted by *Aedes* mosquitos. See: https://www.cdc.gov/zika/index.html (accessed July 6, 2020).

[263] *Britannica*, picornaviruses. The term is derived from "pico" (small) and "rna" (RNA). There are four main types: enteroviruses, rhinoviruses (causing more than 100 varieties of the common cold), echoviruses (from enteric, cytopathogenic, human, orphan), and Coxsackie virus.

Britannica, polio; polio vaccine. The risks and rewards of Oral Polio Vaccine (OPV) are shown in two events which, coincidentally, were reported on the same day. The rewards were emphasized and the risks were minimized in Ruth Maclean, Africa cheers as wild polio is eradicated, *New York Times*, 25 August 2020, A9; and Anon., *Washington Post*, 25 August 2020, B6, for the obituary of John H. Hagar, who contracted polio from the oral dose of vaccine that was administered to his son in 1973, and he remained partially paralyzed until his death from post-polio syndrome in 1997.

[264] *Britannica*, influenza.

[265] *Britannica*, coronavirus: "Club-shaped glycoprotein spikes in the envelope give the viruses a crownlike, or coronal, appearance." MERS, from https://www.cdc.gov/coronavirus/mers/index.html (accessed July 4, 2020): "Middle Ease Respirator Syndrome (MERS) is viral respiratory illness that is new to humans. ... Many have died." "Coronaviruses are enveloped RNA viruses that cause respiratory illnesses of varying severity from the common cold to fatal pneumonia." https://www.merckmanuals.com/professional/infectious-diseases/respiratory-viruses (accessed January 12, 2021). Many common colds, however, are due to adenoviruses, which are DNA viruses (see below).

[266] *Britannica*, hepatitis. The nucleic acid structure of hepatitis viruses is given by Arie J. Zuckerman in "Hepatitis Viruses" (Chapter 70), in Samuel Baron (ed.), *Medical Microbiology* 4th ed. (Galveston, Tex.: University of Texas Medical Branch, 1996), on-line at https://www.ncbi.nlm.nih.gov/books/NBK7864/ (accessed July 5, 2020).

Britannica, cancer: "Three DNA viruses—human papillomaviruses, the Epstein-Barr virus, and the hepatitis B virus—are linked to tumours in humans." Richard J. Whitley adds Kaposi's sarcoma virus (also known as human herpesvirus 8, a DNA virus; see "Herpesvirus," Chapter 68, in Baron, *Medical Microbiology* (op. cit.).

[267] *Britannica*, Ebola: "Ebola is closely related to the Marburg virus, which was discovered in 1967, and the two are the only members of the Filoviridae that cause epidemic human disease."

[268] Ronald B. Johnson, "Viral Diseases" (op. cit., supra), provides a simple classification of DNA viruses as follows: "HAPPy": H = herpes virus (HSV, VZV, CMV, EBV); H = hepadnavirus (hepatitis B); A = adenovirus; P = papovavirus (HPV); P = poxvirus (molluscum, smallpox, Orf, milker's nodule); P = parvovirus B19 (only single-stranded DNA virus): think "slap cheeks with one DNA" (single-stranded).

[269] *Britannica*, smallpox. It was known for several centuries that immunity to smallpox could be achieved with small amounts of smallpox scabs administered to naïve patients, although there was some risk to the treatment, which was called "inoculation." Amy Lynn Filsinger and Raymond Dwek, George Washington and the first mass military inoculation, *Science Reference Services* https://www.loc.gov/rr/scitech/GW&smallpoxinoculation.html (accessed February 2, 2021); Elizabeth Fenn, *Pox Americana: The Great Smallpox Epidemic of 1775-82* (New York: Hill and Wang, 2001); and https://www.history.com/news/smallpox-george-washington-revolutionary-war (accessed February 24, 2021).

[270] Richard J. Whitley, "Herpesviruses," Chapter 68, in Baron, *Medical Microbiology* (op. cit.). Of more than 100 known herpesviruses, 8 are known to infect humans: herpes simplex types 1 and 2; varicella-zoster; cytomegalovirus, Epstein-Barr virus, human herpesvirus 6 and 7; and Kaposi's sarcoma virus (human herpes 8).

Britannica, herpesvirus; Burkitt's lymphoma. Also, Bernard Glemser, *Mr. Burkitt and Africa*.

[271] *Britannia*, Chicken pox. Not stated is that varicella-zoster is a DNA virus (see Whitley, op. cit.), or that zoster vaccine is recommended for adults who have had chickenpox, to prevent late development of shingles.

[272] *Britannica*, adenovirus; and *Merck Manual*: https://www.merckmanuals.com/professional/infectious-diseases/respiratory-viruses/adenovirus-infections (accessed January 12, 2021).

Diseases caused by adenoviruses and coronaviruses may appear to be similar, although adenoviruses are DNA viruses and coronaviruses are RNA viruses. Few studies have been published that compare the two groups of diseases in patients. One of the first compared children who had an adenovirus with those who had COVID-19. Surprisingly, in this small study, the disease was more severe in the patients with adenovirus. See: Kuanrong Li, Ling Li, Xianfeng Wang, et al, Comparative analysis of clinical features of SARS-CoV-2 and adenovirus infection among children, *Virology Journal* 17: 193 (10 December 2020). https://doi.org/10.1186/s12985-020-01461-4. "COVID-19 is an overall less symptomatic and less severe infection at admission compared to HAdV respiratory infection in pediatric population."

[273] *Britannica*, bacteriophage. Phages were discovered in the second decade of the twentieth century and were soon used in failed attempts to control cholera and plague.

[274] Four retroviral infections of humans are listed here. A discussion of the nature of DNA and RNA retroviruses is unnecessary in this essay; for this, see J. M. Coffin, S. H. Hughes, and H. E. Varmus (eds.), *Retroviruses* (Cold Spring Harbor, N.Y.: Cold Spring Harbor Laboratory Press, 1997).

[275] Zuckerman, "Hepatitis Viruses," in Baron, *Medical Microbiology*. Baruch Blumberg "won the Nobel Prize in Medicine for his discovery of the hepatitis B virus. He and his colleagues discovered the virus in 1967, developed the blood test that is used to detect the virus, and invented the first hepatitis B vaccine in 1969." From: https://www.hepb.org/about-us/baruch-blumberg-md-dphil/ (accessed July 5, 2020).

Joan C. M. Macnab and David Onions, "Tumor Viruses," Chapter 47, in Baron, *Medical Microbiology*.

[276] *Britannica*, AIDS. Coffin, et al, *Retroviruses*.

[277] *Britannia*, cancer.

[278] *Britannica*, human papillomavirus (HPV).

F. COVID-19

[279] John Robert McNeill, *Mosquito Empires: Ecology and War in the Greater Caribbean, 1640–1914* (New York: Cambridge University Press, 2010), shows how mosquito-borne diseases like yellow fever and malaria were important in the history of the empires of Spain, Portugal, and Britain in the American continents. He is the son of William McNeill, author of *Plagues and Peoples*, which was cited above.

The "perfect storm" is a metaphor. It was used by Sebastian Junger in his book, *The Perfect Storm: A True Story of Men Against the Sea* (New York: W. W. Norton, 1997), and in a semi-fictionalized movie with the same name (2000), telling of the wreck of a fishing boat, *Andrea Gail*, in a storm in 1991. A pandemic that preceded the Great Influenza of 1918 has largely been forgotten. Jeffrey H. Toney and Stephanie Ishack, A pandemic of confusion, *American Scientist* 108 (Nov-Dec 2020): 344-5, adds that "Confusing, inconsistent public health messages about pandemics are nothing new."

[280] Rochelle P. Walensky and Carlos de Rio, From mitigation to containment of the COVID-19 pandemic: Putting the SARS-CoV-2 genie back in the bottle, *JAMA* 323 (no. 19, May 19, 2020): 1889-90; and Jeffrey F. Addicott, COVID-19 pandemic: policy and legal Issues, *Officer Review, The Military Order of the World Wars* (March-April 2020), 7-9.

In the first two months after patients with COVID-19 were diagnosed in Wuhan, China, the disease spread quickly around the world. The impact of the disease varied greatly. On February 26, the Centers for Disease Control (CDC) reported only 61 cases in the U.S.: https://emergency.cdc.gov/han/2020/han00428.asp (accessed January 9, 2021). This soon changed, "During a 3-week period in late February to early March, the number of U.S. COVID-19 cases increased more than 1,000-fold": https://www.cdc.gov/mmwr/volumes/69/wr/mm6918e2.htm (accessed January 9, 2021). On March 11, 2020, the World Health Organization (WHO) "declared that the COVID-19 outbreak is a pandemic": https://www.alnap.org/help-library/gender-alert-for-covid-19-outbreak-march-2020 (accessed January 9, 2021).

By May 2020, a cost of $500 billion and $30 billion in Medicare and Medicaid expenses due to COVID appeared to be possible, and because of the decrease expected in GDP, "health care would comprise 20% of GDP next year." See Sherry Glied and Helen Levy, The potential effects of coronavirus on national health expenditures, *JAMA* 323 (no. 20, May 26, 2020): 2001-2. The current status of COVID-19 in that month was summarized by Saad B. Omer, Preeti Malani, and Carlos del Rio, The COVID-19 pandemic in the U.S.: A clinical update, *JAMA* 323 (no. 18, May 12, 2020): 1767-8. "The estimated timeline for availability of an initial vaccine is between early and mid-2021."

Poignant comments about COVID patients' deaths and the impact on survivors soon became commonplace in newspapers and magazines. Four examples: Elliot Rosenberg, A case of polio-covid double jeopardy, *Washington Post*, 23 May 2020, A17. Somini Sengupta, Disasters with twice the misery: When global warming collides with a pandemic, *Washington Post* (May 24, 2020), A19. David von Drehle, How to honor our new memories, *Washington Post*, 24 May 2020, A25. Whitney Ellenby, The coronavirus forced me to explain death to my autistic son, *Washington Post*, 26 May 2020, A19. The pandemic caused others to reflect on eschatology and the meaning of life. Roger Cohen, No return to the "Old Dispensation," *Washington Post*, 13 May 2020, A26.

Six months into the pandemic, *JAMA* summarized the problem for patients: Anon., What is COVID-19? *JAMA* 324 (no. 8, August 25, 2020): 816.

Many unintended consequences of COVID-19 have been reported. Two examples are: Jay A. Pandit, Memento mori, *JAMA* 324 (no. 17, November 3, 2020): 1731-2; and Frances Stead Sellers, "Science in real time": From funding to publishing, crisis rewrites the rules, *Washington Post*, 25 October 2020, A23.

[281] Books about COVID-19 began to appear by the end of 2020. Lawrence Wright, *The Plague Year: America in the Time of Covid* (New York: Penguin/Random House, 2021), discussed by Carlos Lozada, Missed opportunities to contain a plague, *Washington Post*, 6 June 2021, B1. See Appendix D for additional comments and references.

Part Two   Health Matters in Human History   Chapter 10

[282] *Health Matters* is a typical example of a person who is looking back at the end of life. This essay is located somewhere between Bill Bryson's entertaining book, *A Short History of Nearly Everything* (New York: Broadway Books, 2003) and what Albert Einstein was working on to develop a Unified Field Theory at the Institute for Advanced Studies in Princeton, N.J. The new world of robots is exemplified by robotic pets. See: Amanda Garrity, These realistic robotic pets that help seniors with dementia have rave reviews on Amazon, *Good Housekeeping* (July 14, 2019). https://www.goodhousekeeping.com/life/pets/a28353484/hasbro-joy-for-all-robotic-pets-for-seniors/ (accessed September 30, 2020).

[283] Summarizing all of these sources, it is fair to say that the Neanderthals (also known as Neandertals, *Homo neanderthalensis* or *Homo sapiens neanderthalensis*) may have originated as early as 430,000 years BCE. They were surely present 130,000 BCE and they became extinct in about 40,000 BCE.

Steve Brusatte, Human Remains: Two new books offer a glimpse into the ruthless, cutthroat world of paleoanthropology, *New York Times Book Review*, 10 January 2010, 10: Review of Kermit Pattison, *Fossil Men: The Quest for the Oldest Skeleton and the Origins of Humankind* (New York: William Morrow, 2020), telling of Tim White and the discovery of *Ardipithecus*; and Meave Leakey with Samira Leakey, *The Sediments of Time: My Lifelong Search for the Past* (Boston: Houghton Mifflin Harcourt, 2020).

History/com (updated October 21, 2019), and slightly edited: "The prehistoric ages: How humans lived before written records: Paleolithic (Old Stone Age), Mesolithic (Middle Stone Age), and Neolithic (New Stone Age), an era marked by the use of tools by early human ancestors (who evolved around 300,000 BCE), and the transformation from a culture of hunting and gathering to farming and food production."

"Australopithecus has a smaller brain size, heavier jaws and larger teeth; compared to Homo." https://www.excellup.com/InterBiology/eleven_history/archaic-humans.aspx (accessed September 13, 2020).

Laura M. MacLatchy, William J. Sanders, and Craig L. Wuthrich, Hominoid origins, *Nature Education Knowledge* 6 (no. 7, 2015): 4. "Although paleoanthropologists are unable to determine the phylogenetic placement of "dental apes" or *Kamoyapithecus* with confidence, there is broad support for the hypothesis that *Proconsul, Afropithecus* and *Morotopithecus* are stem hominoids."
https://www.nature.com/scitable/knowledge/library/hominoid-origins (accessed September 13, 2020).

On https://www.bgs.ac.uk/discoveringGeology/time/timeline/croMagnon.html (accessed September 13, 2020), the British Geological Survey reported that "It is not clear when our species, *Homo sapiens sapiens*, first evolved, but it may have been in Africa about 120 000 or 130 000 years ago." However, anatomically modern humans appear in the fossil record of Africa at least 300,000 years ago, and they co-existed with several other species of our genus for a considerable period of time. Professor Donald Esker called attention to this, citing Jean-Jacques Hublin, et al., "New fossils from Jebel Irhoud Morocco and the pan-African origin of *Homo sapiens*, *Nature* 546 (no. 7657, 7 June 2017): 289-92.

History.com: "The Neolithic Revolution, also called the Agricultural Revolution, marked the transition in human history from small, nomadic bands of hunter-gatherers to larger, agricultural settlements and early civilization. The Neolithic Revolution started around 10,000 B.C. in the Fertile Crescent." Note: History.com refers to hunter-gatherers, agriculturalists, and early settlements as "human history." https://www.history.com/topics/pre-history/neolithic-revolution (accessed September 13, 2020).

Britannica, Hominidae.

[284] The traditional history of law, or of legal systems, usually begins with written laws, such as the Code of Hammurabi. For the tradition history of legal systems and the law, see *Britannica*: legal profession.

[285] *Britannica*, history; science, history of; medicine, history of. These entries in *Britannica* fail to recognize medicine at the beginning of human history. Excerpts from the entries follow, with emphasis added in bold type.
History: "the discipline that studies the chronological record of events (as affecting a nation or people), based on a critical examination of source materials and usually presenting an explanation of their causes."
Science, history of: "Kepler's laws, Newton's absolute space, and Einstein's rejection of the probabilistic nature of quantum mechanics were all based on theological, not scientific, assumptions."
Medicine, history of: "the development of the prevention and treatment of disease from prehistoric and ancient times to the 20th century. ... Magic and religion played a large part in the medicine of prehistoric or early human society." The importance of medicine in both "unwritten history" and in "recorded history" is shown in the entry for "Medicine, history of," in *Britannica*, although "medicine" does not appear at all in the subjects of "History" or "Science, history of."

[286] The Edison effect is "the phenomenon of the flow of electric current when an electrode sealed inside the bulb of an incandescent lamp is connected to the positive terminal of the lamp." https://www.dictionary.com/browse/edison-effect (accessed September 15, 2020).

University of California-Berkeley professor of molecular and cell biology and of chemistry Jennifer Doudna was awarded the 2020 Wolf Prize in Medicine for her discovery of the CRISPR-Cas9 gene-editing tool. https://www.dailycal.org/2020/01/23/uc-berkeley-professor-jennifer-doudna-wins-2020-wolf-prize-in-medicine (accessed September 15, 2020).

A. Human History from the Perspective of Health

[287] My principal sources for the history of medicine and science were given previously. Restated briefly, they are:
For medicine, Roy Porter, *The Greatest Benefit to Mankind*; supplemented by William Bynum, *The History of Medicine*; and Ralph H. Major, *A History of Medicine* (Springfield, Ill.: Charles C Thomas, 1954).
For science, David C. Lindberg, *The Beginnings of Western Science*, supplemented by William Bynum, *A Little History of Science* (New Haven: Yale University Press, 2012). I am also mindful of the warnings in James W. Loewen, *Lies My Teacher Told Me: Everything Your American History Textbook Got Wrong* (New York: Simon & Schuster, [1995], 2007).
For other aspects of history, *Britannica*; Werner Keller (trans. William Neil), *The Bible as History: A Confirmation of the Book of Books* (New York: William Morrow and Company, 1956); and Tim Severin, *The Ulysses Voyage: Sea Search for the Odyssey* (London: Arrow Books, [1987] 1988).

[288] Bill Bryson cogently observed that "We are the only creature that can harm at a distance," in Bryson, *A Short History of Almost Everything* (New York: Broadway Books, 2003), 447.

[289] Quotations from Porter, *Greatest Benefit*, Introduction, 5-13. Italics in original.

[290] Lynn Payer (1945-2001), *Medicine and Culture: Notions of Health and Sickness in Britain, the U.S., France and West Germany* (New York: Macmillan, 1989) says that for a group of symptoms and signs know in America as "the flu," would be treated with decongestants. In England, a similar mild illness would be "constipation," and treated with laxatives. In France, it would be "liver" and in Germany, it would be "the heart." In each of those countries

the treatment would be based on the assumptions shared by patients and physicians. See: Laura Newman, Lynn Payer, *BMJ* 323 (no. 7317, October 13, 2001): 871, and https://www.ncbi.nlm.nih.gov/pmc/articles/PMC1121410/ (accessed January 24, 2021).

B. Developments in Human Health – Topical Viewpoint

[291] The exact mechanism by which digitalis produces beneficial effects on the heart is still incompletely known, but it is likely that it acts, at least in part, through stimulation of the vagus nerve. See Brian F. Hoffman and Donald H. Singer, Effects of digitalis on electrical activity of cardiac fibers, *Progress in Cardiovascular Diseases* 7 (no. 3, November 1964): 226-60. Eugene Braunwald, Effects of digitalis on the normal and the failing heart, *J. Am. Coll. Cardiol.* 5 (May, Suppl A, 1985): 51A-59A.

[292] *Britannica*: nightshade, belladonna, atropine. For scopolamine (hyoscine; burandanga), see "Devil's Breath: Urban Legend or the World's Most Scary Drug," at https://www.drugs.com/illicit/devils-breath.html (accessed October 26, 2020). The manufacture and use of sarin are discussed by Joby Warrick, The Syrian chemical arms master who was a CIA mole, *Washington Post*, 21 February 2021, A1, A6-7. Warrick was the author of *Red Line: The Unraveling of Syria and America's Race to Destroy the Most Dangerous Arsenal in the World* (New York: Doubleday, 2020).

[293] *Britannica*: aspirin, willow. For Bayer, see https://www.bayer.com/en/history/1881-1914 (accessed October 26, 2020). For Reye's syndrome, see: https://www.mayoclinic.org/diseases-conditions/reyes-syndrome/ (accessed October 26, 2020).

[294] Cherry laurel: https://homeguides.sfgate.com/poisonous-cherry-laurel-tree-67400.html (accessed October 24, 2020); and See: https://www.herbal-supplement-resource.com/bay-laurel-benefits (accessed October 26, 2020).

[295] The use of mercury in medicine began with Paracelsus in the 15th century, according to J. G. O'Shea, Two minutes with venus, two years with mercury' – mercury as an antisyphilitic chemotherapeutic agent, *Journal of the Royal Society of Medicine* 83 (June 1990): 392-5. However, Ralph Major (*A History of Medicine*, p. 77) says that many minerals, including mercury, were used by physicians in India long before Paracelsus. Robin A. Bernhoft, Mercury toxicity and treatment: A review of the literature, *J. Environ. Public Health*, 2012. For the long sad story of mercury use and poisoning in humans. See: https://www.ncbi.nlm.nih.gov/pmc/articles/PMC3253456/ (accessed October 31, 2020).

[296] Theodore Gray, For that healthy glow, drink radiation! *Popular Science* (August 18, 2004), at https://www.popsci.com/scitech/article/2004-08/healthy-glow-drink-radiation/ (accessed October 31, 2020); and Kate Moore, *The Radium Girls: The Dark Story of America's Shining Women* (Naperville, Ill.: Sourcebooks, 2017).

[297] *Chang* is a mildly alcoholic beverage, similar to beer, that is made in Nepal from fermented barley. *Chang* can be distilled into *rashki*, a delicious beverage with a higher concentration of alcohol.

[298] Gabriel G. Nahas, Hashish in Islam, 9th to 18th century, *Bull. N.Y. Acad. Med.* 58 (no. 9, Dec. 1982): 814-31. From https://europepmc.org/backend/ptpmcrender.fcgi?accid=PMC1805385&blobtype=pdf (accessed October 20, 2020). Danielle F. Haley and Richard Saitz, The opioid epidemic during the COVID-19 pandemic, *JAMA* 324 (no. 16, 27 October 2020), 1615-17.

Nitrous oxide has now become one of the leading causes of addiction. It is said to be the "10th most popular drug in the world." When NO2 is released into large plastic bags it causes death by asphyxiation. See: Ezra Marcus, "Nitrous Nation," *New York Times*, 31 January 2021, Styles, p.1,8.

"Ayahuasca — also known as the tea, the vine, and *la purga* — is a brew made from the leaves of the *Psychotria viridis* shrub along with the stalks of the *Banisteriopsis caapi* vine, though other plants and ingredients can be added as well." From: https://www.healthline.com/nutrition/ayahuasca (accessed February 6, 2021).

[299] The scope of illegal or improper use of narcotics is estimated in the Medical Encyclopedia of the National Library of Medicine. In 2018, narcotic pain relievers were used by about 11.4 million people without prescriptions during the past year, and about 808,000 people used heroin. See: https://medlineplus.gov/ency/article/000949.htm (accessed October 30, 2020). The American Cancer Society was one of the first organizations to be enticed by agents of Purdue Pharma into sponsoring the use of Oxycontin for cancer pain. Tom Hals and Mike Spector, Where the Purdue Pharm-Sackler legal saga stands, *Reuters.com* (January 29, 2020), https://www.reuters.com/article/us-purdue-pharma-bankruptcy-factbox/where-the-purdue-pharma-sackler-legal-saga-stands-idUSKBN1ZS1H3 (accessed October 30, 2020). *The Man with the Golden Arm* was a film noir which starred Frank Sinatra, Kim Novak, and several other famous actors. It was directed by Otto Preminger. The drug was not identified, but was presumably heroin or morphine.

[300] *The Lost Weekend* starred Ray Milland and Jane Wyman; it was directed by Billy Wilder.

[301] *Britannica*, malaria; quinine. Several species of *Cinchona* produce quinine. Also, Liwang Cui, Sungano Mharakurwa, et al, Antimalarial drug resistance: Literature review and activities and findings of the ICEMR

network, *Am. J. Trop. Med. Hyg.* 93 (3 Suppl., Sep. 2, 2015): 57–68. Arthur Crosby mentions malaria on three pages of *The Columbian Exchange*, but surprisingly he does not mention quinine.

[302] *Britannica*, rubber.

[303] *Britannica*, sugar; sucrose; starch; amylase; ptyalin; senses; sweet. As mentioned previously, taste is one of the principal senses; the taste of sweetness is one of the tastes.

[304] *Britannica*, insulin; diabetes mellitus (from Greek, meaning "copious urination + sweet"). Frederick G. Banting and Charles H. Best isolated insulin in 1921.

Marc Aronson and Marina Budhos, *Sugar Changed the World: A Story of Magic, Spice, Slavery, Freedom, and Science* (New York: Clarion Books, 2010).

My experiences with sugar as an unfortunate caloric substitute for protein and fat were reported in George J. Hill, Manuel G. Herrera-Aceña; Guillermo Arboleda, and Rafael Montoya, Surgical education in a developing country: Participation of a rural community hospital in Colombia, *Arch. Surg.* 106 (1973): 356-8. Also see: Jennie Erin Smith, Patent panela? Really? *New York Times*, 26 January 2021, D1, D8.

[305] This essay is focused on the history of the West, but one of the most important staples of cooking in India is ghee, made from clarified butter. "Removing the milk solids out of butter makes it lactose-free, highly digestible, soothing, anti-inflammatory and increases its smoke point," at https://www.feastingathome.com/how-to-make-ghee/ (accessed January 11, 2021).

For licorice, see https://www.webmd.com/vitamins/ai/ingredientmono-881/licorice (accessed 11/2/2020). For oil of turpentine, see: Vincent Cirillo, Oil of turpentine: Sheet anchor of 19th century therapeutics, to Medical History Society of New Jersey, December 22, 2020, at https://www.mhsnj.org/event-4093300 (accessed January 1, 2021). Oil of turpentine, which comes from the resin of pine trees, was used to ease many symptoms. It is still to be found in Vick's chest rub. It used to be taken as a cure for intestinal parasites, until it was found to be toxic.

[306] The surgeons of Egypt were advised to distinguish between diseases which were treatable and those which would be fatal. The *Smith Papyrus* said that several types of head injuries could be treated, but if the brain is exposed, the surgeon should say, "This disease I will not treat." A fatal outcome after treatment would be sufficient cause to punish the physician severely. See also: Robin Lane Fox, *The Invention of Medicine: From Homer to Hippocrates* (New York: Basic Books, 2020).

For Hippocrates, see: Steven H. Miles, Hippocrates and informed consent, *The Lancet* 374 (no. 9698, 17 October 2009): 1322-3, with image of Hippocrates © 2009 The Bridgeman Art Library. The origin of the aphorism "first do no harm" is uncertain. It does not appear in that form in Hippocrates' works, but Hippocrates wrote in Greek, and "first do no harm" is a reasonable English translation of his warning to physicians. See Anon., First do no harm: The impossible oath, *BMJ* 2019, 366:14734. "The Greek text ὠφελέειν ἢ μὴ βλάπτειν (poorly and inappropriately translated into Latin as primum non nocere) is a passage from the Hippocratic treatise on Epidemics (First book, second part, paragraph 5): 'In illnesses one should keep two things in mind, to be useful rather than cause no harm'."

[307] Atul Gwande, *The Checklist Manifesto: How to Get Things Right* (New York: Henry Holt and Company, 2009).

[308] A technique similar to closure of a duffel coat was used to close a large wound. The sides of the wound were brought together by hand, and a needle was thrust across both sides of the wound. The ends of the needle were joined by a cord which was wrapped around several times and then tied.

[309] *Britannica*, capsaicin, says nothing about the topical use of the powder of the red pepper to stimulate erection in males, and lust when it is applied to female genitals.

[310] For medicine, Roy Porter, *The Greatest Benefit to Mankind*; supplemented by William Bynum, *The History of Medicine*; and Ralph H. Major, *A History of Medicine* (Springfield, Ill.: Charles C Thomas, 1954).

For science, David C. Lindberg, *The Beginnings of Western Science*, supplemented by William Bynum, *A Little History of Science* (New Haven: Yale University Press, 2012).

The list of "Doctors Afield" does not include all of the physicians who were mentioned elsewhere in this essay. For instance, see the reference at a later point in this essay to Dr. Joseph-Ignace Guillotine, who conceived of the notorious French beheading machine.

[311] "Doctors Afield" was published as a series of articles from 1952 to 1969 in the *New England Journal of Medicine* under the general topic of Medical Intelligence. Their names were published in *N Engl J Med* 268 (20 June 1963): 1417. Twenty additional biographies were published by Mary G. McCrea Curran, Howard Spiro, and Deborah St. James, eds., *Doctors Afield* (New Haven, Conn.: Yale University Press, 1999). Curran, et al., credited the title of their work to the series in the *NEJM*.

[312] Quotation abbreviated from Preface to Curran, et al., *Doctors Afield*.

[313] Two examples of "doctors afield" who are still alive are: Jim Whittaker (b. 1929), who on May 1, 1963 became the first American to summit Mt. Everest, and who founded Recreational Equipment Incorporated (REI). He was

originally on this list, but he is still alive. He has inspired thousands of others in his contributions to the environment. Dr. Tenley Albright (b. 1935) won the Gold Medal for figure skating at the 1956 Olympics.

[314] Luke, 1-3: "With this in mind, since I myself have carefully investigated everything from the beginning, I too decided to write an orderly account for you, most excellent Theophilus, so that you may know the certainty of the things you have been taught."

[315] In Luke's narrative of the birth of Jesus, we are given Mary's genealogy (Luke 3:23–38). Probably the best way to interpret verse 23 is like this: Jesus "was thought to be the son of Joseph, the *son-in-law* of Heli." Then the genealogy continues all the way back to David, Abraham, and Adam. This establishes Mary as the physical descendant of David, so it can be stated that Jesus truly was "the Son of David" through the lineage of David's son Nathan. Matthew's genealogy of Jesus (Matt. 1:1–16), from Joseph's perspective, is also important because it clearly demonstrates Jesus' legal right to the throne of David. According to Judaism, Jesus, as the adopted son of Joseph, would have all the legal rights of a biological heir. Joseph descended from David through Solomon, and that was the chosen line of David for someone to be considered king. Hence, the Lord Jesus was the son of David by biological descent through Mary and the king of Israel by legal right through Joseph." From Today in the World: Enter In. Doors and Gates in Scripture, at:https://www.todayintheword.org/issues/2020/march/question-and-answer/question-2/ (accessed March 14, 2021).

[316] *Britannica*: Luke, Evangelist.

[317] Saints, including Luke: https://www.fiamc.org/faith-prayer/saints/physician-saints-of-the-catholic-church/ (accessed March 13, 2021). Luke is not mentioned at all in Bynum, *History of Medicine*, or in Major, *History of Medicine*. Porter, *Greatest Benefit*, mentions Luke briefly (pp. 86-7), as he discusses early Christian theology and practice, in which health and healing were crucial aspects of the ministry of Jesus. "Luke the Evangelist was himself a physician," and "Was not Luke 'the beloved physician?'" Porter continues, "Christ, though he told physicians to heal themselves, gave proofs of his own diving powers by acts of healing? Some thirty-five such miracles are recorded in the Bible."

[318] These images are in the public domain, downloaded from Wikipedia: "Saint Luke," from the Gospel of Saint Riquier (aka Gospel of Charlemagne), manuscript, France ca 800; and "Luke and the Madonna," Altar of the Guild of Saint Luke, Hermen Rode, Lübeck (1484).

[319] Acts 28:16: "And when we came to Rome, the centurion delivered the prisoners to the captain of the guard: but Paul was suffered to dwell by himself with a soldier that kept him." The statement about "one-quarter" of the New Testament is often mentioned. I can verify it from examination of two copies of the King James Version, both published by Oxford University Press, undated but probably c.1939. In one copy, the pages for Luke's Gospel and the Acts total 78/280=27.8%; in the other, it is 67/245=27.3%.

[320] The Hippocratic Oath begins with this contract: "To hold him who taught me this art equally dear to me as my parents, to be a partner in life with him, and to fulfill his needs when required; to look upon his offspring as equals to my own siblings, and to teach them this art, if they wish to learn it, without fee or contract; and the by the set rules, lectures, and every other mode of instruction, I will impart a knowledge of this art to my own sons, and those of my teachers, and to students bound by this contract and having sworn this Oath to the law of medicine, but to no others." The physician abjures giving a lethal drug, and from surgery, unless "trained in this craft." The promise "not to give a woman a pessary to cause an abortion" has usually been taken to mean that Oath prohibits abortion. However, another interpretation is that it is to prevent using an instrument, but would not oppose prescribing an abortifacient, such as ergot. From https://www.nlm.nih.gov/hmd/greek/greek_oath.html (accessed March 14, 2021).

[321] Major, *History of Medicine*, "Medicine in the Roman Empire" (168-222) shows that many of the medical and surgical treatments at that time are similar to those of today. Many of the surgical tools are familiar. Major tells more of the opportunities and challenges that would have been faced by Luke as a physician. There was a never-ending conflict between Greek and Roman physicians. "The lot of the Greek physician in Rome was, at first, a hard one. [However,] the practice of medicine was largely in the hands of Greek physicians during the first centuries of the Roman empire." (p.169). Although the Romans were apt learners, "The Greeks dominated the profession and directed its main stream" (p.178). Antonius Musa (c. 10 A.D.) was a Greek physician of Emperor Caesar Augustus and of the poet Horace. Scribonius Largus (c. 47 A.D.), "possibly a Greek," wrote "a very valuable" collection of medical recipes, dedicated to Emperor Claudius (p. 167). Antonius Cornelius Celsus (25 B.C.–50 A.D.), a Roman, not a Greek, wrote *De re medicina*, which described the history of medicine to that point. His eight books are regarded as "one of the greatest of medical classics" (p.169-72).

[322] The words "fade away," come from the song, "Old Soldiers Never Die," that was quoted in the farewell address to Congress by General of the Army Douglas MacArthur, after he was removed from command by Harry S. Truman in 1951. The words, "pass and be forgotten" come from the Whiffenpoof Song, in the phrase, "Then we'll pass and be forgotten like the rest."

C. Developments in Human Health – Chronological Viewpoint

[323] *Britannica*, Fertile Crescent. This term was coined by James Henry Breasted (1865-1935). It appeared in his article on "Ikhnaton" in the 14th edition of *Encyclopaedia Britannica*.

[324] On a map, the Fertile Crescent is similar to a waning crescent moon, tilted so the horns apparently point to the south-east. See: Bob Berman, The captivating crescent moon: By the light of the slivery moon, *The Old Farmer's Almanac* (20 February 2020), at: https://www.almanac.com/content/captivating-crescent-moon (accessed November 4, 2020).

[325] Keller, *Bible as History*, 6-31, says that Ur had been established before 4000 BCE, but does not give an approximate time for the settlement. Keller says the excavations began with the discovery of a city under Tell al Muqayyar by J. E. Taylor in 1854. *Britannica*, Ur, says that Ur was settled at "some time in the 4th millennium BCE," and that "their occupation was ended by a flood, formerly though to be the one descried in Genesis."

[326] Amy-Jill Levine, What is the difference between the Old Testament, the Tanakh, and the Hebrew Bible? *Bible Odyssey* [on-line] https://www.bibleodyssey.org/en/tools/bible-basics/what-is-the-difference-between-the-old-testament-the-tanakh-and-the-hebrew-bible (accessed November 8, 2020).

[327] *Britannica* does not give a time line for Egyptian history. History.com, "Ancient Egypt": "Around 2630 B.C., the third dynasty's King Djoser asked Imhotep, an architect, priest and healer, to design a funerary monument for him; the result was the world's first major stone building, the Step-Pyramid at Saqqara, near Memphis." https://www.history.com/topics/ancient-history/ancient-egypt (accessed November 6, 2020).

[328] Keller, *Bible as History*, 5.

[329] Major, *History of Medicine*, 33-55; for the Step Pyramid, Major says c.2980, p.40.

[330] Keller, 7; and *Britannica*.

[331] Major, 20-33; Major gives the approximate date of c. 1950 BCE for the Code of Hammurabi. Many dates in this period vary with the source of reference.

[332] Keller, 7; and *Britannica*.

[333] Quotation from *Britannica*, Troy. A recent attempt to recreate the return of Ulysses is told by Tim Severin, *The Ulysses Voyage* (London: Arrow Books, [1987] 1988). Also see Virgil, *The Aeneid*, trans. Robert Fitzgerald (New York: Vintage Classics/Vintage Books/ Random House, [1981] 1990).

[334] Josh. 10:32-38 (KJV), quoted by Keller, 153; Major, 26; Josh. 2:1-24, 6:1-27.

[335] Keller, 183, 193, 202. Hundreds of commandments and laws, with 13 capital crimes, are given in Exodus, Leviticus, and Deuteronomy. See: https://www.biblegateway.com/resources/encyclopedia-of-the-bible/Crimes-Punishments (accessed November 9, 2020). Although there is some doubt about whether some of these were usual punishments, the statement by Jesus, a Jew, "He that is without sin among you, let him first cast a stone at her" (John 8:7), regarding a woman who had committed adultery, shows that adultery was punishable by death. Stephen, the first martyr, also Jewish, was killed by stoning for impiety.

[336] The period known as the Babylonian Exile is mentioned in five books of the Bible: 2 Kings, 2 Chronicles, Ezra, Jeremiah, and Ezekiel. Summarized in https://www.biblestudytools.com/bible-study/topical-studies/who-was-king-nebuchadnezzar-in-the-bible.html (accessed November 7, 2020). However, Keller, 297: "Following [Jeremiah's] well considered advice, the [Jews]sought and found 'the peace of the city' and did not fare at all badly. The exile in Babylon was not to be compared with the harsh existence of the children of Israel on the Nile."

[337] For the *Odyssey*, see Severin, 26; although Major, 33, says ?1102 BC. For Buddha, see *Britannica*.

[338] Herodotus, from Major, 33; other dates from *Britannica*. The Plague of Athens is discussed by Major, *History of Medicine*, 136-9.

[339] *Britannica*; also, Michel Foucault, *The History of Sexuality*, 4 vols., especially vols. 2 and 3, 1976.

[340] *Britannica*, for these people and events.

[341] *Britannica*, Ibid.

[342] *Britannica*, Ibid.

[343] *Britannica*, Ibid.

[344] *Britannica*, Ibid.

[345] *Britannica*, Ibid., and Luke 14:3-4.

[346] https://www.ancient.eu/Attila_the_Hun/ (accessed November 3, 2020). Fall of Rome in 455 from Bynum, *History of Medicine*, 20.

[347] *Britannica* and Order of the Merovingian Dynasty website: http://www.merovingiandynasty.org/ (accessed November 12, 2020).

[348] Ralph Major quotes Sir William Osler as saying that the *Canon* of Avicenna was "the most famous medical textbook ever written." (Major, 244-5). Avicenna's *Canon* is still studied in *madrassas* in the Middle East. Galen's

works total about twenty volumes – varying with the translation and the published editions – and they were the standard medical texts for more than a millennium.

[349] The four kings of England in 1066 were: Edward the Confessor, Edgar the Aetheling, Harold Godwinson, and William I, the Conqueror. The kings of Scotland mentioned were Duncan I, Macbeth, and Malcolm III. St. Margaret of Scotland was Malcolm Canmore's wife, and she was also the sister of Edgar the Aetheling. "Peeping Tom" is said to have gazed at Lady Godiva when she took her bare back ride in Coventry, England, and was punished by blinding.

[350] The oldest universities are said to be in Europe; the University of Bologna (1088; charter granted 1158); University of Oxford (1096); University of Salamanca (1134). See: https://www.mastersavenue.com/articles-guides/good-to-know/the-10-oldest-universities-in-the-world (accessed November 13, 2020), with illustrations. Bynum, *History of Medicine*, 26, gives different dates for the founding of universities in Bologna (c.1180), Paris and Oxford (1200), and Salamanca (c.1218). *Britannica*: university, gives even vaguer dates: Salerno's medical school founded in the 9th century. The universities of Bologna, late in the 11th century; Paris, founded between 1150 and 1170, and Oxford, "well established by the end of the 12th century."

[351] The most interesting and useful book about cathedral construction that I have read is a historical novel set in the 12th century, by Ken Follett, *The Pillars of the Earth* (London: Macmillan, 1989). For views and details of construction, see: https://www.touropia.com/gothic-cathedrals/ (accessed November 12, 2020).

[352] History of the centuries from the 11th to the 16th from http://www.fsmitha.com/time/ce13.htm (accessed November 13, 2020). A recent discussion of the plague proposes that the fleas infected with *Yersinia* spread plague from human to human, without rats. See: Michael Greshko, Maybe rats aren't responsible for the Black Death, *National Geographic* (January 15, 2018), at https://www.nationalgeographic.com/news/2018/01/rats-plague-black-death-humans-lice-health-science/ (accessed November 14, 2020). Major, 323-5 for Anglicus and Bacon.

[353] *Britannica*: syphilis, which mentions that signs of treponema infection have been found in archaeological specimens in Latin America. *Britannica*: yaws. Syphilis is similar in many ways to yaws, which is caused by a bacterium that is identical in appearance to *T. pallidum*, but is not a sexually transmitted disease. For possible exemption of the rat from transmission of plague during the Black Death, see Michael Greshko (see above). The modern form of St. Vitus Dance, due to rheumatic fever, is probably not the same as the Dancing Mania of the Middle Ages. See Major, 266-356, "The Middle Ages: The Late Period." Also, *Britannica*, Chaucer.

[354] 15th Century, 1401-1500, from http://www.fsmitha.com/time/ce15.htm (accessed January 15, 2020).

[355] Vasco da Gama at https://www.biography.com/explorer/vasco-da-gama (accessed January 15, 2020). Crosby, *The Columbian Exchange*, especially smallpox, pp. 42-58. For the impact on Native Americans for more than the next 250 years, see Elizabeth A. Fenn, *Pox Americana: The Great Smallpox Epidemic of 1775-82* (New York: Hill and Wang, 2001).

[356] Bynum, *Medicine*, 35-6 (syphilis)

[357] Bynum, *Medicine*, 34-5 (Paracelsus). Major, *History of Medicine*, pp. 383-93, gives a lengthy assessment of both the useful and useless contributions of Paracelsus, of his alchemy and astrology and other odd directions into which his speculations led. Although he was important in the 16th century, "Historians have pronounced an unfavorable verdict on Paracelsus."

[358] Bynum, *Science*, 58-61 (Copernicus, Brahe, Kepler).
 Britannica: "Copernicus's theory had important consequences for later thinkers of the Scientific Revolution, including such major figures as Galileo, Kepler, Descartes, and Newton."

[359] *Britannica*, Michelangelo; Machiavelli.

[360] *Britannica*, Luther.

[361] *Britannica*, Süleyman I; Henry VIII; Paré. Vesalius, in Bynum, *Science*, 29.

[362] *Britannica*, St. Bartholomew's Day, Massacre.

[363] *Britannica*, Galileo Galilei.

[364] Francis Bacon: Major, *History of Medicine*, 479-80; Bynum, *History of Science*, 74-5.

[365] William Harvey: Major, *History of Medicine*, 494-500: "Harvey's *Exercitatio anatomica de motu codris et sanguinis in animalibus* [1628], which ranks with the *Fabrica* of Vesalius as a milestone in the progress of medicine … It is almost impossible to exaggerate the importance of Harvey's great discovery."

[366] H. N. Segall, William Osler and Thomas Browne, a friendship of fifty-two years; Sir Thomas pervades Sir William's library, *Korot* 8 (nos. 11-12, Summer 1985):150-65. https://pubmed.ncbi.nlm.nih.gov/11614038/ (accessed November 20, 2020). Also: *Britannica*: Sir Thomas Browne.

[367] Bynum, *History of Science*, 75-80; and Russell Shorto, *Descartes' Bones: A Skeletal History of the Between Faith and Reason* (New York: Random House, 2008).

[368] *Britannica*, James I. Ulster was one of the four provinces of Ireland. It is composed of nine counties. Six constitute Northern Ireland, in the United Kingdom; three are in the Republic of Ireland.
Ken Follett, *A Column of Fire* (New York: Penguin Random House, LLC, 2017).
[369] The Lost Colony was the last attempt by English colonists to settle in Virginia before success was achieved at Jamestown. For the causes of the high mortality rate and the impact of demography in Virginia and the Chesapeake Bay area, see: Jean B. Russo and J. Elliott Russo, *Planting an Empire: The Early Chesapeake in British North America* (Washington, D.C: Smithsonian Libraries, 2012).
[370] *Britannica*: gunpowder; dynamite. Potassium nitrate (saltpetre) was originally obtained from bird droppings (guano).
[371] *Britannica*: Bradford, William. This entry credits George Morton as being "Mourt" in *Mourt's Relation*.
[372] For the history of English settlement and comments on health in the colonies of New England, see: David Hackett Fisher, *Albion's Seed: Four British Folkways in America* (New York: Oxford University Press, 1989), which also discusses the group that Fisher calls the Cavaliers of Virginia; Nathaniel Philbrick, *Mayflower: A Story of Courage, Community, and War* (New York: Viking Pilgrim, 2006); John Putnam Demos, *The Unredeemed Captive: A Family Story From Early America* (New York: Vintage, 1994); Demos, *Entertaining Satan: Witchcraft and the Culture of Early New England* (New York: Oxford University Press, 1982); Demos, *A Little Commonwealth: Family Life in Plymouth Colony* (New York: Oxford University Press, 1970); Mrs. Mary Rowlandson, *A True History of the Captivity and Restoration of Mrs. Mary Rowlandson, a Minister's Wife in New England* [1682] (Np.:Createspace, 2017).
[373] Very little is known about medical practice or medicines in colonial New England. The best contemporary account is given by a brilliant but deeply flawed non-physician, Rev. Dr. Cotton Mather, FRS (1663-1728). Cotton Mather, *The Angel of Bethesda: An Essay upon the Common Maladies of Mankind*, ed. Gordon W. Jones ([c.1632] Barre, Mass.: American Antiquarian Society, 1972); and *Britannica*: Mather, Cotton; and variolation.
Variolation was required for potential recruits into the Continental Army in 1777. See: Amy Lynn Filsinger and Raymond Dwek, George Washington and the first mass military inoculation, Smithsonian Reference Services (n.d.): https://www.loc.gov/rr/scitech/GW&smallpoxinoculation.html (accessed November 25, 2020).
For a fine account of the pharmaceuticals used in London in the early 17th century, and then in the Massachusetts Bay Colony, see Anya Seton, *The Winthrop Woman* (London: Hodder & Stoughton, 1958).
[374] For the history of the 17th century, see: http://www.fsmitha.com/time/ce17.htm/ (accessed November 20, 2020). Vienna Pestsäule: https://www.atlasobscura.com/places/vienna-pestsaule-plague-column (accessed November 29, 2020), and Harold Avery, Plague churches, monuments and memorials, *Proceedings of the Royal Society of Medicine*, 59 (no. 2, February 1966):110-16, at https://www.ncbi.nlm.nih.gov/pmc/articles/ PMC1900794/pdf/ procrsmed00186-0033.pdf (accessed November 29, 2020).
[375] Bynum, *History of Medicine*, 37. Sydenham, translated from Latin: J. M. S. Pearce, Sydenham on hysteria, *Eur Neurol* 76 (2016):175-181: "women, except for those who lead a hardy and robust life, are rarely quite free from it; those men who lead a sedentary or studious life are subject to the same complaint; in their case, it is indeed called hypochondria, but this disease is as like hysteria as one egg is like another. Men are less subject to it than women because of their more robust habit of body." From https://www.karger.com/Article/FullText/450605 (accessed April 8, 2021).
[376] Bynum, *History of Science*, 83-6.
[377] *Britannica*, Antonie van Leeuwenhoek.
[378] The term "Scientific Revolution" does not appear as a separate term in the DVD of *Britannica*, although it is mentioned in several places previously cited. A concise definition is given in an essay entitled "Scientific Revolution" in Britannica.com/science/Scientific-Revolution. See: https://www.britannica.com/science/Scientific-Revolution (accessed November 26, 2020).
[379] Britannica: Penn, William. For the Welcome Fleet, see https://www.welcomesociety.org/ancestors.html (accessed November 23, 2020).
[380] *Britannica*: Philadelphia, Pennsylvania. Rhode Island was the first English colony to proclaim freedom of religion for all faiths, but no Roman Catholic Churches were built there in early times. Pennsylvania was unique in its religious tolerance.
[381] *Britannica*: Mather, Cotton. A curious addition to this story was told in a letter to the *New York Times*: "I find it worth mentioning the important role Cotton Mather's slave Onesimus played during the 1721 smallpox epidemic in Boston . . . who suggested the practice of inoculating against smallpox," Mark Weaver, To the Editor, *New York Times Book Review*, 14 June 2020, 6. Gillian Brockell, African roots of inoculation in America go back 300 years, *Washington Post*, 22 December 2020, E4; and Ronald G. Shafer, Abigail Adams faced a "fearsome" inoculation choice, *Washington Post*, 13 December 2020), A14. Shafer quotes Feather Schwartz Foster, *The First Ladies: From*

Martha Washington to Mamie Eisenhower, an Intimate Portrait of the Women Who Shaped America (Naperville, Ill.: Sourcebooks, 2011).

[382] Bynum, *History of Medicine*, 38. Major, *History of Medicine*, 570-3. Boerhaave's volumes are now in the Special Collections at Marshall University, Huntington, W.V. See: https://mds.marshall.edu/sc_finding_aids/344/ + 0789: George J. Hill Collection, 1889-2011 (accessed November 23, 2020).

[383] The Pennsylvania Hospital was built in 1751. It was the first hospital built in the thirteen colonies. Bellevue Hospital was established as an almshouse in New York City in 1736. Charity Hospital in New Orleans, Louisiana, was created in 1751.

Benjamin Franklin's autobiography was composed in parts between 1771 to 1790. It was not in Franklin's lifetime, but it appeared in French as *Mémoires de la vie privée de Benjamin Franklin*. The English text of Franklin's *Autobiography* (first published posthumously in 1791) is the most famous American autobiography.

Also, Walter Isaacson, *Benjamin Franklin: An American Life* (New York: Simon & Schuster, 2003); and Stacy Schiff, *A Great Improvisation: Franklin, France, and the Birth of America* (New York: Henry Holt, 2005).

[384] Bynum, *History of Science:* Franklin, 94-9. *Britannica*: Edison, Thomas. Edison didn't make the grade for Bynum; he is not in the Index of Bynum's *History of Science*.

[385] Bynum, *History of Science*, 109-12, says Linnaeus was a "doctor and naturalist," and that he was "trained in medicine." His name does not appear in Major, *History of Medicine*, so we know nothing about his activities as a physician. However, it is very likely that he had a medical practice of some type. As a professor of botany, he would have had the opportunity to advise and treat patients, if he chose to do so. He sent his students to many parts of the world, looking for specimens. Although "some died" his "followers remained devoted to him." We cannot help but wonder how he felt about the deaths of his students. Did he feel responsible for them?

[386] Major, 596-7: James Lind. Porter, *Greatest Benefit*, 295-6; 556. *Britannia*: Lind, James.

Javier Yanes, James Lind and scurvy: The first clinical trial in history? *Open Mind BBVA* (July 12, 2016). See: https://www.bbvaopenmind.com/en/science/leading-figures/james-lind-and-scurvy-the-first-clinical-trial-in-history/ (accessed November 24, 2020).

[387] *Britannica*: Guillotine.

[388] Major, *History of Medicine*, 598-600. William Withering published *A Botanical Arrangement of all the Vegetables Naturally Growing in Great Britain* (1766).

[389] *Britannica*: Washington, George. See also David Hackett Fisher, *Washington's Crossing* (New York: Oxford University Press, 2004). For perspectives on Patriot/Rebel and Tory/Loyalist, see "Loyalist Trails" of the United Empire Loyalists of Canada (UELAC): http://www.uelac.org/Loyalist-Trails/Loyalist-Trails-index.php (accessed November 27, 2020).

[390] Benjamin Rush is another important physician who failed to make the cut for Bynum's brief *History of Medicine*. Rush has citations on ten pages in Porter, *Greatest Good*. Porter called him the American Hippocrates, said Galen would be proud of him, and cites his work as the "founding father of American Medicine": *Medical Inquiries and Observations upon the Diseases of the Mind* (1812).

[391] *Britannica*: Pott, Percival. Also, Nadia Benmoussa, John-David Rebibo, Patrick Conan, and Philippe Chartier, Chimney-sweeps' cancer – early proof of environmentally driven tumourigenicity, *The Lancet* 20 (no. 3, March 1, 2019): P338. See: https://www.thelancet.com/journals/lanonc/article/PIIS1470-2045(19)30106-8/fulltext#%20 (accessed December 13, 2020). Druin Burch, Astley Paston Cooper (1768-1841): Anatomist, radical and surgeon, *Journal of the Royal Society of Medicine* 103 (no. 12, December 1, 2010): 505-508. https://www.ncbi.nlm.nih.gov/pmc/articles/PMC2996521/ (accessed November 26, 2020).

[392] Jenner, in Ralph Major, *History of Medicine*, 606-9. Also see: *Britannica*: Jenner, William; Porter, *Greatest Benefit*, 176-7; Bynum, *History of Medicine*, 73-4; and Bynum, *History of Science*, 164.

[393] Bynum, *History of Medicine*, 41. Bynum refers to "Enlightenment medical practice" in the 18th century, and he begins his treatment of "Enlightened Medicine?" with Boerhaave (born in 1668). Major, *A History of Medicine*, "The Rise of American Medicine," 717-21; *Britannica*, Morgan; and Elizabeth Fee, The first American medical school: The formative years, *The Lancet* 385 (no. 9981, 16 May 2015): 1917-2014; at https://www.thelancet.com/journals/lancet/issue/vol385no9981 (accessed February 13, 2021).

Britannica: Malthus, Thomas Robert (1766-1834), and the Malthusian Theory, from *Essay on the Principle of Population as It Affects the Future Improvement of Society, with Remarks on the Speculations of Mr. Godwin, M. Condorcet, and Other Writers* (1798), published anonymously.

[394] Bynum, *History of Medicine*, 43 "Mecca," 50-2, 57. Roy Porter, *The Greatest Benefit*, 308-9, et seq. Porter cites Laennec's publication of *Traité de l'auscultation médiate* (1819). The familiar modern stethoscope that is draped around the neck was designed by David Littman, M.D. (1906-1981), a professor at the Harvard Medical School.

[395] Full title: Laurel Thatcher Ulrich, *A Midwife's Tale: The Life of Martha Ballard Based on Her Diary, 1785–1812* (New York: Random House, 1990).

[396] *Britannica*: O'Brian, Patrick.

[397] Timothy Egan, The Next 3 months are going to be pure hell, *New York Times*, 19 December 2020, A26.

[398] *Britannica*: Industrial Revolution. The term was coined by Arnold Toynbee (1852-1883) to describe England's economic development from 1760 to 1840. Also, Lewis Mumford, *Technics and Civilization*. (Chicago: University of Chicago Press, 1934). Mumford showed that many of the same components of England's Industrial Revolution appeared in the United States at a later date, but were ameliorated by differences between England and America.

[399] *Britannica*: Marx, Karl; Engels, Friedrich. Engels, as a sole author, wrote *Die Lage der arbeitenden Klasse in England* (1845; *The Condition of the Working Class in England*). There were attempts made to ameliorate the working conditions in the cotton mills in Scotland, and to educate the children who worked in the mills. See: Ian Donnachie and George Hewitt, *Historic New Lanark: The Dale and Owen Industrial Community since 1785* (Edinburgh: Edinburgh University Press, 1993). See the fictionalized but accurate representation of these conditions in Anthony F. C. Wallace, *Rockdale: The Growth of an American Village in the Early Industrial Revolution* (New York: Alfred A. Knopf, 1978).

[400] The American Civil War was at one time considered to be a war that was fought for State's rights, and that emancipation of enslaved people was a secondary cause of the war. By the 1960s, much of the South still held to that belief, the "Lost Cause," but for most historians, the view changed. Now the reason became emancipation – to free the slaves and prohibit slavery forever in the United States. Many African-Americans look at it from a third perspective: it was all about money – tariffs, cheap labor, and profit – and the battle over slavery was secondary.

Cuba was allowed to become independent in 1902, though it was dominated in many ways by the U.S. until the Cuban Revolution of 1953, which concluded in 1958. The U.S. still occupies a piece of land in Cuba at Guantanamo Bay. The Philippine people initially resisted American occupation of the islands, and the country did not become fully independent until 1946. For Theodore Roosevelt's "splendid little war," see Secretary of State John Hay's letter to Roosevelt in Warren Zimmermann, *First Great Triumph: How Five Americans Made Their Country a World Power* (New York: Farrar, Straus and Giroux, 2002), 310.

[401] *Britannica*: Nightingale, Florence; Barton, Clara. For the ICRC, see: https://www.icrc.org/en/who-we-are/movement (accessed November 27, 2020). For the American Red Cross (ARC), see: Patrick F. Gilbo, *The American Red Cross: The First Century* (New York: Harper and Row, 1981); Foster Rhea Dulles, *The American Red Cross* (New York: Harper and Brothers, 1950); and George J. Hill, *Rolling with Patton: The Letters and Photographs of Field Director Gerald L. Hill, 303rd Infantry Regiment, 97th "Trident" Division, 1943-1945* (Berwyn Heights, Md.: Heritage Books, 2019). The third reference tells of the experiences of an American Red Cross officer in World War II.

[402] Cholera, in Bynum, *History of Medicine*, 77-84 (p.79: "greatest good"), including Chadwick and Snow; John Snow, in Bynum, *History of Science*, 168 (anesthesia for Queen Victoria). Cholera, Chadwick and Snow, in Porter, *Greatest Good*, 409-14; Porter's chapter on "The Enforcement of Health" (420-5). Bynum identified several discoveries in medicine and biology that were not accepted immediately. Thomas Kuhn has shown what he calls paradigm shifts in astronomy, physics, and chemistry in *Scientific Revolutions*.

[403] *Britannica*: anesthesia; Davy, Sir Humphrey; Morton, William; and ether. Dr. John Collins Warren, who performed the first operation with ether anesthesia, does not have a *Britannica* entry. He is profiled at http://collections.countway.harvard.edu/onview/exhibits/show/family-practice/john-collins-warren--1778-1856 (accessed December 13, 2020).

[404] *Britannica*: nitrous oxide, cocaine, chloroform. Renee Tietjen, More to the Dr. Sims story, *Washington Post*, 2 January 2021, A15: Also, Major, *History of Medicine*, 761 (for a biography of Sims).

[405] *Britannica*: Lincoln, Abraham. Sean Wilentz, Paths to abolition: John Brown and Abraham Lincoln chose contrasting methods for ending slavery, *New York Times Book Review*, 13 December 2020, 16; a review of H. W. Brands, *The Zealot and the Emancipator: John Brown, Abraham Lincoln, and the Struggle for American Freedom* (New York: Doubleday, 2020).

[406] The Republican party had strong support for abolition at the start of the Civil War as the result of the immensely popular novel, *Uncle Tom's Cabin*, by Harriet Beecher Stowe (1811-1896). In the White House, Lincoln supposedly told Stowe, "You are the little lady that started this war." The noble character of Uncle Tom has since been mis-appropriated as meaning a Black man who is a sycophant to white people. This reversal is similar to the "ugly American," who was actually only a homely man in this novel who was deeply engaged in helping people in the country, when he was serving as U.S. officer in Vietnam. The "ugly American" has become a meme for an American who does evil things in foreign countries. See: Eugene Burdick and William Lederer, *The Ugly American* (New York: Norton, 1958).

[407] *Britannica*: Reconstruction, in U.S. history.
[408] Reuters Life, "Lincoln came near death from smallpox: researchers," *Healthcare & Pharma* (May 17, 2007), at https://www.reuters.com/article/us-smallpox-lincoln/lincoln-came-near-death-from-smallpox-researchers (accessed December 8, 2020). The 13th Amendment to the U.S. Constitution, which abolished slavery, was passed by Congress on January 31, 1865. On December 6, 1856, it was ratified by the required 27 states of the 36 that comprised the U.S., and it was proclaimed in effect on December 18, 1865.
[409] *Britannica*: Darwin, Charles; Wedgwood, Josiah.
[410] *Britannica*: Lamarck, Jean Baptiste; Lysenko, Trofim.
[411] Mendel, in Bynum, *History of Science*, 210-11.
[412] Galton, in Bynum, *History of Medicine*, 89.
[413] Marvin J. Stone, "Henry Bence Jones and his protein," *Journal of Medical Biography* 6 (Feb 1, 1998):53-57, at: https://journals.sagepub.com/doi/abs/10.1177/096777209800600112?journalCode=jmba (accessed December 13, 2020). *Britannica*, Semmelweis. Puerperal sepsis, "childbed fever," is caused by many different microorganisms.
[414] Bynum, *History of Medicine*, 93-7: Cell theory, and Schleiden, Schwann, Müller, Virchow.
[415] Bynum, *History of Medicine*, 97-101: Pasteur. Bynum points out that Pasteur's disproof of "spontaneous generation" was not immediately accepted. Pasteur's experiment in 1859 used swan-necked flasks ("col de cygnet"). See: https://www.immunology.org/pasteurs-col-de-cygnet-1859 (accessed March 26, 2021).
[416] Bynum, *History of Medicine*, 115-8: Bernard. *Britannica*: Bernard, Claude. He published *Introduction à la médecine expérimentale* (1865; *An Introduction to the Study of Experimental Medicine*). Bernard and Charles Huette, *Illustrated manual of operative surgery and surgical anatomy* (title translated), 1855. Bernard's textbook of surgery was unusual, in that it showed each operation in stages, with illustrations and text on opposite, facing, pages. This format was used by the popular American atlases of surgery, written by Elliot Cutler and Robert M. Zollinger, *Atlas of Surgical Operations* (New York: Macmillan, 1944), and later by Zollinger and Zollinger, Jr., and then Zollinger, Jr. and E. C. Ellison, for the 10th edition (2016). Bernard to Zollinger – 1855 to 2016 – is 161 years.
[417] Bynum, *History of Medicine*, 109-11: Lister. *Britannica*: Lister, Joseph.
[418] Bynum, *History of Medicine*, 103-7: Koch. Also, Bynum, *History of Medicine*, 114-5: Ludwig. Koch proposed four postulates which were necessary to prove that a microorganism was the cause of a disease. The postulates have been modified several times and are still not perfect. Originally stated in German, an English translation is: (1) The microorganism must be found in diseased but not healthy individuals; (2) The microorganism must be cultured from the diseased individual; (3) Inoculation of a healthy individual with the cultured microorganism must recapitulated the disease; and finally (4) The microorganism must be re-isolated from the inoculated, diseased individual and matched to the original microorganism.
[419] *Britannica*: Edison, Thomas Alva; The Edison Laboratory; Edison and the Lumière brothers (from motion picture, history of). Also, Matthew Josephson, *The Robber Barons: The Great American Capitalists, 1861-1901* (New York: Harcourt, Brace and Company, 1934) and *Edison: A Biography* (New York: McGraw Hill, 1959). Josephson co-authored the *Britannica* piece about Edison.
[420] Quotations from George J. Hill, *Edison's Environment: The Great Inventor was Also a Great Polluter*, 3rd ed. (Berwyn Heights, Md.: Heritage Books, 2017).
[421] *Britannica*: Vivaldi, Antonio (1678-1741); Bach, Johann Sebastian (1685-1750); Handel, George Frideric [Georg Friedrich] (1685-1759); Haydn, Joseph (1732-1809); Mozart, Wolfgang Amadeus (1756-1791); Beethoven, Ludwig van (1770-1827); Brahms, Johannes (1833-1897); Mendelssohn, Felix (1809-1847).
[422] *Britannica*: Schubert, Franz; Schumann, Franz; Clara.
[423] *Britannica*: transportation, history of: The rise of the automobile; Daimler; Benz. Automobiles powered by electric batteries preceded the gasoline-powered engines of Daimler and Benz. Also see in *Britannica*, flight, history of. Wendell Willkie, *One World* (New York: Simon & Schuster, 1943). It was the best-selling non-fiction book ever published up to that time.
[424] *Britannica*: Victoria (queen of England); Bismarck, Otto.
[425] *Britannica*: McCormick, Cyrus.
[426] National Resources Defense Council, Flint water crisis, at https://www.nrdc.org/flint (accessed December 5, 2020).
[427] *Britannica*: Sullivan, Sir Arthur; Debussy, *Prélude à l'après-midi d'un faune* (1894; *Prelude to the Afternoon of a Faun*); deism; and freemasonry. Neither entry mentions the other. See: https://www.greatseal.com/symbols/reverse.html; https://greatseal.com/mythamerica/notmasonic.html (accessed December 3, 2020).
[428] *Britannica*: Roosevelt, Theodore.
[429] *Britannica*: Wilson, Woodrow.

[430] *Britannica*: Hoover, Herbert. Hoover's reputation plummeted because the Great Depression occurred when he was president, and the U.S. began to recover during the period that followed, when his successor, FDR, was in office. Hoover's defeat in the election in November 1932 is now commonly believed to have been due to his failure to put an end to the Great Depression, but it was more likely due to the promise that FDR offered to end prohibition.

[431] *Britannica*: Churchill, Winston. Also, Sir Charles Wilson (Lord Moran), *Churchill: Taken from the Diaries of Lord Moran. The Struggle for Survival, 1940-1945* (Boston: Houghton Mifflin Company, 1966). Wilson's previous book, *The Anatomy of Courage* (London: Constable, 1945), was based on the dairy that he wrote while serving as a young physician in the trenches in World War I.

[432] *Britannica*: Stalin, Joseph; Lenin, Vladimir; Trotsky, Leon; Gorbachev, Mikhail (defused the Cold War "powder keg"); Putin, Vladimir. Stalin's prison system's name was given in the 3-volume non-fiction text by Aleksander Solzhenitsyn, *The Gulag Archipelago: An Experiment in Literary Investigation* (1973); originally in Russian. Also see: Solzhenitsyn, trans. Ralph Parker, *One Day in the Life of Ivan Denisovich* (New York: Dutton, 1963); and Boris Pasternak, *Dr. Zhivago* (trans., New York: Pantheon Books, 1957), a novel set in the period, 1905-1945.

[433] *Britannica*: Roosevelt, Franklin Delano.

[434] *Britannica*: Roosevelt, Eleanor.

[435] *Britannica*: Hitler, Adolph [born Schicklgruber, Adolph]. A reader suggested that the number in the Holocaust may be as high as eight million Jews throughout Europe.

[436] Other countries that had significant numbers of Nazi-supporters include Austria (which welcomed *Anschluss* with Hitler's Germany); Western Czechoslovakia (which renamed its German-speaking area as *Sudetenland*); France (with its collaborating government in Vichy, headed by Marshal Philippe Petain and Pierre Laval), and Norway (under Vidkun Quisling, whose surname is now a metaphor for dishonor). There was a significant support for Hitler in England before England came under attack.

[437] *Britannica*: Lamarr, Hedy; which mentions Gene Markey, her second husband; and Porter, Cole. For more on Markey, see Hill, *Proceed to Peshawar*, 66-70, et seq.

[438] *Britannica*; Einstein, Albert; Tesla, Nikola; Marconi, Guglielmo; Curie, Pierre, Marie, and Irène. Health problems seriously affected at least four of these brilliant scientists: Edison nearly died from infections on several occasions, and he was famously deaf. He escaped accidental death in explosions and rock falls, which killed his workers. He also worked with dangerous chemicals, such as lead, mercury, and phenol, which injured and killed some of his workers. His glassblower died of radiation-induced cancer, but Edison also survived that radiation without permanent damage. See Hill, *Edison's Environment*. Tesla had many phobias. Pierre Curie's life was cut short when he fell under the wheels of a horse-drawn cart; Marie died of aplastic anemia that was due to exposure to radiation; and Irène died of leukemia, also due to radiation exposure.

[439] *Britannica*: Osler, Sir William.

[440] *Britannica*: Halsted, William.

[441] *Britannica*: Ehrlich, Paul.

[442] *Britannica*: Freud, Sigmund; and Freud, Anna. His daughter was not a physician, but she was a powerful advocate for children. She introduced the concepts of repression and aggression to control impulses.

[443] *Britannica*: Cannon, Walter; Carrell, Alexis; Lindbergh, Charles; Banting, Frederick; Best, Charles. Dakin is not given his own biographical sketch in *Britannica*. There have been countless studies of diabetes and insulin since Banting and Best made their discovery. For example, E. A. Rasio, George J. Hill, J.S. Soeldner, and Manuel G. Herrera, The effect of pancreatectomy on glucose tolerance and extracellular fluid insulin in the dog, *Diabetes*, 16 (1967): 551-6.

[444] *Britannica*: Van Gogh, Vincent; Picasso, Pablo.

[445] *Britannica*: Cushing, Harvey.

[446] *Britannica*: Pavlov, Ivan; Mayo, William and Charles; Crile, George

[447] *Britannica*: MacArthur, Douglas; Marshall, George; Eisenhower, Dwight.

[448] *Britannica*: Mountbatten, Lord; Rommel, Erwin; Yamamoto, Isoroku.

[449] *Britannica*: Truman, Harry S.

[450] *Britannica*: Lindbergh, Charles.

[451] Annette Gordon-Reed, *Thomas Jefferson and Sally Hemings: An American Controversy* (Charlottesville, Virginia; University of Virginia Press, 1997); and Gordon-Reed, *The Hemingses of Monticello: An American Family* (New York: W. W. Norton & Co., 2008). Angela Serratore, President Cleveland's problem child, *Smithsonian Magazine* (September 26, 2013), at: https://www.smithsonianmag.com/history/president-clevelands-problem-child-100800/ (accessed December 12, 2020). Peter Baker, DNA is said to solve a mystery of Warren Harding's love life, *New York Times*, 12 August 2015), at: https://www.nytimes.com/2015/08/13/us/dna-is-said-to-solve-a-mystery-of-warren-hardings-love-

life.html (accessed December 12, 2020). The University of Arizona Health Science Library, Grover Cleveland - secret surgery, at: http://ahsl.arizona.edu/about/exhibits/presidents/cleveland (accessed December 11, 2020).

[452] Brenda Wineapple, On *All the King's Men* by Robert Penn Warren, *New York Times Book Review*, 13 September 2020, 16. Katie Hafner, A Medical mishap sparks rage at the U.S. Health Care System, review of Timothy Snyder, *Our Malady: Lessons in Liberty from a Hospital Diary* (New York: Crown, 2020)

[453] *Britannica*: Thoreau, Henry David; Gandhi, Mahatma [Mohandas Karamchand]; King, Martin Luther, Jr. For Congressman John L Lewis, see: https://www.biography.com/political-figure/john-lewis (accessed December 15, 2020).

[454] *Britannica*: Doyle, Sir Arthur.

[455] *Britannica*: Stowe, Harriet Beecher; Dickens, Charles; Zola, Émile.

[456] *Britannica*: Dostoyevsky, Fyodor; Tolstoy, Leo; Hardy, Thomas; Conrad, Joseph; Cather, Willa; Joyce, James; Kafka, Franz; Huxley, Aldous; Fitzgerald, F. Scott.; Hemingway, Ernest; Orwell, George.

[457] Some of the great novelists of the frontier are profiled in *Britannica*: Washington Irving, Le Grand Cannon, Jr., Mark Twain (Samuel Clemens) (1835-1910), Owen Wister, Bret Harte, Louis Lamour, and Jack London.

[458] *Britannica*: Verdi, Giuseppe; McMurtry, Larry.

[459] Many events in the period of World War II, in 1943-45, can be recalled from correspondence between a father in service and his family at home. See: Hill, *Rolling with Patton* and *The Home Front*. The cut-off year for "current events" is set arbitrarily as beginning in 1920.

[460] EarthSky: "On October 29, 2020, NASA re-established contact with its Voyager 2 spacecraft, launched from Earth in 1977." See: https://earthsky.org/space/nasa-reestablishes-contact-with-voyager2-spacecraft-oct2020# (accessed December 4, 2020). Voyager 1 and 2 still communicate with Earth.

[461] https://healthcare.utah.edu/healthfeed/postings/2012/12/120212ArtificialHeart30YearsLater.php (accessed March 17, 2021). Sanna Khan and Waqas Jehangir, Evolution of artificial hearts: An overview and history, *Cardio Res* 5 (no. 5, October 2014): 121-25.

Chapter 11　The Health Care Industry　A. Health Care at Home

[462] In *The Greatest Benefit to Mankind* (p.31), Porter wrote that when hunter-gatherers moved into communities, "the family remained the first line of defence against illness."

Well-written fiction provides descriptions of treatment of illness at home in earlier centuries. For example, in James A. Michener's *Chesapeake*, in Virginia and Maryland in the seventeenth and early eighteenth centuries, we have mothers using calomel for indigestion, sassafras tea for fever, "purge" for constipation, and pliers to pull rotten teeth (p. 106); ipecac, laxatives, oil of juniper, saffron, glyster, hot linseed oil, tartar emetic, and laudanum (pp. 274-5); and ginseng drops for flux, Venice treacle for cough, hartshorn for congestion, turmeric for weakness of the blood, and "the bark" [quinine] for fever (p.312). Midwives, shamans, and medicine men were standing by to help. A Native American chief, known as werowance, oversees the work of the indigenous specialists.

[463] A few drops of tincture of iodine would help purify water for a boy's canteen. Gentian violet was known by others, but it was officially pioneered by Robert Aldrich at the Harvard Medical School in the 1930s for treatment of burns. It is a good fungicide, too. See: Jack Arbiser, To look anew, *Harvard Medicine* (winter 2021), 5.

B. The Health Care Industry, 1945-1975

[464] A bit of humor reminds the reader of the difference between law and medicine: It has been said that in a small town, no doctor will welcome another doctor to offer a competing practice. A lawyer, on the other hand, has a hard time making a living until another lawyer comes to town, and they can get to work helping citizens sue each other.

[465] Amy Finkelstein, A tough job of reducing waste in health care, *New York Times* (22 January 2021): "Some red tape is purposeless, but not all of it is."

[466] One of New York's hospitals is emblematic of the new model of health care: In the entrance lobby, a person steps immediately onto an escalator with a conveyor belt.

[467] A reader commented that most of the computers in the world only had 2 numbers for each year, the last two. It was feared that as the date moved from 1999 to 2000 the computers would revert to 1900, with ensuing chaos in travel and financial markets. Programs were written, algorithms installed, and the 'chaos' was minimal.

Part Three – Discussion and Conclusion　Chapter 12 Historiography　A. Three Other Books

[468] *Britannica*: Anthropology, on Darwin.

James George Frazer, *The Golden Bough: A Study in Magic and Religion*, edited with an Introduction and Notes by Robert Fraser (1890. Oxford: Oxford University Press, 2009).

[469] Porter, *The Greatest Benefit to Mankind*, 31-2, for medicine-men, healer-priests, shamans, and others who treated illness in early societies: "they are neither fakes nor mad." Also, Sir Thomas Browne, *Religio Medici* (1643).

[470] Jeff Hardin, Ronald L. Numbers, and Ronald A. Binzley, *The Warfare between Science & Religion: The Idea That Wouldn't Die* (Baltimore: Johns Hopkins University Press, 2018); and Andrew Dickson White, *A History of the Warfare of Science with Theology in Christendom*, 2 vols. (London: Macmillan and Company, 1896).

[471] Nicholas Kristof, Pastor, can white evangelicalism be saved? *New York Times*, 20 December 2020, SR9.

[472] Creation Story in Genesis, including "the earth" at the center. In the 17th century, James Ussher, Archbishop of Armagh and Primate of All Ireland, calculated that the 1st Day of Creation was in 4004 BC ("the entrance of the night preceding the 23rd day of October... the year before Christ 4004").

[473] Brahe is said to have remained unconvinced about Copernicus' theory. "Copernicanism made few converts for almost a century after Copernicus' death" (Kuhn, *Structure of Scientific Revolutions*, 149-54). Kuhn says that Tycho Brahe had an "earth-centered astronomical system" (*Structure*, 155); and that "sun worship helped make Kepler a Copernican ... outside of science" (*Structure*, 151-2). See also Brynum, *Science*, 60-1 (Brahe, Kepler).

[474] Lawrence M. Principe, in Hardin, *Warfare*, 6-19; "obsession with law" (p.13).

[475] Thomas H. Aechtner, in Hardin, *Warfare*, 302-23.

[476] Peter Harrison, in Hardin, *Warfare*, 239-57.

[477] Science never achieves a perfect result. It is always searching.

[478] Protestants in the United States follow the ancient Greek text of the Ten Commandments (the *Septuagint*). "Many of the central concepts of the Mormon religion are laid out in the Articles of Faith, a 13-point list of the Latter-day Saints' most important religious beliefs [including] a belief in the Bible as the word of God." From "The Mormon Faith" at https://www.pbs.org/mormons/faqs/ (accessed December 19, 2020).

[479] Quakers are not required to affirm a belief in God, or that Jesus is divine. Unitarian-Universalists recognize the importance of a spiritual aspect of life, but the way this is defined is left to the individual. Ethical Societies are composed of members who come from different backgrounds, especially Jews and Protestants.

[480] A.F. & A.M. = Ancient Free and Accepted Masons. The Order of the Eastern Star takes its name from the "star in the east" that pointed the way to Jesus' birthplace in Bethlehem (Matthew 2:2). Many Scout meetings conclude with this ecumenical prayer: "May the Great Scoutmaster of all good Scouts be with until we meet again."

[481] Larry Levitt, Trump vs. Biden on health care, *JAMA* 324 (no. 14, 13 October 2020):1384-5.

[482] Kristen Kobes Du Mez, *Jesus and John Wayne: How White Evangelicals Corrupted a Faith and Fractured a Nation* (New York: W. W. Norton, 2020), and her article, Evangelicals: Five myths, *Washington Post*, 24 January 2021: "The National Association of Evangelicals' website says a key tenet of evangelicalism is a belief in the 'infallible' authority of the Bible."

[483] In 2016, Clinton received 65.9M popular votes (48.2% of votes cast) and 227 Electoral College votes. Trump received 63.0M (46.1%) and 304 Electoral College votes. In 2020, Biden received 81.2M (51.3%) popular votes and 306 Electoral College votes. Trump received 74.2M (48.7%) and 232. Trump's percentage of the popular vote fell, but his total vote increased by 11.2M. See: https://abcnews.go.com/Politics/hillary-clinton-officially-wins-popular-vote-29-million/story?id=44354341; and https://www.businessinsider.com/2016-2020-electoral-maps-exit-polls-compared-2020 (accessed December 21, 2010).

The anti-abortion plan in 2021 appears to be to go beyond repeal of *Roe v Wade*, and to plead that fetuses are protected by the Fourteenth Amendment. By Federal law, abortions would thus be completely illegal, and states would not have the right to allow exemptions. XIV (Section 1): "All persons born or naturalized in the United States and subject to the jurisdiction thereof, are citizens of the United States and of the State wherein they reside. No State shall make or enforce any law which shall abridge the privileges or immunities of citizens of the United States; nor shall any State deprive any person of life, liberty, or property, without due process of law; nor deny to any person within its jurisdiction the equal protection of the laws." See: Michelle Goldberg, The authoritarian plan for an abortion ban, *New York Times*, 6 April 6, 2021, A18.

[484] Mychal Denzel Smith, *Stakes is [sic] High: Life After the American Dream* (Hachette Group: Bold Type Books, 2020), quoted in a review by Paul C. Taylor, Delusions, justice, accountability and freedom in America, *Washington Post*, 20 December 2020, B6. The soliloquy by the imaginary Evangelical is fictional, written for *Health Matters*.

[485] Harry Flickinger, We'll take the vaccine, *Washington Post*, 19 December 2020, A18 (Letters to the editor). On LinkedIn, Harry Flickinger is a retired U.S. Assistant Attorney General.

[486] Ian Hacking, "Introductory Essay" in Thomas S. Kuhn, *The Structure of Scientific Revolutions*, 4th edition (Chicago: The University of Chicago Press, 2012), xix. For acronyms that substitute for words, think of TED (Technology, Entertainment, Design), STEM (Science, Technology, Engineering, Mathematics), and CRT (Critical Race Theory). It is now often necessary to use a cellphone to search for the meaning of an unfamiliar acronym when it appears in a newspaper without a definition.

[487] Bill Bryson takes this comprehensive view of history in his book, *A Short History of Almost Everything*.

[488] Kuhn, *Structure*, 150 (quotation from *Origin*), 170-1 (Kuhn, "no goal set either by God or nature"). A prominent life-long opponent to *Origin* was Louis Agassiz (1807-1873).
Britannica, Agassiz: For "life-long opponent of Darwin's theory," https://ucmp.berkeley.edu/history/agassiz.html (accessed December 22, 2020).

[489] Leslie A. Pray, Discovery of DNA structure and function: Watson and Crick, *Nature Education* 1 (no. 1, 2008): 100, at: https://www.nature.com/scitable/topicpage/discovery-of-dna-structure-and-function-watson (accessed December 21, 2020).

[490] Venesection appears in 21 citations in Major, *History of Medicine*, from "primitive" (p.9) to Skoda (p.782). There are references to Chinese, Greek, Hebrew, and later physicians. Bleeding was advised by Hippocrates: "Bleeding and cupping, ancient and accepted therapeutic measures, were to remain an important part of the physician's armamentarium for nearly two thousand years!" Benjamin Rush (1745-1813) "bled to the point of faintness" (p. 727). Francois Magendie (1782-1855) and Josef Skoda (1808-1881) in the late nineteenth century were opposed to bleeding, but they were lone voices. Magendie mocked the practice. Venesection gradually disappeared without additional comment by Major. It is not mentioned in *Britannica*.

[491] The anti-vaccination movement developed new life after Andrew Wakefield published a report in *Lancet* in 1988 that connected development of autism with childhood vaccines containing mercury. The report was challenged and 12 years later, Wakefield lost his medical license, but the anti-vax movement has thrived, nevertheless. See Wakefield's unauthorized biography, reviewed by Saad B. Omer, "The discredited doctor hailed by the anti-vaccine movement," *Nature* 586 (27 October 2020): 668-9.

[492] George J. Hill, Testimony on Laetrile, in "Laetrile: The Commissioner's Decision," HEW publication No. 77-3056 (Superintendent of Documents, U.S. Government Printing Office, Washington, DC 20402, 1977); and in Supreme Court of the United States, United States et al v. Rutherford et al, No. 78-605, p 11, June 18, 1979. "Hill's testimony against Laetrile was cited in the unanimous decision by U.S. Supreme Court which reversed and remanded the decisions by the U.S. District Court and Court of Appeals that had allowed Laetrile to be used in 'terminally ill cancer patients'." Hill is quoted in 442 U.S. 544 (1979), No. 78-605, p. 557, from his longer statement in 42 Fed. Reg. 39768, 39787 (1977).

[493] Drummond Rennie, Thyroid storm, *JAMA* 277 (no. 15, 16 April 1997):1238-1243: Comment by: Ralph T. King, Jr., Long-suppressed thyroid study shows costlier drug isn't better, *Wall Street Journal* (April 16, 1997). At: https://jamanetwork.com/journals/jama/article-abstract/415402, and https://www.wsj.com/articles/SB861137272686553500 (accessed December 22, 2020).

[494] Jeffrey Brainard and Jia You, What a massive database of retracted papers reveals about science publishing's "death penalty," *Science* (25 October 2018) at: https://www.sciencemag.org/news/2018/10/what-massive-database-retracted-papers-reveals-about-science-publishing-s-death-penalty (accessed March 26, 2021): "Ivan Oransky and Adam Marcus, who founded the blog Retraction Watch, based in New York City—to get more insight into just how many scientific papers were being withdrawn, and why. They began to assemble a list of retractions. That list, formally released to the public this week as a searchable database, is now the largest and most comprehensive of its kind. It includes more than 18,000 retracted papers and conference abstracts dating back to the 1970s." For an account of falsified but nevertheless continuously funded experiments, see: Helene Z. Hill, *Hidden Data: The Blind Eye of Science*. 3d ed. (2016. Baltimore, Maryland: Bookwhip, 2019).

[495] In 1990 my lecture at the National Naval Medical Center was entitled "Is p53 an oncogene, or not?" I had studied mutant p53 on sabbatical in 1988 when p53 was considered to be an oncogene.

[496] "communities of perhaps one hundred members," in Kuhn, *Structure*, Postscript, p.117.

[497] A "phage group" is mentioned in Kuhn, *Structure*, Postscript, 177. This would be a "scientific community" that would understand the details of CRISPR-Cas 9, and its use against SARS-CoV-2, the virus that causes COVID-19. Also see many other references in the Index of *Structure* to "communities, scientific."

CRISPRs are DNA sequences found in prokaryotes (bacteria and archaea) that are derived from infections by phages that contained these DNA fragments. The earliest studies of the biological system now known as CRISPR began in 1987. The genome editing technique using CRISPR-Cas9 technology has a wide range of applications. For instance, it has been used to engineer probiotic cultures in yogurt, to immunize industrial cultures against infections, and to improve crop yields. Emmanuelle Charpentier and Jennifer Doudna were awarded the Nobel Prize in Chemistry in 2020 for discovering the application of this technology. It appears that the acquired spacer regions of CRISPR-Cas systems are a form of Lamarckian evolution, in that they are transmitted from acquired mutations. The Cas gene, on the other hand, is an example of Darwinian evolution. CRISPR technology is now being employed in the battle against COVID-19 to produce mRNA vaccines. See also: E. V. Koonin and Y. I. Wolf, Just how Lamarckian is CRISPR-Cas immunity? The continuum of evolutionary mechanisms, *Biology Direct* 11 (no. 1, February 2026): 9. Also: Jennifer

Stratton, CRISPR vs COVID-19: How can gene editing help beat a virus? *Biotechniques* 69 (no. 5, 2 November 2020). At: https://www.future-science.com/doi/ 10.2144/btn-2020-0145 (accessed December 23, 2020).

[498] *Merriam-Webster*, Whig. From www.merriam-webster.com/dictionary (accessed December 28, 2020).

For Whig history of Science, the debate continues. The term "Whig history" was coined by Herbert Butterfield in *The Whig Interpretation of History* (1931). Stephen Weinberg, Eye on the Present – The Whig History of Science, *The New York Review of Books*, 17 December 2015.

[499] Quote from Butterfield in Adrian Wilson and T. G. Ashplant, Whig history and present-centered history, *The Historical Journal*, 31 (no. 1, March 1988): 1–16, p. 10. Also, review of Herbert Butterfield, *The Whig Interpretation of History* (undated) from: https://www.univ.ox.ac.uk/book/the-whig-interpretation-of-history/ (accessed February 23, 2020).

[500] Steven Weinberg, *Third Thoughts: The Universe We Still Don't Know* (Cambridge, Mass.: Harvard University Press/Belknap Press, 2019). Steven Weinberg received the 1979 Nobel Prize in Physics. See Weinberg, Eye on the present—The Whig History of Science," *New York Review of Books* (December 17, 2015): From https://www.nybooks.com/articles/2015/12/17/eye-present-whig-history-science/(accessed February 23, 2020).

Arthur M. Silverstein, comments on Weinberg's article, *New York Review of Books* (25 February 2016), at https://www.nybooks.com/articles/2016/02/25/the-whig-history-of-science-an-exchange/ (accessed February 23, 2020). Silverman is Emeritus Professor, Johns Hopkins Medical School.

Thonyc.wordpress [Thony Christie],"The Renaissance Mathematicus" [blog]: https://thonyc.wordpress.com/2015/08/19/to-explain-the-weinberg-the-discovery-of-a-nobel-laureates-view-of-the-history-of-science/ (accessed February 23, 2020).

B. Telling the Story of History

[501] A contrary view of history can be imputed from the final words of F. Scott Fitzgerald in *The Great Gatsby* (New York: Charles Scribner's Sons, 1925): "boats against the current, borne endlessly into the past." The meaning of these words is endlessly discussed, but there can be no doubt that history itself, like time, is always moving forward.

[502] The two formulas are from Newton's Second Law of Motion. Calculus was described independently by Newton and Gottfried Wilhelm Leibniz. See: Smithsonian: How Things Work, at https://howthingsfly.si.edu/ask-an-explainer/what-difference-between-fma; and https://www.grc.nasa.gov/www/k-12/airplane/newton2c.html (accessed December 30, 2020).

[503] *Britannica*: Napoleonic code.

[504] Emile Zola, *Germinal* (1885) told the story of coal miners in northern France, set in the 1860s. It is rare to see correspondence from both husband and wife in wartime. Exceptions: John Adams and his wife Abigail in the Revolutionary War in America: Charles Francis Adams, *Familiar Letters of John Adams and His Wife Abigail Adams, During the Revolution with a Memoir of Mrs. Adams* (Boston: Houghton Mifflin Company, 1875). Also, books by George J. Hill: in World War II, *Rolling with Patton* and *The Home Front*; and in World War I, *War Letters, 1917-1918*. Charles Dickens tells the story of the lives of poor children in England in the 19th century in many of his books, such as *A Christmas Carol*. They are based on his own childhood.

[505] In 1846 and 1917, the decision was made by the President and a small group of men in Washington, D.C., and then the Congress was persuaded to declare war. It was not a decision made by the American people. They didn't have choices in these matters.

[506] The Declarations of War in 1846 and 1917 were opposed by many Americans. Bernard DeVoto, *The Year of Decision, 1846* (Boston: Houghton Mifflin, 1942). Anon., "George Bancroft, Secretary of the Navy under Polk" at: https://teachinghistory.org/history-content/ask-a-historian/22205 (accessed January 1, 2021). Sidney B. Fay, *The Origins of the World War*; Barbara Tuchman, *The Guns of August*; and Paul Fussell, *The Great War and Modern Memory* (1974. New York: Sterling, 2009).

[507] Some of the ways that lives are suddenly changed and which are reflected in pain are discussed in Hill, *Outpatient Surgery* (Philadelphia: W. B. Saunders Co., 1973), Chapter 27, "Excruciating Pain," 977-93. https://www.mayoclinic.org/healthy-lifestyle/adult-health/in-depth/sleep-aids/art-20047860 (accessed January 2, 2021). Jane E. Brody, Steroids are no help for respiratory issues, *New York Times*, 29 December 2020, D7. Contac: https://www.webmd.com/drugs/2/drug-54534-1096/contac-oral/non-opioid-antitussive-w-decongestant-oral/details (accessed January 2, 2021).

[508] Darnton spoke at a seminar at Drew University in 2000.

C. A Driver of History?

[509] Edward Gibbon, *Decline and Fall*, "As the happiness of a future life is the great object of religion, we may hear without surprise or scandal that the introduction, or at least the abuse of Christianity, had some influence on the decline and fall of the Roman empire" (Chapter 38).

Another example of differing views of history is seen in the ways that the story of Franklin D. Roosevelt's successful campaign in 1932. One view is that FDR's promise of a New Deal led to victory, and he cemented his popularity by successfully enacting the many parts of the New Deal. This view was expressed by Jamelle Bouie, F.D.R. Didn't just fix the economy, a major Opinion article in the *New York Times* (19 April 1930), 19. Bouie quotes Eric Raushway, *Why the New Deal Matters* (New Haven: Yale University Press, 2021), who called the New Deal the "third founding moment in the history of American democracy." Bouie did not mention that many Americans never accepted the New Deal, and that it is still resented by many, especially in the Midwest. They still abhor the taxes which funded WPA, CCC, and Social Security. They still remember that FDR removed the gold standard for currency, which undercut the value of paper money. Also, Bouie never mentions the importance of reversal of prohibition, which the *Times* recognized in November 1932 was the reason that FDR won the election; it was not his promise of a New Deal. Arthur Krock wrote about it in the *Times* as he discussed the election results. See also https://mises.org/library/real-reason-fdrs-popularity (accessed April 28, 2021): "The Real Reason for FDR's Popularity," "FDR had been a 'dry' candidate, but as he built his campaign for the presidency in 1932, he agreed to become a 'wet' in order to receive the Democratic Party nomination at the convention in Chicago. He made a campaign promise to overturn the 18th Amendment and to legalize drinking. He did exactly what he promised to do. The results for liberty and economy were immediate."

D. On the Subject of Intellectual History

[510] Harrison Smith, David Brion Davis, obituary, *The Washington Post*, 17 April 2019, B6; quoting Davis in *American Heritage* magazine, 2005.

Chapter 13 Recent History   The Last 120 Years

[511] The present conflict between Islam and Christianity developed from three unrelated reasons. Although the ancient enmities in the Middle East played a role, the immediate causes of the present conflict developed in the early and middle of the 20th century. They were the unrelated issues of oil in Saudi Arabia, the Jewish resettlement issue in Palestine, and the Cold War between the USSR and its Communist allies versus the non-Communist nations aligned with the North Atlantic Treaty Organization (NATO).

[512] The "American Century" is probably a better expression than the "American Age." The name was given by Fredrik Logevall, *JFK: Coming of Age in the American Century, 1917-1956* (New York: Random House, 2020). David M. Kennedy, The charmer, *New York Times Books* 13 December 2020, 18, says it is the first of "two projected volumes." However, David Brooks assumed that the present period was already known as the American Century. See: Brooks, The case for new optimism, *New York Times*, 21 January 2021: "Donald Trump's patriotism was bloated and fear-based. Biden's is the self-confident patriotism he absorbed by growing up in a certain sort of country during the American century."

[513] Ronald Reagan's words "shining city on a hill" became the motto of the Republican Party. They were derived from Perry Miller's immensely popular work, *Errand into the Wilderness* (1956), in which Miller quoted John Winthrop's sermon of March 21, 1630, "A Model of Christian Charity."

Abram C. Van Engen, *City on a Hill: A History of American Exceptionalism* (New Haven: Yale University Press, 2020). From https://www.neh.gov/article/how-america-became-city-upon-hill (accessed February 6, 2021). A forceful description of the American Empire is given by William H. Lamar IV, Will America finally abandon its racist myth? *Washington Post*, 16 December 2020, A27.

[514] The process has already begun, according to Nicholas Kristof, What are sperm telling us? *New York Times*, 21 February 27, 2021), 7: "Sperm counts are dropping." Citing Shanna H. Swan, *Count Down* (2021), Kristof says that "Swan and other experts say the problem is a class of chemicals called endocrine disruptors … These endocrine disruptors are everywhere: plastics, shampoos, cosmetics, cushions, pesticides, canned foods and A.T.M. receipts. "In some ways, the sperm-count decline is akin to where global warming was 40 years ago." In an eerie prescience to the report of impending infertility of men, the dystopian novel by P.D. James, *The Children of Men*, was set in the year 2021. Our year now!!! In her novel, all men had become infertile, and life on earth was set to come to an end.

[515] The organization known as "Population Connection" has recently been reorganized. The President, John Seager, commented that "Since the era of rapid population growth began around 1800, it's taken more than two full centuries for us to reach current overpopulation levels," *Population Connection* 52 (no. 4, December 2020), 1. The ZPG Society is recognized on pages 8-12. See: https://www.populationconnection.org/ (accessed February 6, 2021).

Chapter 14 Discussion and Conclusion   Final Thoughts

[516] I will restate here the principal references that guided me in this essay about *Health Matters* in history: Alfred Thayer Mahan, *The Influence of Sea Power upon History, 1660-1783* (Cambridge, University Press, 1890); Thomas S. Kuhn, *The Structure of Scientific Revolutions* (Chicago: *University of Chicago Press*, 1962); William H. McNeill, *Plagues and Peoples* (New York: Random House, 1976); Alfred Crosby, Jr. *The Columbian Exchange:*

Biological and Cultural Consequences of 1492 (Westport, Conn.: Greenwood Press, 1972); Hans Zinsser, *Rats, Lice, and History* (London: George Routledge & Sons, 1935); Jared Diamond, *Guns, Germs, and Steel: The Fates of Human Societies* (New York: W. W. Norton & Co., 1997); Roy Porter, *The Greatest Benefit to Mankind: A Medical History of Humanity*. New York: Norton, 1999); Lynn Payer, *Medicine and Culture* (New York: Henry Holt and Company, 1988); C. P. Snow, *The Two Cultures* (Cambridge: Cambridge University Press, 1959), and Paul Starr, *The Social Transformation of American Medicine: The Rise of a Sovereign Profession and the Making of a Vast Industry* (New York: Basic Books, 1984).

Appendix A Death

[517] W. C. Firebaugh, trans., *The Satyricon of Petronius Arbiter*, with an Essay by Charles Whibley (New York: Liveright Publishing Co., n.d. [1922]), 191. The passage continues, "Know that thy head is partly dead this day!" and on p.194: "The very corpse lying there ought to convince you that your duty is to live! *The Oxford Universal Dictionary* does not show "death" and "die" in sex, but see: https://www.urbandictionary.com/define.php?term =The%20Little%20Death (accessed July 13, 2020).

[518] *Britannica, Arrowsmith*. The fictional Dr. Martin Arrowsmith developed an "experimental serum" for plague, although the book actually stated that it was a phage (a bacteriophage).

[519] Berton Rouché, *The Incurable Wound* (Boston, Little Brown, 1958).

[520] Virgil, *The Aeneid*; trans. Robert Fitzgerald (New York: Vintage, 1983): Book IV, line 109 ("need"), 119 ("love"), 142 ("marriage"), 144 ("passion"), 293 ("lust"); 922 ("red blood drenched her hands"); Ed West, *1066 and Before All That: The Battle of Hastings, Anglo-Saxon and Norman England* (New York: Skyhorse Publishing, 2017); and Robert K. Massie, *The Romanovs: The Final Chapter* (New York: Random House, 2012).

Britannica: Genghis Khan, Tamerlane, Babur. Also, Annette Susannah Beveridge, *The Babur Nama* (New York: Alfred A. Knopf, 2020), reviewed by Dwight Garner, When not piling up corpses, a charming sort of fellow, *New York Times Books*, 1 December 2020, C6.

The fate of Napoleon's army was shown in what is said to be the best statistical graph ever drawn. The graph was drawn by Charles Joseph Minard in 1869 (20x9in.); reproduced with comment by Edward R. Tuttle, *The Visual Display of Quantitative Information* (Cheshire, Conn.: Graphics Pres, n.d. [c. 1990]). One of the most terrible incidents occurred on the retreat across the Berenzia River, which was attempted by 50,000 soldiers, of whom 25,000 drowned.

[521] *Britannia*, Frank, Anna; and Arendt, Hannah, who had a romantic relationship with Martin Heidegger before he joined the Nazi party.

[522] Emily Petsko, Reports of Mark Twain's quote about death are greatly exaggerated, *History* (2 November 2018). at https://www.mentalfloss.com/article/562400/reports-mark-twains-quote-about-mark-twains-death-are-greatly-exaggerated (accessed February 21, 2021). One example of the dozens of "false death" claims from COVID-19 was discussed on NBC News Now: Dr. Kavita Patel, The truth about CDC's COVID-19 death rate – and the conspiracies undermining it (29 September 2020), at: https://www.nbcnews.com/think/opinion/truth-about-cdc-s-covid-19-death-rate-conspiracies-undermining-ncna1241343 (accessed February 21, 2021).

My own death was erroneously reported, and then retracted, without explanation: Richard E. Gallagher, In memoriam, George J. Hill, M.D., Ph.D. *Journal of Cancer Education* 29 (2014): 213; and Gallagher, Erratum to: In memoriam, George J. Hill, M.D., Ph.D. *Journal of Cancer Education* 30 (2015): 815.

[523] Paul de Kruif was a silent partner in Lewis' book, *Arrowsmith*.

Books for the general reader which show the effect of infectious diseases on human history are: Hans Zinsser, *Rats, Lice and History: A Study in Biography* (1935. New York: Pocket Books, 1945); Geddes Smith, *Plague on Us* (New York: The Commonwealth Fund, 1940); William H. McNeill (*Plagues and Peoples* (1975. Garden City, N.Y.: Random House, Inc., 1998); Alfred W. Crosby, Jr., *The Columbian Exchange: Biological and Cultural Consequences of 1492* (1973. Westport, Conn.: Praeger Publishers, 2003); Jared Diamond, *Guns, Germs, and Steel: The Fates of Human Societies* (New York: W. W. Norton, 1997); and Frank M. Snowden, *Epidemics and Society: From the Black Death to the Present* (2019. New Haven: Yale University Press, 2020). Also the forthcoming book by Kyle Harper, *Plagues Upon the Earth: Disease and the Course of Human History*. It is based on research for the article by Harper, Ancient Rome has an urgent warning for us, *New York Times* (17 February 2017), A19. This article focuses on the emperor Commodus (ruled A.D. 180-192) and the Antonine Plague which killed "as many as 2,000 Romans a day," a total of seven to 10 million people, 2,000 years ago. The cause is unknown, but Harper says "the likeliest culprit is an ancestor of the smallpox virus."

Zinsser was the chairman of microbiology at Harvard Medical School. He was the author of *A Textbook of Microbiology* (1910); later editions were known as *Zinsser Microbiology*. He was popular as a science writer for the *Atlantic Monthly* magazine – erudite and humorous. His semi-fictional autobiography was entitled *As I Remember*

Him: The Biography of R. S. (1940). *Rats, Lice, and History* is in the same tongue-in-cheek style, which may have diminished its academic impact. The statement on the back cover is correct and devastating: "Typhus, the villain of the piece, has been man's enemy for 1500 years and has played as great a part in the history of civilization as Alexander the Great, Caesar, or Napoleon."

The back cover of *Plagues and Peoples* says that McNeill "explores the political, demographic, and psychological effects of disease on the human race over the entire sweep of human history, from prehistory to the present." He dismisses Zinsser. Whether McNeill failed to read Zinsser carefully, or because he was focused only on the chapters about typhus, he does Zinsser a great disservice.

The back cover of *The Colombian Exchange* states that Crosby makes "a simple point: the most important changes germinated by the voyages of Columbus were not social or political, but biological in nature." Crosby is even more dismissive of Zinsser than was McNeill. He only cites Zinsser in an endnote, without comment. Zinsser's style was intentionally informal and amusing for the lay reader, unlike the style of writing of professional historians such as McNeill and Crosby.

In *Guns, Germs, and Steel*, Diamond argues that Eurasian peoples dominated others because of the advantages they gained through geography and a temperate climate; and that one of the consequences of civilization is recurring epidemics of infectious diseases. Diamond's book had an enormous impact on thoughts about science and history in the late twentieth century. The crucial role of geography in human history was also described by Ed Douglas, *Himalaya: A Human History* (New York, W. W. Norton, 2020), reviewed by Jeffrey Gettleman, The Earth's extremes, *New York Times Book Review*, 10 January 2021, 1, 17. Douglas places the Himalaya (Sanskrit = "abode of snows") at the center of half of the world's population, and they depend on water that flows from these mountains. The 2,000 miles of the Himalaya extend from the Hindu Kush in Kyrgyzstan to Myanmar in the east, and the rivers that flow from this range water the land in India and China, and also Pakistan, Nepal, Bangladesh, and Vietnam. Think of the Indus, the Ganges, the Mekong, and the Yangtze.

Geddes Smith, in *Plague on Us*, says that he "merely set down as clearly as I can some facts and theories about communicable disease that have interested me and, I hope will interest other laymen." Smith used footnotes for "the more important direct quotations," and only a few sources are referenced at chapter endings. *Plague on Us* is a beautifully constructed book for the layman, but it offers no new perspective nor any new sources.

Frank Snowden, in *Epidemics and Society*, presents the hypothesis that "epidemics are not an esoteric subfield for the interested specialist but instead are a more part of the 'big picture' of historical change and development." Snowden uses examples from several important epidemics to show how infectious diseases have influenced human history, in the triad of infectious agents, humans, and the environment. Snowden selected several diseases as examples: plague, smallpox, yellow fever, dysentery, typhus, cholera, tuberculosis, malaria, polio, HIV/AIDS, and "emerging and reemerging diseases." His book was published in 2019, shortly before COVID-19 appeared in Wuhan, China, and which soon spread across the world. Snowden wrote a new Preface to the paperback edition, published in 2020, discussing the COVID-19 and comparing it with other recent viral challenges such as avian flu [H5N1], AIDS, Ebola, MERS, and Zika, which he refers to as "spillovers" from humans' close contact with the original host animals.

[524] *Britannica:* Whitman and Longfellow both remembered tragic deaths in their personal lives – Whitman, as a hospital worker in the Civil War; and Longfellow, whose first wife was fatally burned in a fire in their home.

[525] Lawrence Van Gelder, Vera Lynn, singer whose wartime ballads cheered Britain, is dead at 103, *New York Times*, 19 June 2020, A25. Her most famous World War II songs were "We'll Meet Again," "(There'll Be Bluebirds Over) The White Cliffs of Dover," and "A Nightingale Sang in Berkeley Square." Vera Lynn, CBE, known as the "Forces' Sweetheart," died on June 18, 2020.

[526] *Britannica*, Miller, Arthur, and Sherriff, R[obert]. C[edric].

[527] *Britannica*, Shakespeare, William, and Eliot, T[homas]. S[tearns].

[528] *Britannica. Casablanca.* Dooley Wilson in "As Time Goes By." Bach's "Alle Menschen" (BWV 643), recorded by Fabian Schwarzkopf on the Sauer Organ at Thomaskirche, Leipzig on 12/8/2012, is on YouTube at: https://www.youtube.com/watch?v=77CP5YitoGk (accessed July 18, 2020).

[529] Dr. Sullivan made this statement at the Commencement Address in 1978 at Marshall University in Huntington, W.Va. He remembered his days as an African American boy growing up in Charleston, W.Va. He was later Secretary of Health and Human Services.

[530] *The Methodist Hymnal* (New York: The Methodist Publishing House), 1939.

[531] https://www.navy.mil/navydata/nav_legacy.asp?id=172 (accessed June 10, 2020).

[532] *Britannica*, Verdi, Giuseppe, and Puccini, Giacomo.

[533] *Britannica*, Hitchcock, Alfred; du Maurier, Daphne; Christie, Agatha; Welles, Orson; Lucas, George (*Star Wars*); and Rowling, J[oanne]. K[athleen]. The *New York Times*, 19 July 2020, has an article about the popular music group Dixie Chicks' new release, "Gaslighter," without reference to the origin of the term. The connection appears on the second page of a Google search for "Gaslighting," as https://www.pri.org/stories/2016-10-14/heres-where-gaslighting-got-its-name (accessed July 12, 2020).

[534] *Britannica*, Remarque, Erich Maria; and Hemingway, Ernest. *Paths of Glory* recalls a forgotten comment in Caesar's *Commentaries on the Gallic Wars*, in which Caesar wrote that the last of the Gaul tribesmen to arrive for battle would be killed "as an example to the others." *Pour encourager les autres* was an excuse for execution of innocent men that was said to have been used by the French army in World War I; it has been attributed to Voltaire, but I found it in Caesar's *Commentaries*.

[535] *Britannica*, Collins, Wilkie; and Conan Doyle, Sir Arthur.

[536] *Dunkirk* focused on the British soldiers, and their miseries. It was controversial, because it showed little about the enemy, or why they were fighting.

[537] The Grimm brothers' fairy tales are dated between 1812 and 1858. Hans Christian Anderson's *Fairy Tales* were first published in 1835. *Anderson's Fairy Tales Told in Words of One Syllable*, illustrated by Hart A. Purdy (Akron, Ohio: Saalfield Publishing Co., n.d. [c. 1931]).

[538] *Britannica*, Day of the Dead.

[539] Charles Samuel Addams (1912-1988) was the cartoonist who created the "Addams Family" cartoons.

[540] Stephen D. Stark, The four days that made Tv news, *American Heritage* 48 (no. 3, May/June 1997).

[541] *Britannica*, Hitchcock, Sir Alfred.

[542] *Britannica*, Diana, Princess of Wales; Kelly, Grace. Princess Diana's shocking death was followed by a solemn state funeral with live coverage.

[543] *Britannica*, September 11 attacks (United States [2001]) and September 11 attacks and aftermath in pictures. A map of the flight routes of the four hijacked airplanes is shown in *Britannica*. United Airlines Flight 93 crashed in Shanksville, Pa. A reader pointed out that an additional death toll includes about 1400 who have died of cancer and other causes that are directly related to the products of combustion from the buildings.

Also see: https://www.history.com/topics/21st-century/9-11-attacks (accessed June 15, 2020). The attacks on 9/11 were orchestrated by Osama bin Laden, whose organization, al Qaeda (Arabic = the Base), was reacting to America's involvement in the Middle East.

[544] *Silence of the Lambs* probably based on a true story. See: https://documentarylovers.com/film/silence-of-lambs-true-story/ (accessed July 10, 2020).

[545] INRI (*Iesus Nazarenus Rex Iudaeorum*), The Catholic Miscellany, from https://themiscellany.org/2017/07/22/what-does-inri-stand-for/ (accessed July 10, 2010).

Britannica: Munch, Edvard; and Rodin, Auguste.

[546] *Britannica*: Heinlein, Robert; and Stevenson, Robert Louis. The movie, *2001: A Space Odyssey*, was based on short stories by Arthur C. Clarke.

[547] Elizabeth Kubler Ross and David Kessler, *On Grief and Grieving: Finding the Meaning of Grief Through the Five Stages of Loss* (1969. New York: Scribner's, 2005).

[548] See the Tuskegee study, above. For the Guatemala study, see: The Presidential Commission for the Study of Bioethical Issues, *"Ethically Impossible" STD Research in Guatemala from 1946 to 1948* (Washington, D.C.: [Government Printing Office], www.bioethics.gov: 2011), 93: "Ethically Impossible" is from an article by Waldemar Kaempffert in the *New York Times* in 1947; the leadership of the USPHS immediately realized that their project was in jeopardy.

Ann M. Jacobsen, *Operation Paperclip: The Secret Intelligence Program that Brought Nazi Scientists to America* (Boston: Little, Brown, 2014), 455.

Nicholas D. Kristof, Unmasking horror – a special report: Japan confronting gruesome war atrocity, *The New York Times*, 17 March 1995; Tsuneishi Keiichi (trans. John Junkerman), Unit 731 and the Japanese Imperial Army's biological warfare program, *The Asia Pacific Journal* 3 (no. 11, Nov. 24, 2005); and S. H. Harris, *Factories of Death: Japanese Biological Warfare, 1932—1945, and the American Cover-up* (New York: Routledge, 2002).

Britannica, Mengele, Josef. See below (Plasmodium) for malaria experiments at the NIH.

[549] See Social Connections for an introduction to altruism. The death of an altruistic person may even be as a sacrifice to save the other.

[550] *Britannica*, Scott, Robert Falcon: "At the end of his strength and hoping to aid his companions by his own disappearance, Oates crawled out into a blizzard on March 17, at 79°50′ S." The Eskimo story is from John McPhee, *Coming in to the Country* (New York: Farrar & Straus, 1976).

[551] The subject of death in religion is discussed in more detail in a separate section of this essay. It is simply summarized in this paragraph. Several meanings of "mortal" are given in *Merriam-Webster*, including, as an adjective, 2a: "subject to death," and 5: "human"; and as a noun, "a human being." In Latin, *mors* is a noun; its adjective is *mortalis*. Methuselah, in Genesis 5:27. The ten plagues are in Exodus 7:14-12:36. https://www.livescience.com/58638-science-of-the-10-plagues.html (accessed June 8, 2020). Romans 14:7-8: "We do not live to ourselves, and we do not die to ourselves."

Werner Keller (trans. William Neil), *The Bible as History: A Confirmation of the Book of Books* 13th ed. (1956. New York: William Morrow and Company, 1964), and Keller (trans. Dr. William Neil), *The Bible as History in Pictures* (1963. New York: William Morrow and Company, 1964).

[552] *Britannica*, Sacrifice, sections on Human Sacrifice, and Other Sacrifices (Hindu, pre-historic, pre-Colombian, Roman, etc.). Sacrifice has a religious origin, as the word is derived from "sacred." See Religion (below) for more about Sacrifice and Self-Sacrifice in *Health Matters*.

Genesis 3:1 (KJV): "Now the serpent was more subtil than any beast of the field which the LORD God had made"; Matthew 4:1 (KJV): "Then was Jesus led up of the Spirit into the wilderness to be tempted of the devil."

[553] The estimate of deaths of servicemen in the Civil War, from wounds and non-battle causes, is estimated at 620,000 by the American Battlefield Trust, and at 750,000 by a recent re-evaluation. James McPherson, quoted by Drew Gilpin Faust, estimated that 50,000 civilians died during the Civil War. About 3.2 million were engaged in the war: 2.1M in the North, and 1.1M in the South. See: https://www.battlefields.org/learn/articles/civil-war-casualties (accessed June 13, 2020). Guy Gugliotta, New estimate raises Civil War death toll, *New York Times*, 3 April 2012; and https://www.nps.gov/nr/travel/national_cemeteries/Death.html# (accessed June 13, 2020). American Battlefield Trust, Civil War Facts, at https://www.battlefields.org/learn/articles/civil-war-facts#How%20many%20soldiers%20fought%20in%20the%20Civil%20War? (accessed April 1, 2021).

[554] *Battle Hymn of the Republic* ("Mine eyes have seen the glory of the coming of the Lord") was first published in *The Atlantic Monthly* in February 1862. See https://www.theatlantic.com/entertainment/archive/2010/11/the-battle-hymn-of-the-republic-americas-song-of-itself/66070/ (accessed June 13, 2020).

[555] Booth, John Wilkes, from *Britannica*.

[556] Winston Churchill, *The World Crisis*, vol. 1, *1911-1914*, 2-4, about the crisis that he saw recurring in 1938; and "another Thirty Years War" which ended in 1945 (actually, 31 years), in *The Second World War: The Gathering Storm* (Boston: Houghton Mifflin Co., 1948), iii. Barbara Tuchman, *The Guns of August: The Outbreak of World War I* (New York: Macmillan, 1962).

"75 Years After World War II" Special Section, *New York Times*, 5 September 2020. The Great Influenza caused at least 50 million deaths: https://www.cdc.gov/flu/pandemic-resources/1918-pandemic-h1n1.html (accessed 9/8/2020). Social Sciences at https://www.diffen.com/difference/World_War_I_vs_World_War_II (accessed 9/8/2020), for estimates of deaths in wars. Also, John M. Barry, Keep your mask on. We're not out of this yet, *Washington Post* (15 March 2021), A10; and Barry, *The Great Influenza: The Story of the Deadliest Pandemic in History* (New York: Penguin Random House LLC, [2005] 2018). A reader pointed out that World War II is technically still ongoing, because Japan and the Soviet Union signed an armistice, not a peace treaty. However, one could say the same about the U.S. Civil War, which ended simply because the armies of the Confederacy surrendered. No peace treaty was signed by the United States of America and the Confederate States of America.

Additional references are given in my books of edited letters from World War I and World War II in *War Letters, Rolling with Patton*, and *The Home Front*. See Bibliography for full titles and publication details.

[557] https://www.history.com/topics/vietnam-war/vietnam-war-timeline (accessed June 13, 2020). Aleksandr Solzhenitsyn, *A Day in the Life of Ivan Denisovich*. Trans. by H. T. Willetts (New York: New American Library, 1962).

[558] Stephen Ambrose, *Undaunted Courage: Meriwether Lewis, Thomas Jefferson, and the Opening of the American West* (New York: Simon & Schuster, 1996); Douglas Brinkley, Ranger danger, *The New York Times Book Review*, 14 June 2020, 13, of Doug J. Swanson, *Cult of Glory: The Bold and Brutal History of the Texas Rangers* (New York: Viking, 2020).

[559] Holocaust Museum: https://www.ushmm.org/information/about-the-museum (accessed June 14, 2020); African American History: https://www.smithsonianmag.com/smithsonian-institution/national-museum-african-american-history-and-culture-interactive-museum-tour/ (accessed June 14, 2020).
New Orleans: https://www.nationalww2museum.org/ (accessed June 14, 2020).
Gettysburg: https://www.gettysburgfoundation.org/museum-visitor-center (accessed June 14, 2020).

[560] https://washington.org/visit-dc/must-see-memorials-monuments-national-mall (accessed June 17, 2020).

Also: *Britannica*, cenotaph. Capt. Peter Pennington says that the Cenotaph, built after WWI commemorates the dead of both world wars and British military who died in later wars.

[561] The devastation of the city of Troy in the Trojan War is obscured by many layers of cities that existed on that site. One can look west and imagine the Greeks' ships and their encampment on the plains that surround the ruins, but it now seems bloodless. The *Iliad, Odyssey,* and *Aeneid* are important in order to imagine what happened there.

Britannica, "Memorial Day" ("formerly Decoration Day"). This article states that graves were decorated on various dates during and after the Civil War, but the official date of May 30 was established in 1868 by John Logan, commander of the GAR (Grand Army of the Republic).

The poppy is the Remembrance flower, taken from the sad poem by John McCrae which begins as follows: "In Flanders fields the poppies blow / Between the crosses, row on row."

Henry Wadsworth Longfellow, "Footprints on the Sands of Time" (1838) is usually regarded as a call to action ("Let the dead Past bury its dead! / Act, - act in the living Present!"). However, there is another metaphor in this poem: footprints on a sandy seashore would wash away without a trace in the next high tide. At Yale, a similar lesson is taught in the Whiffenpoof song: "And we'll pass and be forgotten like the rest."

[562] *Britannica,* Plath, Sylvia (1932-1963).

[563] *Britannica,* Socrates (c.470 BCE – 399 BCE); Hitler, Adolph; Braun, Eva; Donovan, William.

[564] *Britannia*, suicide. The suicide bombers on September 11, 2001, followed, probably unknowingly, an example set by a fictional *kamikaze* Japanese Airline pilot who flew a Boeing 747 into the U.S. capitol building in Tom Clancy's novel, *Executive Orders* (1996).

[565] *Britannica*, electromagnetic spectrum; gamma ray: The electromagnetic spectrum ranges from very short gamma and x-rays (about 10^{-10} meters) to radio waves (maximum about 6.7mm).

Amit C. Nathawani, James F. Down, John Goldstone, et al, Polonium-210 poisoning: a first hand account, *The Lancet* 388 (no. 100049, September 10, 2016): 1075-1080, at: https://www.thelancet.com/journals/lancet/article/PIIS0140-6736(16)00144-6/fulltext (accessed July 12, 2020).

For the radiation-induced cancer in Thomas Edison's glassblower, see: Hill, *Edison's Environment*, pp. 285-6. During the Cuban Missile Crisis, mistakes were made that could have been catastrophic. Martin J. Sherwin, *Gambling with Armageddon: Nuclear Roulette from Hiroshima to the Cuban Missile Crisis, 1945-1962* (New York: Alfred A. Knopf, 2020), reviewed by Talmage Boston, Nuclear nightmare, *New York Times Book Review*, 27 December 2019, 19: "[T]he October 1962 near miss of a holocaust" was prevented when "on Day 12 of the crisis, a soviet captain overruled a flawed order to unleash a nuclear missile on American ships blockading Cuba."

[566] The Coconut Grove Fire was the deadliest nightclub fire in history, with 492 deaths. National Fire Protection Association: https://www.nfpa.org/Public-Education/Staying-safe/Safety-in-living-and-entertainment-spaces/Nightclubs-assembly-occupancies/The-Cocoanut-Grove-fire (accessed September 2, 2020). The doors opened inward, and people were trapped as they piled up inside, trying to get out. Massachusetts passed a law requiring all doors in public buildings to open outward.

Halifax explosion: John U. Bacon, *The Great Halifax Explosion: A World War I Story of Treachery, Tragedy, and Extraordinary Heroism* (New York: HarperCollins, 2017), with about 2000 dead, it was the world's largest explosion prior to Hiroshima; https://www.washingtonpost.com/news/retropolis/wp/2017/12/06/two-ships-collided-in-halifax-harbor-one-of-them-was-a-3000-ton-floating-bomb/ (accessed September 2, 2020).

Oklahoma City bombing – History: https://www.history.com/topics/1990s/oklahoma-city-bombing (accessed September 2, 2020). The attack was carried out by Timothy McVeigh, who was radicalized to become an anti-government activist by events known as Ruby Ridge, Idaho, in 1992, and the Branch Davidian/Waco siege in 1993 involving Federal agents.

Beirut: *New York Times*, 8 August 2020, Anger rises after Beirut blast and evidence officials knew of risks, https://www.nytimes.com/2020/08/05/world/middleeast/beirut-lebanon-explosion.html (accessed September 2, 2020).

The New York Times Complete World War II, 1939-1945 (New York: Black Dog & Leventhal, 2013): p. 143: Coventry was bombed on November 15, 1940, with about 2000 casualties, supposedly in retaliation for an RAF bombing of Munich; p. 260: Cologne was bombed on June 1, 1945, in an inferno "almost too gigantic to be real," supposedly in retaliation for Coventry; p. 503: Dresden was destroyed on February 14, 1945, in "one of the greatest night attacks of the war" using 1,400 RAF planes; p. 544-6: Hiroshima (on August 6) and Nagasaki (on August 9, 1945), which came just as the war was ending. Also see John Hersey, *Hiroshima* (New York: Alfred A. Knopf, 1946), a documentary history, but told in a manner similar to that of a novel; and Kurt Vonnegut, *Slaughterhouse Five* or *The Children's Crusade: A Duty-Dance with Death* (New York: Dell Publishing, 1969), a science-fiction novel based on the firebombing of Dresden, which Vonnegut endured as a prisoner of war.

[567] *Britannica,* Little Ice Age (LIA): "It began in the 16th century and advanced and receded intermittently over three centuries in Europe and many other regions. Its maximum development was reached about 1750, at which time glaciers were more widespread on Earth than at any time since the last major ice age ended about 11,700 years ago." Some scientists and historians believe that the eruption of a volcano in the Aleutian Islands one year after the assassination of Julius Caesar contributed to the demise of the Roman Republic. See Katherine Kornei, A far-off volcano and the Roman Republic's end, *New York Times,* 30 June 2020, D1, quoting Joseph Manning, a historian at Yale. See: Joseph G. Manning, Francis Ludlow, Alexander R. Stine, William R. Boos, Michael Sigl and Jennifer R. Marlon, Volcanic suppression of Nile summer flooding triggers revolt and constrains interstate conflict in ancient Egypt, *Nature Communications* 8 (2017). doi:10.1038/s41467-017-00957-y.

Other massive eruptions are said to have occurred during the years preceding the Plague of Justinian in 543 AD, and in the immediately following years. Contrary arguments exist, as in Lee Mordechai, Merle Eisenberg, Timothy P. Newfield, et al, The Justinianic Plague: An inconsequential pandemic? *Proceedings of the National Academy of Sciences* 1116 (no. 51, December 17, 2019), 25546-25554. The sudden eruption in 1980 of Mt. St. Helens, a long-silent volcano in Oregon, is a reminder of the danger of living near a volcano, even one that is supposed to be extinct.

Norman Maclean, *Young Men and Fire* (Chicago: University of Chicago Press, 1992).

[568] Kate Moore, *The Radium Girls the Dark Story of America's Shining Women* (Naperville, Ill.: Sourcebooks, Inc., 2017). See also a great array of natural poisons in Kate Lebo, *The Book of Difficult Fruit: Arguments for the Tart, Tender, and Unruly (with Recipes)* (New York: Farrar, Straus & Giroux, 2021), reviewed by Alex Beggs, Pick your poison: A thorny collection of personal essays on the plant kingdom, *New York Times Book Review* (25 April 26, 2021), 13.

[569] Poison, from *Britannica.* Also see: https://theconversation.com/handle-with-care-the-worlds-five-deadliest-poisons-56089 (accessed July 19, 2020). Thallium was commonly used as a rat poison until Vitamin K antagonists such as Warfarin were discovered. Thallium was the poison used to kill many of the characters in Agatha Christie's novel, *The Pale Horse* (London: Collins Crime Club, 1961). It is said to be tasteless, odorless, and difficult to detect post-mortem.

Antifreeze Poisoning. Healthline.com. https://www.healthline.com/health/antifreeze-poisoning (accessed January 31, 2021). Re: Ethylene Glycol, "It only takes a small amount of antifreeze to poison the human body and cause life-threatening complications." See: Derrick Bryson Taylor, Jenny Gross and Michael Levinson, Soldiers hospitalized after drinking antifreeze, Army says, *Washington Post,* 31 January 2021, 23.

For ricin, see: https://www.rferl.org/a/no-agent-bulgarian-spies-letter-refutes-talk-of-umbrella-murder-victim-markov-as-spy/29772449.html. (accessed July 9, 2020).

Andrew E. Kramer, Poison: easy, and easy to cover your tracks, *New York Times,* 21 August 2020, A9: Writing of "mysterious symptoms that struck Aleksei Navalny, Russia's most prominent opposition politician … as he was on a flight to Moscow," Kramer recounts the poisonings and probably poisonings of five people who displeased the leaders of Russia. Novichuk is an anticholinesterase; the antidote is atropine.

[570] *Britannica,* Second Amendment: "amendment to the Constitution of the United States, adopted in 1791 as part of the Bill of Rights, that provided a constitutional check on congressional power under Article I Section 8 to organize, arm, and discipline the federal militia." *Britannica,* "National Rifle Association of America (NRA): "formed in the United States in 1871. By the early 1990s it claimed a membership of about 3 million target shooters, hunters, gun collectors, gunsmiths, police, and others interested in firearms."

[571] Richard Grant, The King and the conqueror, *Smithsonian* (June 2020), 19-33, about Alexander "the Great" and his father. *Britannica,* Gavrilo, Princip.

[572] *Britannica,* kuru; Donner party. *Soylent Green* was a dystopian movie. Not science fiction, not fantasy, but it was nevertheless troublingly realistic. It was the natural evolution of imagined futures that were foreseen by Aldous Huxley in *Brave New World* (London: Chatto and Windus, 1934), and in George Orwell's novels *Animal Farm: A Fairy Story* (London: Secker and Warburg, 1945) and *Nineteen Eighty-four* (London: Secker and Warburg, 1949).

[573] *Britannica,* AK-47; also called Kalashnikov Model 1947.

[574] Police shootings database. Washingtonpost.com. https://www.washingtonpost.com/graphics/investigations/police-shootings-database/ (accessed January 31, 2021) states that "984 people have been shot by police and killed within the past year."

[575] A few memorable duels were fought by women, including Catherine the Great, Empress of Russia, when she was a young woman. See: 7 duels between women, Mentalfloss.com, https://www.mentalfloss.com/article/75944/7-duels-between-women (accessed January 31, 2021).

Britannica, Hamilton, Alexander, "The Burr quarrel."

[576] *Britannica*, Leopold and Loeb.

[577] Elizabeth Weise, Jury: Hart mothers drugged, killed all six children by driving SUV over California cliff into Pacific Ocean, *USA Today*, 5 April 2019. Tom Reiterman and John Jacobs, *Raven: The Untold Story of Rev. Jim Jones and His People* (New York: E. P. Dutton, 1982). *Britannica*, Manson, Charles.

[578] I am grateful that Dr. Alan Lippman called attention to the problem of medical errors. He wrote, "Medical errors are by far the more serious offense and need to be dealt with in a significantly different manner. I believe these concepts should be more accurately distinguished."

Bill Hathaway, Estimates of preventable hospital deaths are too high, new study shows, *Yale News* (28 January 2020), at: https://news.yale.edu/2020/01/28/estimates-preventable-hospital-deaths-are-too-high-new-study-shows (accessed March 29, 2021): "Previous estimates of preventable deaths of hospitalized patients may be two to four times too high, a new Yale School of Medicine study suggests. The meta-analysis of eight studies of inpatient deaths, published in the *Journal of General Internal Medicine*, puts the number of preventable deaths at just over 22,000 a year in the United States, instead of the oft-cited 44,000-98,000 estimate of a landmark 1999 study by the Institute of Medicine. Other frequently cited studies have placed the number of deaths as high as 250,000 deaths per year, which would make medical error the third leading cause of death, behind cancer and cardiovascular disease. ... The new study also shows that the number of previously healthy people who die every year from hospital error is about 7,150. The remainder of preventable deaths occurred in patients with less than a three-month life expectancy."

[579] *Britannica*, insulin, digitalis, belladonna. *Britannica* does not mention the dangers of large doses of calcium and potassium, whether given intentionally as poisons, or unintentionally, by accident. Curare was the first of the paralytic drugs to be used in anesthesia; it was originally used by indigenous people in South America as a poison on the tip of arrows and spears. Drugs in this class have been synthesized, such as anectine (succinyl choline). A paralytic drug was mixed with the MMR (measles, mumps, rubella) vaccine and caused death of two infants in 2018 in Samoa. Two nurses were found guilty of manslaughter. See: Adam Taylor, Samoa's measles outbreak offers lessons about vaccine availability and use, *Washington Post*, 13 July 2020, A15.

[580] For Laetrile, see https://www.cancer.gov/about-cancer/treatment/cam/hp/laetrile-pdq. (accessed June 20, 2020). See: George J. Hill, Thomas Shine, Helene Z. Hill, and Catherine Miller, Failure of amygdalin to arrest B16 melanoma and BW5147 AKR leukemia, *Cancer Research* 36 (1976): 2102-9; and Helene Z. Hill, R. Backer, and George J. Hill, Blood cyanide levels in mice after administration of amygdalin, *Biopharmaceutics and Drug Disposition*, 1 (1980): 211-20. Testimony by G. J. Hill is quoted in 442 U.S. 544 (1979), No. 78-605, p. 557, from a longer statement in 42 Fed. Reg. 39768, 39787 (1977) which was previously cited in detail.

For Krebiozen, see: https://www.chicagotribune.com/ opinion/commentary/ct-perspec-flashback-cancer-cure-krebiozen-quack-fraud-0930-20180925-story.html (accessed July 9, 2020).

[581] *Encyclopædia Britannica Deluxe Edition* (Chicago: Encyclopædia Britannica, 2013): Burke, William, and Hare, William (Irish criminals).

[582] St. Albans in *Forward Day by Day* (June 2020), 55 (Cincinnati, OH; www.ForwardMovement.org; accessed June 22, 2020). For the guillotine and Dr. Guillotin, see: Macleod Yearsley, Joseph Ignace Guillotin, *Proceedings of the Royal Society of Medicine*, 8 (1915):1-6; Ciaran F. Donegan, Dr Guillotin – Reformer and humanitarian, *Journal of the Royal Society of Medicine*, 83 (no. 10, 1990): 637–639; and Naomi Russo, the death-penalty abolitionist who invented the guillotine, *The Atlantic*, (25 March 2016).

[583] *Britannica*, Cromwell, Oliver.

[584] *Britannica*, Vlad III Dracula.

[585] Mike Winchell, *The Electric War: Edison, Tesla, Westinghouse, and the Race to Light the World* (New York: Henry Holt and Co., 2019); Adam Kline, *The Current War: A Battle Story Between Two Electrical Titans, Thomas Edison and George Westinghouse* (CreateSpace, 2017); and George J. Hill, *Edison's Environment: The Great Inventor Was Also a Great Polluter*. 3d edition (Berwyn Height, Md.: Heritage Books, 2017).

[586] . *Britannica*, Salem witch trials; Hale, Nathan.

[587] *Britannica*, witchcraft; Joan of Arc.

[588] The Equal Justice Initiative, founded by Byran Stevenson, has documented 2,000 lynchings of black people in the 12-year period of Reconstruction and more than 4,400 lynchings in the 74 years since the end of Reconstruction. See: Campbell Robertson, Report documents over 2,000 lynchings in 12-year period after Civil War, *New York Times*, 17 June 2020, A19; and Stevenson, *Just Mercy: A Story of Justice and Redemption* (New York: Spiegel & Grau, 2014). The Tulsa Race Massacre on May 31-June 1, 2021, is said to have been the worst incident of racial violence in American history. See: DeNeen Brown, Tulsa plans to dig for suspected mass graves from a 1921 race massacre, *Washington Post*, 4 February 2020.

Appendix B Parasitology and Microbiology

[589] Plasmodium, from World Health Organization: https://www.who.int/news-room/fact-sheets/detail/malaria (accessed June 28, 2020). Donald G. McNeil, Jr., Malaria mystery is partly solved in Mali, *New York Times*, 10 November 2020, D5. Justin M. Andrews, Griffith E. Quinby, and Alexander D. Langmuir, Malaria eradication in the United States, *American Journal of Public Health* 40 (Nov., 1950): 1405-10; references include James S. Simmons, American mobilization for the conquest of malaria in the United States, *J. Nat. Malaria Soc.* 3 (1944):7-11. Vivax malaria is not a benign disease. Complications from vivax malaria were described above in two articles from the NIH-NIAID by George J. Hill, et al.

[590] Leishmaniasis, from World Health Organization: https://www.who.int/news-room/fact- sheets/detail/leishmaniasis (accessed June 28, 2020).

[591] Chagas disease, from Centers for Disease Control (CDC): https://www.cdc.gov/parasites/chagas/gen_info/detailed.html (accessed June 29, 2020).

[592] *Britannica*, schistosomiasis.

[593] Google Images show many photographs of these unfortunate men, and also cartoons which illustrates the wheelbarrow and scrotum as a warning. William S. Burroughs commented about "some elephantiasis victim with his distended testicles in a wheelbarrow" in Burroughs, *Word Virus: The William S. Burroughs Reader* (New York: Grove/Atlantic, Inc., 2007), 348; from https://www.azquotes.com/quote/1336316 (accessed July 17, 2020). The photographs of men with scrota in wheelbarrows were probably scrubbed from Google Images as being pornographic.

[594] Treatment is usually successful, but reinfections are common.

[595] William M. Stauffer, Jonathan D. Alpern, and Patricia F. Walker, COVID-19 and dexamethasone: A potential strategy to avoid steroid-related *Strongyloides* hyperinfection," *JAMA* (30 July 2020). doi:10.1001/ jama.2020.

[596] Hookworm, from CDC: https://www.cdc.gov/dpdx/hookworm/index.html (accessed June 29, 2020).

[597] William C. Campbell, in The Nobel Prize in Physiology or Medicine 2015: https://www.nobelprize.org/prizes/medicine/2015/press-release/ (accessed June 29, 2020).

[598] "Human prototothecosis is a rare infection caused by members of the genus *Prototheca*." from Cornelia Lass-Florl and Astrid Mayr, "Human prototothecosis, *Clin. Microbiol. Rev.* 20 (no. 2, April 2007): 230-242, at https://www.ncbi.nlm.nih.gov/pmc/articles/PMC1865593/ (accessed June 18, 2020).

[599] *Britannica*, fungi; baking. For Fungal Disease in humans, the best source of information is from the Centers for Disease Control, at https://www.cdc.gov/fungal/diseases/ (accessed July 18, 2020).

[600] *Aspergillus* infections in various body organs may occur in patients with depressed immunity, or after inhalation of a large number of spores.

[601] Amphotericin B been the treatment of choice for systemic fungal diseases for more than 60 years.

[602] *Candida auris* is an emerging fungus that presents a serious global health threat, because it is often resistant to many drugs that are commonly used to treat Candida infections, and it is difficult to diagnose.

[603] Coccidioidomycosis due to *C. neoformans* was the most common fungal disease that was being studied at the NIH in 1961, and it was probably the most common systemic fungal disease in the U.S. at that time. Meningeal and brain infection was very resistant to treatment, probably because of the "blood-brain" barrier. *C. gatti* has since emerged as a recent threat.

[604] *Britannica*, ergot. Ergot is a powerful, illegal, and dangerous abortifacient (a potion used to cause a miscarriage).

[605] The pulmonary nodule is called a histoplasmoma.

[606] *Britannica*, antibiotic; and Biology LibreTexts: https://bio.libretexts.org/Bookshelves/Microbiology/Book%3A_Microbiology_(Boundless)/13%3A_Antimicrobial_Drugs/13.3%3A_Commonly_Used_Antimicrobial_Drugs/13.3D%3A_Antibiotics_from_Prokaryotes (accessed February 1, 2021).

[607] The discovery of the action of *Penicillium notatum* was made in 1928 by Alexander Fleming, and the responsible ingredient was isolated by Ernst Chain and Howard Florey in the late 1930s. Penicillin was very scarce before 1945; it was first used in America in 1942: George Will, A year [1942] as disruptive as 2020, *Washington Post*, 26 July 2020, A23.

[608] U.S. government websites give additional information about the problem: About Antibiotic Use in Food Animals. From https://www.cdc.gov/drugresistance/food.html (accessed August 22, 2020).
The Effects on Human Health of Subtherapeutic Use of Antimicrobials in Animal Feeds. From https://www.ncbi.nlm.nih.gov/books/NBK216502/ (accessed August 22, 2020).

[609] *Clostridium perfringens* has gone through several changes in name, among them being *Clostridium welchii*. It is said to have complicated 6% of open fractures and 1% of all open wounds in World War I. Equine antitoxin is effective in treatment. https://emedicine.medscape.com/article/217943-overview (accessed September 2, 2020).

Specific antitoxin raised in horses and serum from convalescent patients (immune serum) is also used in treatment of rabies, tetanus, botulism, anthrax, and diphtheria. E. E. Ballantyne, Gas gangrene antitoxin production, *Canadian Journal of Comparative Medicine* 3 (no. 4, April 1944): 109-110, at: http://europepmc.org/backend/ptpmcrender.fcgi?accid=PMC1660816&blobtype=pdf (accessed September 9, 2020).

[610] Before there was a vaccine to prevent diphtheria, the disease was treated with convalescent plasma. As explained by Victoria Harden, director emerita of the History and Stetten Museum at the National Institutes of Health, in a letter to the *Washington Post*, August 2020, p. A26.

[611] "Herd immunity" is not discussed in *Britannica*. For herd immunity, see: Gypsyamber D'Souza and David Dowdy, What is herd immunity and how can we achieve it with COVID-19? From https://www.jhsph.edu/covid-19/articles/achieving-herd-immunity-with-covid19.html (accessed July 18, 2020).

[612] In the laboratory, *Proteus* is easily recognized. It grows rapidly in a Petri dish, displaying a unique quality known as swarming, and it exhibits a unique slimy surface. *Proteus* is named for Proteus, a minor Greek god of the ocean, who had the ability to change shape and escape. The Proteus syndrome, first described in 1976, is now believed to be one possible cause of the condition of Joseph (aka John) Merrick, the so-called "Elephant Man" of London in the nineteenth century. Jonathan Sanger, *Making the Elephant Man: A Producer's Memoir* (Jefferson, N.C.: McFarland & Co., 2016).

[613] Typhoid Mary, in *Britannica*. Byname of Mary Mallon (1869-1938).

[614] Thomas Butler, *Plague and Other Yersinia Infections* (New York: Plenum Publishing Corp., 1983). Barbara E. Murry, et al., Destroying the life and career of a valued physician-scientist who tried to protect us from plague: Was it really necessary?" *Clinical Infectious Diseases* 40 (no. 11, 1 June 2005): 1644-1648. At: https://academic.oup.com/cid/article/40/11/1644/446159 (accessed February 21, 2021).

[615] George J. Hill, *Leprosy in Five Young Men* (Boulder: Colorado Associated University Press, 1970). This book is based on research conducted at the National Institutes of Health in 1962-63.

[616] Filterable virus: Any of the infectious agents that pass through a filter of diatomite or unglazed porcelain with the filtrate and remain virulent and that includes the viruses and various other groups (such as the mycoplasmas and rickettsias) which were originally considered viruses before their cellular nature was established (from Merriam-Webster, https://www.merriam-webster.com/dictionary/filterable%20virus (accessed July 2, 2020).

[617] *Britannica*, mycoplasma. Unlike other bacteria, mycoplasmas are "filterable agents" (see next section). A new disease described by Monroe Eaton in 1944, known as Eaton Agent Pneumonia, was later shown to be due to mycoplasma. Maurice A. Mufson, Michael A. Manko, James R. Kingston, et al, "Eaton agent pneumonia – Clinical features," *JAMA* 178 (no. 4, 1961): 369-74.

[618] *Britannica*, Rickettsia. "Except for *Coxiella burnetii*, the cause of Q fever, [Rickettsia] are intracellular parasites, most of which are transmitted to humans by an arthropod carrier such as a louse or tick. *C. burnetii*, however, can survive in milk, sewage, and aerosols and can be transmitted to humans by a tick or by inhalation, causing pneumonia in the latter case."

[619] *Rickettsia. prowazekii* is transmitted to humans by the body louse and causes epidemic typhus, with a high mortality rate, and Brill-Zinsser disease in recurring cases. From: https://www.encyclopedia.com/people/medicine/medicine-biographies/hans-zinsser (accessed February 8, 2021).

Frank M. Snowden's description of typhus in the French army in Russia in 1812 is based on the assumption that it was epidemic typhus; he mentions only louse-borne typhus, although no specific organism was identified. Snowden never mentions the existence of human typhus due to rats and fleas. Snowden, *Epidemics and Society*, 160-66. R. Tello-Martin, K. Dzul-Rosado, J. Zavala-Castro, and C. Lugo-Caballero, Approaches for the successful isolation and cell culture of American *Rickettsia* species, *Journal of Vector Borne Diseases*, 55 (no. 4, 2018): 258-64. *R. rickettsia* is transmitted by ticks and causes Rocky Mountain spotted fever. *R. conorii* is transmitted by the dog tick and causes Boutonneuse fever. The disease known as Tsutsugamushi fever (scrub typhus) is caused by *R. tsutsugamushi*, which is transmitted from a rodent host on a chigger mite.

[620] *Britannica*, prion. Dr. Donald Matson, a neurosurgeon in Boston, died in 1969 at the age of 55 after a long period of slowly progressing dementia. Eben Alexander, Jr., Donald Darrow Matson" [obituary], *Journal of Neurosurgery* 31 (no. 3, Sept 1969): 249-50; and Roberta Rehder, Subash Lohani, and Alan R. Cohen, Unsung hero: Donald Darrow Matson's legacy in pediatric neurosurgery, *J. Neurosurg. Pediatr.* 16 (no. 5, Nov 2015): 483-94.

Appendix C   More Doctors Afield

[621] I first became aware of the doctor as actor (as in the theatre) when two articles on this subject were published in *The Lancet*. I cannot locate those articles, but this topic was the subject of a paper in *JAMA* in 2005: Eric B. Larson and Xin Yao, Clinical empathy as emotional labor in the patient-physician relationship, *JAMA* 293 (no. 9, 2 March

2005): 1100-1106. "We focus on physicians as professionals [who] engage in such emotional labor through deep acting [which is] similar to the method-acting tradition used by some stage and screen acting, surface acting (i.e., forging empathetic behaviors toward the patient, absent of consistent emotional and cognitive reactions), or both.

I admit to having aspired to be an actor since I was on stage in eighth grade. I enjoyed learning to ad lib, memorize lines, overcome stage fright, follow cues, to choose either to pretend or to immerse myself in a role (method acting), and – as my instructor Carrie Babcock taught me at her Fred Astaire Dance Studio – "If you fall, make it part of the act."

[622] Alan Cowell, Nawal el Saadawi, advocate for women in the Arab world, is dead at 89, *Washington Post* (22 March 2021), A19. Some of her many books were translated into English, including *The Hidden Face of Eve: Women in the Arab World* (1977) trans. Sherif Hetata (New York: Zed Books, 1980).

[623] Claire L. Wendland, Physician anthropologists, *Annual Review of Anthropology* 48 (2020): 187-205, at: https://www.annualreviews.org/doi/abs/10.1146/annurev-anthro-102218-011338?journalCode=anthro (accessed March 15, 2021). "Physician anthropologists have contributed extensively to the anthropology of biomedicine, as well as to other aspects of medical anthropology." See: Francine Saillant and Serge Genest, *Anthropologie médicale. Ancrages locaux, défis globaux (Medical anthropology. Local roots, global challenges)*. In French. (Quebec: Les presses de l'Université Laval: 2005); and Ibid., *Medical Anthropology: Regional Perspectives and Shared Concerns* (Malden, Mass.: Blackwell, 2007); and Paul Farmer, *Infections and Inequalities: The Modern Plagues* (Berkeley, University of California Press, 1999) and Farmer, *Pathologies of Power: Health, Human Rights, and the New War on the Poor* (Berkeley, University of California Press, 2003). Charles S. Bosk, *Forgive and Remember: Managing Medical Failure* (Chicago: University of Chicago Press, 1979), was a ground-breaking study of the surgical profession in America.

[624] I have chosen the classification of Author to include physician-writers. In the *New England Journal of Medicine*, they are usually called "writers." Walter B. Cannon, *The Way of an Investigator: A Scientist's Experiences in Medical Research* (New York: W. W. Norton & Company, Inc., 1945).

[625] William Osler, *The Principles and Practice of Medicine: Designed for the Use of Practitioners and Students of Medicine* (New York: Appleton and Company, 1899); and *Aequanimitas* (Philadelphia: P. Blakiston's Son & Co., 1914). Harvey Cushing, *The Life of Sir William Osler*, 3vols. (Oxford: Oxford University Press, 1926); and *From a Surgeon's Journal, 1915-1918* (Boston: Little Brown and Co., 1936). A definitive, though hagiographic, biography is John Farquhar Fulton, *Harvey Cushing A Biography* (Springfield, Illinois: Charles C Thomas, 1946). A shorter but more balanced view of Cushing's personal life is Elizabeth H. Thomson, *Harvey Cushing: Surgeon, Author, Artist* (New York: Henry Schuman, 1950).

[626] The Johnson & Johnson – Janssen one dose vaccine to protect against COVID-19 was released for use in the United States in March 2021. One of the first scientific publications about this vaccine was Kathryn E. Stephenson, Mathieu Le Gars, Jerald Sadoff, et al., Immunogenicity of the Ad26.COV2.S vaccine for COVID-19, *JAMA* (11 March 2021). The authors concluded that, "This randomized, double-blind, placebo-controlled phase 1 clinical trial of Ad26.COV2.S enrolled 25 participants. Antibodies were detected in vaccine recipients by day 8 and were observed in all vaccine recipients by day 57 after a single immunization. T-cell responses were also generated in vaccine recipients."

The Sackler family was profiled by Patrick Radden Keefe, An empire of pain, *The New Yorker* (23 October 2017): "The Sackler dynasty's ruthless marketing of painkillers has generated billions of dollars – and millions of addicts. Litigation continues in many jurisdictions with the Sackler family and Purdue Pharma as defendants, and as of March 2021, there is not yet an end in sight for the epidemic of drug overdoses and deaths in the United States. Also: Keefe, *Empire of Pain: The Secret History of the Sackler Dynasty* (New York: Doubleday, 2010), reviewed by John Carryrou, Kingpins, *New York Times Book Review*, 25 April 2021, 1-20. On 16 March 2021, ABC news reported that "Sackler family to pay $4.2 billion toward opioid lawsuit settlement, documents show. Under the restructuring, the Sacklers would relinquish control of the company," at: https://abcnews.go.com/US/sackler-family-pay-42-billion-opioid-lawsuit-settlement/story?id=76485141 (accessed March 16, 2021). For oxycodone, see: https://medlineplus.gov/druginfo/meds/a682132.html (accessed March 16, 2021) and https://www.dea.gov/factsheets/oxycodone (accessed March 16, 2021).

Summary of lawsuits, Sackler family pledges extra opioid payout, *Washington Post* (17 March 2017), A30: "In a bid to resolve thousands of lawsuits stemming from the opioid epidemic, the Sackler family pledged to contribute $1.5 billion more than previously promised, roughly $4.3 billion paid out over nine years from their personal fortune [because] many suing the company blame the Sackler family, in part, for the opioid epidemic that has killed more than 450,000 people in the past two decades."

[627] Physician-criminals, selected from Linda Girgis, Top 14 most evil doctors of the last two centuries, *Physicians Weekly* (25 October 2019) at https://www.physiciansweekly.com/top-14-most-evil-doctors-of-the-last-two-centuries/ (accessed March 16, 2021).

Three physicians who are still alive committed heinous crimes that were enabled by their positions as doctors of medicine. Two committed serial assaults against women, and the other was a serial killer and poisoner. Cecil B. Jacobson, M.D. (b. 1936), who impregnated patients with his own sperm in the 1980s, fathered more than 70 children. He said he was a "fertility specialist," and he was, in a bizarre way. He was only sentenced to five years in prison. Dr. Michael Swango (b. 1954) had a macabre career, killing patients in medical school and in other places in residency training, poisoning friends and colleagues, changing names several times, dodging the law, and slipping away. He pleaded guilty to crimes in the U.S. in order to avoid a death sentence in Zimbabwe, and is imprisoned for life at the ADX Supermax Federal Prison. Dr. Larry Nassar (b. 1963) was sentenced to 40-125 years in prison for sexual assaults on scores of young women as the team sports physician for USA Gymnastics. See: Naveed Saleh, 10 notorious doctors in history, *MDlinx* (24 February 2019) at https://www.mdlinx.com/article/ 10-notorious-doctors-in-history/lfc-3448 (accessed March 16, 2021).

[628] Simon Winchester, *The Professor and the Madman A Tale of Murder, Insanity and the Making of the Oxford English Dictionary* (New York: HarperCollins, 1998).

[629] Thomas Harris, *The Silence of the Lambs* (New York: St. Martin's Press, 1988), was the basis for the movie of the same name, starring Jodie Foster and Anthony Hopkins. It was the fifth-highest grossing film of 1991.

[630] The quote about "the most successful spies" paraphrases a comment made to me by a movie producer, the late Harvey Rochman. My lecture on October 13, 2006, to the National Reconnaissance Office entitled "Master and Commander, Surgeon and Spy," was videotaped and marked "Unclassified." My comments about matters other than the fictional Captain Aubrey and Dr. Maturin were redacted.

Patrick O'Brian, *Master and Commander* (Philadelphia: Lippincott, 1969) was the first in the Aubrey-Maturin series of 17 novels. *The Far Side of the World* (London: Collins, 1984) was the tenth. The movie, *Master and Commander*, was based primarily on the novel, *The Far Side of the World*, and the location was changed to the Galapagos, and the enemy was France instead of the United States.

[631] Howard I. Kushner, Medical historians and the history of medicine, *The Lancet* 374 (no. 9698, 17 October 2009): 1322-3: "Critical of internalist narratives, academic historians insisted that production of scientific and medical knowledge was framed within the context of wider political, intellectual, and cultural factors including race, gender, and class."

[632] Three names are of current interest, who are still alive:
Fillmore Buckner, MD, JD, is the author of two books about physicians who had distinguished themselves in other fields: *Versatile Physicians* and *Versatile Physicians II* (Heritage Books). Dr. Buckner, a specialist in obstetrics and gynecology, was president of the American College of Legal Medicine in 2002. See: https://www.aclm.org/Past-Presidents.

A well-known professor of law and medicine is George Annas, who has a J.D. and M.P.H., but he is not a physician. Dr. Fred Jacobs, a pulmonologist, retired as an executive in the Saint Barnabas Medical Center, Livingston, N.J. He was a physician who earned the J.D. at a late stage in his career. Dr. Jacobs used his knowledge of both fields effectively on behalf of the hospital and in service as Chairman of the New Jersey State Board of Medical Examiners.

For additional information about Dr. Annas, see: https://www.quora.com/Are-there-people-who-are-both-lawyers-and-doctors (accessed March 16, 2021). George J. Annas, Doctors and lawyers and wolves, *Lancet* 371 (no. 9627, 31 May 2008): 1832-3. Annas is the William Fairfield Warren Distinguished Professor and chair of the Health Law, Bioethics & Human Rights Department of Boston University School of Public Health. He is also a professor in the Boston University School of Medicine and the School of Law. He is the cofounder of Global Lawyers and Physicians, a transnational professional association of lawyers and physicians working together to promote human rights and health. He has degrees from Harvard College (AB economics, '67), Harvard Law School (JD '70) and Harvard School of Public Health (MPH '72).

For more about Dr. Jacobs, see: "SHORT HILLS, NJ – After a four-decade career at Barnabas Health, Fred M. Jacobs, M.D., J.D., has announced that he will retire as Executive Vice President and Director of the Barnabas Health Quality Institute as of Dec. 31, and will serve as a consultant for one year. Jacobs, who lives in Short Hills, has been associated with Saint Barnabas Medical Center and then Saint Barnabas Health Care System since 1969." From https://www.tapinto.net/towns/livingston/sections/health-and-wellness/articles/jacobs-retiring-after-long-career-with-saint-barn (accessed March 16, 2021).

[633] https://www.fiamc.org/faith-prayer/saints/physician-saints-of-the-catholic-church/ (accessed March 13, 2021).

G. Androutsos, A. Diamantis, and L. Vladimiros, The first leg transplant for the treatment of a cancer by Saints Cosmas and Damian, *J. Buon* 13 (no. 2, April-June 2008): 297-304. At: https://pubmed.ncbi.nlm.nih.gov/18555483/ (accessed March 13, 2021).
Also: https://www.jewishgen.org/databases/Holocaust/0065_Polish_Martyred_Physicians.html (accessed March 12, 2021). "Polish Martyred Physicians": "This database contains information about 2,465 Polish-Jewish physicians who perished during the Holocaust."

[634] Dr. John Potts' career was summarized by Susan Evans McCrobie, Chirurgian, phisique and the sicke: The art and history of Jamestown medicine, *Jamestowne Society Magazine* 45 (no. 1, Spring 2021): 23-4. It was based on Thomas Proctor Hughes, *Medicine in Virginia, 1607-1689* (Hamburg: Trendition Classics, 2012). David Owen (b. 1938), 1st Baron Owen, was Foreign Minister of United Kingdom from 1977-1979. He was one of the youngest to serve in that office. His tenure is generally regarded as having been successful, although there was a hint of scandal in connection with contaminated blood that was purchased by the government. One of the other physicians to become head of state is Bashir al-Assad (b. 1965), who has been the controversial president of Syria since 2000. Of several others who have been head of state, and are still alive, Michelle Bachelet (b. 1951), M.D., should be mentioned. She was the courageous President of Chile and was re-elected in 2013.

A list of 16 physicians who became Head of State is given by Richard Lilford's Friday Blog, at https://richardlilfordsfridayblog.wordpress.com/2013/07/19/doctors-and-natural-scientists-who-became-head-of-state/ (accessed March 15, 2021). This list is useful, but it is incomplete. It does not show Georges Clemenceau or Pope John XXI, who was Pope, briefly, in 1276. He died when construction in the Papal Palace collapsed on him. See: D. Blanchard, Pope John XXI, ophthalmologist, *Doc Ophthalmol*. 89 (no. 1-2, 1995): 75-84.

[635] Sinclair Lewis, *Main Street* (New York: Harcourt, Brace & Co., 1920); and *Arrowsmith* (New York: Harcourt Brace & Co., 1925). Jürgen Thorwald, trans., *The Century of the Surgeon* (New York: Pantheon Books, 1957). Boris Pasternak, *Dr. Zhivago*, trans. (New York: Pantheon Books, 1957).

[636] Hermann Hagedorn, *Leonard Wood: A Biography* (New York: Harper & Brothers, 1931). The concluding phrase in Latin can be translated as "Thus passes worldly glory."

[637] Although he is dead, Michael Crichton continues to be enormously influential in Hollywood. His "Star Rating" on IMDbPro has ranged over the past year from a high of 1,900 in October 2020 to 10,148 in March 2021. To put this into perspective, Ed Asner's was 2,681 on March 12, 2021. Asner was still alive. Star Ratings of others that were posthumous on that date were Sean Connery (817) and Clark Gable (2,990). Some of Crichton's publications and movies: *The Andromeda Strain* (1969); *Five Patients* (1970); *The Andromeda Strain* (1971); *The Great Train Robbery* (1978); and *Jurassic Park* (1990).

Also see: Tyler D. Barrett, Five patients in 50 years: Revisiting the speculations of Michael Crichton's medical school nonfiction, *The Pharos* (winter, 2021): 8-14.

Appendix E   Hippocratic Oath

[638] Translated by Michael North, National Library of Medicine, 2002. From https://www.nlm.nih.gov/hmd/greek/greek_oath.html (accessed April 24, 2021).
Merriam-Webster spelling is Hygeia. From ancient Greek: Ὑγιεία or Ὑγεία, Latin: Hygēa or Hygīa.
Another spelling in the internet is Hygiea. This version was used as the Oath given to Harvard Medical School students in the 1950s.

[639] This version of the Hippocratic Oath is from Ludwig Edelstein, *The Hippocratic Oath: Text, Translation, and Interpretation* (Baltimore: Johns Hopkins Press, 1943).
From https://www.medicinenet.com/hippocratic_oath/definition.htm (accessed April 24, 2021).

[640] The modern version of the Hippocratic Oath was written in 1964 by Louis Lasagna, Dean of the School of Medicine at Tufts University.
From https://www.medicinenet.com/hippocratic_oath/definition.htm (accessed April 24, 2021).

Index

80 Years War, 121
Aachen, 113
Abel, 107
Abraham the Patriarch, 106
Achilles, 108
Acts, Book of, 103-5, 112
Adam and Eve, 28, 37, 43-4, 47, 66, 158
Adams, Abigail, 123
Adams, John, 32, 123
Adams, John Quincy, 123
Addison's Disease, 154
ADHD, 69
Adonis, 51
Adriatic Sea, 116
Aechtner, Thomas H., 159
Aedes, 67, 84, 86
Aeneas, 80
Aeolus, 17
Aesculapius, 96
Aetna, 143
Affordable Care Act (ACA), 144, 161, 179
Afghan War, 2d (British), 144
Afghanistan; Afghan, 29, 95, 99, 110, 113, 128, 139, 144, 176
Africa; African; Afrika, 25, 35, 43-4, 86-8, 90-1, 101, 113, 116, 120, 128, 138-9, 142, 154, 157, 161, 163, 165, 176-9
African Union, 177
Afropithecus, 90
Agamemnon, 108
Age of Discovery or Exploration, 116, 175
Age of Modern Warfare, 175
Akkad, 108
Alaska, 20, 49, 145, 162
Albert, Prince of England, 31
Albucasis of Cordoba (Abu'l-Qasim), 102, 114
Alexander III of Macedon, "the Great," 29, 74, 110, 170, 179
Alexandria, Egypt, 106
al-Khwarizm, Muhammad ibn Musa, 114
Allah, 52, 63, 158
Alps Mountains, the, 49
Al-Qaeda, 66, 175
al Razi, Abu Bakr Muhammad ibn Zakariya (see Rhazes)
Alsace-Lorraine, 128, 136
Altman, Lawrence, 67
Alzheimer's Disease, 11, 69, 76, 78, 87, 177

Amazon River, 24, 43, 91, 138
Ambrose, Stephen, 68
Amenemhet I, 108
America (see United States)
America First movement, 34, 143, 175
America(s), the, 13, 14, 22, 25, 27, 30-6, 40, 42, 46, 49, 50, 53-4, 65-8, 74, 78-9, 85-6, 92-3, 99, 100-1, 106, 117, 120, 122-6, 134-48, 152-3, 157, 161-2, 165-6, 171-3, 176, 179
American Age, 175-6
American Cancer Society, 79, 153
American College of Surgeons, 153
American Dream, 176
American Expeditionary Force, 143
American Medical Association, 153
American Red Cross (also see Red Cross), 127, 129, 153
American Society of Clinical Oncology, 153
Ammon, 29
Amorites, 108
Amsterdam, 64, 115, 122
Amur Darya River, 113
Anatolia, 106, 112-3
Andes Mountains; Andean, 70, 100, 130, 171
Anemoi, 17
Anglicus, Bartholomaeus, 115
Anglo-Saxon (see England)
Anopheles, 84
Antarctica, 39, 43
Antonine Plague, 81
Antony, Mark, 29, 110
Aphrodite, 51
Apollo, 102
Appalachia, 30, 128
Appleton, Fanny, 137
Appomattox, 131
Arab; Arabic, 66, 98-9, 102, 106, 108, 111, 113-14 116, 175
Ararat, Mount, 107
Arbella ship, and Lady Arbella, 120
Arecibo, Puerto Rico, 146
Aristotle, 110, 170
Arizona, 82
Ark, the, 22, 62, 107
Arlington Cemetery, 54
Arlington (Pentagon), Virginia, 175
Armstrong, Neil, 171
Army of Northern Virginia, 131

Army of the Potomac, 131
Art Nouveau, 138, 146
Arthur, King, 29
Asia Minor (see Middle East)
Asia, 13, 24, 29, 30, 42, 45, 49, 50, 54, 56, 63, 81, 86-7, 93-9, 105-10, 113-5, 129, 138-9, 142, 163-5, 170-1, 175-9
Asperger, 41, 69
Assyria, 108
Athens, 81, 109-10, 116
Atilla the Hun, 113
Atlanta, Georgia, 136
Atlantic Ocean, 50, 113, 127, 143, 176
Atomic Age, 146
Aubrey, Captain Jack, 127
Augustus (Octavian), Emperor (Caesar), 110-11
Auschwitz, 54, 64
Australia, 18, 24, 46, 93, 165
Australopithecus, 90
Averroës (Ibn Ruischd), 114
Avicenna (Ibn Sina), 114
Avignon, France, 27, 115
Axis Powers, 140
Ayyubid Dynasty, 114
Azores, 165
Aztec, 171
Baal, 65
Babel, Tower of, 38
Babylon; Babylonia, 90, 93, 107-10, 143, 146, 179
Bacchus, 102
Bach, Johann Sebastian, 135
Bacon, Francis, 119
Bacon, Roger, 115
Baghdad, Iraq, 29
Balboa, Nunez de, 117
Balkans, 107, 116, 118
Ballard, Martha, 127
Baltic Sea, 93
Baltimore, Maryland, 69, 131, 137
Band-Aids, 150
Banting, Sir Frederick, 141, 171
Barnard, Christian, 147
Bartlett, Robert, 147
Barton, Clara, 38, 127, 129
Bath, England, 23, 136
Bathsheba, 109
Bauchner, Howard, 88
Bavaria, Germany, 116
Baylor St. Luke's Medical Center, 154
Beethoven, Ludwig van, 135, 170-1

Belgium, 138
Bell, Alexander Graham, 171
Bence Jones, Henry, 132
Benedict X, Pope, 115
Bentham, Jeremy, 129
Benz, Karl, 135
Bergey, David, 85
Berkeley, Gloucestershire, England, 126
Berlin, Germany, 140
Berlioz, Hector, 92
Bermuda, 121
Bernard, Claude, 133
Best, Charles, 141
Bethlehem, 111
Bible, Holy, 4, 15-18, 21-3, 27-9, 34, 39, 43-6, 51-2, 61-4, 67, 69, 76, 79, 80, 93, 104, 106, 108, 111-12, 116-7, 119, 132, 138, 150, 158-65
Biden, Joseph Robinette, Jr. (Joe Biden), 33, 144, 161-2
Big Bang, 18, 165-6
bin Laden, Osama, 66
Birmingham, 124
Bismarck, Otto von, 136, 170-1
Black Death (Black Plague), 81, 115, 121
Black Hawk War, 131
Blue Cross / Blue Shield, 143
Boeotia, Greece, 105
Boer War, 139, 144
Boerhaave, Herman, 123
Bohemia(n), 138, 149
Boleyn, Ann, Queen of England, 30, 118
Bolivia, 100
Bologna, Italy, 115
Bolshevik, 139
Booth, John Wilkes, 131-2
Boraxo, 149
Boreas, 17
Borrelia burgdorferi, 84
Boston, Massachusetts, 30, 41, 120-3, 129, 136
Boy Scouts of America, 20, 64, 103, 161
Boyle, Robert, 121-2
Boylston, Zabadiel, 123
Bradford, William, 120
Brahe, Tycho, 118, 158
Brahms, Johannes, 135
Braintree, Massachusetts, 123
Brazil, 39, 74
Bremerhaven, Germany, 26
Brighton, England, 82
Bristol, England, 126

Britain; British (also see England), 29, 31-2, 51, 99, 107, 124-5, 127-9, 136, 139, 144, 152, 161, 169, 172, 176
Britannica, Encyclopedia, 4, 17, 82, 104-5, 137, 139, 157
Broad Street pump, London, 129
Bronze Age, 47, 107
Brooklyn Bridge, 137, 171
Brooklyn, N.Y., 137
Brown, John, 31
Browne, Sir Thomas, 119, 157
Browning, Elizabeth Barrett, 51
Bruno, Giordano, 66
Brutus, 29, 110
Buck, Carrie, 34
Budapest, Hungary, 132
Buddha; Buddhist, 12, 15, 22, 37, 45, 52, 62, 64, 67, 109, 111-2, 161, 170
Buffalo, N.Y., 79
Bullfinch, Thomas, 123
Burkitt, Denis, 87
Burma, 109
Bush, George Herbert Walker, 33
Bush, George Walker, 33
Butterfield, Sir Herbert, 169-70
Bynum, William, 126
Byrd, Admiral Richard E., 39
Byzantine Plague, 81
Byzantium, 112
Cabot, John, 117
Caesar (see others by first name)
Caesar, Julius, 29, 105, 110-11, 119, 170
Cain, 107
Cairo, Egypt, 106
California, 29, 162
Calliope, 42
Camelot, 29, 32
Camilla, Duchess of Cornwall, 31
Campho-Phenique, 149
Canaan, 48, 65
Canada, 82, 84, 125, 141, 163
Canary Islands, 165
Cannon, LeGrand, Jr., 145
Cannon, Walter B., 23, 44, 133, 141
Canterbury Tales, 30, 116
Cape Horn, 116
Capp, Al, 73
Caribbean Sea, 101
Carolina(s) (see also North and South Carolina), 31, 120, 122
Carrell, Alexis, 141, 143, 147
Carroll, Lewis (Charles Dodson), 28
Carson, Rachel, 13, 23, 84, 171
Carter, James E., Jr., "Jimmy," 32
Carter, Rosalynn, 32
Carter's Little Liver Pills, 149
Carthage, 80, 108
Cassandra, 40
Cassius, 110
Castleman, Benjamin, 103
Cather, Willa, 145
Catherine the Great, Empress of Russia, 33, 38
Catskill Mountains, 145
Center for Medicare and Medicaid Services (CMS), 144
Central Intelligence Agency, U.S. (CIA), 176
Chadwick, Edward, 129
Chagas Disease, 83
Charlemagne; Carolingian, 66, 113, 170
Charles I, King of England, 119, 121
Charles II, King of England, 119, 121-2
Charles, Prince of Wales, 31
Charleston, South Carolina, 130
Chaucer, Geoffrey, 30, 102, 116, 171
Chesapeake Bay, 120, 137
China; Chinese, 13, 14, 33, 38, 42, 56, 67, 78, 81, 99, 100, 106, 113-5, 120, 129, 132, 163, 177
Christ, Jesus; Christian(s)(ity), 22, 29, 33, 40, 45-6, 49, 52, 61-7, 76, 102-23, 138, 158-63, 171, 175-7
Christmas, 111, 144, 152
Churchill, Sir Winston, 139, 142, 170
Circe, 28
Civil War (U.S.), 31, 127-31, 145, 163, 172, 175
Clark, Barney, 147
Clark, William, 68, 117, 127
Cleopatra VII, the last Ptolemy, 29, 33, 38, 110, 119, 170
Cleveland Clinic, 142
Cleveland, Grover, 32, 143
Cleveland, Ohio, 142
Clinton, Hillary, 33, 162
Clinton, William J. "Bill," 33
Clio, 42
Clovis I, 113
Cold War, 78, 139, 176
Collins, Francis, 159
Colombia, 76, 97, 100
Colosseum, 112
Colossians, 105
Columbian Exchange, 117, 178

Columbus, Christopher, 42, 117, 161 (Knights), 165, 170-1, 178
Comanche, 146
Commonwealth of Independent States (CIS), 177
Commonwealth of Nations (British), 176
Communism; Communist, 38-9, 112, 128, 132, 139
Confederate States of America; Confederate; Confederacy, 130-2; 140
Conference on Security and Cooperation in Europe (CSCE), 176
Connecticut, 26, 121
Conrad, Joseph, 145
Constance, Council of, 116
Constantine, 112, 116
Constantinople, 105, 115-6
Constitution, U.S., 124, 130-2, 161-2
Cooper, Kenneth, 58
Cooper, Sir Astley Paston, 126
Copernicus; Copernican, 69, 117-9, 121, 158, 164, 168, 170-1
Cordova (Cordoba), Spain, 102, 114
Cornell University, 159
Cornwall, 119
Corps of Discovery, 68, 127
Cos, Island of, 102
COVID-19, 14, 16, 20, 39, 42, 62, 69, 73-5, 80-1, 87-8, 136, 147, 152, 160-3, 170, 179
CPR (Cardio-Pulmonary Resuscitation), 75-6
Crete, 80, 107
Crichton, Michael, 103
Crick, Francis, 166, 168
Crile, George, 142
Crimean War, 128-9
Crisco, 148
CRISPR, 168
Cromwell, Oliver, 121
Crosby, Arthur, 117, 178
Crusades, 115
Cuba, 67, 101, 129
Cupid, 51
Curie, Irène (Joliot-Curie), 38, 141
Curie, Marie (née Sklodowska), 38, 141, 170
Curie, Pierre, 38, 141
Cushing, Harvey, 141
Cyprus, 106
Czech(s); Czechoslovakia, 23, 116, 136, 163
da Vinci, Leonardo (see Leonardo da Vinci)
Daimler, Gottlieb, 135
Dakin, Henry Drysdale, 141

Dalai Lama, 109
Dalton, John, 127-8, 164
Daniel, the Prophet, 109
Dardanelles, 108
Dark Ages, 113, 116
Darnton, Robert, 3, 173
Darwin, Charles; Darwinism, 28, 33, 41, 52, 56, 62, 64, 82, 132, 165-8
Darwin, Erasmus, 132
Darwin, Robert, 132
David, King of Israel, 54, 69, 104, 109, 163
Davis, David Brion, 174
Davis, Nancy (see Reagan)
Davy, Humphrey, 130
D-Day, 73, 138
DDT, 13, 84, 167
Dead Sea, 66, 106
Death Valley, 82
DeBakey, Michael E., 154
DeBakey Veterans Affairs Medical Center, 154
Debussy, Claude, 138
Declaration of Independence, 124-5
DEET, 84
Defense Intelligence Agency, U.S., (DIA), 176
Delaware River, 122, 135-6
Delaware, 82, 122
Delilah, 29
Democrat(s), U.S., 32, 69, 131, 140, 161-3
Denmark, 26
Department of Health and Human Services, U.S (see HHS)
Descartes, René, 11, 119, 170
Deuteronomy, 23
DeVries, William, 147
Diamond, Jared, 178
Diana, Princess of Wales, 31
Dias, Bartolomeu, 116
Dickens, Charles, 144, 171
Dickinson, Emily, 42
Digitalis, 97
DNA, 35, 77, 82-3, 86-8, 92, 132, 166-8
Doctors without Borders, 105
Dodson, Charles (see Carroll)
Domagk, Gerhard, 171
Donne, John, 74
Donner-Reed group, 68
Dostoyevsky, Fyodor, 145
Down syndrome, 2, 41, 59, 69, 70
Doyle, Sir Arthur Conan, 144
Draper, William, 159
Dreyfuss, Alfred, 145

Durant, Will and Ariel, 170
Dutch (also see Netherlands), 30, 64, 120-1, 128, 160
Dvořák, Antonin, 138
East Indies, 113
East River, New York, 137
Ebers Papyrus, 107
Ebola River, Congo, 79, 87
Ecuador, 100
Edinburgh, Scotland, 26, 124
Edison, Thomas, 19, 92, 124, 134-5, 171
Edward VII, King of England, 31
Edward VIII, King of England, 31, 34
Egypt, 29, 38, 50, 62, 80, 86, 90, 93, 96, 102, 106-14, 170
Ehrlich, Paul, 141
Einstein, Albert, 141, 170-1
Eisenhower, Dwight D., 32, 73, 142, 154
Elamitic, 107
Electoral College, U.S., 130, 162
Elgar, Sir Arthur, 138
Elizabeth I, Queen of England, 30-1, 33, 38, 118-9, 170
Elizabeth II, Queen of England, 31, 142
Elizabeth, New Jersey, 136
Ellis, E. Earle, 104
Emancipation Proclamation, 132
Empedocles, 15
Encyclopedia Britannica, see *Britannica*
Engels, Friedrich, 112, 128
England; English (also see Britain), 12, 23, 26, 29-31, 34, 38, 53, 65-6, 70, 73, 82, 97, 101-2, 104, 112, 114-33, 138-45, 161, 169
Enlightenment, 10, 119, 122, 175
Entamoeba, 83
Epimetheus, 47
Equator, 18, 19, 61, 94, 165
Eros, 29, 51
Eskimo, 24
Essex County, Massachusetts, 123
Esther, 33, 38
Ethiopia, 91
Etruscans, 108
Euclid, 110, 170
Eugenics, 33-4, 77, 132
Euglena, 16
Euphrates River, 106
Europe; European, 24-6, 29, 32, 42, 45, 50, 57, 81, 86, 90, 93, 97-9, 101-2, 108-29, 134-42, 146, 162, 165, 170-2, 175-6
European Union (EU), 176

Evangelist (see Matthew, Mark, Luke, John)
Evans, John H., 159
Eve (see Adam and Eve)
Everest, Mount, 37, 67
Exodus, 52, 80
Extra-corporeal membrane oxygenator (ECMO), 147
Fairfax, Lord, and wife Sally, 32
falciparum, 100
Far East, 99, 120, 142, 166
Faraday, Michael, 128, 171
Ferdinand and Isabella, King and Queen of Spain, 116
Fertile Crescent (see Middle East)
Ficus, 27, 100
Fitzgerald, F. Scott, 145
Flavivirus, 86
Fleming, Sir Alexander, 171
Flickinger, Harry, 164
Flint, Michigan, 137
Florida, 82
Follett, Ken, 115, 120
Ford, Betty, 32
Ford, Gerald, 32
Fort Lauderdale, Florida, 82
Fossett, Steve, 68
France; French, 12-13, 16, 24, 27, 29-30, 56-7, 66, 73, 82, 85, 101, 107, 110, 112-5, 118, 120, 123, 125-8, 133-4, 136, 138-9, 142-3, 145, 171-2
Franciscan (see St. Francis)
Franco-Prussian War, 128, 136
Frank, Anne, 64
Franks, 113
Franklin, Benjamin, 123-4, 143, 164, 170
Frazer, James George, 157, 159, 178
French and Indian War, 125
Freud, Anna, 141
Freud, Sigmund, 28, 41, 141
Fuller, Matthew, 121
Fuller, Samuel, 120-1
Gaia, 12
Galapagos Islands, 127
Galen, 81, 112, 114, 117, 168
Galilei, Galileo, 92, 118, 158, 170
Gallipoli, Turkey, 139
Galton, Sir Francis, 33, 132
Gandhi, Mahatma, 46, 144, 171
Ganesh, Lord, 63
Ganges River, 22, 54
Gaul (see France)

Gay Nineties, 146
General Electric Co. (formerly Edison General Electric), 134
Genesis, 4, 17-18, 21, 38, 43, 45, 47, 52, 69, 94, 106, 158, 163
Geneva Convention, 129
Genghis Khan, 29, 115, 170
George IV, King of England, 125
George V, King of England, 31
George VI, King of England, 31
Georgia, U.S., 136
Georgia, USSR, 139
German; Germany, 23, 26, 34, 40, 49, 56-7, 65, 85, 97, 107, 112-3, 117-8, 122, 126-9, 134-43, 160-1, 163, 169, 171-2
Gettysburg, Pennsylvania, 131
Giardia, 83
Gibbon, Edward, 173
Gibbon, John, 147
Gibraltar, Straits of, 113
Gilbert, A. C. (Gilbert Chemistry Set), 120
Gilbert, W. S., 138
Gilded Age, 146, 175
Gilgamesh, 108
Glorious Revolution, 38, 122
GNP (Gross National Product), 78
God; god, 7, 12, 17, 21-3, 28-30, 47-8, 51-2, 59, 61-6, 80, 94, 96, 102, 104, 106-,7 111-13, 118, 149-50, 158, 160-6, 179
Golden Age of Arabic Civilization, 102, 114
Golden Age of Greece, 96, 109-10
Golden Rule, 36
Goliath, 69, 109
Gorbachev, Mikhail, 139
Gospel, 104-5, 111-2 (also see Evangelist)
Gram stain, 85
Granada, 116
Grand Army of the Republic, 131
Grant, Ulysses S., 131
Great Depression, 176, 179
Great Flood, 22, 107-8
Great Influenza (1918-19), 81, 87-8, 141
Great London Fire, 121
Great Migration, 121
Greece; Greeks, 12, 15, 17, 29, 40-1, 47, 51-2, 61, 63, 80, 96, 102, 104-5, 107-13 116, 143, 161, 168, 170
Green Revolution, 25
Greenland, 50
Gregory IX (Pope); Gregorian, 115, 118
Gross, Robert E., 147

Guillotin, Joseph-Ignace, 124
Guinevere, Queen, 29
Gunga Din, 68
Gutenberg, Johannes, 116
H1N1 virus, 81, 87
Hacking, Ian, 164, 166
Hades, 63, 108
Hadith, 113
Hagar the Egyptian, 106
Haiti, 81, 161
Hallowe'en, 61
Halsted, William Stewart, 141
Hamburg, Germany, 26
Hammurabi, King, 107-8
Handel, George Frideric, 135
Hapsburg(s), 121
Hardin, Jeff, 158-9
Harding, Warren G., 143
Hardy, Thomas, 145
Harken, Dwight E., 147
Harris, Jean, 31
Harrison, Peter, 159
Harte, Bret, 145
Harvard, 10, 58, 103, 129, 142, 147
Harvey, William, 53, 119, 121, 141, 168, 170
Hastings, Battle of, 29
Hatshepsut, Pharoah, 33, 38
Hawaii, 45, 128-9, 165
Hawthorne, Nathaniel, 30
Haydn, Joseph, 135
Hayes, Rutherford B., 131
Hazda, 58
Health Care Industry, 88, 148, 151-4, 179
Health Insurance Portability and Accountability Act (HIPPA), 152
Heaven, 12, 23, 51, 61-2, 66, 76, 117-8, 158
Hebrew(s) (see Jews)
Heisenberg, Werner, 170
Helen of Troy, 27-8
Helicobacter pylori, 10
Hell, 62-3, 108 (Hades)
Hemingway, Ernest, 18, 145, 171
Henrich, Joseph, 11
Henry VIII, 27, 30, 37, 118
Henry, Prince of Portugal, "the Navigator," 116, 166
Hero of Alexandria, 47
Herod, 111
Herodotus, 109
Hevea brasiliensis, 100

HHS (U.S. Department of Health and Human Services), 79
Hickok, Lorena, 140
Hildegard of Bingen, 115
Himalaya Mountains, 99, 109
Hindu Kush Mountains, 99
Hindu(s), 22, 30, 40, 62, 66, 99, 109, 161
Hippocrates; Hippocratic, 53, 57, 76, 102-3, 105, 110, 117, 121, 170-1
Hiroshima, Japan, 142
Hitler, Adolph, 33-4, 139-43, 169-70, 175
Ho Chi Minh, 125
Hollywood, California, 19, 32, 34
Holmes, Oliver Wendell, 33
Holocaust, 41, 140, 169
Holocene, 49-50
Homer, 28, 108-9, 170-1
Homo sapiens, 6, 14, 44, 46, 90, 124, 157, 176
Hong Kong, 81
Hooke, Robert, 121
Hoover, Herbert, 139
Hospital Corporation of America (HCA), 143
Houston Methodist Hospital, 154
Houston, Texas, 154-5
Hubble telescope, 146
Hubei Province, China, 14, 177
Hudson River, 12, 120, 135-6, 145
Hudson, Henry, 120
Huguenot, 118
Hun; Huns, 113
Hungary, 132
Hunter, John, 125-6
Hunter, Kim, 145
Hunter, William, 126
Huntington's chorea, 59
Hus, Jan, 116
Huxley, Aldous, 145
Hygeia, 96
Iberia, 113
Ice Age, 25, 49-50, 93, 115 (Little),
Iceland, 22-3
Illinois, 131
Inca, 61, 171
India, 24-5, 33, 42, 45, 63, 74, 78, 99, 106, 109-13, 116, 120, 128, 136, 139, 142, 144, 163, 166
Indian Ocean, 110, 113
Indonesia, 45
Industrial Revolution, 127-8, 171
Insulin, 101, 141, 171
Iowa, 74, 139, 161
Iran (see Persia)

Iraq, 93, 106, 176
Ireland; Irish, 119, 121, 128, 142, 161-3, 172
Irish Republican Army, 142
Iron Age, 47, 91
Irving, Washington, 145
Isaac, son of Abraham, 106
Ishmael, son of Abraham, 106, 113
Islam (see Muslim)
Issachar Fund, 158
Istanbul, Turkey, 116, 129 (also see Constantinople)
Italy; Italian, 24, 57, 80, 101, 105, 108, 114-16, 126, 143, 146, 163
Ivory soap, 150
Iwo Jima, 179
Jacob, son of Isaac, 29, 107
Jain, 24, 62
Jamaica, 101
James I, King of England (also, James VI of Scotland), 30, 51, 53, 63, 119-20, 158, 160
James II, King of England, 122
Jamestown, Virginia, 120
Japan; Japanese, 15, 22, 45, 56, 65-6, 86, 101, 109, 129, 139, 142-3, 175-7
Jarvik, Robert, 147
Jefferson, Thomas, 32, 127, 143
Jello, 148
Jenner, Edward, 87, 123-6
Jephthah's daughter, 66
Jeremiah, the Prophet, 109
Jericho, 93, 106, 108
Jerusalem, 62-3, 66, 106, 109, 114-5, 146
Jesus (see Christ)
Jews; Hebrews, 22, 41, 51, 54, 62-6, 79-80, 102-18, 122, 138, 140, 146, 158, 161-3, 177
Joan of Arc, Saint, 33, 38, 66, 116
John the Baptist, 45
John the Evangelist, 104
John, King of England, 115
Johns Hopkins University, 141
Johnson, Andrew, 131
Johnson, Lady Bird, 32
Johnson, Lyndon B., 32, 179
Joint Commission, 57
Joliot, Frédéric, 38, 141
Joseph, father of Jesus, 29, 45, 104-5, 111, 163
Joseph, son of Jacob, 45, 107, 163
Joyce, James, 145
Judah, 45
Judea, 105, 111
Julian Calendar, 118

Justinian Plague, 81
Kafka, Franz, 26, 145, 171
Kaiser-Permanente, 143
Kalahari, 24, 43, 91
Kant, Immanuel, 17
Kazakhstan, 113
Kellogg, John Harvey, 53, 98
Kelly, Colin, 66
Kennedy, Jacqueline, 32
Kennedy, John F., 32, 154
Kennedy, Joseph P., 68
Kentucky, 40, 131
Kenya, 162
Kepler, Johannes, 118, 158, 164
Key, Francis Scott, 31
Key, Philip Barton, II, 31
Khan (see Genghis, Ogedei, Kublai)
Khan family, 29
Khumbu region, Nepal, 37
King Philip's War, 121
King, Martin Luther, Jr., 19, 144, 171
Kinsey, Albert, 27
Kipling, Rudyard, 68
Kitty Hawk, North Carolina, 135
Koch, Robert, 85, 134
Kolkata (Calcutta), India, 33
Koran; *Qur'an*, 52, 64, 113
Korea; Korean, 129, 139
Korean War, 139
Kotex, 150
Krebiozen, 167
Ku Klux Klan (KKK), 131
Kublai Khan, 115
Kuhn, Thomas, 3, 164-9, 178
L'Amour, Louis, 145
Lacks, Henrietta, 77
Laennec, René T. H., 126-7
Laetrile, 167
Lamarck, Jean Baptiste, 132
Lamarr, Hedy, 140
Lancelot, Sir, 29
Languedoc, France, 113
Latin America, 129
Latin, 12, 17, 26, 29, 38, 40-1, 49, 57, 88, 97, 103-4, 108, 110, 112, 114, 116-7, 121-3, 133
Lauris, 97
Lavoisier, Antoine, 16, 164
League of Nations, 129
Leah, 29
Lebanon, 113
Lee, Harper, 35

Lee, Robert E., 131
Leeuwenhoek, Antonie van, 85, 92, 122
Leishmania, 83
Lenin, Vladimir, 128, 139, 170
Leonardo da Vinci, 116, 170
Letheon, 130
Leviticus, 24, 63
Lewinsky, Monica, 33
Lewis and Clark expedition, 68, 117, 127
Lewis, John L., Congressman, 144
Lewis, Meriweather, 68, 117, 127
Leyden jar, 124
Lhasa, 63
Libya, 113
Lieberman, Daniel, 57-8
Life-Boy soap, 150
Lincoln, Abraham, 127, 130-2, 163, 170
Lincoln, Robert Todd, 131
Lind, James, 124
Lindbergh, Charles, 34, 141-3, 175
Lindbergh, Charles, Jr., 143
Linnaeus, Carl, 124
Lisbon, Portugal, 118
Lister, Joseph, 1st Baron, 134
Listerine, 149
Lloyd's of London, 143
Locke, John, 121
London, England, 13, 18, 26, 39, 41, 81, 101, 114, 121-2, 125-6, 129, 132, 143-4
London, Jack, 48-9, 145
Long Island Sound, 137
Longfellow, Henry Wadsworth, 137
Lot, 29, 107, 163
Louisiana Purchase, 127
Lovelock, James, 12
LSD, 32, 70, 99
Ludwig, Carl, 134
Luke, Saint (see St. Luke the Evangelist)
Luther, Martin; Lutheran, 25-6, 63, 118, 138, 160, 170
Luxor, Egypt, 106
Lyme Disease, 81, 84
Lysenko, Trofim, 132
M.D. Anderson Cancer Center, 154
Maass, Clara, 67
MacArthur, Douglas, 142
Macedonia, 110, 112
Machiavelli, Niccolò, 118
Machu Picchu, 61
Macroglossus minimus, 13
Madeira School, 31

Madison, Dolley, 37
Madison, James, 37
Magdeburg, Germany, 26
Magna Carta, 115
Mahan, Alfred Thayer, 3, 173, 178
Maimonides (Musa ibn Mainun), 114
Maine, 121, 127
Mainz, Germany, 118
Major, Ralph, 105, 108, 119, 126
Make America Great Again; MAGA, 162-3, 175
Malakand, Pakistan, 139
Mallory, George, 67
Malthus, Thomas, 15, 42, 126, 176
Mandan, 117
Manhattan Island; Borough, 120, 137
Manheim, Germany, 135
Manifest Destiny, 176
Mannerism, 164
Marco Polo, 115
Marconi, Guglielmo, 141, 171
Marcus Aurelius, Emperor, 112
Margaret, Princess, 31
Margulis, Lynn, 4, 12
Marienbad, Czechoslovakia, 23, 136
Mark the Evangelist, 45, 104
Markey, Gene, 140
Marriott's Brighton Gardens, 153
Mars, planet, 12
Marseilles, France, 81
Marshall, George, 142
Marx, Karl, 39, 112, 128, 170
Mary II, Queen of England, 38, 122
Mary, Queen of Scots, 119
Mary, Virgin, 29, 33, 38, 104, 111, 160
Maryland, 69, 120, 137
Masada, 66
Mason jar, 149
Mason; Masonic Order, 138, 161
Massachusetts General Hospital, 103, 129
Massachusetts, 30, 120-1
Mather, Rev. Cotton, 123
Matthew, Gospel writer, 23, 45, 52, 104
Maturin, Stephen, 127
Maya(n); Mayans, 171
Mayflower, 30, 120
Mayo Clinic, 142
Mayo, Charles, 142
Mayo, William, 142
McCormick, Cyrus, 137
McMurtry, Larry, 146
McNeill, William, 178

Mecca, 41, 62, 113, 126
Medal of Honor, 138
Medawar, Sir Peter, 58
Medicaid, 144
Medical Society of New Jersey, 152
Medicare, 144, 154, 162, 179
Medina, 113
Mediterranean Sea, 42, 44, 80, 93, 96, 102, 106, 110, 113-4, 171, 179
Meier, Golda, 33
Melpomene, 42
Melville, Herman, 145
Memorial Hermann (Houston, Texas), 154
Memphis, Egypt, 106
Mendel, Gregor, 132
Mendelssohn, Felix, 135
Mentholatum, 149
Mercer, Hugh, 125
Mercer, Lucy, 140
Merkel, Angela, 33
Merovee; Merovingian, 113
Merriam-Webster, 4, 27, 51
Mesa Verde, Colorado, 27
Meso America(n), 179
Mesopotamia, 87, 106-8, 113
Metacom (see Philip, King; and King Philip's War)
Mexican War (U.S. vs Mexico), 145, 172
Mexico; Mexican(s), 98, 139, 143-5, 162-3, 167-8, 172
Michelangelo, 118
Michigan State University, 71
Michigan, 71, 137, 147
Midas, 52, 56
Middle Ages (Medieval Period), 29, 42, 98-9, 102, 104, 108, 112, 114, 116, 151, 161, 164
Middle East, 28-9, 65, 80, 87, 90, 93, 99, 102, 106, 112, 165
Milky Way, 18, 146
Miller, Arthur, 162
Milton, John, 162
Minnesota, 84, 142
Minoa, 107
Mississippi, 35, 145 (River)
Missouri River, 127
Moab, 29
Modern; Modernity, 3, 6, 7, 10, 24, 42, 53, 60, 77, 93, 98, 102, 104, 113-18, 123, 127, 129, 138, 151, 159, 165, 175, 178
Mohammed, 170 (also see Muhammad)
Mohave Desert, 82

Mondino d'Liuzzi, 115
Mongol; Mongolia, 29, 109, 113, 115
Monmouth, New Jersey, 125
Monroe Doctrine, 129
Moon, the, 12, 18, 55, 69, 94, 96, 106-7, 112, 146, 158, 171
Moravia(n), 132
Mormon(s); Church of Jesus Christ of Latter Day Saints; LDS, 160
Morrow, Ann (m. Lindbergh), 143
Morse, Samuel F. B., 39, 171
Morton, George (of "Mourt's Relation"), 120
Morton, William T. G., 117, 129-30
Moscow, 128
Moses, 21-2, 52, 80, 108-9, 160
Mountbatten, Lord Louis, 142
Mozart, Wolfgang Amadeus, 135
Muhammad the Prophet, 113
Mukherjee, Siddhartha, 79
Müller, Johannes, 133
Mumford, Lewis, 2, 12
Murray, Joseph E., 147
Mus, 50
Museum of Modern Art, 116
Muslim, 22, 33, 37, 41, 46, 55, 61-4, 66, 96, 109, 112-8, 129, 161-2. 175, 177
Mussolini, Benito, 170
Mussorgsky, Modest, 138
Myanmar, 33, 109
Mycenae, 107-8
Mycobacterium leprae, 85
Mycobacterium tuberculosis, 85
Nader, Ralph, 136
Nagasaki, Japan, 142
Nantucket Island, 121
Napoleon Bonaparte, Emperor 74, 127-8, 170-1, 175
Napoleonic Period, 175
NASA (National Aeronautics and Space Administration, U.S.), 72
Nassar, Larry, 71
National Cancer Act, 79, 154
National Cancer Institute, 79
National Institutes of Health (NIH), 79, 80, 153, 160, 167
National Security Agency, U.S. (NSA), 176
Native American(s), 39, 53, 117, 120-2, 128, 130, 145-6, 161
Navy, Japanese, 66, 142
Navy, Royal (British), 124, 132, 142
Navy, U.S., 46, 48, 68, 139, 142

Nazareth, 66, 111
Nazi; National Socialist Party, 54, 65, 140
Near East (see Middle East)
Nebuchadnezzar II, 108-9, 146
Neolithic (see Stone Age)
Nepal, 15, 33, 37, 98, 109
Nero, 29, 112
Netherlands, the (also see Dutch), 76, 101, 138
Neutragena, 150
Nevada, 68
New Amsterdam, 30
New England, 30, 36, 66, 95, 121-2
New Guinea, 24, 43, 73, 91, 157
New Hampshire, 20, 121, 125, 145
New Haven, Connecticut, 26, 136
New Jersey, 67, 76, 82, 110, 125, 136-7, 143, 152, 161
New Testament (see Bible)
New York City, 31, 79, 122, 136-7, 141, 143, 175
New York state, 122, 145, 162
New Zealand, 50, 74
Newark, New Jersey, 143
Newport, Rhode Island, 26
Newton, Isaac, 122, 170-1
Nightingale, Florence, 38, 129
Nile River, 86, 93, 106-7, 165
Nixon, Patricia "Pat," 32
Nixon, Richard M., 32
Noah, 23, 29, 63, 107
Nobel, Alfred; Nobel Prize, 38, 67, 120, 138-9, 141, 147, 166, 169, 172
Normandy, France, 29, 138-9
North Atlantic Treaty Organization (NATO), 176
North Carolina, 31
North Pole, 83
Norway, 83
Nuclear Age, 139, 146
Nuremberg, Germany, 116
O'Brian, Patrick, 127
Obama, Barack, 33, 144, 162
Occam's Razor, 16
Ogedei Khan, 115
Ohio River, 49, 128
Ohio, 142
Old Kingdom of Egypt, 107
Old Testament (see Bible)
Old World, 24-5, 42, 100, 117
Olympias, Queen of Macedonia, 110
Oncology Nursing Society, 153

Opioid, 2, 25, 32, 57, 70-1, 99-100, 167
Organization of American States (OAS), 176
Origin of Species, The, 28, 33, 52, 132, 165
Orwell, George, 145
Osler, Revere, 141
Osler, Sir William, 96, 119, 141
Ottoman, 116, 118
Oxford, 119, 125
OxyContin (also see Sackler family), 99, 32, 70, 99
p53, 77, 168
Pacific Ocean, 34, 132, 139, 143, 145
Pakistan, 25, 113, 139
Palestine, 114
Panacea, 96
Panama Canal, 86
Panchen Lama, 109
Pandora, 47
Papua New Guinea (see New Guinea)
Paracelsus, Theophrastus von Hohenheim, 117
Paré, Ambroise, 118
Paris, France, 34, 41, 113, 124, 127, 133-4, 137, 143
Paris, Prince of Troy, 28
Parkinson's Disease, 11, 76
Parthenon, 109
Passover, 111
Pasteur, Louis, 20, 85, 133-4, 145, 149, 170
Pathan, 139
Pauling, Linus, 166
Pavlov, Ivan, 11, 142
Payer, Lynn, 179
Pearl Harbor, Hawaii, 142
Pediculus humanus, 84
Penelope, 28
Penn, William, 122, 170
Pennsylvania Hospital, 124
Pennsylvania, 30, 67, 122-4, 131, 147, 175
Pentagon, the, 175
Pepto Bismol, 37, 149
Pequot, 121
Pergamum, 80, 112
Persia, 29, 38, 102, 106-7, 113-4
Persian Gulf, 106, 113
Peru, 100, 121, 124
Peruvian bark (quinine), 121, 124
Peter Bent Brigham Hospital, 147
Petronius the Arbiter, 29
Pharisees, 111
Pharaoh, 29, 33, 38, 80, 108
Philadelphia Contributorship, 143

Philadelphia, Pennsylvania, 86, 122-4, 136, 143
Philemon, 105
Philip II, King of Macedonia, 110
Philip, "King" (Metacom), 121
Philip, Prince, Duke of Edinburgh, 142
Philippines, 128-9
Philistines, 80
Phoenix, Arizona, 82
PHS (U.S. Public Health Service), 79-80
Physick, Philip Syng, 126
Picasso, Pablo, 141
Pilate, Pontius, 111
Pilgrim, 30, 120-1
Pinkham, Lydia, 149
Plague Monuments, 121
Planck time, 18
Plasmodium, 83
Plato, 51, 109-10
Pleistocene, 49, 176
Plymouth Colony (now Massachusetts), 120-1
Poland, 65, 116
Polyhymnia, 42
Pontus (Greek god), 12
Poor Law Commission, 129
Porter, Cole, 141
Porter, Roy, 92-3, 152, 157, 179
Portugal; Portuguese, 113, 116-8, 128, 165, 171
Potsdam Conference, Germany, 142
Pott, Sir Percival, 125
Priam, King of Troy, 108
Priestly, Joseph, 16, 164
Princeton University, 173
Princeton, New Jersey, 125, 173
Principe, Lawrence M., 158-9
Proctor, John, 66
Prometheus, 47, 63
Proverbs, 4
Prudential Insurance Co. 143
Prussia, Germany, 128, 136
Psalm, 45
Pthirus pubis, 84
Ptolemaic Dynasty, 110 (also see Cleopatra)
Ptolemy I Soter, 29, 110
Ptolemy XIV, 29
Ptolemy, Claudius Ptolemaeus (astronomer), 112, 159, 164
PTSD, 65, 69
Public Health Service, U.S., 35, 79
Puccini, Giacomo, 38
Puerto Rico, 129, 146
Pulitzer Prize, 127, 141

Puritan, 30, 46, 95, 120-3
Putin, Vladimir, 139
Pyrenees Mountains, 66
Pythagorean theorem, 165
Q-tips, 150
Quaker, 30, 46, 66, 122-4, 138-9, 161
Quebec, Canada, 120
Quran; *Qur'an* (see Koran)
Rabelais, François, 30
Rachel, 29, 163
Rahab, 108
Raleigh, Sir Walter, 30
Raleigh, North Carolina, 31
Ramadan, 61
Rawlinson, George, 107
Reagan, Nancy Davis, 33
Reagan, Ronald, 32-3
Rebecca (movie), 145
Reconstruction, 131
Red Crescent, International Society, 129
Red Cross, American; and International Society, 127, 129
Red Sea, 113
Redford, Robert, 20
Redgrave, Vanessa, 145
Reed, Walter, 67, 86
Reformation, 63, 118, 122, 175
Reisman, David, 40
Renaissance, 102, 104, 116, 122, 164, 175
Republican(s); Republican Party, 32, 69, 74, 130, 138, 161-3
Revelation, Book of, 15, 112
Revolutionary War, American, 123-5, 129, 145
Rhazes (al Razi, Abu Bakr Muhammad ibn Zakariya), 114
Rhine River, 110, 113, 122
Rhode Island, 26, 30, 121
Rice Krispies, 148
Richmond, Virginia, 132
Rickettsia prowazekii, 84
Rio de Janeiro, Brazil, 39
Riviera, 82
Roanoke, Lost Colony (now North Carolina), 120
Roaring Twenties, 176
Rochester, Minnesota, 142
Rockefeller Institute, 141, 143
Rockefeller, Nelson, 31
Rocky Mountains, 68, 84, 145
Roe v Wade, 162-3
Roebling, Emily, 137
Roebling, John, 137
Roebling, Washington, 137, 170
Rohingya, 109
Roland, 66
Rome; Roman, 23, 28-9, 33-4, 42-3, 51, 61-3, 66, 81, 93, 96-8, 105, 108-15, 117-8, 122, 136, 138, 143, 159-61, 170, 173, 177
Rommel, Erwin, 142
Roncevaux Pass, Spain, 66
Roosevelt, Alice, 32
Roosevelt, Eleanor, 32-3, 140
Roosevelt, Franklin Delano, 32-3, 68, 139-40, 170, 179
Roosevelt, Quentin, 139
Roosevelt, Theodore, 32-4, 68, 128, 138-9, 171-2
Roosevelt, Theodore, Jr., 139-40
Rosetta Stone, 107
Rouen, France, 66
Roxanna, wife of Alexander of Macedon, 29
Royal College of Physicians, 102, 119
Royal College of Surgeons, 102
Royal Navy, 132, 142
Royal Society, the, 85, 119, 122, 126
Rush, Benjamin, 86, 125
Russia; Russian, 38, 115, 128, 136, 138-40, 142, 177
Russo-Japanese War, 142
Sacagawea, 68
Sachs, Oliver, 11
Sadducees, 76
Sagan, Carl, 4
Sagan, Dorian, 4
Sahara Desert, 27, 113
Saint Barnabas Health Care System – Robert Wood Johnson, 143
Sakkara, Egypt, 107
Saladin, Sultan, 114
Salem, Massachusetts, 30, 66, 123, 145
Salerno, Italy, 114
Salix, 97
Saltin, Bengt, 58
Salvarsan, 141, 166, 177
Samarkand, Uzbekistan, 63, 115
Samuel, 80
Sarah, wife of Abraham, 106
Sarbanes-Oxley Act, 152
Sardinia, 107
SARS-CoV-2, 14, 42, 69, 81, 87-8, 152, 160, 177
Saudi Arabia, 113

Saxony, Germany, 135
Schleiden, Matthias, 133
Schubert, Franz Peter, 135
Schumann, Clara, 135
Schumann, Robert, 135
Schuylkill River, 122, 136
Schwann, Theodor, 133
Scientific Revolution(s), 3, 38, 122, 127, 164-6, 169, 178
Scotland; Scots, 18, 31, 114-5, 119, 125, 128, 161
Scouts (see Boy Scouts)
SEAL, 68
Second Amendment, 163
Semmelweis, Ignaz, 132-3
September 11, 2001, 66, 175
Shakespeare, William, 8, 19, 20, 27, 29-30, 51, 110, 116, 118-19, 162, 170-1
Sheba, Queen of, 33, 109
Sherpa, 33, 37, 109
Shinto, 66, 109
Shrewsbury, England, 132
Shriners, the, 161
Shriners Hospital, Houston, Texas, 154
Shropshire, England, 125
Sicily, 116
Sickles, Daniel, 31
Sierra Nevada Mountains, 68
Sikh, 27, 62
Silk Road, 99, 115
Simpson, Wallis, 31
Sinai Desert, 106, 108-9
Singapore, 109
Smith Papyrus, 107
Smith, Adam, 39
Smith, John (Captain), 120
Smith, Joseph (of LDS), 160
Smyrna, Turkey, 116
Snow, Charles Percy (C. P.), Baron Snow, 38, 74, 179
Snow, John, 129
Social Security, 154, 163
Socialism, 39, 112, 163
Society of Surgical Oncology, 153
Socrates, 109-10
Sodom, 29, 107, 163
Solomon, King, 109
Somalia, 163
SOS (Morse Code), 39
South America, 100, 106, 130, 132, 139, 157
South Carolina, 130

South Dakota, 69, 74, 82, 117
South East Asia Command (SEAC), 142
South-East Asia Treaty Organization (SEATO), 176
Soviet Union (see Union of Soviet Socialist Republics; USSR)
Space Age, 146, 175
Spain; Spanish, 31, 56-7, 81, 87, 101-2, 112-4, 116, 121, 128, 138, 146, 175
Spanish-American War, 101, 128, 138
Sparta, Greece, 109
Spencer, Diana (see Diana, Princess of Wales)
Spencer, Herbert, 41
Springfield, Illinois, 131
St. Francis of Assisi; Franciscan, 52, 56, 115
St. George's Hospital, 125
St. Helens, Mount, 12
St. Ignatius of Loyola, 56
St. Joan of Arc (see Joan of Arc)
St. Louis, Missouri, 104
St. Luke the Evangelist, 103-5, 111, 154
St. Martin of Tours, 45, 52
St. Paul the Apostle, 104-5
St. Teresa (see Teresa, Mother)
St. Vitus Dancing Mania (Sydenham's chorea), 115, 121
Stalin, Josef, 132, 139, 142, 170
Starbucks, 101
Stark, Rodney, 159
Starr, Paul, 152, 179
Starzl, Thomas, 147
Stewart, Jimmy, 65
Stewart, Rod, 39
Stone Age (Neolithic Period), 46-50, 91, 107
Stonehenge, 107
Stowe, Harriet Beecher, 144
Stroud, Robert Franklin, 40
Structure of Scientific Revolutions, The, 3, 164-9, 178
Stryker, Homer Hartman, 53
Sturgis, South Dakota, 39-40
Stuttgart, Germany, 135
Styx, River, 63, 108
Suez, 106
Süleyman I, Sultan, 118
Sullivan, Sir Arthur, 138
Sumer; Sumerian(s), 108, 170
Sumter, Fort, 130
Suu Kyi, Aung San, 33
Svalbard, Norway, 83
Sweden; Swedish, 73, 83, 122, 124

Switzerland, 68
Sydenham, Thomas, 121, 123
Syria, 113-4
Tamar, 45
Tanzania, 58
Tarnower, Herman, 31
Tashkent, Uzbekistan, 115
Tay-Sachs disease, 59
Tchaikovsky, Pyotr Ilyich, 138
Tehran, Iran, 114, 139-40
Tennessee, 131
Tennyson, Alfred Lord, 51
Teresa, Mother, 34, 52, 74
Terra, 12
Tesla, Nikola, 141
Texas Heart Institute, 154
Texas Medical Center (TMC), 154, 156
Texas; Texans, 146, 154-6, 163, 172
Thailand, 109
Thames, 129
Thatcher, Margaret, 33
Thebes, Egypt, 106
Thebes, Greece, 105
Theophilus, 103-4
Thessaly, Greece, 110
Third Millennium, 154
Thoreau, Henry David, 144, 171
Thucydides, 81, 109
Tibet, 15, 67, 109
Tierra del Fuego, 46
Tigris River, 106
Tijuana, Mexico, 167
Till, Emmett, 35
Timothy, 52, 105
Timur (Tamerlane), 29, 115-6, 170
TMC Library, 154
Todd, Mary, 131
Tolstoy, Leo, 145, 171
Torah, 52, 62, 109, 162
Tory; Tories (English colonists), 125
Tory; Tories (English political party), 169
Trafalgar, 128
Trenton, New Jersey, 125, 136
Tribal (see Native American)
Tri-Care, 144
Trichinella spiralis, 83
Tris, 48
Trotsky, Leon, 139
Troy; Trojans, 27-8, 40, 80, 108-9
Truman, Harry S, 32, 142-3, 179
Trump, Donald J., 33-4, 154, 161-3, 175

Trypanosoma cruzi, 83
Tse-tung, Mao (Zedong), 132
Turkey; Turks, 80, 99, 108, 112, 116, 139
Turkmenistan, 113
Tuskegee experiment, 35
Tutankhamun, King "Tut," 108
Twain, Mark (Samuel Clemens), 145, 171
U.S. Agency for International Development (USAID), 176
U.S. Military Academy (West Point), 142
Ukraine; Ukrainians, 139
Ulysses, 28, 108
Union of Soviet Socialist Republics; USSR, 132, 139, 176
Unitarian(s), 138, 161
United Kingdom (see England)
United Nations; UN, 78, 129, 140, 175-6
United States (see also America[n]), 14-16, 27, 32, 35-6, 40-2, 55, 68-9, 74, 76-81, 85, 99, 101, 116, 123, 125, 128-31, 134, 138, 140, 142, 145, 152, 154, 159-60, 162, 169, 172, 175-6
University of Wisconsin-Madison, 158
Upjohn, William E., 53
Ur of the Chaldees, 106-7
Uranus, 12
Uriah, 109
Utah, 147
Uzbekistan, 113, 115
Van Gogh, Vincent, 141
Vasco de Gama, 116
Vaseline, 149
Vatican, 63, 118
Venice, Italy, 81, 115-6, 121
Venus, Greek god, 28, 51
Venus, planet, 107
Verdi, Giuseppe, 146
Versailles, Treaty of, 138, 175
Vesalius, Andreas, 118, 170
Vespucci, Amerigo, 117
Victoria, Queen, 31, 46, 129, 136, 175
Victorian Age, 175
Vienna, Austria, 115, 118, 121
Vietnam War, 139
Vietnam, 14, 45, 57, 109, 125, 139
Virchow, Rudolf, 133
Virgil, 28, 80, 108
Virginia Military Institute, 142
Virginia, 30-1, 34, 120, 122, 131-2, 142, 145, 175 (Pentagon)
Visigoths, 112-3
Vitamin C, 124

Vitamin D, 18
Vivaldi, Antonio, 135
Voyager 1 and 2, 146
Wales, 31, 34, 119
Wallace, Henry, 179
Wallace, William, 115
Wampanoag Indian Tribe, 121
Wappinger Confederacy, 120
War of 1812, 127-8, 138
Warren, John Collins, 129-30
Warren, John, 129
Warren, Joseph, 129
Washington, D.C., 19, 31-2, 42, 63, 67, 127, 131, 142
Washington, George, 31, 37, 125
Washington, Martha Custis, 31, 37
Watson, James; Watson-Crick, 166, 168
Watts, Isaac, 171
Wedgwood, Josiah, 132
Weinberg, Steven, 169
Weisse, Allen, 67
Welcome, ship, and Welcome Fleet, 122
Wesley, John, 161
Westminster Abbey, 132
Westphalia, Peace of, 121
Wheaties, 148
Whig history; Whiggish history, 60, 164, 169-72
Whig political party, 170
White, Andrew Dickson, 158-9
Whitman, Walt, 127
Wiccans, 161
Wilde, Oscar, 27
William II (Prince of Orange) and Mary II, King and Queen of England, 122
William I, King of England and Duke of Normandy, 29, 139, 170
Wilson, Edith Bolling, 37
Wilson, Woodrow, 32, 37, 138
Winthrop, John, 120
Wisconsin Glacial Episode, 49
Wister, Owen, 145
Withering, William, 124-5
Wittenberg, Germany, 118
Women's Christian Temperance Union (WCTU), 161
World Bank, 53, 176
World Court, 176
World Health Organization (WHO), 14, 42, 53, 78, 88, 129, 176
World Trade Center, 67
World War I, 136, 138-43, 172, 175-6

World War II, 15, 54, 64-6, 115, 129, 136, 138-43, 152, 175-6, 179
World Wars, 31 years, 175
World, New (see America)
World, Old, (see Old World)
Wood, Leonard, 103
Wright, Orville, 135
Wright, Wilbur, 135
Wuhan, China, 14, 42, 81, 177
Wyoming, 162
Yale University, 103, 142
Yamamoto, Isoroku, 142
Yangtze River, 14, 177
Yellowstone Park, 22-3
Yersinia pestis, 80
York, enslaved by William Clark, 127
Yorktown, Virginia, 125
Younger Dryas, 49
Zero Population Growth (ZPG), 177
Zeus, 47, 51
Zhengli, Shi, 14
Zinsser, Hans, 178
Zola, Émile, 144, 171-2
Zoroastrian, 22, 63, 113, 161

Heritage Books by George J. Hill:

*American Dreams: Ancestors and Descendants of John Zimmermann and
Eva Katherine Kellenbenz, Who Were Married in Philadelphia in 1885*

*"Dearest Barb": From Karachi, 1943–1945, Letters and Photographs in the World War II Papers
of a Naval Intelligence Officer, Lieutenant Albert Zimmermann, USNR*

Edison's Environment: The Great Inventor Was Also a Great Polluter

Four Families: A Tetralogy Reader's Guide to Western Pilgrims, Quakers and Puritans, Fundy to Chesapeake, *and*
American Dreams; *Synopsis of 481 Immigrants and First Known Ancestors in America from Northern Europe
in the Families of George J. Hill and Jessie F. Stockwell, William T. Shoemaker and Mabel Warren,
William H. Thompson and Sarah D. Rundall, John Zimmermann and Eva K. Kellenbenz,
with Outlines of Their Descent from the Immigrants*

*Fundy to Chesapeake: The Thompson, Rundall and Allied Families; Ancestors and Descendants of
William Henry Thompson and Sarah D. Rundall, Who Were Married in Linn County, Iowa, in 1889*

Health Matters: A New View of Human History

*Hill: The Ferry Keeper's Family, Luke Hill and Mary Hout, Who Were Married in Windsor,
Connecticut, in 1651 and Fourteen Generations of Their Known and Possible Descendants*

John Saxe, Loyalist (1732–1808) and His Descendants for Five Generations

Prairie Daughter: Stories and Poems from Iowa by Essie Mae Thompson Hill

*Quakers and Puritans: The Shoemaker, Warren and Allied Families; Ancestors and Descendants of
William Toy Shoemaker and Mabel Warren, Who Were Married in Philadelphia in 1895*

*Rolling with Patton: The Letters and Photographs of Field Director Gerald L. Hill,
303rd Infantry Regiment, 97th "Trident" Division, 1943–1945*

*The Home Front in World War II: From the Letters of
Essie Mae Hill to Field Director Gerald L. Hill*

*War Letters, 1917–1918: From Dr. William T. Shoemaker, A.E.F.,
in France, and His Family in Philadelphia*

*Three Men in a Jeep Called "Ma Kabul," Script for a Movie:
A True Story of High Adventure by Three Allied Intelligence Officers in World War II*

*Western Pilgrims: The Hill, Stockwell and Allied Families; Ancestors and Descendants of
George J. Hill and Jessie Fidelia Stockwell, Who Were Married
in Wright County, Iowa, in 1882*

About the Author

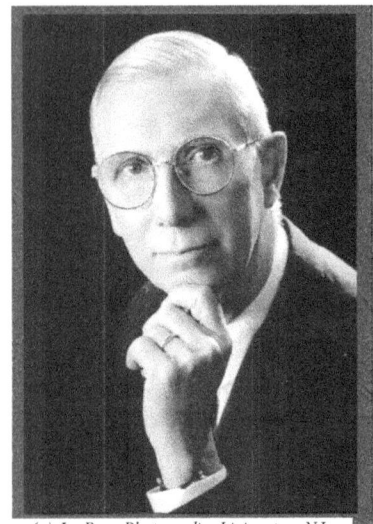

George J. Hill is a fifth-generation Iowan. He graduated from high school in Sac City, Iowa, and then attended Yale University, where he majored in history. He graduated from Harvard Medical School, and after forty years as a practicing surgeon, he is now Emeritus Professor of Surgery at Rutgers-New Jersey Medical School. He served in the U.S. Marine Corps and the U.S. Public Health Service, and he was awarded the Meritorious Service Medal upon retirement as a Captain, Medical Corps, in the U.S. Navy. Dr. Hill also earned an M.A. in history at Rutgers University and a D.Litt. in history from Drew University. He has written or edited more than 20 books on medicine and surgery, family history and genealogy, environmental history and international relations.

(c) JanPressPhotomedia, Livingston, NJ

Other Books by the Author

Medicine and Science

Leprosy in Five Young Men
Outpatient Surgery (3 editions; 2 translated into Spanish as *Cirugia Menor*)
Clinical Oncology, with John Horton

History

Edison's Environment (3 editions)
Intimate Relationships: The U.S. and Liberia, 1917-1947 (3 editions)
Proceed to Peshawar

www.ingramcontent.com/pod-product-compliance
Lightning Source LLC
Chambersburg PA
CBHW081758300426
44116CB00014B/2163